Percutaneous Renal Surgery

John D. Denstedt · Evangelos N. Liatsikos

Editors

Percutaneous Renal Surgery

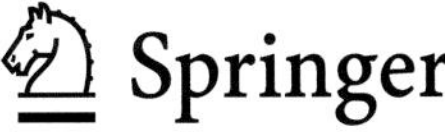 Springer

Editors
John D. Denstedt
Western University
London, ON, Canada

Evangelos N. Liatsikos
University Hospital of Patras
Patras, Greece

ISBN 978-3-031-40544-0   ISBN 978-3-031-40542-6 (eBook)
https://doi.org/10.1007/978-3-031-40542-6

This Springer imprint is published by the registered company Springer Nature Switzerland AG
The registered company address is: Gewerbestrasse 11, 6330 Cham, Switzerland

Paper in this product is recyclable.

Contents

Contents

This History of Percutaneous Nephrolithotomy

Gregory Mullen, David Hoenig, and Arthur Smith

Abstract Previously, the standard treatment for patients with renal calculi was open nephrolithotomy, which was associated with significant morbidity. The need for a minimally invasive procedure to remove renal stones was ultimately met by the establishment of percutaneous nephrostomy, which became popular in the 1950s with the advent of X-ray. The first true percutaneous nephrolithotomy was performed in 1973 by Fernström and Johansson at the Karolinska Institute in Sweden, which required a prolonged hospital stay due to serial dilation and maturation of the nephrostomy tract. At the 1980 AUA meeting, Dr. Arthur Smith and colleagues presented new techniques using a percutaneous renal approach in a poster titled "Endourology." In the 1980s, percutaneous nephrolithotomy underwent modifications including rapid dilation, which was aided by the development of a variety of new medical devices. Percutaneous techniques were subsequently disseminated at educational courses and with the founding of the Endourological Society. Percutaneous nephrolithotomy is now the gold standard for treatment of large renal calculi and continues to undergo innovations.

Keywords Percutaneous nephrolithotomy history · Endourology history

1 Open Stone Surgery

Up until the 1950s, the standard treatment for patients with renal calculi was open nephrolithotomy. This was done via either the avascular plane made popular by Hyrtl and Brödel, or via pyelolithotomy, first done by Czerny. These procedures

G. Mullen · D. Hoenig · A. Smith (✉)
The Arthur Smith Institute for Urology, Northwell Health, New York, NY, USA
e-mail: asmith0733@gmail.com

G. Mullen
e-mail: gmullen1@northwell.edu

D. Hoenig
e-mail: dhoenig@northwell.edu

© The Author(s), under exclusive license to Springer Nature Switzerland AG 2023
J. D. Denstedt and E. N. Liatsikos (eds.), *Percutaneous Renal Surgery*,
https://doi.org/10.1007/978-3-031-40542-6_1

required large incisions and were associated with significant morbidity including pneumothorax, hemorrhage, urinary leakage, loss of renal parenchyma, and even death (Pettersson 2000). The need for a highly successful minimally invasive procedure to remove renal stones was ultimately met by the establishment of percutaneous nephrostomy. Like most innovations, its origins are fascinating to explore.

2 The First Percutaneous Nephrostomy

The first recorded percutaneous nephrostomies were performed by Thomas Hillier in the 1860s. Dr. Hillier was caring for a four-year-old boy with presumed ureteropelvic junction obstruction and hydronephrosis causing difficulty ambulating and breathing. In attempt to alleviate the boy's suffering, Dr. Hillier performed multiple percutaneous aspirations over the course of several years in an attempt to create a permanent fistula to the skin, however, the nephrostomy sites repeatedly closed and the child eventually died at the age of eight (Bloom et al. 1989). Percutaneous nephrostomy did not become widely accepted for almost another 100 years, aided by the development of X-ray and a few opportune accidents.

3 Image Guided Nephrostomy

Wilhelm Röentgen discovered X-ray in 1895 which later earned him the Nobel Prize. Over the next 50 years, innovations in X-ray technology paved the way for modern fluoroscopy, which expanded the possibilities for diagnostic and therapeutic procedures (Seibert 1995). Willard Goodwin was a urology trainee at Johns Hopkins in the 1940s with an interest in angiography. During an attempted percutaneous arteriogram for a nonfunctioning kidney, Dr. Goodwin instead punctured a hydronephrotic kidney. Unsure of what to do, he removed his needle and hoped there would be no untoward consequences (there weren't any). A few years later, now the chair of the urology department at UCLA, Dr. Goodwin was presented with a similar scenario. William Casey, a urology resident at UCLA under the watchful eye of Dr. Goodwin, was attempting to perform a percutaneous renal biopsy when he too punctured a hydronephrotic kidney. This time though, Dr. Goodwin injected contrast and performed one of the first recorded antegrade pyelograms. Sensing the potential of this procedure, Casey and Goodwin began performing antegrade pyelograms on patients with hydronephrosis. Their presentation at the 1954 American Urological Association meeting (which was awarded first prize in the essay competition) generated excitement, and paved the way for modern percutaneous nephrostomy. They described their experience and technique in 55 patients, with the optimal puncture site usually being "about five fingerbreadths lateral to the midline and at a level where

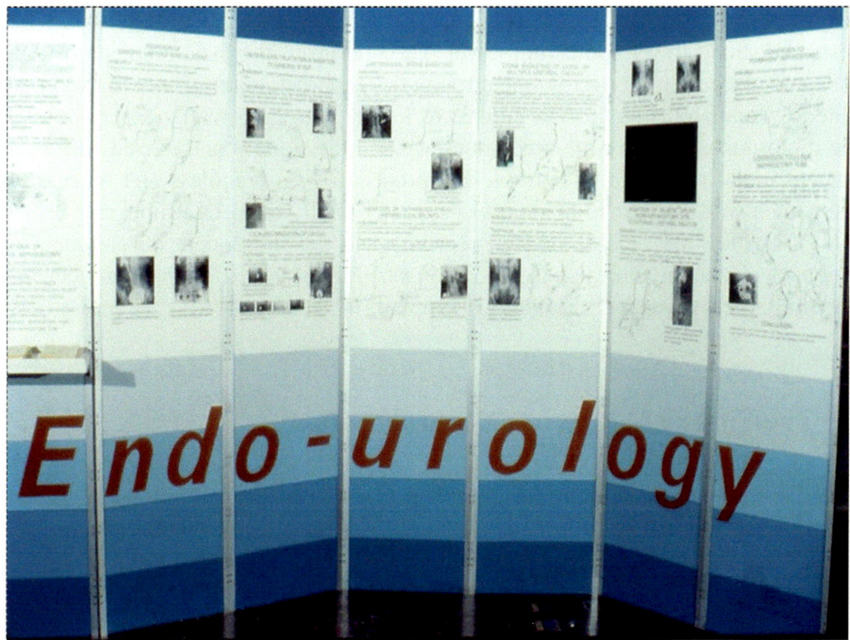

Fig. 1 Endourology Poster at 1980 AUA. Arthur Smith personal collection

a 13th rib would be". Their follow up study of percutaneous nephrostomy tube placement in 16 patients was a natural progression of antegrade pyelography and highlighted the safety of the procedure with notably minimal bleeding risk (Goodwin
1991; Casey and Goodwin 1955; Goodwin et al. 1955). Over the next 20 years,
percutaneous nephrostomy become more widely used. At the same time ultrasound
technology advanced significantly and in 1974 Pedersen reported on the first use
of ultrasound guided percutaneous nephrostomy (Seibert 1995; Pedersen 1974).
With percutaneous nephrostomy now well established, the next logical progression was to utilize a percutaneous nephrostomy to eventually perform percutaneous
nephrolithotomy (Fig. 1).

4 The First Percutaneous Stone Extraction

Believe it or not, the first percutaneous renal stone extraction actually predated
Dr. Goodwin's percutaneous nephrostomy. In 1941, Rupel and Brown performed a
nephrectomy on a 44-year-old woman with a nonfunctioning, infected right kidney.
Notably, her left kidney had a large nonobstructing stone. One month after her right
nephrectomy, the woman returned with anuria and an open nephrostomy tube was
emergently placed on the left side after retrograde catheter placement failed. After

two weeks recovery, Drs. Rupel and Brown contemplated open nephrolithotomy, but instead decided to try something novel. They removed the patient's nephrostomy tube and placed a rigid cystoscope through the nephrostomy tract where they were able to visualize the stone. The stone was too large to grab with graspers through the cystoscope, so the scope was withdrawn and the stone was removed with rigid forceps under radiographic control. The procedure was bloodless and successful; the patient was discharged home four days later totally tubeless (Rupel and Brown 1941). Despite the success of the procedure and the subsequent development of percutaneous nephrostomy in the 1950s, it wasn't until the 1970s that percutaneous nephrolithotomy was more formally attempted.

5   The First Percutaneous Nephrolithotomy

The first true percutaneous nephrolithotomy was performed in 1973 by Fernström and Johansson at the Karolinska Institute in Sweden. They adapted an established technique to percutaneously remove common bile duct stones at their institution to treat three patients with recurrent renal stones. First, a percutaneous nephrostomy was performed at a suitable site for eventual stone removal. Next, the nephrostomy tract was serially dilated by 0.5 mm each day until the caliber of the tract was large enough for stone extraction. Prior to stone extraction, the nephrostomy tract was left to mature with a nephrostomy tube for 14 days. Stones were extracted with either a Dormia stone basket or rigid grasping forceps. After stone extraction, a nephrostomy tube was maintained for at least three days until the patient was radiologically free of stone and had no evidence of obstruction (Fernström and Johansson 1976). While the procedure required a prolonged hospital stay with multiple interventions, the morbidity associated with it was far less than open nephrolithotomy. Over the next several years, percutaneous nephrolithotomy became more common and a variety of other percutaneous renal procedures were developed.

6   The Birth of Endourology

Arthur Smith was a practicing urologist in South Africa in the 1970s when percutaneous renal procedures became popular. At that time in South Africa, it was common practice for urologists to perform percutaneous aspiration and sclerotherapy of renal cysts. When he emigrated from South Africa to the United States to work at the VA Hospital in Minnesota, he discovered that radiologists commonly performed these procedures in America. This led to a collegial relationship with an interventional radiologist, Dr. Robert Miller, who together with Dr. Smith started performing a variety of new percutaneous renal procedures (Smith 2002). Their first collaboration was to treat a patient with an anastomotic leak after a ureteral reimplantation. Because Gibbons stents were the only available stents at the time, and were difficult to place after reimplantation, they devised a technique to pull the Gibbons stent up from the kidney. They placed an angiographic catheter through a percutaneous nephrostomy, maneuvered the angiographic catheter antegrade down the ureter into the bladder, connected the angiographic catheter to the Gibbons ureteral stent, and finally pulled the Gibbons stent up into the desired position (Smith et al. 1978). Using similar principles, Drs. Smith and Miller published a variety of techniques including percutaneous ureteral stone removal in a patient with an ileal conduit, percutaneous dilation of a ureteroileal anastomotic stricture, percutaneous antegrade ureteral meatotomy, conversion of a percutaneous nephrostomy to a U-loop nephrostomy, and percutaneous dissolution of cystine, uric acid, and struvite stones, to name a few. These procedures convinced Dr. Smith that percutaneous nephrostomy gave more direct access to the kidney and ureter than retrograde access did, allowing for many novel treatments. At the 1980 AUA meeting, Dr. Smith and colleagues presented many of these new techniques in a poster titled "Endourology," which was then defined as "closed controlled manipulation within the genitourinary tract" (Smith 2002).

During this same 1980 American Urological Association meeting, Peter Alken presented his German groups initial experience with percutaneous nephrolithotomy. Like Fernström and Johansson, Dr. Alken described serially dilating percutaneous nephrostomy tracts over the course of several days after which a nephrostomy tube was left in place for several more days to mature the nephrostomy tract prior to stone extraction (Alken et al. 1981). Over the next few years, the progression of percutaneous nephrolithotomy was enhanced both in Europe and America, notably by Dr. Alken's group in Germany, Michael Marberger's group in Vienna, John Wickham's group in London, Dr. Smith's group at Long Island Jewish Medical Center, Joseph Segura's group at the Mayo Clinic and Ralph Clayman at the University of Minnesota.

7 Medical Devices for Percutaneous Nephrolithotomy

Around this time, Dr. Smith moved from the Minnesota VA Hospital to the University of Minnesota campus where he began working with two other interventional radiologists, Drs. Kurt Amplatz and Wilfrido Castaneda-Zuniga. Together, they performed rapid dilation of the nephrostomy tract in a single procedure for percutaneous nephrolithotomy (Castaneda-Zuniga et al. 1982a). Dr. Amplatz oversaw a lab that would eventually manufacture many devices still used for percutaneous renal procedures today. Initially they attached a filiform follower to the end of a 5 Fr angiographic catheter to dilate the tract, but this proved too difficult. Instead, they designed dilators to fit over the angiographic catheter, however, the tip of the dilator was not easily distinguished via X-ray causing potential for overdilation and damage to the ureteropelvic junction. This led to creation of a dilator with a radiopaque metal band at the tip for easy radiologic identification. Various different tract sizes were tried, up to 50 Fr, but ultimately the size of a standard tract was set to be 30 Fr, as it would allow for intact removal of a 1 cm stone. The initial sheaths produced by Dr. Amplatz's lab were simply round tubes which had a tendency to adhere to the tissue when suction was applied, so the tips were cut at oblique angles which were less likely to adhere to tissue (Fig. 2) (Smith 2002; Castaneda-Zuniga et al. 1982b).

A variety of different medical devices were developed to further facilitate percutaneous nephrolithotomy. Initially, percutaneous tracts were dilated with Couvelaire catheters and tapered plastic dilators (Fernström and Johansson 1976). Over time, these dilators were placed by polyurethane, metallic, and balloon dilators still used today (Alken et al. 1981; Castaneda-Zuniga et al. 1982a, b; Clayman et al. 1983). When percutaneous nephrolithotomy began, rigid cystoscopes limited the ability of stone removal to various baskets, graspers, or chemolysis. The introduction of the offset nephroscope in the 1980s provided a straight working channel allowing for the treatment of bigger, more complex stones using larger, rigid instruments as such electrohydraulic and ultrasound lithotripters (Alken et al. 1981; Castaneda-Zuniga et al. 1982a, b; Clayman et al. 1983). After completing percutaneous stone extraction, patients were typically left with nephrostomy tubes of various sizes. Dr. Smith's group preferred a Malecot nephrostomy tube, which was modified so that it could be flattened to fit through a narrow tract. Further modifications led to the addition of a ureteral tail which crossed the ureteropelvic junction and allowed for easy reentry into the collecting system should a second stage procedure be needed.

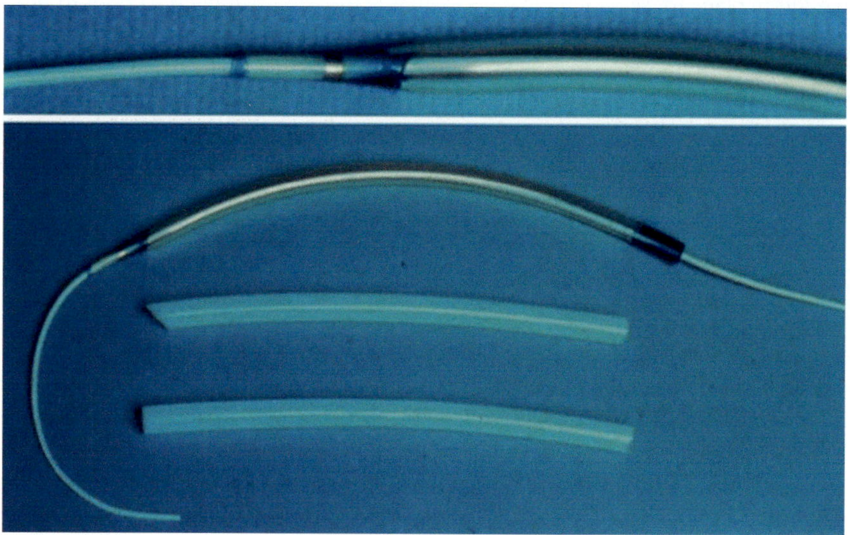

Fig. 2 Original dilators and nephrostomy sheaths (Smith 2002)

8 Dissemination of Percutaneous Nephrolithotomy

In 1982, Dr. Smith moved to New York to become chair at Long Island Jewish Medical Center. That year, Ralph Clayman organized the first course in Endourology at the University of Minneapolis. The goal was to teach general urologists the new methods of performing percutaneous renal procedures, which was aided by the use of a novel porcine model. The course was a great success and was the beginning of a slew of courses offered by the American Urological Association at many centers throughout the United States (Fig. 3) (Smith 2002).

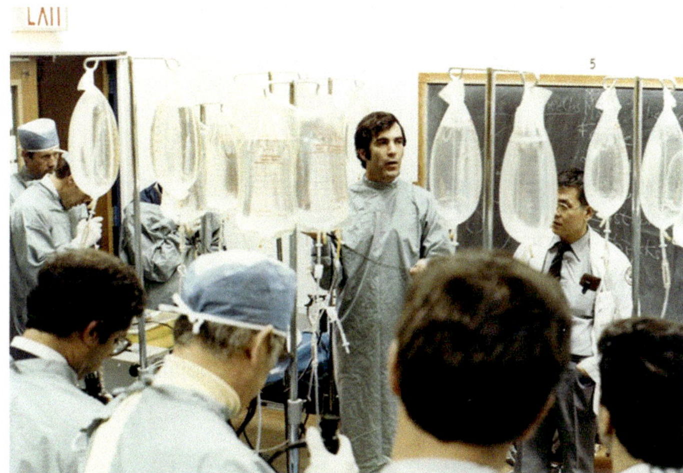

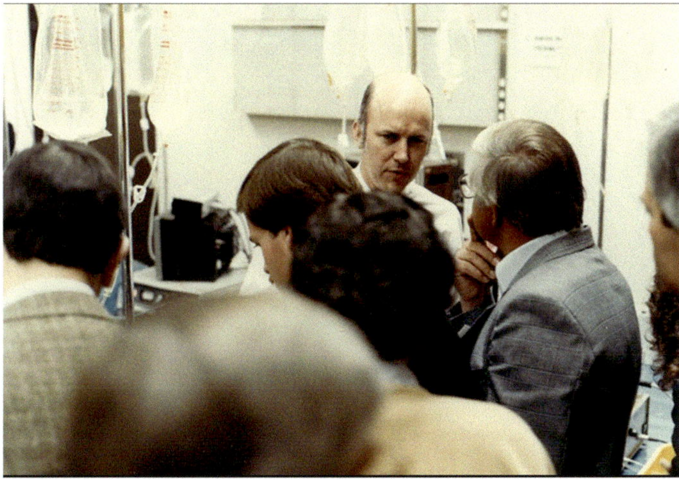

Fig. 3 Pioneers teaching the first course on Percutaneous Nephrolithotomy. Arthur Smith personal collection

                                                    G. Mullen et al.

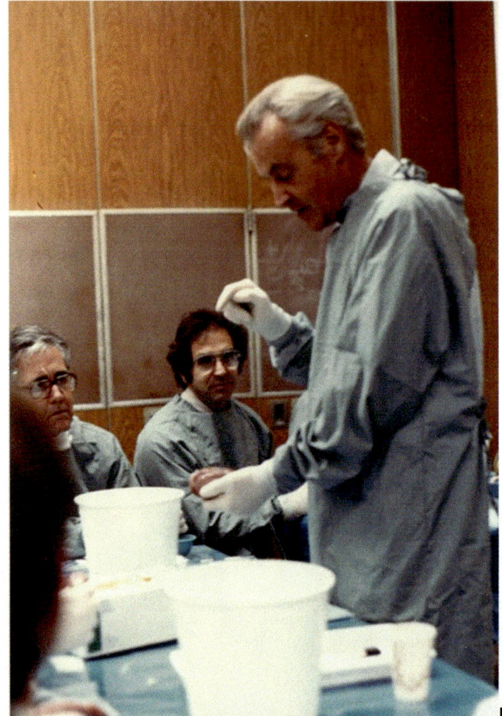

Kurt Amplatz

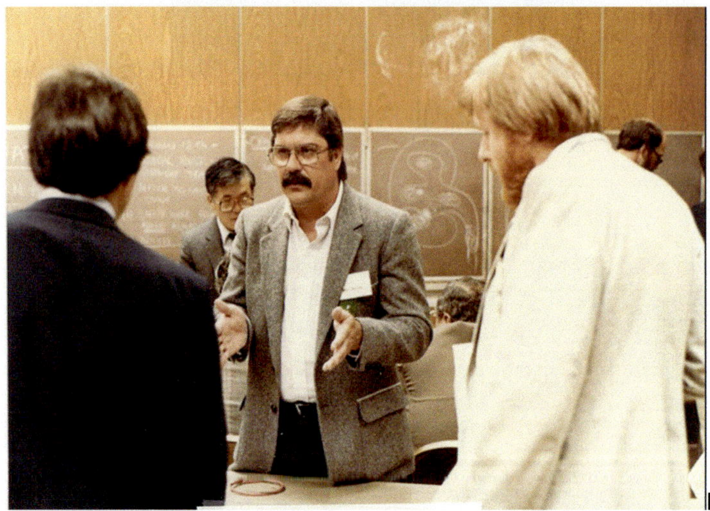

Robert Miller

Fig. 3 (continued)

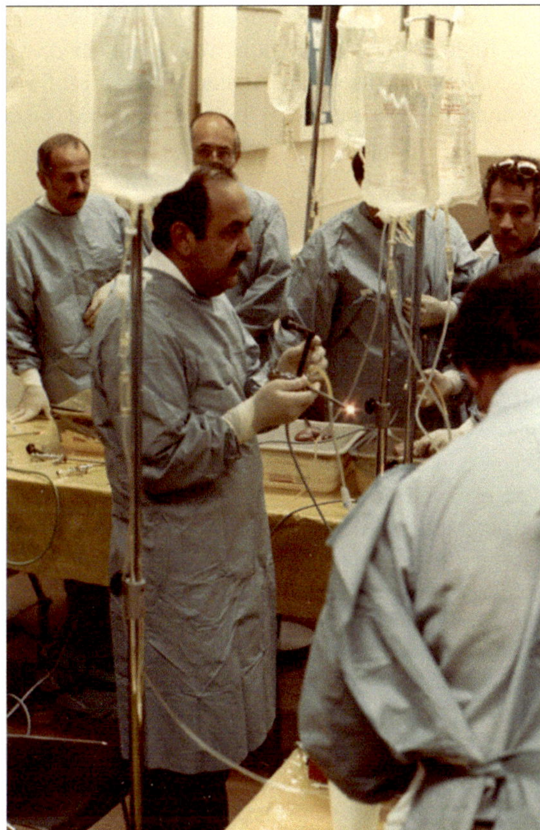

Fig. 3 (continued)

In 1983 John Wickham arranged the first World Congress on Percutaneous Renal Surgery in London, which engendered great enthusiasm. At this meeting, it was decided that Dr. Alken would host the second World Congress and Dr. Smith the third. Shortly after the meeting, Dr. Smith formed the Endourological Society along with Joseph Segura as vice-president, Ralph Clayman as secretary, and Gopal Badlani as treasurer. The guiding principles of the society were to encourage international collaboration, develop and train younger urologists, establish and maintain high quality fellowships, and exchange ideas at yearly international meetings. It was decided that this would not be an exclusive society, but rather all-inclusive with the goal to propagate minimally invasive techniques for the benefit of all patients. Members throughout the world were encouraged to develop their own branches of the Endourological Society, to have local meetings, and to attend the World Congress. A few years after the creation of the Endourological Society, Mary Ann Liebert persuaded Drs. Clayman and Smith to become co-editors and founders of the Journal of Endourology. Initially there were six issues per year, which rapidly increased to monthly issues and has since been in press for over 40 years (Smith 2002). Shortly thereafter, Endourology fellowships were established, which have since trained almost 600 fellows in the United States, over 40% of whom have remained in academic medicine, further advancing the field (Patel and Nakada 2022).

9 Percutaneous Nephrolithotomy Innovations

Percutaneous nephrolithotomy has remained the gold standard treatment for large renal calculi and has undergone dramatic improvements in the fifty years that have passed since the first percutaneous nephrolithotomy. Dr. Wickham's group was the first to report on the omission of a nephrostomy tube after percutaneous renal stone extraction, instead opting for a 'totally tubeless' approach in some patients (Wickham et al. 1984). Gary Bellman and colleagues were the first to study the 'tubeless' approach, which involved leaving a double J stent instead of a nephrostomy tube at the conclusion of the procedure (Bellman et al. 1997). Aside from innovative exit strategies, additional modifications have been proposed as well. Whereas most percutaneous renal procedures were performed in the prone position, José Gabriel Valdivia Uría and his group in Spain were the first to report on the safety and efficacy of performing percutaneous nephrolithotomy in the supine position (Valdivia Uría et al. 1987). Years later, Guohua Zeng and colleagues in China were one of the first groups to report on reducing the tract size for percutaneous nephrolithotomy (Zeng et al. 2013). More recently, percutaneous nephrolithotomy has been performed as an ambulatory procedure with low rates of complications (Chong et al. 2021). Finally, and as should be expected, as percutaneous nephrolithotomy evolved, so too have the number and type of percutaneous renal procedures.

10 Other Percutaneous Renal Procedures

Dr. Smith's presentation of various endourology procedures at the 1980 American Urological Association meeting certainly inspired the development of future percutaneous renal procedures. A few years later at the first World Congress in 1983, Dr. Wickham introduced his experience performing percutaneous incision of a uretero-pelvic junction obstruction, which he termed "pyelolysis" (Wickham and Kellet 1983). Dr. Smith subsequently published a series on percutaneous full-thickness incision of the ureteropelvic junction followed by stenting which he termed "endopyelotomy," a name that has remained (Badlani et al. 1986). Shortly thereafter, Stevan Streem at the Cleveland Clinic published the first reports of percutaneous treatment of upper tract urothelial carcinoma, which is now recognized by the National Comprehensive Cancer Network as an acceptable treatment option for select patients (Streem and Pontes 1986; National Comprehensive Cancer Network 2022). The number of percutaneous renal procedures now offered is even greater, and all trace their roots back to the first percutaneous nephrostomy of the 1860s.

11 Conclusion

Percutaneous nephrolithotomy remains the gold standard for removal of large and complex renal stones. While its origins can be traced, one cannot underestimate the incredible vision which ensured its development. From clinical trials to technological development to education and dissemination of the techniques to all parts of the world, the history of endourology is a marvel. The legacy of the pioneers of percutaneous nephrolithotomy continue to live on at endourology meetings, fellowships, and international collaborative research settings.

References

Alken P, Hutschenreiter G, Günther R, Marberger M. Percutaneous stone manipulation. J Urol. 1981;125(4):463–6.

Badlani G, Eshghi M, Smith AD. Percutaneous surgery for ureteropelvic junction obstruction (endopyelotomy): technique and early results. J Urol. 1986;135(1):26–8.

Bellman GC, Davidoff R, Candela J, Gerspach J, Kurtz S, Stout L. Tubeless percutaneous renal surgery. J Urol. 1997;157(5):1578–82.

Bloom DA, Morgan RJ, Scardino PL. Thomas Hillier and percutaneous nephrostomy. Urology. 1989;33(4):346–50.

Casey WC, Goodwin WE. Percutaneous antegrade pyelography and hydronephrosis; direct, intrapelvic injection of urographic contrast material to secure a pyeloureterogram after percutaneous needle puncture and aspiration of hydronephrosis. J Urol. 1955;74(1):164–73.

Castaneda-Zuniga WR, Smith AD, Rusnak B, Herrera M, Amplatz K. Single-step dilation of nephrostomy tract. J Urol. 1982a;127(2):341.

Castaneda-Zuniga WR, Clayman R, Smith A, Rusnak B, Herrera M, Amplatz K. Nephrostolithotomy: percutaneous techniques for urinary calculus removal. Am J Roentgenol. 1982b;139(4):721–6.

Chong JT, Dunne M, Magnan B, Abbott J, Davalos JG. Ambulatory percutaneous nephrolithotomy in a free-standing surgery center: an analysis of 500 consecutive cases. J Endourol. 2021;35(12):1738–42.

Clayman RV, Castaneda-Zuniga WR, Hunter DW, Miller RP, Lange PH, Amplatz K. Rapid balloon dilatation of the nephrostomy track for nephrostolithotomy. Radiology. 1983;147(3):884–5.

Fernström I, Johansson B. Percutaneous pyelolithotomy. A new extraction technique. Scand J Urol Nephrol. 1976;10(3):257–59

Goodwin WE. A memoir of percutaneous access to the kidney (antegrade pyelography and percutaneous nephrostomy). J Endourol. 1991;5:185–9.

Goodwin WE, Casey WC, Woolf W. Percutaneous trocar (needle) nephrostomy in hydronephrosis. JAMA. 1955;157(11):891–4.

National Comprehensive Cancer Network (2022) Bladder cancer (version 2.2022). https://www.nccn.org/professionals/physician_gls/pdf/bladder.pdf Accessed 2022.

Patel SR, Nakada SY. Quantifying the educational history of the endourological society fellowship programs in the United States. J Urol. 2022;207.

Pedersen JF. Percutaneous nephrostomy guided by ultrasound. J Urol. 1974;112(2):157–9.

Pettersson S. Incisional surgery for renal stones. In: Novick AC, Marberger M, editors. Atlas of clinical urology. London: Current Medicine Group; 2000.

Rupel E, Brown R. Nephroscopy with removal of stone following nephrostomy for obstructive calculus anuria. J Urol. 1941;46:177–82.

Seibert JA. One hundred years of medical diagnostic imaging technology. Health Phys. 1995;69(5):695–720.

Smith AD. A personal perspective on the origins of endourology and the endourological society. J Endourol. 2002;16(10):705–8.

Smith AD, Lange PH, Miller RP, Reinke DB. Introduction of the Gibbons ureteral stent facilitated by antecedent percutaneous nephrostomy. J Urol. 1978;120(5):543–4.

Streem SB, Pontes EJ. Percutaneous management of upper tract transitional cell carcinoma. J Urol. 1986;135(4):773–5.

Valdivia Uría JG, Lachares Santamaría E, Villarroya Rodríguez S, Taberner Llop J, Abril Baquero G, Aranda Lassa JM. Nefrolitectomía percutánea: técnica simplificada (nota previa) [Percutaneous nephrolithectomy: simplified technic (preliminary report)]. Arch Esp Urol. 1987;40(3):177–80.

Wickham JE, Kellet MJ. Percutaneous pyelolysis. Eur Urol. 1983;9(2):122–4.

Wickham JE, Miller RA, Kellett MJ, Payne SR. Percutaneous nephrolithotomy: one stage or two? Br J Urol. 1984;56(6):582–5.

Zeng G, Zhao Z, Wan S, Mai Z, Wu W, Zhong W, Yuan J. Minimally invasive percutaneous nephrolithotomy for simple and complex renal caliceal stones: a comparative analysis of more than 10,000 cases. J Endourol. 2013;27(10):1203–8.

Indications for PCNL Including Guidelines

Victoria Jahrreiss, Robert Geraghty, Lazaros Tzelves, Christian Seitz, Andreas Skolarikos, and Bhaskar Somani

Abstract Percutaneous nephrolithotomy (PCNL) is a well-established procedure for the management of renal and upper ureteric stones. The European Association of Urology (EAU) and the American Urological Association (AUA) provide guidelines on the indications for PCNL. Determining factors are related to size, stone composition and stone location, patient factors as well as failure of other treatment modalities. According to these guidelines, PCNL is recommended as first treatment choice for stones in the kidney, stones larger than 2 cm and stones in patients with anatomical abnormalities. For stones in patients with poor general health or previous failed extracorporeal shock wave lithotripsy (ESWL), PCNL may be considered. The decision to perform PCNL should be made with the patient's unique medical history in mind and individual clinical judgment. Guidelines provide useful information for urologists and can serve as a general reference for the indications for PCNL.

Keywords PNL · PCNL · Indications · Guidelines · Urolithiasis · Kidney stone disease · Kidney calculi

V. Jahrreiss · B. Somani (✉)
Department of Urology, University Hospital Southampton, Southampton, UK
e-mail: bhaskarsomani@yahoo.com

R. Geraghty
Department of Urology, Newcastle Upon Tyne Hospital, Newcastle, UK

L. Tzelves
Department of Urology, University College of London, London, UK

C. Seitz
Department of Urology, Medical University of Vienna, Vienna, Austria

A. Skolarikos
Department of Urology, University of Athens, Athens, Greece

© The Author(s), under exclusive license to Springer Nature Switzerland AG 2023
J. D. Denstedt and E. N. Liatsikos (eds.), *Percutaneous Renal Surgery*,
https://doi.org/10.1007/978-3-031-40542-6_2

1   Introduction

Percutaneous nephrolithotomy (PCNL) has a predominant role in the management of large volume and complex upper urinary tract stones. As a result of technological advances within the last decades, indications for PCNL have changed over the years since the procedure has first been implemented in 1976 by Fernström and Johansson (1976).

In the beginning patients were referred for PCNL if they were not suited for open stone removal. The introduction of new treatment modalities like shock wave lithotripsy (SWL) and ureteroscopy (URS), developments in lithotripsy technology and increasing surgical experience has led to changes in the indications for PCNL towards larger and more complex renal stones (Sabler et al. 2018). The field of PCNL is constantly evolving, with ongoing research aimed at improving the procedure and reducing the risk of complications. One area of focus is the development of less invasive techniques through miniaturization of instruments, which led to further expansion in the role of PCNL (Wright et al. 2016).

However, the introduction of new laser technologies has expanded the feasibility of treating larger stones with retrograde intrarenal surgery (RIRS), which is a less invasive alternative to PCNL. RIRS is associated with fewer risk of major complications and shorter hospital stay compared to PCNL. Although PCNL remains the preferred method for stones greater than 2 cm in diameter.

Recent advancements in laser technology and the development of new minimally invasive PCNL procedures have expanded the treatment options for large renal and upper ureteric stones (Skolarikos et al. 2023; Assimos et al. 2016; Preminger et al. 2005). Guidelines from international expert societies such as the European Association of Urologists (EAU) or the American Urological Association (AUA) offer a framework for urologist to find the best treatment modality for their patients, however these guidelines are only recommendations, and the final decision of patient selection should be made on a case-by-case basis, taking also into consideration the needs, and social or occupational patient requirements.

1.1   EAU Guidelines

According to the EAU Guidelines for urolithiasis (Skolarikos et al. 2023), indications for active removal of renal calculi include obstruction, infections, other symptoms caused by stones, stone growth, stones larger than 15 mm or smaller than 15 mm if observation is not the option of choice, stones in high-risk patients as well as patient related factors like patient preference, comorbidities and patient social situation.

PCNL is still considered the standard procedure for large renal calculi. It is the gold standard and primary treatment option for renal calculi >20 mm. PCNL is an alternative to RIRS and SWL in calculi between 20 and 10 mm due to its higher stone free rates (SFR) although there is a higher risk of bleeding and prolonged hospital

Table 1 Treatment recommendations for renal stones according to EAU guidelines

Stone size	Recommendation
Treatment recommendations for renal stones according to EAU guidelines	
All stones but lower pole stones 10–20 mm	
>20 mm	1. PCNL 2. RIRS or SWL
10–20 mm	SWL or RIRS/PCNL
<10 mm	1. SWL or RIRS 2. PCNL
Lower pole stones 10–20 mm	
No unfavorable factors for SWL	ESWL or RIRS/PCNL
Unfavorable factors for SWL	1. RIRS/PCNL 2. ESWL

stay. PCNL or RIRS is the first choice in lower pole stones between 10 and 20 mm in cases with unfavorable factors for SWL. In lower pole stones PCNL and RIRS can be considered even for stones <10 mm.

According to the EAU guidelines, contraindications for PCNL include ongoing therapy with anticoagulants, untreated urinary tract infections, tumors in the access tract area, potentially malignant kidney tumors and pregnancy (Skolarikos et al. 2023) (Table 1).

1.2 AUA Guidelines

Similar to the EAU guidelines, AUA guidelines state that PCNL should be offered as first line treatment in symptomatic patients with a renal stone burden of >20 mm. Percutaneous nephrolithotomy is considered the first-line treatment for patients with staghorn stones. PCNL can be considered for lower pole stones >10 mm since SFRs are higher, even though morbidity is also higher. In patients with symptomatic caliceal stones PCNL is considered one of the preferred treatments. PCNL may be offered as a treatment option for patients with ureteral stones who are unlikely to have successful treatment with SWL and/or RIRS (Assimos et al. 2016).

It is important to note that these guidelines are intended to serve as a general reference and not as a substitute for individual clinical judgment. Ultimately, the decision to perform PCNL should be made on a case-by-case basis and in conjunction with the patient's unique medical history and needs (Table 2).

Table 2 Treatment recommendations for renal stones according to AUA guidelines

Stone size	Recommendation
Treatment recommendations for renal stones according to AUA guidelines	
Non lower pole <20 mm	SWL or RIRS
All renal stones >20 mm	PCNL
Lower pole stones <10 mm	SWL or RIRS
Lower pole stones >10 mm	PCNL recommended

1.3 Stone Size

Stone size is one of the main factors guiding the choice of treatment in patients with kidney stone disease. The EAU guidelines recommend that stones larger than 2 cm should be treated with PCNL, as other minimally invasive procedures such as ureteroscopy and SWL may be less effective for stones of this size (Skolarikos et al. 2023). Similarly, the AUA guidelines state that PCNL should be offered for stones larger than 20 mm (Assimos et al. 2016). Furthermore PCNL is considered the gold standard in the treatment of staghorn stones due to higher SFRs and less need for multiple treatments (Preminger et al. 2005; Ucer et al. 2022). A recent prospective controlled study compared SFRs in patients with renal stones between 20 and 40 mm treated with RIRS or PCNL. The SFR in patients treated with PCNL was 94%, while the SFR for patients treated with RIRS was 73% ($p < 0.01$). The authors found no significant statistical differences in minor complication rates and operating times. Hospital stay for patients treated with PCNL and RIRS was 2.9 days and 1.13 days, respectively ($p < 0.05$) (Ucer et al. 2022).

Although stone size is an important factor in determining the optimal treatment option for patients with kidney stone disease, it is important to note that stone size is not the only factor that should be considered in the decision to perform PCNL. Other factors, such as the patient's medical history, anatomy, and the composition of the stones, should also be taken into account.

1.4 Stone Composition

The chemical composition of the urinary stone determines its hardness which has a direct effect on the ability of shockwaves to fragment a stone. Therefore understanding stone composition is an important factor in determining the most appropriate treatment for patients with kidney stone disease (Gücük and Uyetürk 2014). Evaluation of stone density utilizing non contrast computed tomography can help assess the success rates of SWL and consequently the need for PCNL (Shah et al. 2010; El-Nahas et al. 2007). The European Association of Urology (EAU) and the American

Urological Association (AUA) both include stone composition as a factor in their guidelines for the management of ureteral and renal stones.

Stones with a higher density, measured by Hounsfield Units on non-contrast CT scans such as brushite, calcium oxalate monohydrate, or cystine stones are particularly hard and known to be resistant to SWL (El-Nahas et al. 2007; Lee et al. 2016). Both the AUA and the EAU guidelines recommend the utilization of PCNL or RIRS for the treatment of these SWL-resistant large kidney stones (Skolarikos et al. 2023; Assimos et al. 2016). Although stone free is the goal of treatment, this is especially important in certain type of stones such as struvite and cystine stones (Skolarikos et al. 2023; Assimos et al. 2016; Preminger et al. 2005).

1.5 Stone Location

The treatment of lower pole stones can be challenging due to the complex anatomy of the lower pole calyces, their low likelihood of passing fragments spontaneously and possible difficulties in accessing these with RIRS. PCNL is considered a safe and effective option for the treatment of lower pole stones, especially when other minimally invasive methods are not feasible or have been unsuccessful.

According to the EAU guidelines PCNL, RIRS and SWL should be considered for the treatment of lower pole stones between 10 and 20 mm. However, in cases with unfavorable factors like steep infundibular pelvic angle and long infundibular length and narrow infundibular width, SWL is not the treatment of choice due to its low efficacy. In lower pole stones PCNL and RIRS can be considered for stones smaller than 10 mm (Skolarikos et al. 2023). According to the AUA guidelines PCNL can be offered in lower pole stones larger than 10 mm (Assimos et al. 2016).

In a recent systematic review and meta-analysis comparing PCNL, RIRS and SWL for lower pole stones, SWL was shown to achieve lower complication rates when compared to PCNL with OR 0.40 (95% CI 0.24–0.65) ($p = 0.0002$). On the other hand, PCNL and RIRS had higher SFR compared to SWL with OR 6.7 (95% CI 4.35–10.31) ($p < 0.00001$). Therefore, the authors recommend PCNL or RIRS to be the treatment of choice to accomplish stone free status with a minimal number of sessions in lower pole stones. However, the optimal treatment option for each patient should be determined individually depending on anatomy, comorbidities and patients' preference (Kallidonis et al. 2020).

1.6 Anatomical Anomalies

Urinary tract anomalies can be accompanied by impaired urine drainage and stone formation. The variation in collecting system architecture as well as vascular differences presented in patients with renal abnormalities makes PCNL a challenging procedure (Prakash et al. 2017). In anatomically normal kidneys, the renal pelvis lies medially, and the calyces are located posteriorly, making renal puncture easier. In a malrotated kidney on the other hand, the puncture becomes challenging as the pelvis rotates anteriorly, and the calyces are found postero-laterally. In the case of ectopic pelvic kidney, where the bowel lies in close proximity to the kidney, a laparoscopic assistance may be required to access the kidney percutaneously. In a duplex system, stones located in upper calyx cannot be managed by accessing a lower pole calyx and vice versa. All these complicating factors make PCNL quite difficult and challenging.

1.7 Calyceal Diverticular Stones

The treatment of calyceal diverticular stones can be challenging due to the complex anatomy of the diverticulum and difficulty in accessing stones within the calyx. While there is no clear consensus on the need to treat calyceal calculi, indications for treatment include pain, de novo obstruction, associated infections and stone growth (Brandt et al. 1993; Andersson and Sylvén 1983). The presence of symptomatic calyceal diverticular stones is widely recognized as an indication for active stone removal by both EAU and AUA guidelines.

For the treatment of calyceal diverticular stones, higher success rates were previously demonstrated with PCNL when compared to SWL. Percutaneous approach has many advantages when compared to intrarenal approach. It offers an improved access to larger and complex stones especially when they are located posteriorly within the kidney.

Through percutaneous approach fulguration or incision of the diverticular neck is also possible, which is essential in preventing further stone formation within the diverticulum (Nakada et al. 1999). In another review, PCNL was defined as the most suitable approach for posteriorly located mid- to lower-pole stones and it has the advantage to directly ablate the diverticulum. PCNL is also a feasible option for upper pole calyceal diverticular stones, but it bears the risk of pulmonary complications. Therefore, the some authors recommend the implication of subcostal access strategies such as triangulation or renal displacement (Waingankar et al. 2014).

In another retrospective study Srivastava et al. reported their 10 years of experience in 44 cases with calyceal diverticular stones. PCNL showed a total stone clearance of 90%. In about 80% of the cases the diverticula were dilated and stented and in 20% fulguration was the method of choice. If the guide wire could be passed through the neck of the diverticula, the surgeons dilated and stented it. If the neck of the diverticula could not be found, they fulgurated the diverticular walls. Complications occurred in only 3(6.8%) of 44 patients. The postoperative imaging showed obliteration of diverticula in seven patients and improved drainage in 37 patients. Patients were followed for an average of 2 years where 41 (93.18%) patients remained asymptomatic and only two (4.5%) patients developed recurrent stones (Srivastava et al. 2013).

1.8 Horseshoe Kidney

With an incidence of 1/400, Horseshoe kidney (HSK) is the most common renal fusion anomaly (Evans and Resnick 1981). Due to the malrotation of the kidney and collecting system complexity, PCNL in HSK is a challenging procedure for RIRS or SWL (Skolarikos et al. 2023; Assimos et al. 2016; Preminger et al. 2005). In patients with HSKs, even smaller stone volume can be treated through a percutaneous approach. An infra-costal puncture aiming at the posterior upper calix, which is typically in a more medial and caudal location than the normal kidney, should be preferred in HSKs. This method will deliver a safe access and success rates quoted is about 92% for PCNL in HSKs. Auxiliary procedures may be however be needed in order to achieve this stone free rates (Purkait et al. 2016).

In their study Satav et al. performed PCNL on 23 patients with HSKs. Mean stones size was 22 mm, and a complete stone clearance was achieved in 88% of the patients. Post operatively, two renal units with residual stone >8 mm were cleared with ESWL. No significant intra- or postoperative complications were observed (Satav et al. 2018).

Another important aspect to consider in HSKs is the increased length of the access tract which might require the usage of flexible instruments and intracorporeal lithotripsy devices in order to achieve a better stone clearance as rigid nephroscopes can be size-limiting to work with.

1.9 Ectopic or Fused Kidneys

In ectopic and fused kidneys PCNL can be performed either using the standard approach or with the utilization of laparoscopic-assisted transabdominal puncture. In their small series with eight patients, Matlaga et al. reached a 100% SFR with primary and second look PCNL without any complications (Matlaga et al. 2006).

2   Patient Factors

2.1 Occupation

In certain group of patients even asymptomatic kidney stones poses a threat to their safety or occupation. For example, civilian and military pilots or soldiers who are on active duty cannot take the risk of developing a renal colic when performing their tasks. In these patients' indication for PCNL can be justified due to the higher one procedure SFR when compared to ESWL or RIRS. In their multicenter study analyzing treatment outcomes of aircraft pilots with kidney stones, Zeng et al. (2002) demonstrated SWL to be the least likely treatment modality to render the patients stone free (35%) after the initial treatment, and has resulted in the longest work-lost interval (4.7 weeks). On the other hand, PCNL showed an SFR of 100% after the first intervention and a work-loss interval of only 2.6 weeks.

2.2 Obesity

With an increasing body mass index (BMI) of above 30 kg/m² any surgical or interventional procedure becomes more challenging. The number of obese patients in the western world has increased in the past years due to unhealthy lifestyle and poor eating habits. Obesity can hinder SWL mostly due to technical issues. Limitation of the SWL tables with regard to the weight they can support, bad imaging resolution due to access fat and lower impact of shock waves due to a longer skin to stone distance can alter success rates after SWL. For example, obesity was shown to diminish the success rate of SWL from 79 to 57% when the skin to stone distance is greater than 9 cm (Perks et al. 2008).

A higher BMI does not appear to hinder the success rates after PCNL with regards to SFR, complications, cost or length of hospital stay. In morbidly obese patients, alterations and minor modifications to the working instruments or technique may be necessary. PCNL can also be performed under conscious sedation with local anesthesia, which can minimize the cardiovascular and pulmonary impact of the prone position in morbidly obese patients (Kanaroglou and Razvi 2006).

2.3 Patients with Urinary Diversions

Urinary stones are a common long-term complication in patients with ileum conduits (12%). In these patients retrograde access can be quite challenging due to the anatomical alterations. PCNL has been reported to deliver higher SFR (75–100%) and lower complication rates (12%) in patients with urinary diversions (Méndez Probst et al. 2009). Another important factor that favorizes the utilization of PCNL in patients with urinary diversion is their tendency to build struvite stones, which require a complete stone clearance in order to prevent rapid recurrent stone formation.

2.4 Skeletal Anomalies

In cases of severe scoliosis or body contractures, SWL positioning and effective coupling with the shockwave head may be limited; thus, this subgroup of patients may be better treated with RIRS or PCNL (Méndez Probst et al. 2009). However, such orthopedic limitations my also hinder the percutaneous approach and limit the utilization of PCNL.

2.5 *Encrusted Foreign Objects*

Foreign bodies within the upper urinary tract such as ureteral stent fragments, nonabsorbable sutures, and dilation balloon fragments may be best removed through a percutaneous access if the retrograde approach fails. It is important to remove all foreign bodies out of the renal system as they serve as a nidus for stone formation and urinary tract infections (Méndez Probst et al. 2009).

2.6 *PCNL in Paediatric Patients*

With the popularization of minimally invasive PCNLs, it is now gaining more popularity in the paediatric age group (Jones et al. 2017). It should a low risk of major complications, with a high SFR suggesting that a smaller tract size is much better in this age group.

2.7 *Future Directions for PCNL*

With the introduction of super pulsed thulium laser technology, a new era began in the treatment of kidney stones. The indications for RIRS have been expanded for even larger stones. A recent systematic review on renal calculi larger than 20 mm found a cumulative SFR for RIRS of 91% with 1.45 procedures needed per patient (Geraghty et al. 2015). However, the data on the feasibility of RIRS for treating large stones is still limited. PCNL remains to be the first option for stones larger than 20 mm however with more data emerging there might be a shift towards RIRS in the coming years. In the recent years we have also seen a miniaturization of PCNL instruments resulting in SFRs comparable to standard PCNL with lower perioperative complication rates especially in term of bleeding. There seems to be a wider use of suction with PCNL procedures, and it might help to achieve better SFR and minimize recurrences (Chen et al. 2022). PCNL will definitely remain as a very important technique in the urological armamentarium in the future.

References

Andersson L, Sylvén M. Small renal caliceal calculi as a cause of pain. J Urol. 1983;130(4):752–3.

Assimos D, Krambeck A, Miller N, Monga M, Murad M, Nelson C. Surgical management of stones: AUA/endourology society guideline. 2016.

Brandt B, Ostri P, Lange P, Kvist Kristensen J. Painful caliceal calculi. The treatment of small nonobstructing caliceal calculi in patients with symptoms. Scand J Urol Nephrol. 1993;27(1):75–6.

Chen J, Cai X, Wang G, et al. Efficacy and safety of percutaneous nephrolithotomy combined with negative pressure suction in the treatment of renal calculi: a systematic review and meta-analysis. Transl Androl Urol. 2022;11(1):79019.

El-Nahas AR, El-Assmy AM, Mansour O, Sheir KZ. A prospective multivariate analysis of factors predicting stone disintegration by extracorporeal shock wave lithotripsy: the value of high-resolution noncontrast computed tomography. Eur Urol. 2007;51(6):1688–93; discussion 93–4.

Evans WP, Resnick MI. Horseshoe kidney and urolithiasis. J Urol. 1981;125(5):620–1.

Fernström I, Johansson B. Percutaneous pyelolithotomy. A new extraction technique. Scand J Urol Nephrol. 1976;10(3):257–59.

Geraghty R, Abourmarzouk O, Rai B, Biyani CS, Rukin NJ, Somani BK. Evidence for ureterorenoscopy and laser fragmentation (URSL) for large renal stones in the modern era. Curr Urol Rep. 2015;16(8):54.

Gücük A, Uyetürk U. Usefulness of hounsfield unit and density in the assessment and treatment of urinary stones. World J Nephrol. 2014;3(4):282–6.

Jones P, Bennett G, Aboumarzouk OM, Griffin S, Somani BK. Role of minimally invasive percutaneous nephrolithotomy techniques—Micro and ultra-mini PCNL (<15F) in the pediatric population: a systematic review. J Endourol. 2017;31(9):816–24.

Kallidonis P, Ntasiotis P, Somani B, Adamou C, Emiliani E, Knoll T, et al. Systematic review and meta-analysis comparing percutaneous nephrolithotomy, retrograde intrarenal surgery and shock wave lithotripsy for lower pole renal stones less than 2 cm in maximum diameter. J Urol. 2020;204(3):427–33.

Kanaroglou A, Razvi H. Percutaneous nephrolithotomy under conscious sedation in morbidly obese patients. Can J Urol. 2006;13(3):3153–5.

Lee JY, Kim JH, Kang DH, Chung DY, Lee DH, Do Jung H, et al. Stone heterogeneity index as the standard deviation of Hounsfield units: a novel predictor for shock-wave lithotripsy outcomes in ureter calculi. Sci Rep. 2016;6:23988.

Matlaga BR, Kim SC, Watkins SL, Kuo RL, Munch LC, Lingeman JE. Percutaneous nephrolithotomy for ectopic kidneys: over, around, or through. Urology. 2006;67(3):513–7.

Méndez Probst CE, Denstedt JD, Razvi H. Preoperative indications for percutaneous nephrolithotripsy in 2009. J Endourol. 2009;23(10):1557–61.

Nakada SY, Streem S, Preminger GM, Wolf JS Jr, Leveillee RJ. Controversial cases in endourology. Caliceal diverticular calculi. J Endourol. 1999;13(2):61–4.

Perks AE, Schuler TD, Lee J, Ghiculete D, Chung DG, Honey RJDA, et al. Stone attenuation and skin-to-stone distance on computed tomography predicts for stone fragmentation by shock wave lithotripsy. Urology. 2008;72(4):765–9.

Prakash G, Sinha RJ, Jhanwar A, Bansal A, Singh V. Outcome of percutaneous nephrolithotomy in anomalous kidney: Is it different? Urol Ann. 2017;9(1):23–6.

Preminger GM, Assimos DG, Lingeman JE, Nakada SY, Pearle MS, Wolf JS, Jr. Chapter 1: AUA guideline on management of staghorn calculi: diagnosis and treatment recommendations. J Urol. 2005;173(6):1991–2000.

Purkait B, Sankhwar SN, Kumar M, Patodia M, Bansal A, Bhaskar V. Do outcomes of percutaneous nephrolithotomy in horseshoe kidney in children differ from adults? A single-center experience. J Endourol. 2016;30(5):497–503.

Sabler IM, Katafigiotis I, Gofrit ON, Duvdevani M. Present indications and techniques of percutaneous nephrolithotomy: What the future holds? Asian J Urol. 2018;5(4):287–94.

Satav V, Sabale V, Pramanik P, Kanklia SP, Mhaske S. Percutaneous nephrolithotomy of horseshoe kidney: our institutional experience. Urol Ann. 2018;10(3):258–62.

Shah K, Kurien A, Mishra S, Ganpule A, Muthu V, Sabnis RB, et al. Predicting effectiveness of extracorporeal shockwave lithotripsy by stone attenuation value. J Endourol. 2010;24(7):1169–73.

Skolarikos A, Neisius A, Petřík A, Somani BS, Tailly T, et al. EAU guidelines on urolithiasis. 2023.

Srivastava A, Chipde SS, Mandhani A, Kapoor R, Ansari MS. Percutaneous management of renal caliceal diverticular stones: ten-year experience of a tertiary care center with different techniques to deal with diverticula after stone extraction. Ind J Urol. 2013;29(4):273–6.

Ucer O, Erbatu O, Albaz AC, Temeltas G, Gumus B, Muezzinoglu T. Comparison stone-free rate and effects on quality of life of percutaneous nephrolithotomy and retrograde intrarenal surgery for treatment of renal pelvis stone (2–4 cm): a prospective controlled study. Curr Urol. 2022;16(1):5–8.

Waingankar N, Hayek S, Smith AD, Okeke Z. Calyceal diverticula: a comprehensive review. Rev Urol. 2014;16(1):29–43.

Wright A, Rukin N, Smith D, De la Rosette J, Somani BK. Mini, ultra, micro'—nomenclature and cost of these new minimally invasive percutaneous nephrolithotomy (PCNL) techniques. Ther Adv Urol. 2016;8(2):142–6.

Zheng W, Beiko DT, Segura JW, Preminger GM, Albala DM, Denstedt JD. Urinary calculi in aviation pilots: what is the best therapeutic approach? J Urol. 2002;168(4 Pt 1):1341–3.

Training and Simulation Models in PCNL

Christopher Wanderling, Ashley Li, Aaron Saxton, Domenico Veneziano, and Ahmed Ghazi

Abstract Urolithiasis have become an increasingly common medical problem. While urologists have many tools in their armamentarium for treatment, percutaneous nephrolithotomy (PCNL) remains a first-line treatment for large (≥ 2 cm) or challenging stones. PCNL bolsters high stone-free rates, but it remains a complex procedure with many nuances. One of the most challenging steps is percutaneous access. Meticulous preparation is involved for PCNL, as surgeons plan the most ideal needle access path. If perfect access is achieved in an efficient manner, this significantly reduces the risks of complications and increases the chance of rendering patients stone-free. Many simulation training modalities exist for PCNL ranging from low-fidelity benchtop models to high-fidelity, validated immersion simulation. In this chapter we review the available simulation platforms for training PCNL procedure.

Keywords Simulation · Training · Percutaneous neprolithotomy (PCNL) · Augmented reality (AR) · Virtual reality (VR) · Immersive · Patient-specific

Abbreviations

PCNl	Percutaneous nephrolithotomy
PRA	Percutaneous renal access
SBE	Simulation-based education
VR	Virtual reality
AR	Augmented reality
MR	Mixed reality

C. Wanderling · A. Li · A. Saxton
University of Rochester Medical Center, Rochester, NY, USA

D. Veneziano
The Smith Institute of Urology, Northwell Health, New York, NY, USA

A. Ghazi (✉)
Brady Urological Institute, Johns Hopkins University, Baltimore, MD, USA
e-mail: ahmed_ghazi@urmc.rochester.edu

© The Author(s), under exclusive license to Springer Nature Switzerland AG 2023   25
J. D. Denstedt and E. N. Liatsikos (eds.), *Percutaneous Renal Surgery*,
https://doi.org/10.1007/978-3-031-40542-6_3

TEC	Thiel's-embalmed cadaver
US	Ultrasound
PCS	Pelvicalyceal collecting system
PVA	Polyvinyl alcohol
SFR	Stone-free rates
SIL	Simulation Innovation Laboratory
IP	In person

1   Section 1: Introduction

The most crucial step of percutaneous nephrolithotomy (PCNL) is obtaining percutaneous renal access (PRA), which is also the most challenging. Given the close proximity of the kidney to vital structures, incorrect placement of the needle may lead to complications such as bleeding, pneumothorax, hydrothorax, or injury to surrounding organs. According to the largest PCNL database, the major complications included significant bleeding (7.8%), renal pelvis perforation (3.4%), and hydrothorax (1.8%). Blood transfusion was administered in 5.7% of patients, and fever >38.5 °C occurred in 10.5% of patients. At 30-day follow-up, the stone-free rate (SFR) was 75.7%, and 84.5% of patients did not need additional treatment (Rosette et al. 2008). Obtaining PRA independently gives urologists more flexibility and ability for procedural optimization, including the timing of surgery and optimizing PRA tract location. A retrospective single center study demonstrated improved surgical outcomes of PCNL when PRA was obtained by the urologist rather than by an interventional radiologist. However, a prior survey of urologist practice patterns demonstrated that only 11% of those performing PCNL obtained PRA themselves whom were more likely trained on the procedure during residency. A significant difference in annually performed percutaneous renal procedures (14 $\pm$ 4 vs. 3.3 $\pm$ 1.7, $p = 0.02$) was also demonstrated in urologists formally trained versus those untrained in obtaining PRA. Furthermore, in order to maintain competence, it is suggested that a urologist should perform a minimum of 14–16 PCNLs annually. Gaining proficiency in PCNL can be difficult given its steep learning curve. To track the learning curve for PCNL, there are several surrogate markers of surgical competence including SFR, complication rate, operation time, and fluoroscopy time. It has been recognized that operative time for new surgeons decreases to a plateau at 60 cases, but the duration of fluoroscopy and radiation dose improved to a plateau level after 115 cases. Therefore, it was reasonable to conclude that competency is achieved at 60 cases and excellence is obtained after 115 cases (Patterson 2022).

Training for PCNL was traditionally performed under the Halsted apprenticeship model of "see one, do one, teach one". Surgical skills were traditionally acquired over a long period of time under direct supervision, requiring a large investment of time, effort, and resources for the mentor and trainee. With the work hours restriction, increased procedural complexity, limited operative time, and increased medical litigation, there has been a shift away from this apprentice model. To address these concerns, simulation and skills laboratories found ways to provide efficient and effective modes of learning in a controlled and safe setting. The role of simulation-based education (SBE) is to create an artificial environment that mimics a real-life scenario in order to train and evaluate an individual to that particular scenario (Kozan et al. 2020).

2 Section 2: Types of Simulation

2.1 *Generic Simulation*

SBE is a method of interactive training that can replace or support education; this can be achieved with simulators of any kind. The benefit of SBE is the ability to practice in a safe environment without supervision. Since errors and mistakes are more common in a novice surgeon, it is important to allow for practice to improve skills to reduce the incidence. SBE has been accepted by Graduate Medical Education (GME) as an effective adjunct to surgical training and has been adopted into many residency curriculums. There are several SBEs in urology residency training such as suprapubic catheter insertion, cystoscopy, and circumcision with routine items (ex. surgical gloves or sponges). With improved technology, there have been recent advancements in PCNL SBE including virtual reality (VR), augmented reality (AR), and mixed reality (MR) platforms as well as patient specific simulation, which will be highlighted in this chapter (Kozan et al. 2020).

For SBE to be valuable for training, it must be validated. Validity is "the property of a test being true, correct, and in conformity with reality". There are several standards to evaluate the validity of a test, although now outdated face validity, content validity, contrast validity, concurrent validity and predictive validity remain the most common reported parameters. Face validity is typically determined by experts, who evaluate whether the test will measure what it is supposed to measure. Content validity is a detailed review of each of the test items and its relevance and cohesiveness in the test. Construct validity is the ability to discern individuals of different performance levels in a given task (ex. expert vs. novice). Concurrent validity is the evaluation of the new test in comparison to the "gold standard" assessment. Predictive validity is how the scores of the test will be predictive of actual performance. Predictive validity is likely the most clinically meaningful but also the less commonly demonstrated, while the other validity types focus on the elements of the test itself.

Fidelity refers to how realistic and exact a SBE is to the real-life situation that it is designed to emulate (Kozan et al. 2020). These are based on physical, psychosocial, and conceptual characteristics including the environment, equipment, specific scenario and mental processes the learner must use in the SBE. Low-fidelity models (ex. foam, surgical glove, vegetable models) are mostly used to train particular skills or techniques, such as suturing and knot tying, with the advantage of drastically reducing the cost and widespread of education. On the other hand the more expensive and less democratized high-fidelity models (ex. biologic models, cadaver/animal models, VR/AR/MR SBE) practice more detailed steps of a procedure and may feel more realistic. Typically, a learner starts with low-fidelity models and transfer the acquired skills to high-fidelity models. If learners begin their training with a high-fidelity model with no prior acquisition of the prerequisite skillset yet, they may feel overwhelmed and slower in their learning.

2.2 Physical Simulation

Physical SBE exists as many domains. These include basic bench models, 3D printed models, animal models, and cadaveric SBE. One of the purest benefits of physical SBE is the ability to provide haptic feedback. Surgery is an art that takes hundreds of hours to achieve competence and years to master. As the focus of SBE surrounds technology, many advanced SBEs rely on AR or VR. While these modalities possess clear benefit, they lack the haptic feedback necessary to refine technical skills, which in this specific field may be critical in order to achieve the expected goals.

Cadaveric Models

Human cadavers are considered the "gold standard" for surgical training as they are the ultimate anatomical simulation. Cadavers provide many opportunities for SBE, ranging from open to minimally invasive cases and endoscopic procedures. Human cadavers can be preserved in several methods. The most common are fresh frozen cadavers, Thiel's embalmed cadavers (TEC), and formalin-fixed cadavers. While fresh frozen cadavers are the most realistic, they are also the most difficult to maintain and store and can decay rapidly. Formalin-fixed cadavers are more cost effective yet the formalin stiffens the tissue. TECs carry lower storage cost and more supple tissues, however, require the tedious embalming process and do not allow tissue perfusion (Ghazi et al. 2022). Though human cadavers may be the most anatomically accurate to patients, they carry a high cost, limited supply, dedicated environments, challenging tissue perfusion, and difficulties preserving natural color and texture of tissue notably with repeat usage.

There is a paucity of literature evaluating PCNL SBE in human cadavers (Patterson 2022). Fresh frozen cadavers have been validated for face and content for various procedures. Veys et al. evaluated TECs for ultrasound (US) guided PCNL access simulation and training. 13 urologists evaluated the platform via a questionnaire (5-point Likert scale). US images, kidney puncture and dilatation were deemed very realistic and useful as a training tool. PCS anatomy and consistency were similar to real life. Quality and satisfaction of TEC in US-guided supine endoscopic was good to excellent and comparable to a real-life procedure. Overall appropriateness of the TEC model was considered excellent for both initial and advanced supine

PCNL training. Drawbacks included difficulty in incising skin compared to living patients and inconsistency among cadavers in ability to distend the collecting system (Patterson 2022; Kozan et al. 2020).

Animal Models

Live animal models are able to maintain tissue perfusion allowing for trainees to manage hemorrhage and hemostasis. Porcine model is the most common animal model in urology due to similar renal anatomy, however the kidneys are often smaller with narrower pelvicalyceal collecting system (PCS). An *in vivo* biological model for PCNL also takes into account the movement of the kidney with respirations, which is difficult to simulate in other platforms. Several animal models have been evaluated but only realism was established (Kozan et al. 2020). A modular training scheme on anesthetized pigs has been developed prior to performing PCNL independently on patients (Kallidonis et al. 2015). However, the use of animal models can carry high costs correlated to the raise of the animal, its management in dedicated facilities, veterinarian support in addition to extensive ethical concerns (Fig. 1).

As a result of imperfect anatomic correlation to humans and financial and ethical concerns surrounding anesthetized animal models, more focus of animal models has been on obtaining the kidneys from previously slaughtered animals and incorporating them as *ex vivo* biologic bench models. An example of an *ex vivo* biologic model is the porcine kidney inserted into a chicken carcass. On this model, with US or fluoroscopic guidance, subjects were able to perform PRA, wire manipulation, tract dilation, and pyelography. This model has established content and construct validity (Vijayakumar et al. 2019). Klein, et al. also used porcine kidneys as an *ex vivo* model but instead implanted into ballistic gel. This model was able to utilize US

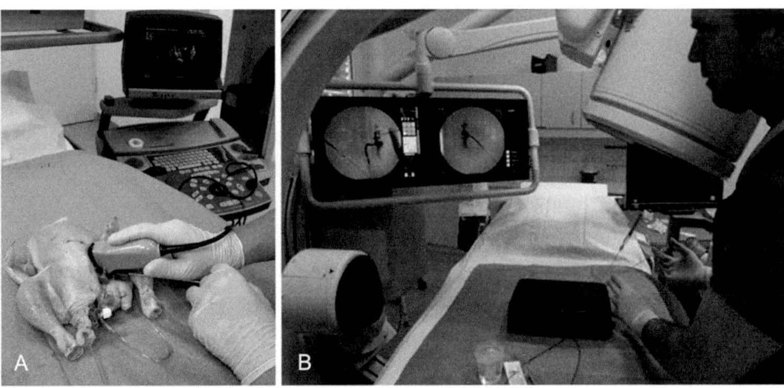

Fig. 1 Animal models for PCNL simulation (**A**) *Ex vivo* porcine kidney in chicken carcass with US guided access (Hacker et al. 2007). (**B**) *Ex vivo* porcine kidney in ballistic gel with fluoroscopic guided access (Klein et al. 2018)

and fluoroscopic-guided PRA. This model was able to establish face, content, and construct validity (Klein et al. 2018).

The widely accepted PERC Mentor (discussed below) was compared to a porcine model by Mishra, et al. In this study, 24 experts attempted PRA on the anesthetized pig and then on the PERC Mentor simulator. These experts rated the porcine model as more realistic overall in comparison with the PERC Mentor. The PERC mentor was rated better for needle aspiration and repetitive performance. Results were similar regarding tactile feedback. This porcine model established content validity (Mishra et al. 2010).

Limitations applied to the use of ex-vivo biologic models have to be considered anyway in the evaluation of such experimental simulators, which are often not easily spreadable on a large scale.

Bench Simulators

Bench simulators may be characterized as biologic or non-biologic. The difference is that the biologic models may contain animal or cadaveric components (ex. porcine or bovine kidneys) while non-biologic models do not contain any animal or cadaveric components (ex. 3D printed, silicon or hydrogel models). Recently, several high-fidelity benchtop non-biological models have been fabricated with realism comparative to human tissue that allow for the practice of multiple steps or even a complete procedure (Fig. 2).

An example of such a high-fidelity bench model is the CAT (C-Arm Trainer), created by a group from the University of Minnesota. This SBE simulates fluoroscopic-guided PRA by utilizing a silicone block containing a synthetic kidney model with 2 cameras on a miniature 3D printed C-arm simulating fluoroscopy. 14 novice urology residents attempted 2 PRA sticks. 92.3% of participants classified the CAT at least equal to the PERC Mentor. Face and content validity were established with this SBE; predictive validity was not established (Veneziano et al. 2015). One of the downsides of this devices is that it focuses on fluoroscopy-guided access and does not bolster the capability for US-guided access.

Ghazi, et al. established face, content, and construct validity an immersive simulation fabricated using 3D printing and hydrogel casting at the Simulation Innovation laboratory (SIL), containing a watertight PCS with a calcium carbonate stone. Data from mechanical testing of cadaveric specimens was utilized to formulate hydrogel polymer for sufficient tissue realism of each abdominal layer. 10 novices and 5 experts participated in this study and performed PRA, tract dilation, and stone lithotripsy. They found that experts used less fluoroscopy and required fewer attempts to achieve PRA in addition to less needle repositioning and fewer complications (Ghazi et al. 2017).

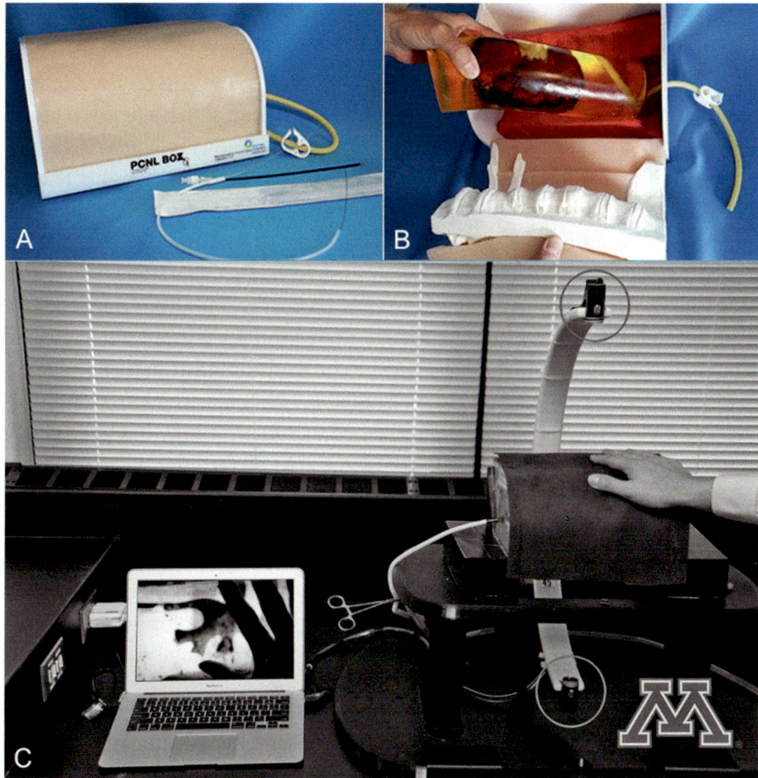

Fig. 2 Benchtop models of PCNL SBE. (**A**, **B**) PCNL Box consisting of interchangeable kidney cartridges and bony landmarks (https://encoris.com/pcnl-kidney-trainer/). (**C**) SimPORTAL fluoroless PCNL trainer using two mounted cameras on a silicone flank model (Veneziano et al. 2015)

Advances in Bench Top Simulators- US-Guided Access

Traditionally, fluoroscopic PRA was the mainstay approach, however as US technology has improved, more attention has been dedicated to US-guided PRA. The advantages of US-guided PRA are the ability to visualize the PCS and surrounding anatomy in real time, there is no need for contrast with reduced radiation exposure. Biologic models have previously been described for US-guided PRA. Unfortunately, there are only few reported bench physical models for US-guided PRA- the, SIL model, PCNL Box trainer (Encoris), Perc Trainer (Mediskills), and PCNL trainer LS40 (Samed GmbH Dresden) (Patterson 2022; Mu 2020). Regardless of the modality utilized, gaining familiarity with the US imaging is crucial. It has been recognized that competence is achieved after approximately 60 US-guided PRA cases while increased SFR and decreased complications occur at approximately 120 cases. Near-perfection is thought to be achieved after 180 cases (Song et al. 2015).

One consideration is that elevated BMI/obesity can complicate the success of PRA and prolong the learning curve, thus these simulations need to adapt to that.

The PCNL Box trainer (Encoris) has been produced and can be used to simulate all aspects of PCNL procedures. This model boasts material that is said to accurately simulate human skin and tissue. The trainer contains radio-opaque ribs and spine beneath the artificial skin layer. The kidney is encased in an exchangeable cartridge and may simulate a variety of calculus pathology. The PCS can be filled to simulate hydronephrosis. It can be used to train US- or fluoroscopic guided PRA. Although one study did not explicitly state their use of the PCNL Box (the images in their study depict the PCNL Box), they established face and construct validity. One benefit of this model is said to be the cost-effectiveness as each simulation can withstand multiple punctures before the skin or cartridge need to be replaced (Sarmah et al. 2017).

The PCNL trainer LS40 produced by Samed (GmbH Dresden) does not have any published studies, however, it has been reported that face validity has been confirmed (Patterson 2022). Additionally, the Perc Trainer (Mediskills) has been reported in the literature but no validation has been achieved.

Ghazi et al., modified their SIL high-fidelity, non-biohazardous hydrogel PCNL simulator to adopt an US-guided approach to PCNL using a consensus-based educational approach. Consensus (>80% agreement) was reached on a high-fidelity PCNL simulator with 12 international experts using a Delphi methodology over three rounds in 31.3% of 284 questions (categorized into overall utility, anatomical components, tissue fidelity, and assessment of surgical performance). The prone PCNL simulator included anatomical landmarks (11th and 12th rib, iliac crest), realistic external and US appearance with appropriate tactile properties, and a water tight, distensible PCS with a stone for laser lithotripsy and retrograde ureteroscopy. A weighted evaluation checklist was also developed via consensus. Experts agreed that >89.2% of prototype and checklist components conformed to the consensus statement. 28 Novices and 20 experts from 5 centers were graded for US-guided lower pole access, with statistically significant differences for checklist score ($42.3 \pm 19.0\%$ vs. $93.4 \pm 4.6\%$, $P < 0.001$). Furthermore, novices significantly improved both lower pole and upper pole access score ($P < 0.01$, $P < 0.001$) respectively with repeated ($\times 5$) training sessions.

2.3 Virtual Reality and Augmented Reality

These technologic SBEs allow for trainees to practice a specific step or an entire procedure depending on the specific simulator. Although these technologies have large costs upfront and can be involved to get the simulations established, once the simulator and software has been purchased and departments gain familiarity, the investment over the long term becomes increasingly cost-effective and the simulations are able to be started in a timelier manner. Additionally, many of these simulators provide feedback which is arguably the most important aspect of training.

Virtual Reality

VR relies completely on a virtual environment and is described as the use of computer modeling and simulation that enables one to interact with an artificial 3D sensory environment. While VR SBEs have been shown to improve trainee performance, they lack haptic feedback.

PERC Mentor

The PERC Mentor was the first VR simulator created for fluoroscopic-guided PRA training for both normal and obese patients. It includes a mannequin that represents the virtual patient's torso approached from the back. Two interchangeable cartridges fitted with life-like layers of epidermis and underlying tissue combined with simulated ribs that provide the haptic perception and provide the physical system for PRA puncturing. It gives the opportunity to practice PRA with various procedural steps such as (1) puncturing the PCS, (2) aspiration from the puncture needle using a virtual syringe, (3) injecting a contrast medium through a virtual ureteral catheter, (4) monitoring the anatomy of the PCS, planning the puncture, and following the progress of the puncture needle into the PCS while the kidney is moving up and down with respiration, using biplanar VR C-arm controlled using a foot pedal, and (5) providing feedback on performance parameters such as procedure time, fluoroscopy time, number of attempts for PCS puncture, number of vascular injuries, number of PCS perforations, number of rib collisions, and the amount of contrast medium used during antegrade and/or retrograde urography.

Multiple studies have validated the PERC Mentor for face, construct, content, and skill validity as a quality SBE modality (Mishra et al. 2010). This simulator has modules with varying difficulty which allows for a graduated training regimen. It has a sensor-embedded needle to track needle access positioning which can be passed through the mannequin torso that simulates human tissue, a C-arm simulator that can be controlled with a foot pedal; additionally, respiration SBE is a feature that provides more realism that makes the trainee account for rib positioning and kidney motion. The biggest downside of the PERC Mentor is the size and cost ($100,000 USD) (Mu 2020).

SimPCNL

Tai, et al. developed an AR simulation (SimPCNL) and compared this to the commercially available simulation trainer, PERC Mentor. The SimPCNL SBE consists of a computer, Hololens visor (Microsoft, Redmond), and 2 PHANTOM omni with a stylus which are controlled with the subject's hands—once acts as the needle/instrument while the other is free hand for palpation. Images for the simulation are obtained from intraoperative fluoroscopy or patient CT scans and uploaded via mesher software to the simulator. This team evaluated the validity of the SimPCNL simulator by enrolling 36 novices and 18 experts; face, content, construct, criterion, and improvement validation were established. This simulator provides real-time visual and haptic feedback. This simulator demonstrated improvements for novice trainers for fluoroscopy time, puncture attempts, and overall surgical time.

Additionally, the SimPCNL has also shown advantages such as portability, low-cost, and is reusable. The SimPCNL was compared to the commercially available PERC Mentor and has also shown some advantages such as being portable, low-cost (cheaper than the PERC Mentor), and reusable without limited wastage. Additionally, experts valued the SimPCNL as useful as the PERC Mentor. Compared with PERC Mentor, specialists believed the SimPCNL as being a quality instrument for urology trainees based on the face and content performances. One of the great benefits of this SBE is the quality of haptic feedback for PRA attempts. One of the downsides of this devices is that it focuses on fluoroscopy-guided access and does not bolster the capability for US-guided access; however given how advanced the program is, there exists the potential of this adaptation (Mu 2020).

Augmented Reality

AR is different, allowing the visualization of the real world with superimposed images. AR may be used to allow for the transposition of an image over a physical model (or patient), with the ultimate goal of providing haptic feedback (Ferraguti 2020).

Muller, et al. evaluated an AR SBE bench model utilizing an iPad. They constructed a phantom model consisting of two porcine kidneys embedded in a ballistic gelatin mold. Radio-dense skin markers were placed on the surface of the model and a CT was completed on the model with contrast instilled in the PCS. The 2D CT scan was then converted into a 3D image and with specific software, the 3D image was then transitioned to the iPad. The skin markers from the CT scan were correlated with skin markers on the model and the AR image was transposed over the model. This study did not validate the AR system. They did find that the AR decreased fluoroscopy time for both experienced and novice participants. Interestingly, there was a decreased time for PRA with AR for novices whereas there this time was increased for experienced participants (Muller et al. 2013).

2.4 Immersive Simulation

Immersive SBE is a high-fidelity training modality that simulates a full experience. While the immersive simulation can allow for practice of specific surgical steps, the true benefit is the complete experience of simulating an entire procedure. Immersive simulations be in the form of physical reality or may incorporate AR, VR, or MR.

A novel 3D immersive simulation is the Marion K181 PCNL simulator. The user wears a headset which simulates a VR OR which is connected to a device that the user controls and is provided haptic feedback. It simulates a VR OR and provides haptic feedback. The trainee is able to practice fluoroscopic-guided PRA and proceed through a complete case. The Marion K181 PCNL simulator is able to provide feedback such as total operative time, fluoroscopy time, tissue damage, number of puncture attempts, total path length, and an overall pass/fail rating. This SBE was found to be validated and rates comparably to a biologic porcine kidney model as well as the PERC Mentor (Farcas et al. 2021). Studies have established face, content, and construct validity of the Marion K181 PCNL simulator (Farcas et al. 2021). The benefits of this trainer are that it simulates a VR procedure inclusive of all steps of the PCNL with haptic feedback with no radiation exposure. One unique feature is that the software contains varying modules for the trainee to practice on. This simulator even permits the upload of patient CT scans allowing for practice on specific calculus pathologies or for patient-specific rehearsal. One shortcoming of this simulator though is that it does not provide US-SBE.

3   Section 3: Patient-Specific Simulation

The benefit of SBE in surgical training is widely recognized. PCNL requires extensive pre-operative planning which is classically done by reviewing the patient's pre-operative CT scan and then using the surgeon's cognitive skills and training PRA via fluoroscopic or US guidance.

Patient-specific simulations not only assess one's technical skills but also evaluate their surgical planning and approach that can be directly translated to the OR. Both physical skills and cognitive approaches to surgery are tested in a safe setting. A thorough understanding of patient anatomy allows for the creation of a concision surgical plan, decreasing surgical time and radiation (Ryu et al. 2017). With the continued advancement in technology, we are able to translate patient data into simulations useful for surgical training and pre-operative preparation/rehearsal. The benefit of patient-specific simulation is that it takes the 2D patient images and translates this into a 3D model (virtual or physical). This allows for thorough assessment of patient anatomy which in turn improves pre-operative planning. Both AR and physical reality patient-specific SBE rely on patient imaging (MRI or CT). The quality of medical imaging has improved, yielding expeditious model prototyping in a more cost-effective manner (Ryu et al. 2017). Patient-specific SBE for PCNL has proven the ability to decrease the number of required needle sticks to achieve PRA, reduce fluoroscopy time, improve SFR, and a reduce surgical complications. It is also hypothesized that surgical times are reduced due to improved surgeon knowledge of patient anatomy (Ghazi et al. 2022).

Creation of patient-specific models

The process of generating the patient-specific model is similar when considering the AR model and the physical model. The specific process varies depending on the study and department/hospital system/lab.

In summary, DICOM data from CT or MRI (with or without contrast) from patients planning to undergo PCNL are obtained. These images are segmented to isolate the kidney, PCS, and stone. Depending on individual preferences and technology, local anatomy may be included (bowel, spleen, liver, ribs, spine). If a physical-reality/3D model is to be created, from the patient image, a 3D mesh/virtual rendering can be created [computer-assisted design (CAD)]. These CAD designs are transferred to the 3D printer to create the 3D physical model or phantom molds. These models can be utilized as an isolated organ model or combined into more anatomically complete models to execute more steps of the procedure. When considering AR, the patient image should be performed in the surgical positioning (ex. prone PCNL should have prone CT completed) with anatomic/fiducial markers placed on the skin. Patient anatomy is then segmented in a different software program (ex. MITK—Medical Interaction Tool Kit, Blender). This information can then be transparently superimposed over the patient on the image device (ex. tablet/iPad, Hololens) with anatomic markers to recognize the appropriate positioning for the AR (Ghazi et al. 2022; Rassweiler-Seyfried et al. 2020; Ryu et al. 2017; Checcucci et al. 2022; Parkhomenko et al. 2019; Li et al. 2013; Porpiglia et al. 2022). Currently two types of simulations exist for Patient-Specific PCNL.

3.1 Augmented Reality Patient-Specific PCNL

AR allows for visualization of the all relevant anatomy, unlike fluoroscopic or US guided access. This is especially beneficial during PRA. One further aspect of AR is that the image can be rotated or manipulated to appreciate the relevant anatomy in real time (Parkhomenko et al. 2019). While the cost of the equipment may be an impedance for broader adaptation, one of the benefits of AR is that once the patient imaging data has been acquired, it will remain and would not have to be replicated or reproduced. A simulation could be repeated as many times as desired at no additional cost (Parkhomenko et al. 2019). One concern is that for some adaptations of AR, the patients must undergo a contrast-enhanced CT scan or endure additional phase, leading to the possibility of increased radiation exposure or contrast-induced toxicities. Additionally, when completing the CT scan, the patient may have to complete the imaging in the prone/surgical position with fiducial markers adherent to the skin. If the markers are inaccurate between the CT scan and procedure, this may detract from the precision of the AR image; along with the inaccuracy, the superimposed image is not a real-time image, thus respirations could alter the precision of the image overlay (Li et al. 2013; Rassweiler et al. 2012).

SimPCNL is an AR simulation and Marion K181 PCNL immersive simulator (Chi et al. 2022) are both of which have been previously discussed, use a headset which simulates a virtual OR and connected to a device that the user controls and is provided haptic feedback. Images for the simulation are obtained from patient CT scans and uploaded via mesher software to the simulator for practice of the procedure. Li, et al. reported a study of 15 patients, patient-specific SBE was utilized by overlaying the AR imaging via iPad intraoperatively. Not only were they able to achieve a SFR of 93%, but the surgeon also expressed more confidence and comfort with PRA as a result. Validation was not demonstrated with this study (Li et al. 2013) (Fig. 3)

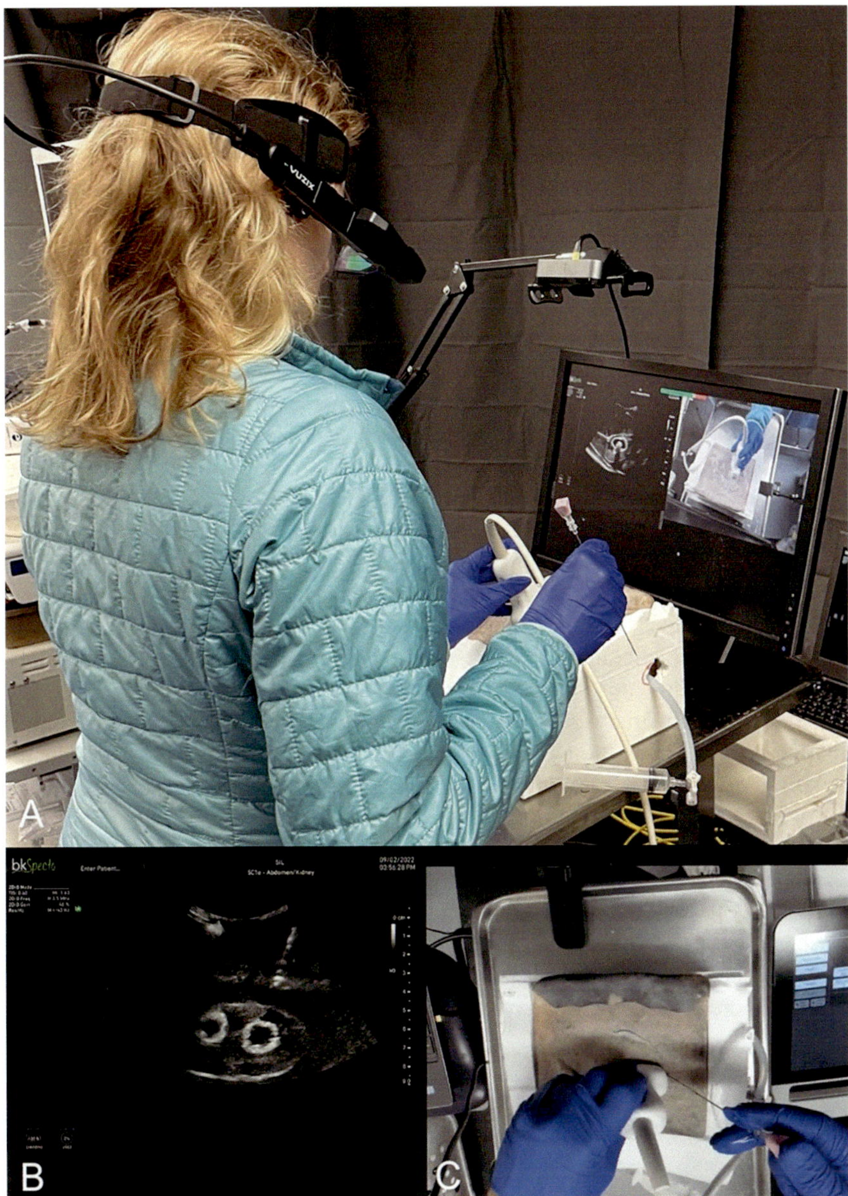

Fig. 3 VR SBEs for PCNL. (**A**) Comparison of real surgery with PERC Mentor and SimPCNL (Mu 2020) (**B**) Marion K181 Simulator with user wearing VR headset and operating haptic device while undergoing VR PCNL (Farcas et al. 2021)

Rassweiler et al. also utilized iPad-assisted AR patient-specific simulation (Fig. 4). Initially in their 2011 study on 2 patients, they used the iPad to overlay the AR image onto the patients in surgery. For both patients, they were able to obtain access to the desired calyx on their first stick (Rassweiler et al. 2012). This group built upon their initial study to evaluate 22 patients undergoing AR access with the iPad and compare them to 22 patients who had previously undergone standard PRA. Interestingly, both the fluoroscopy time and puncture time was longer for the AR group in comparison with the standard fluoroscopy or US group. The authors concluded that the results could be attributed to the lack of experience with AR (Rassweiler-Seyfried et al. 2020). Parkhomenko, et al. evaluated the Oculus Rift VR headset system in a study of 25 patients. They evaluated 4 experienced surgeons who examined the standard 2D CT scan of a patient and then the virtual model. A questionnaire was answered following each step. The results of these 25 patients were compared to 25 patients from a PCNL database. This study found that the VR-prepared surgeons had 50% less blood-loss, fewer needle access sticks, less fluoroscopy time. This study was validated by the surgeons participating in the study, however did not specify what validity was confirmed. They did note that the early models took 6–9 h to prepare (Parkhomenko et al. 2019). Porpiglia, et al. utilized 3D AR models from 10 patients and compared this with 10 patients from their PCNL database. They constructed a 3D hologram of each patient's kidney and surrounding anatomy and utilized this for pre-operative planning and for intraoperative assistance (projected transparently via Hololens). While this study was not validated, it was found to be effective as it lowered the intra-operative fluoroscopy time (however the pre-operative CT required an additional phase and thus increased radiation), improved PRA via reproducing the planned access tract, and improved first-stick success for PRA. It should be recognized, however that the time to PRA was longer in the AR group (27 min vs. 12 min) (Porpiglia et al. 2022).

While AR is gaining traction for SBE, its broad benefit is yet to be recognized. Studies have been performed evaluated pre-operative planning and intraoperative assistance for PRA. While these studies support the added benefit of AR, the conclusive evidence is lacking. As we gain more familiarity with this technology and it becomes more affordable, we may see its broader adoption (Ferraguti 2020).

3.2 Patient-Specific Physical Reality Simulation

While the benefits of patient-specific AR SBEs are apparent as described previously, it is important to consider benefits of physical reality SBE. The patient-specific 3D models allow for SBE of individual pathology which improves pre-operative planning as the models were adapted directly from patient imaging. This allows for more concise decision-making and could potentially alter the surgeon's approach. Patient-specific 3D models allow for the haptic feedback that AR may not accurately provide. The 3D models provide patient-specific pathology and anatomy that generic models (cadavers, bench models) cannot provide (Ryu et al. 2017). Some studies with

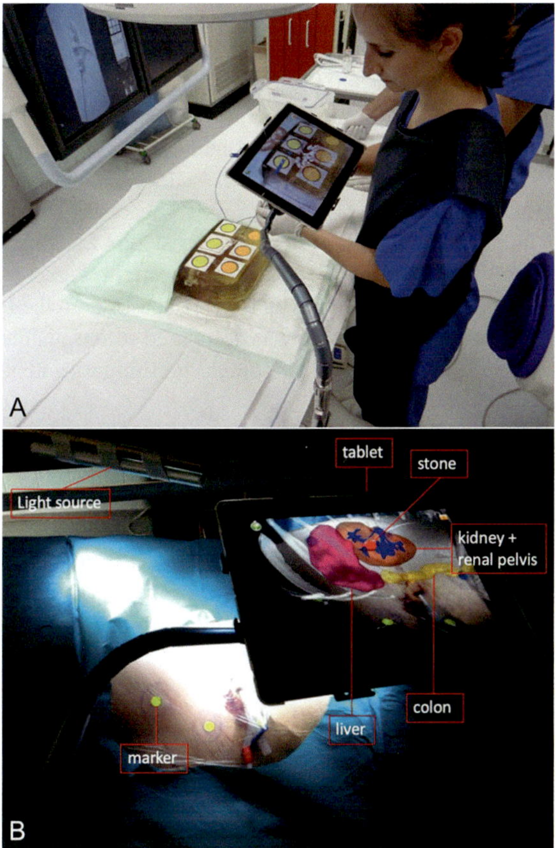

Fig. 4 Use of iPad with computer-based AR system to assist in PRA in (**A**) SBE (Muller et al. 2013) and (**B**) intra operatively (Rassweiler-Seyfried et al. 2020)

3D models have been mechanically validated to accurately simulate human tissue (Ghazi et al. 2022, 2017).

The SIL at the University of Rochester, NY, expanded upon their previous generic model to validate a patient-specific model developing a high-fidelity, realistic, PCNL simulator. This SBE possessed a kidney with a complete PCS and an artificial staghorn calculus. The model was constructed using a combination of 3D printing and hydrogel polymer polyvinyl alcohol (PVA) and mechanically tested to ensure the adequate tissue realism. The models were tested to confirm anatomic accuracy to the original CT scan (Ghazi et al. 2017). A fellowship-trained endourologist performed 20 consecutive PCNL cases at an academic referral center. For the first 10 patients, only standard review of patient imaging was completed. For the next 10 patients, patient imaging was utilized to fabricate patient-specific models. Full procedural rehearsals were completed 24–48 h before the real case. Surgical metrics and patient outcomes from both groups (rehearsal vs. standard) were compared. Significant improvements in mean fluoroscopy time, PRA attempts, complications, and additional procedures were significantly lower in the rehearsal group (184.8 vs. 365.7 s, $p < 0.001$; 1.9 vs. 3.6 attempts, $p < 0.001$; 1 vs. 5, $p < 0.001$; and 1 vs. 5, $p < 0.001$ respectively). There were no differences in SFR, mean patient age, body mass index, or stone size between the two groups. Additionally, the cost of the patient-specific SBE was $242 for each participant ($100 in material, $80 in personnel, and $162 in consumables) (Ghazi et al. 2022, 2017).

Checcucci, et al. developed a MR system that assisted in PRA. A route for needle placement was identified on a 2D CT scan from a patient. Next, a 3D model was printed with the simulated needle route which was visualized on the Hololens during puncture. The angle of needle puncture was compared to the planned one and was found to be accurate in 10/10 patients. This study is preliminary and not yet published at this time (Checcucci et al. 2022).

These SBEs have demonstrated decreased operative times, decreased complication rates, improved SFR for PCNL (Ghazi et al. 2017, 2022). In summary patient-specific SBE is a new frontier with a plethora of opportunity. These technologies have the potential to improve surgical planning as well as reduce surgical time and complications particularly in patients with complex anatomy (ex. horseshoe or malrotated kidney).While the benefits are apparent, there are some short-comings. These can be an expensive technology and require training to utilize. While it can assist in access, if the image overlay is not precise, it has the potential to lead a surgeon astray (Rassweiler-Seyfried et al. 2020; Li et al. 2013; Rassweiler et al. 2012).

4 Section 4: Advances for Training in PCNL Simulation

4.1 Advances in Training-Remote Proctoring

One of the most recent advances in SBE is remote proctoring. In a preliminary study by Ghazi at the SIL, 12 novices were randomized into either an in-person (IP) or MR training session to practice US-guided PRA on a high-fidelity, 3D hydrogel model (Fig. 5).

During IP sessions, the instructor proctored similar to a traditional learning environment. During MR sessions, the participants shared their first-person perspective using the Vuzix M4000 smart glasses with installed a cloud-based MR software that fuses two camera feeds. The instructor interacted with the live-feed of the participant through hand gestures and 3D printed US and 3D printed kidney replicas using a webcam directed at their hands over a white tabletop. The instructor also annotated directly on the shared US screen through Zoom. The IP group scored better on the pre-test as well as demonstrated fewer PRA attempts with a comparable time to access. A mid-test evaluation was completed and demonstrated a greater improvement in PRA attempts and time to access. A final questionnaire of trainees found that 66.7% of trainees found MR training to be similar to in-person training regarding

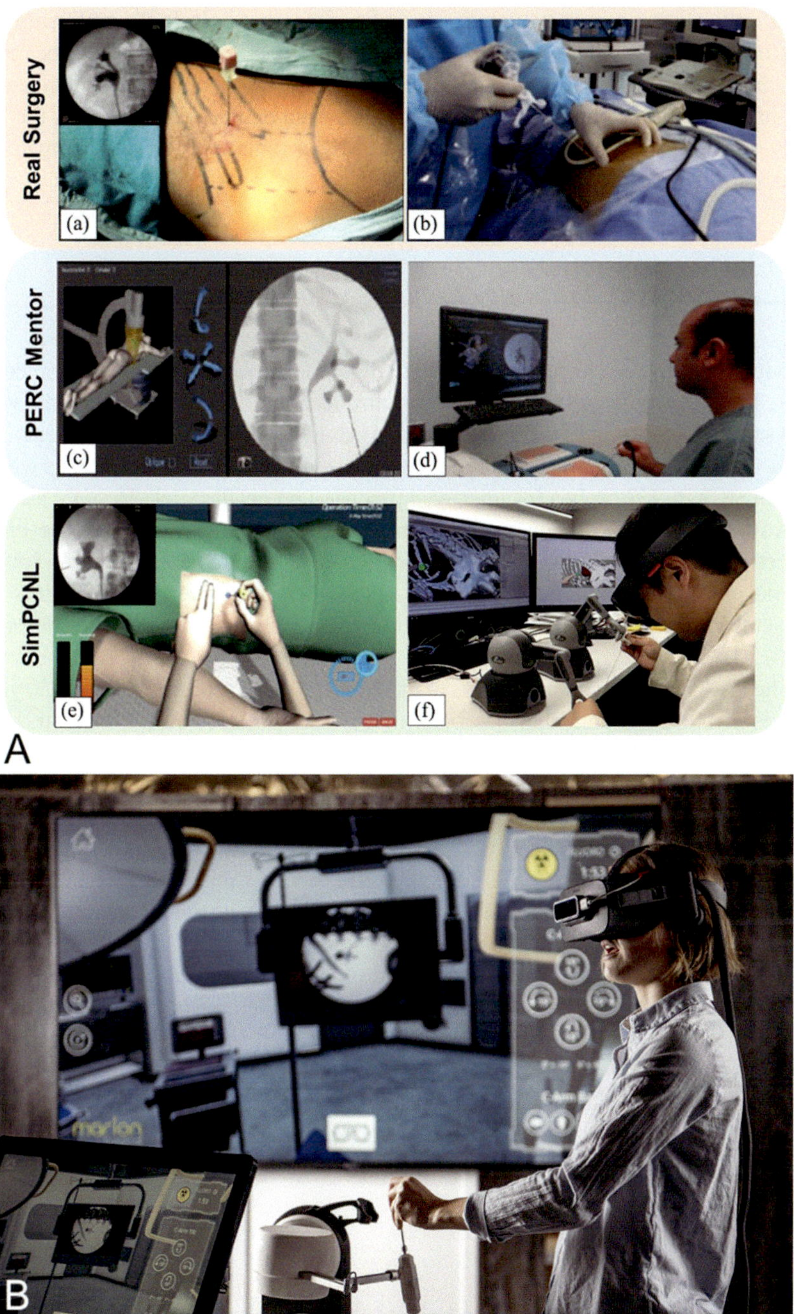

Fig. 5 Immersive simulation with hydrogel model created by SIL. (**A**) Trainee performs US guided access while receiving live virtual feedback through headset. (**B**) Real time videos of the PRA on the ultrasound and (**C**) the hydrogel model are broadcasted to the mentor (Ghazi et al. 2022, 2017)

usefulness, clarity, accuracy, timeliness and quantity but only 8.3% preferring MR (Saxton et al. 2023). This study demonstrated the potential of remote proctoring, especially for SBE training in PCNL. Further studies are necessary to elucidate the true impact of this technology as there is scarce data on this matter. This is the first study demonstrating similar effectiveness of MR or remote proctoring compared to IP proctoring during PCNL SBE.

4.2   Advances in Training- Robotic Assistance

As with other procedures in urology, there exists potential for robotic assistance for PRA. The first robotic device for PRA was introduced in 1998. This device achieved a high success of first-attempt PRA, however it was too costly for wide implementation. Many robotic systems are focused to facilitate needle positioning for PRA as well as coordinate with US probes for improved precision on needle stick. Robotic assisted PRA may improve accuracy and shorten the learning curve for PRA. One of the concerns regarding robotic assistance for PRA is how much autonomy the robotic component would maintain. If the robotic assistance is too overwhelming, this will detract from the trainees ability to learn how to obtain PRA on their own (Ferraguti 2020).

The PAKY (Percutaneous Access to the Kidney) system, developed over 20 years ago, is a robotic system that has been created for precise PRA. Ferraguti, et al. evaluated a combination of AR with PAKY robot. The surgeon wears an AR headset and is able to manually direct the robot to achieve PRA; this system had previously been validated. The patient's CT scan is converted appropriately so the AR image is transposed through the headset. This study was able to validate the registration, performance, and usability of this combined AR-robotic simulation (Ferraguti 2020).

Another, novel robotic- assisted device for PCNL is the Monarch Platform (Ethicon, Auris Health Inc.). In a preliminary study, Chi, et al. evaluated the Monarch Platform on a porcine model. Two endourologists performed 12 PCNL and 12 ureteroscopy procedures on 24 porcine kidneys. They demonstrated no safety issues during the use of the Monarch Platform. They found that, while not significant, there was a trend towards improved ease of task completion (ex. renal access). They concluded that the Monarch Platform was safe and demonstrated a comparable usability profile to standard PCNL and ureteroscopy (Chi et al. 2022).

References

Checcucci E, Amparore D, Volpi G, Piramide F, De Cillis S, Piana A, et al. Percutaneous puncture during PCNL: new perspective for the future with virtual imaging guidance. World J Urol. 2022;40(3):639–50.

Chi T, Hathaway L, Chok, R et al. Robotic-assisted percutaneous nephrolithotomy and ureteroscopy with the monarch® platform, urology compares favorably against conventional techniques. J Urol 2022;e638.

de la Rosette JJ, Laguna MP, Rassweiler JJ, Conort P. Training in percutaneous nephrolithotomy—A critical review. Eur Urol. 2008;54(5):994–1001.

Farcas M, Reynolds LF, Lee JY. Simulation-based percutaneous renal access training: evaluating a novel 3D immersive virtual reality platform. J Endourol. 2021;35(5):695–9.

Ferraguti F. Augmented reality and robotic-assistance for percutaneous nephrolithotomy. In: EEE robotics and automation letters: IEEE; 2020. p. 4556–563.

Ghazi A, Campbell T, Melnyk R, Feng C, Andrusco A, Stone J, et al. Validation of a full-immersion simulation platform for percutaneous nephrolithotomy using three-dimensional printing technology. J Endourol. 2017;31(12):1314–20.

Ghazi A, Melnyk R, Farooq S, Bell A, Holler T, Saba P, et al. Validity of a patient-specific percutaneous nephrolithotomy (PCNL) simulated surgical rehearsal platform: impact on patient and surgical outcomes. World J Urol. 2022;40(3):627–37.

Hacker A, Wendt-Nordahl G, Honeck P, Michel MS, Alken P, Knoll T. A biological model to teach percutaneous nephrolithotomy technique with ultrasound- and fluoroscopy-guided access. J Endourol. 2007;21(5):545–50.

Kallidonis P, Kyriazis I, Vasilas M, Panagopoulos V, Georgiopoulos I, Ozsoy M, et al. Modular training for percutaneous nephrolithotripsy: the safe way to go. Arab J Urol. 2015;13(4):270–6.

Klein JT, Rassweiler J, Rassweiler-Seyfried MC. Validation of a novel cost effective easy to produce and durable in vitro model for kidney-puncture and percutaneous nephrolitholapaxy-simulation. J Endourol. 2018;32(9):871–6.

Kozan AA, Chan LH, Biyani CS. Current status of simulation training in urology: a non-systematic review. Res Rep Urol. 2020;12:111–28.

Li H, Chen Y, Liu C, Li B, Xu K, Bao S. Construction of a three-dimensional model of renal stones: comprehensive planning for percutaneous nephrolithotomy and assistance in surgery. World J Urol. 2013;31(6):1587–92.

Mishra S, Kurien A, Ganpule A, Muthu V, Sabnis R, Desai M. Percutaneous renal access training: content validation comparison between a live porcine and a virtual reality (VR) simulation model. BJU Int. 2010;106(11):1753–6.

Mu Y. Development and validation of augmented reality training simulator for ultrasound guided percutaneous renal access. Electronic Thesis and Dissertation Repository. Canada: The University of Western Ontario; 2020.

Muller M, Rassweiler MC, Klein J, Seitel A, Gondan M, Baumhauer M, et al. Mobile augmented reality for computer-assisted percutaneous nephrolithotomy. Int J Comput Assist Radiol Surg. 2013;8(4):663–75.

Parkhomenko E, O'Leary M, Safiullah S, Walia S, Owyong M, Lin C, et al. Pilot assessment of immersive virtual reality renal models as an educational and preoperative planning tool for percutaneous nephrolithotomy. J Endourol. 2019;33(4):283–8.

Patterson JM. Simulation in percutaneous nephrolithotomy (PCNL). In: Practical simulation in urology. Cham: Springer; 2022.

Porpiglia F, Checcucci E, Amparore D, Peretti D, Piramide F, De Cillis S, et al. Percutaneous kidney puncture with three-dimensional mixed-reality hologram guidance: from preoperative planning to intraoperative navigation. Eur Urol. 2022;81(6):588–97.

Rassweiler JJ, Müller M, Fangerau M, Klein J, Goezen AS, Pereira P, et al. iPad-assisted percutaneous access to the kidney using marker-based navigation: initial clinical experience. Eur Urol. 2012;61(3):628–31.

Rassweiler-Seyfried MC, Rassweiler JJ, Weiss C, Muller M, Meinzer HP, Maier-Hein L, et al. iPad-assisted percutaneous nephrolithotomy (PCNL): a matched pair analysis compared to standard PCNL. World J Urol. 2020;38(2):447–53.

Ryu WHA, Dharampal N, Mostafa AE, Sharlin E, Kopp G, Jacobs WB, et al. Systematic review of patient-specific surgical simulation: toward advancing medical education. J Surg Educ. 2017;74(6):1028–38.

Sarmah P, Voss J, Ho A, Veneziano D, Somani B. Low versus high fidelity: the importance of 'realism' in the simulation of a stone treatment procedure. Curr Opin Urol. 2017;27(4):316–22.

Saxton A, Shepard L, Holler T, Wanderling C, Schuler N, Lee A, et al. Evaluation of mixed reality (MR) technologies for remote guidance during ultrasound (US)-guided percutaneous renal access simulation: a prospective, randomized comparative trial. AUA; 2023.

Song Y, Ma Y, Fei X. Evaluating the learning curve for percutaneous nephrolithotomy under total ultrasound guidance. PLoS ONE. 2015;10(8): e0132986.

Veneziano D, Smith A, Reihsen T, Speich J, Sweet RM. The SimPORTAL fluoro-less C-arm trainer: an innovative device for percutaneous kidney access. J Endourol. 2015;29(2):240–5.

Vijayakumar M, Balaji S, Singh A, Ganpule A, Sabnis R, Desai M. A novel biological model for training in percutaneous renal access. Arab J Urol. 2019;17(4):292–7.

Preoperative Patient Preparation and Imaging in PCNL

Nicole Miller, Amy Reed, Anne Hong, and Damien Bolton

Abstract The decision to proceed to percutaneous nephrolithotomy (PCNL) is always undertaken after due consideration of the individual circumstances of the patient. This includes a detailed assessment of previous medical history and concurrent pharmaceutical therapy, in particular anticoagulant use, plus optimal imaging of the stone burden and location in order to determine the most appropriate positioning of the patient and puncture site. Contingency plans should also be developed in case of intraoperative difficulty achieving complete stone clearance, and these will usually be based upon evaluation of cross sectional imaging studies using contrast agents. Such PCNL complexity can be graded preoperatively using nephrolithotomy scores.

Keywords PCNL · Opiods · Fusion imaging · Nephrolithometry · CT imaging

1 Introduction

A thorough preoperative patient evaluation is necessary to reduce operative risks and potential complications of surgical intervention for urolithiasis. Initial assessment starts with a complete history and physical to ensure patients are appropriately selected for percutaneous nephrolithotomy (PCNL). This evaluation should include prior medical and surgical history, age, stone characteristics, renal anatomy, and patient preference.

Patients with high-risk medical co-morbidities and/or prior surgical history may pose a higher perioperative surgical risk. On physical exam, special attention should be paid to anatomic factors that may require intraoperative modification including obesity, surgical scars, contractures and scoliosis. Appropriate preoperative laboratory and radiographic studies can be used to mitigate risk. Complex patients or

N. Miller · A. Reed
Vanderbilt University Medical Center, Nashville, TN, USA

A. Hong · D. Bolton (✉)
Department of Surgery, Olivia Newton-John Cancer Research Institute, University of Melbourne, Austin Health, Melbourne, VI, Australia
e-mail: damien.bolton@unimelb.edu.au

J. D. Denstedt and E. N. Liatsikos (eds.), *Percutaneous Renal Surgery*,
https://doi.org/10.1007/978-3-031-40542-6_4

those with significant risk factors may benefit from evaluation by internal medicine, cardiology and/or anesthesia for optimization prior to surgery.

Finally, the patient and surgical team must engage in shared decision making to obtain informed consent. This discussion should cover the risks, benefits and alternatives to PCNL and the patient and family members should be given ample opportunity to ask clarifying questions.

2 Patient History

2.1 Anticoagulation

PCNL is contraindicated in patients unable to hold anticoagulants and antiplatelet agents, other than low dose aspirin, or who have an uncorrectable bleeding disorder or coagulopathy. The reported incidence of blood transfusion after PCNL ranges from 3 to 24% (Ganpule et al. 2014; MacDonald et al. 2022; Tayeb et al. 2015; Nasseh et al. 2022; Said et al. 2017; Rosette et al. 2011). Therefore, it is important to identify which patients are at increased risk of bleeding prior to undergoing surgery. Several scoring systems have been developed. The HAS-BLED score, for example, takes into account risk factors in atrial fibrillation patients such as age over 65, chronic kidney disease, stroke, hypertension, liver dysfunction, coagulation disorders, history of bleeding or high alcohol and drug use. A HAS-BLED score greater than three is predictive of future bleeding events (Doherty et al. 2017).

Perioperative management of anticoagulation should be a shared decision between the surgeon and prescribing provider. The American College of Cardiology published perioperative management guidelines for anticoagulation use in nonvalvular atrial fibrillation patients (Doherty et al. 2017). For vitamin K antagonists (VKA) like warfarin, the guidelines recommend checking an INR 5–7 days preoperatively. For most patients, VKAs can be held 5 days preoperatively for patients with normal INR who are undergoing low risk surgery. For patients at a high risk of VTE, such as those with CHADSVASC score >7, consideration should be given to bridging with low molecular weight heparin. While patients with a low risk of postoperative bleeding can restart VKAs after 24 h, patients with a higher risk of bleeding, including PCNL, should restart after 48–72 h without the need for bridging. In contrast, direct-acting oral anticoagulation (DOACs) can be held for shorter periods due to shorter drug half-lives. Newer reversible agents are also now available. DOACs should be held for 4–5 half-lives and adjusted for a patient's renal function. For surgeries with low bleeding risk, DOACs can be held for 24 h preoperatively and held for 48 h for higher risk surgeries. Longer intervals may be needed for patients with impaired renal function. DOACs can typically be restarted 24 h after surgery for low-risk surgeries and, after higher risk surgery like PCNL, they can be restarted after 48–72 h or at the surgeon's discretion.

Antiplatelet agents should also be held prior to surgery. Due to the irreversible binding to platelets, P2Y12 inhibitors like clopidogrel should be held for five days to allow bleeding time and platelet aggregation to return to normal (Muluk UpToDate). However, continuing low dose aspirin (81 mg) perioperatively is not associated with an increase in complications, difference in hemoglobin or higher transfusion rate after PCNL (Pan et al. 2022). Therefore, low dose aspirin (81 mg) may be able to be safely continued perioperatively.

2.2   Contrast Allergies

There are no formal guidelines for management of patients with allergies to iodinated intravenous contrast. A large retrospective study by Blackwell et al. reported very low rates of adverse reactions with intraluminal contrast (0.48%), however, 3–4% of surveyed urologists have seen a serious reaction with contrast use during PCNL (Blackwell et al. 2017; Dai et al. 2018). Perioperative management of contrast allergies is variable among surveyed urologists and up to a third of respondents premedicate patients prior to PCNL with steroids or antihistamines (Dai et al. 2018; Mohapatra et al. 2019). With the lack of supporting evidence to guide practice patterns, urologists should be cautious with patients who have a history of anaphylaxis to iodinated contrast and could consider premedicating prior to PCNL. In addition, maintaining low intrarenal pressure to prevent pyelovenous backflow is prudent.

2.3   Anatomic Considerations

Certain anatomic factors may require additional preoperative evaluation or modification of operative technique. Prior intrarenal surgery, for example, can cause scar tissue in the collecting system, renal parenchyma, or perirenal fascia of the retroperitoneum that can increase the difficulty of percutaneous renal access and tract dilation. In these situations, specialty equipment may be necessary such as the use of a high-pressure balloon dilator or fascial incising needle. Prior abdominal surgery may cause scar tissue or adhesions around the kidney that can alter the location of adjacent organs. Specifically, the position of the colon can be variable and move with changes in position. Colon injury can be a serious complication with a reported incidence of 0.3% of cases (El-Nahas et al. 2006). Avoiding this complication begins with identifying higher risk patients based on patient demographics, access site and colon anatomy. El-Nahas et al. reported complicated lower pole access, especially in older patients, was associated with colon injury (El-Nahas et al. 2006). With respect to the kidney, a posterolateral colon extends beyond the posterior calyceal border and a retrorenal colon is completely posterior to the kidney. A colon in one of these orientations is also at higher risk of injury during percutaneous renal access. However, anatomy may be hard to predict because patients are often in different positions during imaging studies versus in the operating room. For example, Hur et al. demonstrated 15% of patients had posterolateral or retrorenal colons when imaged supine but increased to 25% of patients when they were imaged prone (Hur et al. 2021). Retrorenal colon is more common with older age and lower BMI with decreased perirenal fat. Intraoperative adjuncts like ultrasound guidance during access can help locate adjacent structures to decrease the risk of injury.

Complex renal and patient anatomy related to obesity, spinal cord injury and spina bifida may complicate intraoperative positioning and renal access. Malrotated, horseshoe, ectopic or transplanted kidneys increases complexity of percutaneous renal access. Positioning spina bifida patients is challenging due to severe spinal curvature, contractures of upper and lower extremities and restricted joint movement. In particular, the concave aspect of spinal curvature can limit the distance between the ribs and iliac crest, limiting renal access and altering the anatomic relationships of adjacent structures. In these patients, additional preoperative contrasted CT imaging may be needed to provide detailed renal and ureteral anatomy and to better define the collecting system (Assimos et al. 2016). It may also be beneficial to use a combination of ultrasound and fluoroscopic guidance and, in some cases, may require interventional radiology consultation for CT guided access.

Obese or morbidly obese patients present several intraoperative challenges. Special consideration must be given to patient positioning to avoid injuries. Prone positioning can increase intrathoracic pressure which can lead to decreased tidal volumes and difficult ventilation. Truncal obesity can make it difficult to identify bony landmarks and, as tissues shift once in the prone or supine position, there may be an increase in the skin to stone distance. Operative teams need access to extra-long PCNL equipment if proceeding with surgery in patients with an increased skin to stone distance. However, despite these considerations, overall outcomes, complications and stone free rates are comparable in morbidly obese and lower BMI patients after PCNL (Torrecilla Ortiz et al. 2014; Zhou et al. 2017).

3 Laboratory and Radiographic Evaluation

3.1 *Urinalysis and Urine Culture*

Preoperative urinalysis is mandated by the AUA guidelines prior to proceeding with stone surgery and urine cultures are, at a minimum, required for clinical or laboratory signs of infection (Assimos et al. 2016). Untreated urinary tract infection is an absolute contraindication to PCNL. Thirty percent of patients have a positive preoperative midstream urine culture (Liu et al. 2021) and have a higher rate of SIRS (12%) and urosepsis (5%) postoperatively, even when treated prior to surgery (Tang et al. 2021). Culture speciation and sensitivity results should be used to select perioperative antibiotics. The ideal timing between obtaining urine culture and surgery is not completely clear. In a retrospective study, Akkas et al. did not find increased rates of postoperative sepsis when urine cultures were collected more than ten days prior to surgery compared to within ten days (Akkas et al. 2021). Adequate antibiotic coverage based on urine culture results is imperative, therefore, a minimum of 10 days is recommended to allow for culture results and treatment of a positive culture.

Intraoperative renal pelvis and stone cultures are recommended as patients with positive cultures are four times more likely to have postoperative sepsis (Mariappan et al. 2006). Stone and renal pelvis cultures are more reliable than midstream urine in predicting postoperative sepsis as well as the causative organism to direct postoperative antibiotic therapy (Liu et al. 2021; Castellani et al. 2022). Midstream urine cultures have been shown to have poor diagnostic accuracy in predicting renal pelvis or stone cultures (Castellani et al. 2022). Mariappan et al. found that, in patients with negative preoperative midstream cultures, 11% of patients had positive intraoperative bladder urine cultures, 20% had positive renal pelvis cultures and 35% had positive stone cultures. Only 5.6% of patients had positive bladder cultures with positive upper tract cultures (Mariappan et al. 2005). Similarly, Korets et al. reported 33% of patients with a positive intraoperative renal pelvis culture and 48% of patients with a positive stone culture had negative preoperative midstream urine cultures (Korets et al. 2011). In addition, positive midstream cultures have been reported to be discordant in 55% of patients with positive renal pelvis cultures and 30% of stone cultures, complicating antibiotic selection (Korets et al. 2011). This data underscores the benefit of renal pelvis and stone cultures in the management of patients undergoing PCNL.

3.2 Laboratory Data

AUA stone guidelines recommend obtaining serum electrolytes and creatinine if there is a concern for reduced renal function (Assimos et al. 2016). Renal function can dictate choice and dosage of perioperative medications. There is no evidence that PCNL worsens renal function long term and often improves renal function after treating obstructing stones (Reeves et al. 2020). When a chronically obstructed kidney is suspected to be nonfunctional, nuclear renogram should be considered prior to PCNL (Assimos et al. 2016).

Hematologic evaluation including CBC, coagulation panel and type and screen should be obtained before surgeries where there is a significant risk of bleeding or in patients with a history of anemia or coagulopathies (Assimos et al. 2016). The reported incidence of postoperative blood transfusion ranges from 3 to 24% and reported incidence of embolization ranges 0.5–1.8% (Ganpule et al. 2014; MacDonald et al. 2022; Tayeb et al. 2015; Nasseh et al. 2022; Said et al. 2017; Rosette et al. 2011). Given this, an updated type and screen and consent for blood products should be completed prior to surgery. An elevated white blood cell count, abnormal coagulation studies or low platelet count may require further hematologic investigation to minimize complications.

Platelet lymphocyte ratio (PLR) and neutrophil lymphocyte ratio (NLR) can be helpful adjuncts as they are easily calculated from routine CBC and have been shown to be independent risk factors for postoperative sepsis (Kriplani et al. 2022). PLR and NLR have been utilized in other inflammatory, cardiovascular and metabolic conditions as a marker of systemic inflammation. It has also been shown to be elevated in some stone formers (Tang et al. 2021). Proinflammatory molecules found in the renal papilla of stone formers is thought to promote crystallization through oxidative stress and release of reactive oxygen species (Tang et al. 2021; Kriplani et al. 2022; Khan et al. 2021). The inflammatory immune response can promote Randall's plaque and calcium stone formation (Khan et al. 2021). Increased neutrophils triggered by inflammation leads to an exaggerated inflammatory response that suppresses the immune response of lymphocytes, T cells and NK cells (Tang et al. 2021). Platelets can also release proinflammatory agents that can perpetuate inflammatory conditions and reactions (Gasparyan et al. 2019). Therefore, NLR and PLR can be used as markers of an ongoing inflammatory reaction and, thus, can be used as predictors of postoperative sepsis following PCNL (Tang et al. 2021; Kriplani et al. 2022). PLR is calculated by dividing the absolute platelet count by the absolute lymphocyte count. Similarly, NLR is calculated by dividing the absolute neutrophil count by the absolute lymphocyte count. Special consideration should be given to patients with preoperative PLR (>110) and NLR (>2.03) as they may be at higher risk for postoperative sepsis (Tang et al. 2021; Kriplani et al. 2022; Sen et al. 2016).

3.3 Electrocardiogram and Chest X-Ray

The American Academy of Family Practice preoperative guidelines recommend an electrocardiogram (EKG) for high-risk surgery or for intermediate risk surgery with patient risk factors such as cardiac history, chronic kidney disease or diabetes (Preoperative 2002). Chest x-rays are not routinely indicated but may be needed for symptomatic patients. Most patients do not require routine EKG or chest x-ray prior to PCNL unless significant risk factors or symptoms are present.

4 Patient Preparation

4.1 Antibiotics

Historic reported incidence of postoperative sepsis after PCNL ranges from 0.8 to 3% and SIRS occurs in as high as 30% of cases (O'Keeffe et al. 1993; Bag et al. 2011; Segura 1984). AUA perioperative antibiotic guidelines recommend antibiotic coverage for gram negative bacteria, enterococci and skin flora including S. aureus (Lai and Assimos 2016). First line antibiotics should be first or second generation cephalosporins followed by an aminoglycoside with metronidazole or clindamycin and continued for less than 24 h postoperatively. However, the AUA guidelines do not specifically address the role of empiric or directed preoperative antibiotics.

Preoperative antibiotic regimens should be tailored according to patient risk factors and preoperative cultures. Risk factors include stone size, hydronephrosis, foreign bodies, indwelling drainage tubes, recurrent UTI, struvite stone formers, and or urinary diversion. For low-risk patients with negative urine cultures, Zeng et al. reported no difference in sepsis rates based on preoperative antibiotic duration (Zeng et al. 2020). These findings were confirmed by a prospective multi-institutional randomized controlled trial (RCT) conducted by the Endourology Disease Group for Excellence (EDGE) Consortium. Sepsis rates were similar between low-risk patients with negative preoperative cultures who received seven days of nitrofurantoin versus patients who just received perioperative antibiotics (Chew et al. 2018).

Patients with risk factors may develop postoperative sepsis even with a negative preoperative urine culture. Specifically, patients with hydronephrosis and stones over 2cm in size are more likely to have postoperative sepsis even with negative midstream urine cultures (Mariappan et al. 2005). When these patients were treated with one week of preoperative antibiotics (ciprofloxacin 250 mg twice daily), they were three times less likely to have postoperative SIRS compared to no empiric antibiotics (Mariappan et al. 2006). Bag et al. also reported decreased postoperative SIRS (19% vs. 49%) in these patients when treated with one week of nitrofurantoin (100 mg twice daily) preoperatively (Bag et al. 2011).

Positive urine cultures should be treated preoperatively but antibiotic management is highly variable. Decreased SIRS rates (21% vs. 40%) have been reported when patients are treated with greater than 7 days of preoperative antibiotics compared to less than six days (Zeng et al. 2020; Xu et al. 2022). To elucidate this further, the EDGE Consortium prospectively compared 2 days versus 7 days of antibiotics for high-risk patients defined as either positive urine culture or presence of indwelling drainage tube. Patients treated for 7 days preoperatively had decreased rates of sepsis compared to those treated for a shorter duration (Chew et al. 2018). The AUA guidelines do not recommend the routine use of antibiotics postoperatively as they have not been shown to decrease sepsis rates (Yu et al. 2020).

Patients at higher risk for infectious complications such as those with struvite nephrolithiasis, positive stone culture, chronic indwelling catheters urinary diversion, hydronephrosis or large stone burden should be treated with an antibiotic regimen that is individually tailored to cover risk factors.

4.2   Anesthesia

The majority of PCNL cases are completed under a general anesthetic. This allows for continuous airway protection during positioning, improved pain control intraoperatively and allows for adjunctive measures such as breath holding during access. In select cases, PCNL can be successfully performed under regional anesthesia.

Selection of an anesthetic approach depends on patient anatomy, comorbidities and planned surgical approach and should be a discussion between the urology and anesthesia teams. Spinal anesthesia involves injecting anesthetic medication into the intrathecal space to create motor and sensory blockade. For patients who are appropriate candidates, a spinal is commonly placed at L4 and then the patient is placed in Trendelenburg position until the anesthetic reaches the T6-T7 level. Conversion to a general anesthetic occurs in 5–10% of cases due to incomplete spinal blockade (Mehrabi et al. 2013). In a prospective RCT, patients who underwent PCNL under a spinal anesthetic had a shorter operative time and decreased narcotic requirement postoperatively (Mehrabi et al. 2013).

In addition, the anesthesia team can be consulted for perioperative nerve blocks. Intercostal, paravertebral and peritubular nerve blocks have all been proposed as analgesic adjuncts. Intercostal nerve blocks are performed by injecting local anesthetic at the inferior margin of the 10th, 11th and 12th ribs at the posterior axillary line. With this technique, care must be taken to avoid injury to the neurovascular bundle during needle placement. The peritubular nerve block involves injecting local anesthetic along the nephrostomy tube if left at the end of the case. Proposed technique by Jonnavithula et al. involves image guidance of the needle into the renal capsule adjacent to the nephrostomy tube and then local anesthetic infiltration along the nephrostomy tract as the needle is removed (Jonnavithula et al. 2017). The paravertebral block can be completed by visualizing the T10 paravertebral space under ultrasound guidance and instilling local anesthetic into this space. This can create a nerve block along the T7-L1 dermatomes (Baldea et al. 2020). Paravertebral nerve blocks have been shown to improve subjective pain scores and significantly decreased opioid use postoperatively (Baldea et al. 2020; Borle et al. 2014) Comparative studies between peritubular and intercostal nerve blocks found that intercostal nerve blocks were superior and had lower pain scores and decreased PACU opioid requirements (Jonnavithula et al. 2017).

4.3   Tranexamic Acid

Tranexamic acid is a synthetic derivative of lysine and inhibits fibrinolysis by blocking the conversion of plasminogen to plasmin. Intraoperative use of TXA has been shown to decrease perioperative blood loss in gynecology, orthopedic and general surgery cases with minimal complications (Tanaka et al. 2001; Gungorduk et al. 2011; Massicotte et al. 2011). TXA has also been adapted to urologic cases, including PCNL. Several prospective randomized controlled trials have uniformly reported decreased change in hemoglobin, decreased intraoperative blood loss and decreased transfusion rates (Mokhtari et al. 2021; Batagello et al. 2022; Kumar et al. 2013; Siddiq 2017; Bansal and Arora 2017). Several different TXA regimens have been proposed. The majority of protocols include 1g given intravenously at induction (Mokhtari et al. 2021; Siddiq 2017) and some give an additional dose of 500 mg three times over the following 24 h (Kumar et al. 2013). Bansal et al. also propose adding

TXA in the irrigant fluid in lieu of giving it intravenously. Currently, there are no comparative studies to identify the optimal dosing regimen but a meta-analysis found decreased blood loss, decreased transfusion rates and shorter operative times across all dosing regimens. Patients who have a higher risk of VTE should be excluded from use including active smokers, known coagulopathies, uses of oral contraceptives, use of anticoagulation or antiplatelets, history of VTE or impaired renal function. With an established favorable safety profile and low cost, TXA should be considered during PCNL for eligible patients.

5　Imaging

The development of Percutaneous Nephrolithotomy (PCNL) enabled for the first time the successful treatment of large, complex renal calculi in a minimally invasive manner. Even very large, very hard and very complex calculi can be treated with very high stone clearance rates. However over time the expectations of outcomes from such surgery have increased substantially, and now the goal of achieving a stone free, complication free patient with minimal intervention has become the standard to which all endourologists aspire. An essential component of such an outcome is the appropriate imaging and evaluation of the patient prior to surgery being undertaken. This should be undertaken with the lowest radiation dose and the least invasiveness possible, but with the utilization of more complex investigation whenever likely to be required.

5.1　CT Imaging

CT imaging, also known as computed tomography, is the best practice imaging methodology in the preoperative assessment and planning of treatment of urinary calculi by PCNL (Lipkin and Ackerman 2016). This technology utilizes X-rays and computer algorithms to generate detailed cross-sectional images and of the body that can then be reconstructed into any plane. CT imaging provides excellent visualization of urinary stones, allowing for precise assessment of stone size, location, and composition. It also enables evaluation of surrounding structures, such as the renal parenchyma, collecting system, vasculature and adjacent organs, aiding in treatment planning and identification of potential complications (see Fig. 1).

While non-contrast CT scans are the most common study in preoperative assessment of urinary stone disease, contrast-enhanced CT urography is routinely utilized for evaluating upper urinary tract stone burden and renal collecting system anatomy. Such CT imaging also assists in determining stone complexity and composition, guiding surgical planning including nephrostomy placement and choice of equipment based on the post-processing determination of Hounsfield density of the calculus.

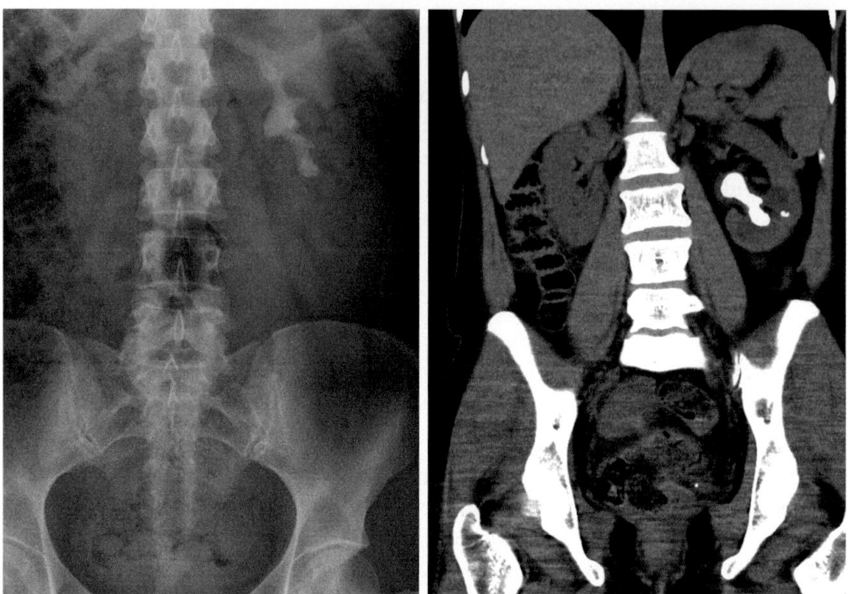

Fig. 1 Comparison of respective images from plain abdominal X ray (left) and CT KUB (right) reconstruction, showing greater detail of lower pole calyceal anatomy for where puncture is planned, including additional fragment separate to main calculus which will also require extraction

While CT imaging provides valuable diagnostic information, radiation exposure is a concern, particularly in younger patients or those requiring repeated imaging studies. Radiation reduction techniques, such as low-dose protocols, iterative reconstruction algorithms, and dose modulation, should be employed wherever possible to minimize radiation exposure without compromising image quality (Lipkin and Ackerman 2016).

Traditional CT imaging does however entertain specific limitations. A major disadvantage is its inability to provide real-time imaging, limiting its use during dynamic procedures. Additionally the use of iodinated contrast agents can pose risks to patients with renal insufficiency or contrast allergies. Moreover technical considerations such as beam hardening or patient motion may affect image quality and interpretation. These limitations highlight the importance of a multidisciplinary approach, considering other imaging modalities and clinical data to make informed decisions.

5.2 Ultrasound Imaging

Ultrasound imaging utilizes high-frequency sound waves to generate real-time images of the body's structures, and is widely used in urology due to its safety, cost-effectiveness, portability, and ability to provide dynamic imaging. Ultrasound imaging does not involve ionizing radiation or contrast agents, making it ideal for repeated evaluations, pediatric patients, pregnant patients, and individuals with contraindications to other imaging modalities.

In preoperative assessment of patients prior to PCNL, ultrasound aids in the evaluation of renal size, shape, and stone location, identifying abnormalities such as hydronephrosis, concurrent renal masses, or cysts. Doppler ultrasound can assess renal blood flow and detect vascular abnormalities. Most importantly in patients due to undergo ultrasound guided puncture of the collecting system it enables familiarity with what will be apparent at the time of surgery.

The sensitivity and specificity of ultrasonography is lower than CT imaging for urolithiasis (Ray et al. 2010). This is particularly apparent in situations such as obese patients or in patients with bowel gas interference. Its operator-dependent nature can also lead to variability in image quality and interpretation. Additionally, ultrasound is not as effective as CT imaging in evaluating stone composition or complex stone burden.

5.3 Fusion Imaging

Fusion imaging combines different imaging modalities such as CT or MRI with real-time ultrasound imaging, providing a comprehensive and detailed visualization of the urinary tract. It combines the strengths of each modality, such as the anatomical information from CT or MRI and the real-time guidance of ultrasound. Fusion imaging may potentially enhance the accuracy of stone localization, aid in needle guidance during procedures, and improve outcomes by allowing for precise targeting and minimizing damage to surrounding structures.

There are various techniques for fusion imaging, including software-based registration of preoperative CT or MRI images with real-time ultrasound, or hardware-based systems that use electromagnetic or mechanical tracking to merge the imaging data. In percutaneous nephrolithotomy this technology has been reported to facilitate more precise needle placement and reduced procedure time. Like routine ultrasound, fusion imaging also enables real-time monitoring during interventions, enhancing safety and minimizing complications.

Despite these advantages, fusion imaging also has certain limitations and challenges. The registration accuracy between different imaging modalities can be affected by organ deformation, patient movement or technical limitations. The complexity and cost of fusion imaging systems may limit their widespread use. Operator expertise and training are crucial to ensure optimal image fusion and interpretation. Ongoing advancements in technology and further research are necessary to address these limitations and expand their clinical utility.

5.4 Advanced Imaging Modalities: Virtual Image Guidance, 3D Imaging and 3D Printed Modelling

Newer software and processing techniques have allowed reconstruction of CT images into 3D models of the renal stone (Hubert et al. 1997; Li et al. Dec 2013) or the renal pelvis (Durutović et al. 2022). 3D models may be used to plan for the puncture trajectory. More recently virtual image guidance has been piloted, where the 3D model was translated on the skin of the lumbar area to enable the planned puncture trajectory. This technique was able to reduce the duration of fluoroscopy time required to obtain a successful puncture (Durutović et al. 2022) and may also reduce the number of puncture attempts. While promising, the major limitation to the utility of these techniques lies in the lack of supporting research to this point.

Syngo Dyna-CT (Siemens), also called the C-arm CT, is a form of imaging comprising a mounted biplanar X-ray system and a carbon-based operating table. It was initially used in angiography and supported vascular interventions. With adjusted protocols specific for urology, real time acquisition of cross-sectional imaging of the renal pelvis and calyces can be achieved. The images obtained can further undergo 3-dimensional reconstruction allowing for accurate visualisation of the collecting system.

There are major advantages in the utility of Dyna-CT for PCNLs. Firstly, the 3-dimensional image reconstructions may improve accuracy during puncture planning. Further guidance is provided with a laser crosshair on the detector, which can aid in planning trajectory fluoroscopic needle provide further control of the puncture process (Ritter et al. Nov 2015). Secondly, at the conclusion of the treatment, an on-table scan may be performed to examine for any missed stones or to confirm stone clearance (Ritter et al. Nov 2015). This is particularly helpful in avoiding repeated treatments after an incomplete PCNL.

Consideration needs to be given to radiation dose. Dyna-CT is currently used uncommonly in urology, and as such there is limited research on radiation doses. It has been shown to have mildly less radiation than a non-contrast multi-slice CT (7.04 mSv vs. 8.23 mSv) (Bai et al. Nov 2012). There are no studies comparing Dyna-CT with the more commonly used fluoroscopic images intraoperatively. However, this comparison using the C-arm CT system has previously been examined in neuro-surgical intervention, with results demonstrating that a single 3-dimensional CT scan can equate to up to 132 fluoroscopic images' worth of radiation exposure (Naseri et al. 2020). As such, strict radiation safety protocols need to accompany Dyna-CT use. As an extension of the 3D reconstructed images, printed 3D models show promise in preparation for complex cases. 3D printed models of patient kidneys have been used as part of doctor–patient communication in addition to surgical planning, and have been demonstrated to improve both the patient experience and stone clearance rates (Liu et al. 2022; Cui et al. 2022).

Finally, a pilot study for the 3D printing of a patient specific needle access guide to aid puncture has demonstrated 100% success rate with a single puncture (Keyu et al. 2021). Despite positive results to date, barriers still exist to the wider adoption of 3D printing in PCNL planning. 3D printing imposes an additional financial burden to the healthcare system, plus clinicians often lack the technical skills to process radiology images and render 3D printing files (Manning et al. Apr 2018), and outsourcing of this task may be required.

5.5 *Skin-to-Stone Distance (SSD)*

Skin-to-stone distance (SSD) is the measurement from the skin surface to the location of a urinary stone within the body, and is the key parameter in the planning and execution of percutaneous puncture of the collecting system prior to PCNL. SSD helps determine the optimal puncture site and approach, influencing the success and safety of the procedure, and should be considered before any percutaneous puncture is undertaken (see Fig. 2).

SSD can be measured using either ultrasound or CT. It is influenced by several factors, including patient body habitus, the position of the kidney, and the location and size of the stone. The position of the kidney, whether it is ectopic in a lower

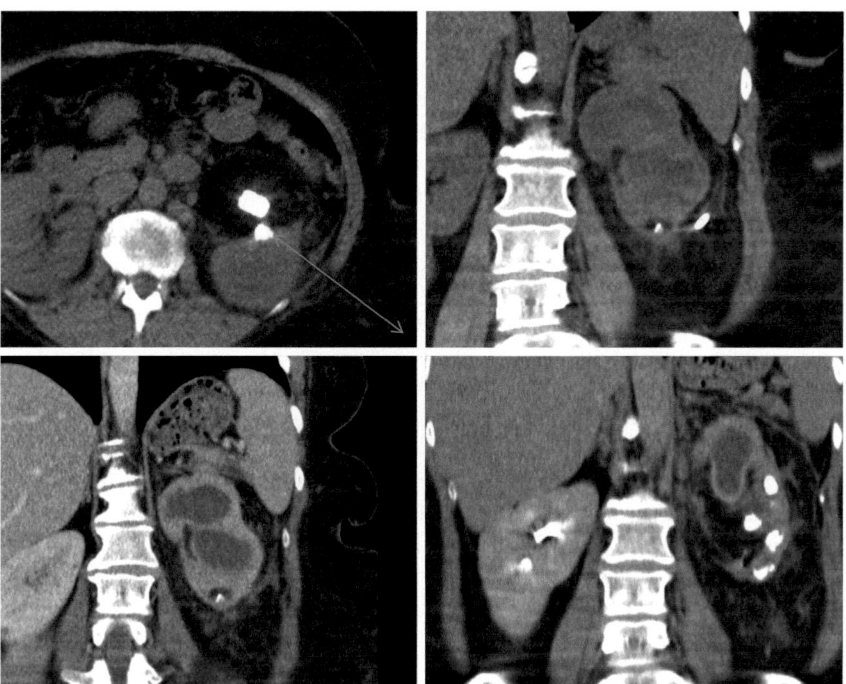

Fig. 2 Multiplanar CT demonstrating extensive abdominal wall adipose tissue with skin stone distance 19.1 cm with patient lying supine. Accordingly decision was made to treat the patient prone

or higher position, also affects SSD. The size and location of the stone within the kidney determine the optimal calyx for puncture, and consequent needle trajectory.

SSD plays a significant role in the success and safety of PCNL. A shorter SSD allows for a more direct access to the stone, usually reducing the need for multiple puncture attempts and minimizing the risk of injury to adjacent structures. However, a very short SSD may increase the risk of complications such as bowel injury or pleural injury if the kidney is unusually high or lateral. For this reason SSD is best calculated in conjunction with careful appraisal of individual anatomy with the patient in the orientation in which their procedure will be undertaken eg. with the CT scan being undertaken in the prone position for a patient having a prone PCNL and in the supine position for a supine puncture. The integration of SSD measurement with other imaging parameters and clinical data ensures the optimal needle tract and the best possible patient outcomes.

5.6 Grading PCNL Complexity and Outcomes

Four prognosticating tools have been reported in literature aiming to predict stone free rates after a PCNL, and pre-operative imaging is necessary to use these tools. These are the Guy's stone score, CROES nomogram, S.T.O.N.E nephrolithometry score and the Seoul National University Renal Stone Complexity (S-ReSC) score.

The Guy's stone score was first described in 2011 and comprises four grades of increasing anatomical and renal calculi related complexities (Thomas et al. 2011). The major advantage of this score include it being the only one aiming to predict for complications as well as stone free rates. In addition, its simplicity lends to ease of use. However multiple other patient factors and surgeon factors are not taken into consideration.

The CROES (Clinical Research Office of the Endourological Society) nomogram resulted from multinational data. It accounts for the number of stones, stone position, stone volume, prior treatment, and surgeon experience to predict stone free rates after PCNL (Smith et al. 2013). It is the only scoring system accounting for surgeon experience, however this metric has been subjectively rather than objectively assessed (Wu and Okeke 2017).

The S.T.O.N.E. nephrolithometry score was developed using variables identi-fied in literature reviews that can affect PCNL outcomes. The acronym S.T.O.N.E. represents these factors: stone **s**ize, **t**ract length, degree of **o**bstruction, **n**umber of involved calyces, and stone **e**ssence (i.e. density) (Okhunov et al. 2013). On the basis of these factors, a score of 5–13 may be calculated, with increasing scores representing decreasing stone free rates. A strength of this particular score is that factors are chosen solely based on published data, whereas the remainder were based at least in part on expert opinion.

The S-ReSC score was first presented in 2013, where cases were assigned scores from 1 to 9 based on the number of sites involved: in the renal pelvis (#1), superior major calyceal groups (#2), inferior major calyceal group (#3), anterior and posterior minor calyceal groups of the superior (#4–5), middle (#6–7), and inferior calyx (#8–9) (Jeong et al. 2013). The S-ReSC score takes into account the anatomy of the patient and the renal calculi, and like Guy's stone score it is simple to use. The authors also demonstrated a relationship between the S-ReSC score and complication rates; however, the correlation failed to reach statistically significance.

With several scoring systems available, the question of whether any single system is superior to another often falls to operator preference. Several comparison studies have been performed; however no single score has consistently proven more accurate in predicting outcomes after PCNL (Withington et al. Jan 2016; Jaipuria et al. 2016; Kumar et al. 2016; Noureldin et al. 2015).

5.7 Imaging Considerations for Supine Versus Prone Percutaneous Nephrolithotomy (PCNL)

Traditionally PCNL was performed with the patient in the prone position, which provided excellent access to the renal collecting system. In recent years there has been a shift toward performing PCNL in the supine position due to potential advantages such as improved patient comfort (Goumas-Kartalas and Montanari Jul 2010), shorter operative times (Yuan et al. 2016; Liu et al. 2010), and suggested easier access to lower pole stones. The choice between supine and prone PCNL depends on several factors, including stone characteristics, patient anatomy, and surgeon preference.

For both approaches to PCNL the puncture is usually performed using fluoroscopic guidance based on preoperative imaging. Choice of approach should be individualised, and based on the use of contrast enhanced imaging to optimize access to all calyces. Ideally the pre-operative contrast CT should have been performed with the patient in the position proposed for the puncture.

5.8 Imaging Considerations for Size of the PCNL Tract

There can be considerable morbidity associated with the PCNL tract, including urine extravasation, renal haemorrhage and need for transfusions, renal parenchymal loss and post-operative pain (Michel et al. 2007; Tailly and Denstedt Dec 2016). In attempt to reduce these risks, there has been a trend towards smaller tract sizes. Standard PCNL utilises outer sheath sizes of 24Fr or greater (Kallidonis et al. Jan 2021), while mini-PCNL utilises outer sheath sizes of 22 Fr or smaller (DiBianco and Ghani 2021).

Despite these trends and research, mini-PCNL did not show the anticipated improvements in the observed complication domains. The positive outcomes favouring mini-PCNL were reduced blood loss and reduced blood transfusion rates (Giusti et al. 2007). Additionally, mini-PCNL equipment has been used to gain access in cases where standard PCNL access was unable to be achieved (Hennessey et al. May 2017). Parenchymal loss has been examined (Traxer et al. May 2001), and mini-PCNL made no statistically significant improvement. Furthermore, higher intrarenal pressures are demonstrated in mini-PCNL (Tepeler et al. Jun 2014), and this has been associated with higher rates of bacteraemia and septic complications (Loftus et al. Apr 2018). Finally, mini-PCNL operative time has been reported as significantly longer than standard PCNL at 155.5 vs 106.6 min respectively (Giusti et al. 2007). As such standard PCNL with standard tract sizes remains the mainstay of percutaneous management of urolithiasis in many departments.

5.9 Calyceal Diverticula

Calyceal diverticula are pouch-like cavities arising from the calyces of the collecting system within the kidney. They are often congenital and can be classified as either true diverticula, which involve all layers of the calyx, or false diverticula, which only involve the mucosal layer. Calyceal diverticula are typically located in the upper or lower pole of the kidney and can vary in size and shape. They may be asymptomatic or present with symptoms such as recurrent urinary tract infections, hematuria, or stone formation.

Where calculi are present and requiring of treatment in calyceal diverticulae, delayed phase imaging (Stunell et al. Oct 2010) on CT or even magnetic resonance urography (MRU) can provide more detailed information regarding the size, location, orientation and characteristics of the diverticula. Detailed assessment of the calyceal anatomy can assist in determining whether marsupialization is an appropriate option for consideration in association with stone extraction.

5.10 Ectopic Kidney

An ectopic kidney is a congenital condition in which the kidney is located in an abnormal position instead of the normal retroperitoneal space due to a developmental anomaly. The prevalence of ectopic kidneys is relatively rare, estimated to occur in approximately 1 in 1000 live births (Chavis et al. Nov 1992), and where PCNL is contemplated these kidneys are usually located in the pelvis or across the midline of the abdomen.

Imaging techniques play a crucial role in identifying and characterizing ectopic kidneys. CT scans or MRI with intravenous contrast are commonly employed, because almost by definition the vascular supply will be anomalous. Visualization of the vascular supply is critical preoperatively in order to avoid injury to associated vessels during puncture and nephrostomy tract dilation. As the kidney's shape is often abnormal, and there is greater potential for additional associated congenital anomalies including ureteropelvic junction obstruction (Eid et al. 2018), CT urography is particularly valuable in evaluating the optimal approach to any calyx where a calculus may be present. Punctures for nephrostomy tube placement in such kidneys are often more vertical than normal due to failure of the kidney to lodge into the relatively deep renal fossa during arrestation of its development, and consequently it is essential to optimize preoperative imaging—often by the use of 3D reconstructions that can show the orientation of calyces and identify any overlying structures such as the colon. This is particularly pertinent to the presence of a Horseshoe kidney where the collecting system lies especially close to the midline of the abdomen.

5.11 Paediatric Stones

The incidence of paediatric stones varies across different regions and populations, but has been noted to increase over the past 2 decades. Various factors contribute to the formation of stones in children, including metabolic disorders, urinary tract abnormalities, dietary habits, genetic predisposition and inadequate fluid intake. The greater availability of ultrasonography has also no doubt made possible the more frequent diagnosis of this pathology (Jobs et al. 2018).

Imaging techniques based around ultrasound are more commonly used as initial diagnostic modalities due to the lack of radiation (Jobs et al. 2018). However the disadvantages of ultrasound in general remain applicable in the paediatric population, therefore, in complex cases CT scan or occasionally intravenous pyelography (IVP) may be necessary for more appropriate, detailed evaluation (Jobs et al. 2018) (Table 1).

Preoperative Checklist
- History and Physical
- Medical clearance
- Appropriate laboratory and radiographic testing
  - Urine Culture
  - CBC
  - BMP
  - Coagulation Panel
  - Type and Screen
  - Non contrasted CT abdomen and pelvis
- Discussion of anesthetic options and pain control adjuncts
- Obtain informed consent

Table 1 Perioperative antibiotic regimens

		Antibiotic regimen	Duration	Study findings
Low risk: Negative preoperative culture and no risk factors				
Zeng et al. (2020)	Review	Guideline based	Single Dose	No difference in postop sepsis
Chew et al. (2018)	Prospective RCT	Nitrofurantoin 100 mg versus No antibiotics	7 days	No difference in postop sepsis (12% v 14%)
Intermediate risk: Negative urine cultures with risk factors (hydronephrosis and stones >2 cm)				
Mariappan et al. (2006)	PCT	Ciprofloxacin 250 mg BID	7 days	3 times less likely to have SIRS (RR 2.9)
Bag et al. (2011)	PCT	Nitrofurantoin 100 mg BID	7 days	Decreased postoperative SIRS (19% v 49%)
High risk: Positive urine cultures, large stone size, hydronephrosis, foreign bodies, indwelling drainage tubes, recurrent UTI, struvite stone, and or urinary diversion				
Xu et al. (2022)	Review	Culture specific	>7 days versus <6 days	Decreased SIRS (21% v 40%)
Zeng et al. (2020)	Review	Culture specific	>7 days versus <3 days	Decreased SIRS (8% v 28%)
Sur et al.	Prospective RCT	Culture specific	2 days versus 7 days	Decreased sepsis in the 7-day group

RCT Randomized controlled trial, *PCT* Prospective controlled trial, *SIRS* Systemic inflammatory response syndrome

References

Akkas F, Karadag S, Haciislamoglu A. Does the duration between urine culture and percutaneous nephrolithotomy affect the rate of systemic inflammatory response syndrome postoperatively? Urolithiasis. 2021;49(5):451–6. https://doi.org/10.1007/s00240-021-01245-7.

Assimos DKAMN, et al. Surgical management of stones: American urological association/ endourological society guideline, part II. J Urol. 2016;196:1161.

Bag S, Kumar S, Taneja N, Sharma V, Mandal AK, Singh SK. One week of nitrofurantoin before percutaneous nephrolithotomy significantly reduces upper tract infection and urosepsis: a prospective controlled study. Urology. 2011;77(1):45–9. https://doi.org/10.1016/j.urology.2010.03.025.

Bai M, Liu B, Mu H, et al. The comparison of radiation dose between C-arm flat-detector CT (DynaCT) and multi-slice CT (MSCT): a phantom study (in eng). Eur J Radiol. 2012;81(11):3577–80. https://doi.org/10.1016/j.ejrad.2011.09.006.

Baldea KG, Patel PM, Delos Santos G, et al. Paravertebral block for percutaneous nephrolithotomy: a prospective, randomized, double-blind placebo-controlled study. World J Urol. 2020;38(11):2963–9. https://doi.org/10.1007/s00345-020-03093-3.

Bansal A, Arora A. A double-blind, placebo-controlled randomized clinical trial to evaluate the efficacy of tranexamic acid in irrigant solution on blood loss during percutaneous nephrolithotomy: a pilot study from tertiary care center of North India. World J Urol. 2017;35(8):1233–40. https://doi.org/10.1007/s00345-016-1980-6.

Batagello CA, Vicentini FC, Monga M, et al. Tranexamic acid in patients with complex stones undergoing percutaneous nephrolithotomy: a randomised, double-blinded, placebo-controlled trial. BJU Int. 2022;129(1):35–47. https://doi.org/10.1111/bju.15378.

Blackwell RH, Kirshenbaum EJ, Zapf MAC, et al. Incidence of adverse contrast reaction following nonintravenous urinary tract imaging. Eur Urol Focus. 2017;3(1):89–93. https://doi.org/10.1016/j.euf.2016.01.009.

Borle AP, Chhabra A, Subramaniam R, et al. Analgesic efficacy of paravertebral bupivacaine during percutaneous nephrolithotomy: an observer blinded, randomized controlled trial. J Endourol. 2014;28(9):1085–90. https://doi.org/10.1089/end.2014.0179.

Castellani D, Teoh JY, Pavia MP, et al. Assessing the optimal urine culture for predicting systemic inflammatory response syndrome after percutaneous nephrolithotomy and retrograde intrarenal surgery: results from a systematic review and meta-analysis. J Endourol. 2022;36(2):158–68. https://doi.org/10.1089/end.2021.0386.

Chavis CV, Press HC Jr, Gumbs RV. Fused pelvic kidneys: case report (in eng). J Natl Med Assoc. 1992;84(11):980–2.

Chew BH, Miller NL, Abbott JE, et al. A randomized controlled trial of preoperative prophylactic antibiotics prior to percutaneous nephrolithotomy in a low infectious risk population: a report from the EDGE consortium. J Urol. 2018;200(4):801–8. https://doi.org/10.1016/j.juro.2018.04.062.

Cui D, Yan F, Yi J et al. Efficacy and safety of 3D printing-assisted percutaneous nephrolithotomy in complex renal calculi. Sci Rep. 2022;12(1):417. https://doi.org/10.1038/s41598-021-03851-2

Dai JC, Brisbane WG, Chang HC, Hsi RS, Harper JD. Anaphylactoid reactions after instillation of contrast material into the urinary tract: a survey of contemporary practice patterns and review of the literature. Urology. 2018;122:58–63. https://doi.org/10.1016/j.urology.2018.08.029.

de la Rosette J, Assimos D, Desai M, et al. The clinical research office of the endourological society percutaneous nephrolithotomy global study: indications, complications, and outcomes in 5803 patients. J Endourol. 2011;25(1):11–7. https://doi.org/10.1089/end.2010.0424.

DiBianco JM, Ghani KR. Precision stone surgery: current status of miniaturized percutaneous nephrolithotomy (in eng) Curr Urol Rep. 2021;22(4):24. https://doi.org/10.1007/s11934-021-01042-0

Doherty JU, Gluckman TJ, Hucker WJ, et al. 2017 ACC expert consensus decision pathway for periprocedural management of anticoagulation in patients with nonvalvular atrial fibrillation: a report of the american college of cardiology clinical expert consensus document task force. J Am Coll Cardiol. 2017;69(7):871–98. https://doi.org/10.1016/j.jacc.2016.11.024.

Durutović O, Filipović A, Milićević K, et al. 3D imaging segmentation and 3D rendering process for a precise puncture strategy during PCNL—A pilot study (in eng). Front Surg. 2022;9: 891596. https://doi.org/10.3389/fsurg.2022.891596.

Eid S, Iwanaga J, Loukas M et al. Pelvic kidney: a review of the literature (in eng) Cureus. 2018;10(6):e2775. https://doi.org/10.7759/cureus.2775

El Tayeb MM, Knoedler JJ, Krambeck AE, Paonessa JE, Mellon MJ, Lingeman JE. Vascular complications after percutaneous nephrolithotomy: 10 years of experience. Urology. 2015;85(4):777–81. https://doi.org/10.1016/j.urology.2014.12.044.

El-Nahas AR, Shokeir AA, El-Assmy AM, et al. Colonic perforation during percutaneous nephrolithotomy: study of risk factors. Urology. 2006;67(5):937–41. https://doi.org/10.1016/j.urology.2005.11.025.

Ganpule AP, Shah DH, Desai MR. Postpercutaneous nephrolithotomy bleeding: aetiology and management. Curr Opin Urol. 2014;24(2):189–94. https://doi.org/10.1097/MOU.000000000 0000025.

Gasparyan AY, Ayvazyan L, Mukanova U, Yessirkepov M, Kitas GD. The platelet-to-lymphocyte ratio as an inflammatory marker in rheumatic diseases. Ann Lab Med. 2019;39(4):345–57. https://doi.org/10.3343/alm.2019.39.4.345.

Giusti G, Piccinelli A, Taverna G et al. Miniperc? No, thank you! (in eng) Eur Urol. 2007;51(3):810–14; discussion 815. https://doi.org/10.1016/j.eururo.2006.07.047

Goumas-Kartalas I, Montanari E. Percutaneous nephrolithotomy in patients with spinal deformities (in eng). J Endourol. 2010;24(7):1081–9. https://doi.org/10.1089/end.2010.0095.

Gungorduk K, Yıldırım G, Asıcıoğlu O, Gungorduk OC, Sudolmus S, Ark C. Efficacy of intravenous tranexamic acid in reducing blood loss after elective cesarean section: a prospective, randomized, double-blind, placebo-controlled study. Am J Perinatol. 2011;28(3):233–40. https://doi.org/10. 1055/s-0030-1268238.

Hennessey DB, Kinnear NK, Troy A et al. Mini PCNL for renal calculi: does size matter? (in eng). BJU Int. 2017;119(Suppl 5):39–46. https://doi.org/10.1111/bju.13839

Hubert J, Blum A, Cormier L et al. Three-dimensional CT-scan reconstruction of renal calculi. a new tool for mapping-out staghorn calculi and follow-up of radiolucent stones (in eng). Eur Urol. 1997;31(3):297–301. https://doi.org/10.1159/000474471

Hur KJ, Moon HW, Kang SM, Kim KS, Choi YS, Cho H. Incidence of posterolateral and retrorenal colon in supine and prone position in percutaneous nephrolithotomy. Urolithiasis. 2021;49(6):585–90. https://doi.org/10.1007/s00240-021-01272-4.

Jaipuria J, Suryavanshi M, Sen TK. Comparative testing of reliability and audit utility of ordinal objective calculus complexity scores. Can we make an informed choice yet? BJU Int. 2016;118(6):958–68. https://doi.org/10.1111/bju.13597

Jeong CW, Jung JW, Cha WH, et al. Seoul national university renal stone complexity score for predicting stone-free rate after percutaneous nephrolithotomy (in eng). PLoS ONE. 2013;8(6): e65888. https://doi.org/10.1371/journal.pone.0065888.

Jobs K, Rakowska M, Paturej A. Urolithiasis in the pediatric population—Current opinion on epidemiology, patophysiology, diagnostic evaluation and treatment (in eng). Dev Period Med. 2018;22(2):201–08. https://doi.org/10.34763/devperiodmed.20182202.201208

Jonnavithula N, Chirra RR, Pasupuleti SL, Devraj R, Sriramoju V, Pisapati MVLN. A comparison of the efficacy of intercostal nerve block and peritubal infiltration of ropivacaine for post-operative analgesia following percutaneous nephrolithotomy: a prospective randomised double-blind study. Ind J Anaesth. 2017;61(8):655–60. https://doi.org/10.4103/ija.IJA_88_17.

Kallidonis P, Liourdi D, Liatsikos E, et al. Will mini percutaneous nephrolithotomy change the game? (in eng). Eur Urol. 2021;79(1):122–3. https://doi.org/10.1016/j.eururo.2020.10.010.

Keyu G, Shuaishuai L, Raj A et al. A 3D printing personalized percutaneous puncture guide access plate for percutaneous nephrolithotomy: a pilot study. BMC Urol. 2021;21(1):184. https://doi. org/10.1186/s12894-021-00945-x

Khan SR, Canales BK, Dominguez-Gutierrez PR. Randall's plaque and calcium oxalate stone formation: role for immunity and inflammation. Nat Rev Nephrol. 2021;17(6):417–33. https:// doi.org/10.1038/s41581-020-00392-1.

Korets R, Graversen JA, Kates M, Mues AC, Gupta M. Post-percutaneous nephrolithotomy systemic inflammatory response: a prospective analysis of preoperative urine, renal pelvic urine and stone cultures. J Urol. 2011;186(5):1899–903. https://doi.org/10.1016/j.juro.2011.06.064

Kriplani A, Pandit S, Chawla A, et al. Neutrophil-lymphocyte ratio (NLR), platelet-lymphocyte ratio (PLR) and lymphocyte-monocyte ratio (LMR) in predicting systemic inflammatory response syndrome (SIRS) and sepsis after percutaneous nephrolithotomy (PNL). Urolithiasis. 2022;50(3):341–8. https://doi.org/10.1007/s00240-022-01319-0.

Kumar S, Randhawa MS, Ganesamoni R, Singh SK. Tranexamic acid reduces blood loss during percutaneous nephrolithotomy: a prospective randomized controlled study. J Urol. 2013;189(5):1757–61. https://doi.org/10.1016/j.juro.2012.10.115.

Kumar S, Sreenivas J, Karthikeyan VS et al. Evaluation of CROES nephrolithometry nomogram as a preoperative predictive system for percutaneous nephrolithotomy outcomes. J Endourol. 2016;30(10):1079–83. https://doi.org/10.1089/end.2016.0340

Lai WS, Assimos D. ProPhylactic management update the role of antibiotic prophylaxis in percutaneous nephrolithotomy. Rev Urol. 2016;18(1):10–4. https://doi.org/10.3909/riu0699A.

Li H, Chen Y, Liu C, et al. Construction of a three-dimensional model of renal stones: comprehensive planning for percutaneous nephrolithotomy and assistance in surgery (in eng). World J Urol. 2013;31(6):1587–92. https://doi.org/10.1007/s00345-012-0998-7.

Lipkin M, Ackerman A. Imaging for urolithiasis: standards, trends, and radiation exposure. Curr Opin Urol 2016;26(1). Available https://journals.lww.com/co-urology/Fulltext/2016/01000/Imaging_for_urolithiasis__standards,_trends,_and.12.aspx

Liu M, Chen J, Gao M, et al. Preoperative midstream urine cultures. J Endourol. 2021;35(10):1467–78. https://doi.org/10.1089/end.2020.1140.

Liu Y, Song H, Xiao B, et al. PCNL combined with 3D printing technology for the treatment of complex staghorn kidney stones (in eng). J Healthc Eng. 2022;2022:7554673. https://doi.org/10.1155/2022/7554673.

Liu L, Zheng S, Xu Y et al. Systematic review and meta-analysis of percutaneous nephrolithotomy for patients in the supine versus prone position. J. Endourol. 2010;24(12):1941–946. https://doi.org/10.1089/end.2010.0292

Loftus CJ, Hinck B, Makovey I, et al. Mini versus standard percutaneous nephrolithotomy: the impact of sheath size on intrarenal pelvic pressure and infectious complications in a porcine model (in eng). J Endourol. 2018;32(4):350–3. https://doi.org/10.1089/end.2017.0602.

MacDonald M, Ilie G, Power L, et al. Effect of tranexamic acid on bleeding outcomes after percutaneous nephrolithotomy: a systematic review and meta-analysis of randomized controlled trials. J Endourol. 2022;36(5):589–97. https://doi.org/10.1089/end.2021.0762.

Manning TG, O'Brien JS, Christidis D, et al. Three dimensional models in uro-oncology: a future built with additive fabrication (in eng). World J Urol. 2018;36(4):557–63. https://doi.org/10.1007/s00345-018-2201-2.

Mariappan P, Smith G, Bariol SV, Moussa SA, Tolley DA. Stone and pelvic urine culture and sensitivity are better than bladder urine as predictors of urosepsis following percutaneous nephrolithotomy: a prospective clinical study. J Urol. 2005;173(5):1610–4. https://doi.org/10.1097/01.ju.0000154350.78826.96.

Mariappan P, Smith G, Moussa SA, Tolley DA. One week of ciprofloxacin before percutaneous nephrolithotomy significantly reduces upper tract infection and urosepsis: a prospective controlled study. BJU Int. 2006;98(5):1075–9. https://doi.org/10.1111/j.1464-410X.2006.06450.x.

Massicotte L, Denault AY, Beaulieu D, Thibeault L, Hevesi Z, Roy A. Aprotinin versus tranexamic acid during liver transplantation: impact on blood product requirements and survival. Transplantation. 2011;91(11):1273–8. https://doi.org/10.1097/TP.0b013e31821ab9f8.

Mehrabi S, Mousavi Zadeh A, Akbartabar Toori M, Mehrabi F. General versus spinal anesthesia in percutaneous nephrolithotomy. Urol J. 2013;10(1):756–61. https://www.ncbi.nlm.nih.gov/pubmed/23504678

Michel MS, Trojan L, Rassweiler JJ. Complications in percutaneous nephrolithotomy (in eng). Eur Urol. 2007; 51(4):899–906; discussion 906. https://doi.org/10.1016/j.eururo.2006.10.020

Mohapatra A, Hyun G, Semins MJ. Trends in the usage of contrast allergy prophylaxis for endourologic procedures. Urology. 2019;131:53–6. https://doi.org/10.1016/j.urology.2019.05.010.

Mokhtari MR, Farshid S, Modresi P, Abedi F. The effects of tranexamic acid on bleeding control during and after percutaneous nephrolithotomy (PCNL): a randomized clinical trial. Urol J. 2021;18(6):608–11. https://doi.org/10.22037/uj.v18i.6505

Muluk V, Cohn S, Whinney C. Perioperative medication management. UpToDate.

Naseri Y, Hubbe U, Scholz C et al. Radiation exposure of a mobile 3D C-arm with large flat-panel detector for intraoperative imaging and navigation—An experimental study using an anthropomorphic Alderson phantom. BMC Med Imaging. 2020;20(1):96. https://doi.org/10.1186/s12880-020-00495-y

Nasseh H, Mokhtari G, Ghasemi S, Biazar G, Kazemnezhad Leyli E, Gholamjani MK. Risk factors for intra-operative bleeding in percutaneous nephrolithotomy in an academic center: a retrospective study. Anesth Pain Med. 2022;12(4): e126974. https://doi.org/10.5812/aapm-126974.

Noureldin YA, Elkoushy MA, Andonian S. Which is better? Guy's versus S.T.O.N.E. nephrolithometry scoring systems in predicting stone-free status post-percutaneous nephrolithotomy (in eng) World J Urol. 2015;33(11):1821–825. https://doi.org/10.1007/s00345-015-1508-5

O'Keeffe NK, Mortimer AJ, Sambrook PA, Rao PN. Severe sepsis following percutaneous or endoscopic procedures for urinary tract stones. Br J Urol. 1993;72(3):277–83. https://doi.org/10.1111/j.1464-410x.1993.tb00717.x.

Okhunov Z, Friedlander JI, George AK et al. S.T.O.N.E. nephrolithometry: novel surgical classification system for kidney calculi (in eng). Urology. 2013;81(6):1154–159. https://doi.org/10.1016/j.urology.2012.10.083

Pan Y, Xu M, Kang J, Wang S, Liu X. The safety of continuing low-dose aspirin therapy perioperatively in the patients had undergone percutaneous nephrolithotomy: a systematic review and meta-analysis. Urol J. 2022;19(4):253–61. https://doi.org/10.22037/uj.v19i.7170

Karnath BM. Preoperative cardiac risk assessment, vol. 15. 2002. www.aafp.org/afpAMERICANFAMILYPHYSICIAN1889

Ray AA, Ghiculete D, Pace KT, et al. Limitations to ultrasound in the detection and measurement of urinary tract calculi (in eng). Urology. 2010;76(2):295–300. https://doi.org/10.1016/j.urology.2009.12.015.

Reeves T, Pietropaolo A, Gadzhiev N, Seitz C, Somani BK. Role of endourological procedures (PCNL and URS) on renal function: a systematic review. Curr Urol Rep. 2020;21(5):21. https://doi.org/10.1007/s11934-020-00973-4.

Ritter M, Rassweiler MC, Michel MS. The uro dyna-CT enables three-dimensional planned laser-guided complex punctures (in eng). Eur Urol. 2015;68(5):880–4. https://doi.org/10.1016/j.eururo.2015.07.005.

Said SH, Al Kadum Hassan MA, Ali RH, Aghaways I, Kakamad FH, Mohammad KQ. Percutaneous nephrolithotomy; alarming variables for postoperative bleeding. Arab J Urol. 2017;15(1):24–9. https://doi.org/10.1016/j.aju.2016.12.001.

Segura JW. Endourology. J Urol. 1984;132(6):1079–84. https://doi.org/10.1016/s0022-5347(17)50041-5.

Sen V, Bozkurt IH, Aydogdu O, et al. Significance of preoperative neutrophil-lymphocyte count ratio on predicting postoperative sepsis after percutaneous nephrolithotomy. Kaohsiung J Med Sci. 2016;32(10):507–13. https://doi.org/10.1016/j.kjms.2016.08.008.

Siddiq A, Khalid S, Mithani H, Anis S, Sharif I, Shaikh J. Preventing Excessive Blood Loss During Percutaneous Nephrolithotomy by Using Tranexamic Acid: A Double Blinded Prospective Randomized Controlled Trial. J Urol Surg. 2017;4(4):195–201.

Smith A, Averch Timothy D, Shahrour K et al. A nephrolithometric nomogram to predict treatment success of percutaneous nephrolithotomy. J Urol. 2013;190(1):149–56. https://doi.org/10.1016/j.juro.2013.01.047

Stunell H, McNeill G, Browne RF, et al. The imaging appearances of calyceal diverticula complicated by uroliathasis (in eng). Br J Radiol. 2010;83(994):888–94. https://doi.org/10.1259/bjr/22591022.

Tailly T, Denstedt J. Innovations in percutaneous nephrolithotomy (in eng). Int J Surg. 2016;36(Pt D):665–72. https://doi.org/10.1016/j.ijsu.2016.11.007.

Tanaka N, Sakahashi H, Sato E, Hirose K, Ishima T, Ishii S. Timing of the administration of tranexamic acid for maximum reduction in blood loss in arthroplasty of the knee. J Bone Joint Surg Br. 2001;83(5):702–5. https://doi.org/10.1302/0301-620x.83b5.11745.

Tang Y, Zhang C, Mo C, Gui C, Luo J, Wu R. Predictive model for systemic infection after percutaneous nephrolithotomy and related factors analysis. Front Surg. 2021;8: 696463. https://doi.org/10.3389/fsurg.2021.696463.

Tepeler A, Akman T, Silay MS, et al. Comparison of intrarenal pelvic pressure during micropercutaneous nephrolithotomy and conventional percutaneous nephrolithotomy (in eng). Urolithiasis. 2014;42(3):275–9. https://doi.org/10.1007/s00240-014-0646-3.

Thomas K, Smith NC, Hegarty N et al. The guy's stone score—Grading the complexity of percutaneous nephrolithotomy procedures. Urology. 2011;78(2):277–81. https://doi.org/10.1016/j.urology.2010.12.026

Torrecilla Ortiz C, Meza Martínez AI, Vicens Morton AJ, et al. Obesity in percutaneous nephrolithotomy. Is body mass index really important? Urology. 2014;84(3):538–43. https://doi.org/10.1016/j.urology.2014.03.062

Traxer O, Smith TG 3rd, Pearle MS, et al. Renal parenchymal injury after standard and mini percutaneous nephrostolithotomy (in eng). J Urol. 2001;165(5):1693–5.

Withington J, Armitage J, Finch W, et al. Assessment of stone complexity for PCNL: a systematic review of the literature, how best can we record stone complexity in PCNL? (in eng). J Endourol. 2016;30(1):13–23. https://doi.org/10.1089/end.2015.0278.

Wu WJ, Okeke Z (2017) Current clinical scoring systems of percutaneous nephrolithotomy outcomes. Nat Rev Urol. 2017;14(8):459–69. https://doi.org/10.1038/nrurol.2017.71

Xu P, Zhang S, Zhang Y, et al. Preoperative antibiotic therapy exceeding 7 days can minimize infectious complications after percutaneous nephrolithotomy in patients with positive urine culture. World J Urol. 2022;40(1):193–9. https://doi.org/10.1007/s00345-021-03834-y.

Yu J, Guo B, Chen T, et al. Antibiotic prophylaxis in perioperative period of percutaneous nephrolithotomy: a systematic review and meta-analysis of comparative studies. World J Urol. 2020;38(7):1685–700. https://doi.org/10.1007/s00345-019-02967-5.

Yuan D, Liu Y, Rao H et al. Supine versus prone position in percutaneous nephrolithotomy for kidney calculi: a meta-analysis. J Endourol. 2016;30(7):754–63. https://doi.org/10.1089/end.2015.0402

Zeng T, Chen D, Wu W, et al. Optimal perioperative antibiotic strategy for kidney stone patients treated with percutaneous nephrolithotomy. Int J Infect Dis. 2020;97:162–6. https://doi.org/10.1016/j.ijid.2020.05.095.

Zhou X, Sun X, Chen X, et al. Effect of obesity on outcomes of percutaneous nephrolithotomy in renal stone management: a systematic review and meta-analysis. Urol Int. 2017;98(4):382–90. https://doi.org/10.1159/000455162.

Anatomy of the Renal Surgery

Francisco J. B. Sampaio ⓘ

Abstract A thorough understanding of the relevant anatomy is essential for the successful execution of percutaneous renal surgery. Percutaneous renal surgery is a minimally invasive procedure that requires precise knowledge of the anatomical structures within the kidney and surrounding areas. This abstract highlights the key anatomical considerations crucial for percutaneous renal surgery. The anatomy of the kidney encompasses various structures such as the renal cortex, renal medulla, renal pelvis, renal calyces, renal papilla, renal pyramids, and the renal hilum. The renal vessels, including the renal artery and renal vein, play a vital role in maintaining blood supply to the kidney. Additionally, the collecting ducts, ureter, urinary bladder, renal parenchyma, renal capsule, renal sinus, and renal fascia contribute to the overall anatomy and function of the kidney. Accurate knowledge of these structures is crucial for appropriate patient positioning, precise localization of the target area, and safe access during percutaneous renal surgery. Understanding the three-dimensional anatomy and spatial relationships is essential to minimize the risk of complications and maximize the efficacy of the procedure. This abstract emphasizes the significance of comprehensive knowledge of renal anatomy in percutaneous renal surgery. It underscores the importance of preoperative evaluation, imaging modalities, and anatomical landmarks for optimal patient outcomes. By mastering the relevant anatomy, urologists can confidently navigate the complexities of percutaneous renal surgery, ensuring successful interventions and improved patient care.

Keywords Kidney anatomy · Renal anatomy · Nephron · Renal cortex · Renal medulla · Renal pelvis · Renal calyces · Renal papilla · Renal pyramids · Renal hilum · Renal vessels · Renal artery · Renal vein · Collecting ducts · Ureter · Urinary bladder · Renal parenchyma · Renal capsule · Renal sinus · Renal fascia

---

F. J. B. Sampaio (✉)
Urogenital Research Unit, Satate University of Rio de Janeiro, Rua Siqueira Campos 30, sl 1101, Copacabana, Rio de Janeiro 22031-072, Brazil
e-mail: Sampaio.uerj@gmail.com

J. D. Denstedt and E. N. Liatsikos (eds.), *Percutaneous Renal Surgery*,
https://doi.org/10.1007/978-3-031-40542-6_5

1   Pelviocalyceal System: Endourological Implications

1.1   Anatomical Background

To assist endourologists in making a mental image of the collecting system in three dimensions and learning the exact spatial position of the calices, in 40 cases, before obtaining pelviocalyceal system corrosion endocasts, an iodinated contrast material was injected into the ureter to opacify the collecting system in order to obtain a pyelogram. After radiography, the contrast material was removed and the collecting system was filled with a polyester resin to obtain a three-dimensional endocast. These 40 kidneys enabled a comparative study between the radiographic images and their corresponding three-dimensional endocasts.

1.2   Findings and Clinical Implications

The comparative study between pyelograms and three-dimensional endocasts of the collecting system enabled a perception of some remarkable anatomical aspects of the kidney collecting system that are very important to be considered by endourologists during the endourologic procedures.

Presence of Perpendicular Minor Calices. In 11.4% of the cases (16/140 casts) we found a perpendicular minor calyx draining directly into the renal pelvis or into a major calyx (Fig. 1). The minor calices perpendicular to the surface of the collecting system, which are seen in the casts, can be superimposed on other structures. Because of this fact, visualization of these calices radiographically can be difficult. Stones in such minor calices can be seen on standard anteroposterior radiographic images as if they were placed in the pelvis or in a major calyx. Thus, one must consider this anatomical detail in cases of stones that do not alter the renal function and that apparently are in the renal pelvis or in a major calyx. In this situation, a complementary radiological study with lateral and oblique films must be done to determine accurately the position and extent of the stones (Sampaio and Mandarim-de-Lacerda 1988a; Sampaio 1993a).

When a stone is located in a perpendicular minor calyx (Fig. 1) its removal presents additional difficulties for both extracorporeal shock wave lithotripsy (SWL) and percutaneous nephrolithotripsy (PCNL). Patients with stones in such calices are not good candidates for SWL because these calices invariably present narrow infundibula (smaller than 4 mm in diameter), therefore, the discharge of the disintegrated stone fragments will be difficult (Sampaio and Aragao 1992; Sampaio 2001, 2007). Regarding the percutaneous removal, direct access into the calyx containing the stone is an easy approach; nevertheless, it involves a puncture performed without considering the arterial and venous anatomical relationships to the collecting system. This kind of puncture carries a great risk of injuring a vascular structure (Sampaio

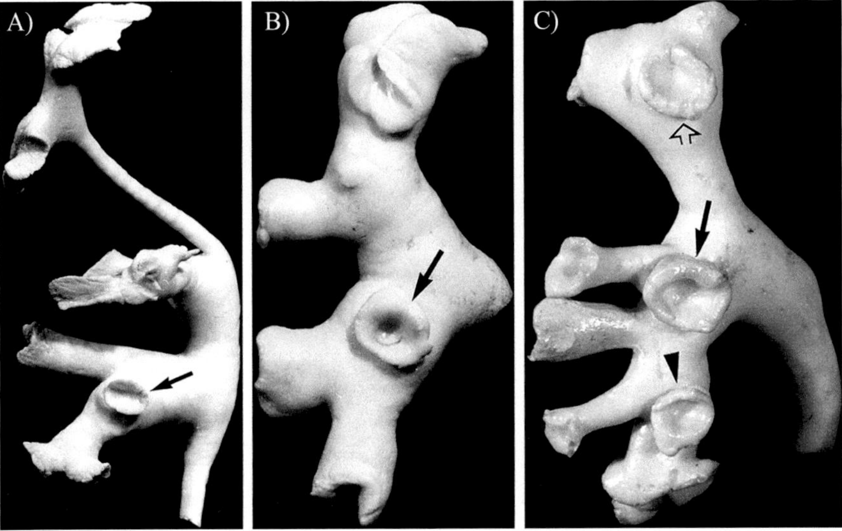

Fig. 1 (A) Anterior view of right pelviocalyceal endocast reveals perpendicular minor calyx draining into the inferior calyceal group (arrow) (B) Anterior view of right pelviocalyceal endocast reveals perpendicular minor calyx draining into the inferior calyceal group (arrow) very close to the renal pelvis. (C) Anterior view of right pelviocalyceal endocast reveals perpendicular minor calyx draining into the renal pelvis (arrow). This cast also shows a perpendicular minor calyx draining into the superior calyceal group (open-arrow) and a perpendicular minor calyx draining into the inferior calyceal group (arrowhead)

1993a). Therefore, in cases of stone in such calices, a variety of safe and refined accesses, techniques and instruments should be used.

Position of the Calices Relative to the Lateral Kidney Margin. In 39 of 140 casts (27.8%), the anterior calices had a more lateral (peripheral) position than the posterior calices (Fig. 2A). In 27 casts (19.3%), the posterior calices were in a more lateral position than the anterior calices (Fig. 2B). Nevertheless, in the majority of the cases (74 casts; 52.9%) the anterior and posterior calices had varied positions: superimposed or alternately distributed (in one region the most lateral were the anterior calices and in another region the most lateral were the posterior calices) (Fig. 2C).

Since the place of choice to access the collecting system is through a posterior calyx, much effort has been dispensed in an attempt to determine preoperatively which calices are anterior and which calices are posterior. Previous studies have presented contradictory results and have led to misunderstanding of this subject (Kaye and Reinke 1984). Since we described a kind of kidney collecting system, found in the majority of the endocasts, on which the calices are disposed in varied positions (superimposed or alternately distributed), we may affirm that the position of the calices cannot be defined as more lateral or more medial. Considering the large variation of the calices (more than 50% in varied positions), we believe that precise determination of calyceal position becomes difficult with the common radiological

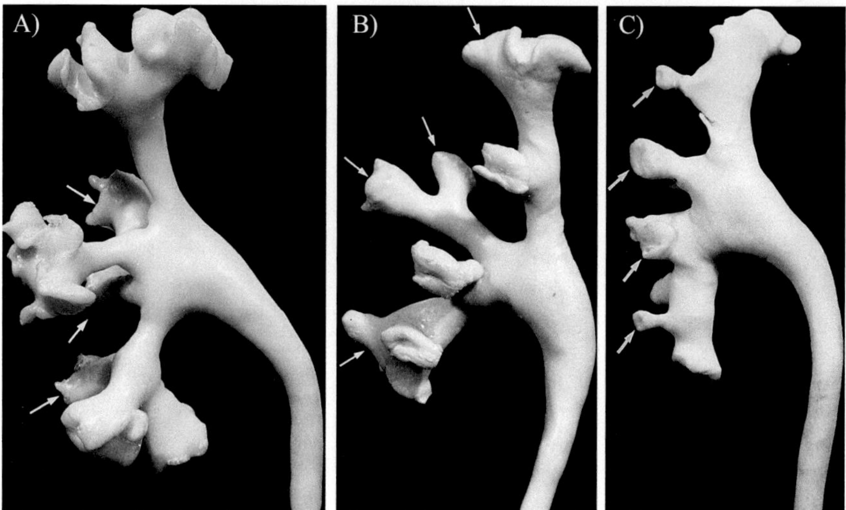

Fig. 2 Position of the calices related to lateral margin of the kidney. A) Anterior view of right pelviocalyceal cast. This cast reveals that the anterior calices have a more lateral (peripheral) position than posterior calices (arrows). It means that the posterior calices are placed medially. B) Anterior view of right pelviocalyceal cast. This cast reveals that the posterior calices (arrows) have a more lateral (peripheral) position than anterior calices. C) Anterior view of right pelviocalyceal cast. This cast reveals that the calices in the anterior plane (arrows) are placed alternately relative to the lateral margin of kidney. In one region they are more lateral and in another region they are more medial

methods, even using oblique and lateral views (Sampaio and Mandarim-de-Lacerda 1988a, 1988b). To solve this problem quickly and inexpensively, during endourological procedures, with the patient in the prone position, injection of room air into the collecting system will rise to the more posterior portions of the collecting system, determining which calices are placed posteriorly (radiolucent contrast) (Sampaio and Mandarim-de-Lacerda 1988a; Sampaio 1993a; Weyman 1986).

Position of the Calices Relative to the Polar Regions and to the Kidney Mid-zone. The superior pole was drained by a midline calyceal infundibulum in 98.6% of the cases (Fig. 3). The midzone (hilar) was drained by paired calices that were arranged in two rows (anterior and posterior) in 95.7% of the cases (Fig. 3). The inferior pole was drained by paired calices arranged in two rows in 81 casts (57.9%) (Fig. 3A) and by a single midline calyceal infundibulum in 59 casts (42.1%) (Fig. 3B).

Concerning the calyceal drainage of the kidney polar regions, many investigators affirmed that there usually is only one calyceal infundibulum draining each pole (Sampaio 2001, 2000; Kaye and Goldberg 1982). In our study the superior pole was drained by only one midline calyceal infundibulum in 98.6% of the cases. However, the inferior pole was drained by paired calices arranged in two rows in 81 of 140 cases (57.9%) and by one midline calyceal infundibulum in 59 cases (42.1%) (Fig. 3). These results are important to endourology; it will be easier to access endoscopically a polar region drained by a single infundibulum, which usually has suitable diameter,

Fig. 3 Position of calices related to the polar regions and kidney midzone. A) Lateral view of a left pelviocalyceal cast. The superior pole is drained by a single midline calyceal infundibulum (arrowhead). The midzone (hilar) is drained by paired calices arranged in two rows (short arrow); anterior and posterior. The inferior pole is drained by paired calices arranged in two rows (long arrow). B) Lateral view of a right pelviocalyceal cast. The superior pole is drained by a single midline calyceal infundibulum (arrowhead). The midzone is drained by paired calices arranged in two rows (short arrow); anterior and posterior. The inferior pole is drained by only one midline calyceal infundibulum (long arrow)

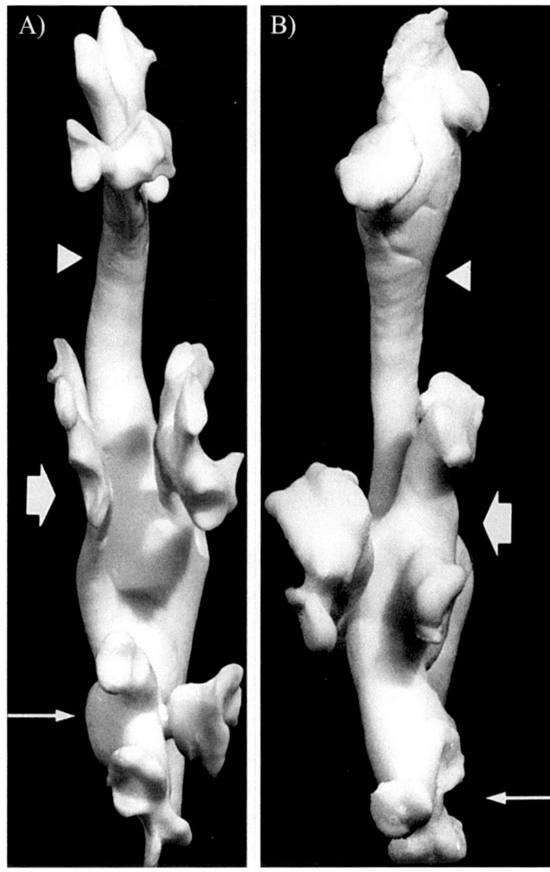

rather than a polar region drained by paired calices (Fig. 3). Because the inferior pole is drained by paired calices in 57.9% of the cases, one must keep in mind this anatomical detail, both to plan and perform the intrarenal access and the endoscopic procedures in the inferior pole. The calyceal drainage of superior and inferior poles is also of utmost importance in SWL and was fully discussed in previous papers (Sampaio and Aragao 1992; Sampaio 2000). Concerning the kidney midzone (hilar) drainage, our results show that this region is drained by paired calices arranged in two rows (anterior and posterior) in 95.7% of the cases (Fig. 3). These results should also be retained by endourologists to access and work in the mid-kidney.

2 Anatomic Relationships of Intrarenal Vessels (Arteries and Veins) with the Kidney Collecting System

2.1 I—Relevance for the Intrarenal Access by Puncture

Percutaneous procedures are relatively invasive and complications may occur. One of the most significant complications is vascular injury that occurs when the urologist is obtaining intrarenal access. This problem may have several cumbersome consequences, including intraoperative hemorrhage, hypotension, loss of functioning renal parenchyma, arteriovenous fistula, and pseudoaneurysm (Segura 1989; Clayman et al. 1984a; Lee et al. 1987; Sampaio et al. 1992; Sampaio 1993b).

The goal of this item is to offer an anatomical depiction of refined details concerning intrarenal vessels and their relationships to the collecting system, showing how to perform safe percutaneous intrarenal access by keeping as many renal vessels as possible intact during puncture.

2.2 Material Studied for the Anatomical Background

We analyzed 62 retrograde pyelograms and the corresponding three-dimensional polyester resin corrosion endocasts of the kidney collecting system together with the intrarenal arteries and veins, obtained from fresh cadavers.

The kidneys were punctured under fluoroscopic guidance and the endocasts obtained with the needles positioned in the place of puncture (Fig. 4). For comparative analysis, we studied kidneys that had been punctured through a calyceal infundibulum and kidneys punctured through a calyceal fornix.

2.3 Intrarenal Access Through an Infundibulum

Superior Pole. Puncture is most dangerous through the upper pole infundibulum because this region is surrounded almost completely by large vessels (Fig. 5). Infundibular arteries and veins course parallel to the anterior and posterior aspects of the upper pole infundibulum. In our series, injury to an interlobar (infundibular) vessel was a common consequence of puncturing the upper-pole infundibulum (67% of kidneys) (Fig. 6); the injured vessel was an artery in 26% of those cases.

The most serious vascular accident in upper infundibulum puncture is a lesion of the posterior segmental artery (retropelvic artery). This event may occur because this artery crossed and is related to the posterior surface of the upper infundibulum in 57% of the cases (Fig. 7A) (Sampaio and Aragao 1990a). Figure 7B and C show an upper infundibulum puncture in which the needle tract produced complete laceration of the posterior segmental artery. Because the posterior segmental artery (retropelvic artery)

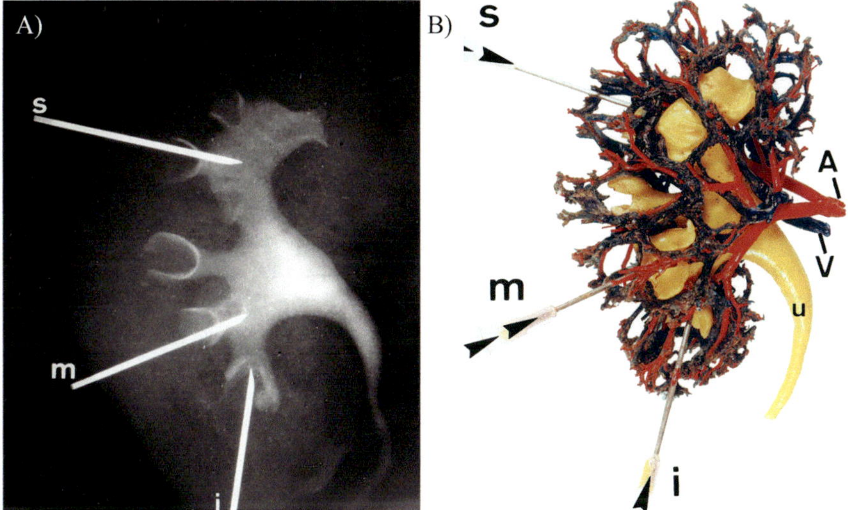

Fig. 4 A) Anterior view of a retrograde pyelogram from a right kidney shows superior pole (s), mid-kidney (m), and inferior pole (i) punctures. These punctures were performed after polyester resin injections into the arterial and venous systems, while the resins were still in the gel state. Note that the injected resins are not opaque to x-rays. B) Anterior view of the corresponding corrosion endocast obtained after contrast removal and pelviocalyceal system injection with resin. The needles are maintained in their original places. s = superior pole puncture; m = mid-kidney puncture; i = inferior pole puncture. The arrowheads point out the tracts of the needles. A = renal artery; V = renal vein; u = ureter

may supply up to 50% of the renal parenchyma, injury to it may result in significant loss of functioning renal tissue, in addition to causing hemorrhage (Sampaio et al. 1993).

Middle Kidney. Intrarenal access through the mid-kidney infundibulum produced arterial lesion in 23% of kidneys studied. The middle branch of the posterior segmental artery was injured more often than any other vessel.

Inferior Pole. The posterior aspect of the lower-pole infundibulum is widely presumed by endourologists and interventional radiologists to be free of arteries. It is considered, therefore, to be a safe region through which to gain access to the collecting system and to place a nephrostomy tube. In about 38% of the kidneys examined, however, an infundibular artery is found in this region (Sampaio and Aragao 1990a). Thus, significant complications may develop as a consequence of a posterior approach through the supposedly vessel-free lower infundibulum (Clayman et al. 1984a; Sampaio 1993b, 1994). In fact, we found an arterial injury in 13% of kidneys in which we had made a puncture through the lower pole infundibulum.

Concerning the veins, in many kidneys that we studied, we found large venous anastomoses—similar to collars—around the calyceal infundibula (the so-called calyceal necks) (Sampaio and Aragao 1990b). Puncture through the lower pole infundibulum therefore also risks injury to a venous arcade. A venous lesion usually

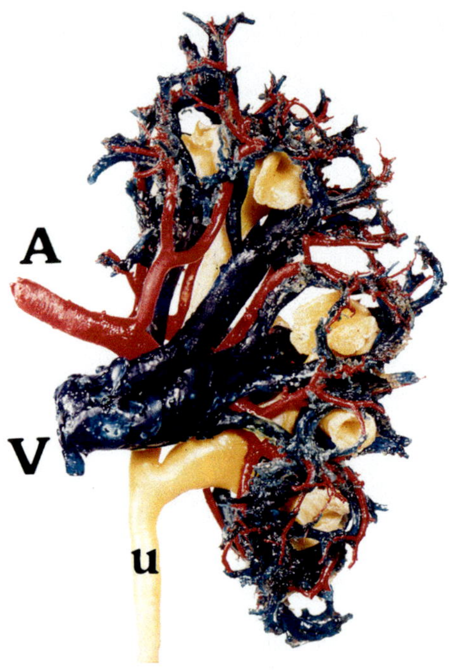

Fig. 5 Oblique medial view of an endocast of arterial (A), venous (V), and pelviocalyceal systems from a left kidney reveals the upper infundibulum almost completely encircled by infundibular arteries and veins. This anatomic arrangement makes the upper pole infundibular puncture especially dangerous. u = ureter

heals spontaneously, but consequent hemorrhage may be cumbersome during the procedure.

Our findings clearly demonstrate that percutaneous nephrostomy through an infundibulum of a calyx is not a safe route, because this type of access poses an important risk of significant bleeding from interlobar (infundibular) vessels.

Infundibular puncture also creates the hazard of through-and-through (two-wall) puncture of the collecting system (Fig. 6). Because major segmental branches of the renal artery, as well as major tributaries of the renal vein, are positioned on the anterior surface of the renal pelvis, marked hemorrhage may occur as a result of an anterior through-and-through perforation. In addition, effective tamponade of anterior vessels that have been injured is difficult because they lie distantly in the nephrostomy tract (Sampaio et al. 1992; Sampaio 1994; Clayman et al. 1984b).

Although the infundibular access is feasible in some circumstances and must be considered in specific situations (some difficult anatomical cases for example), the surgeon must evaluate the risk of an arterial lesion, primarily in the superior pole and in the mid-kidney (Sampaio et al. 1992).

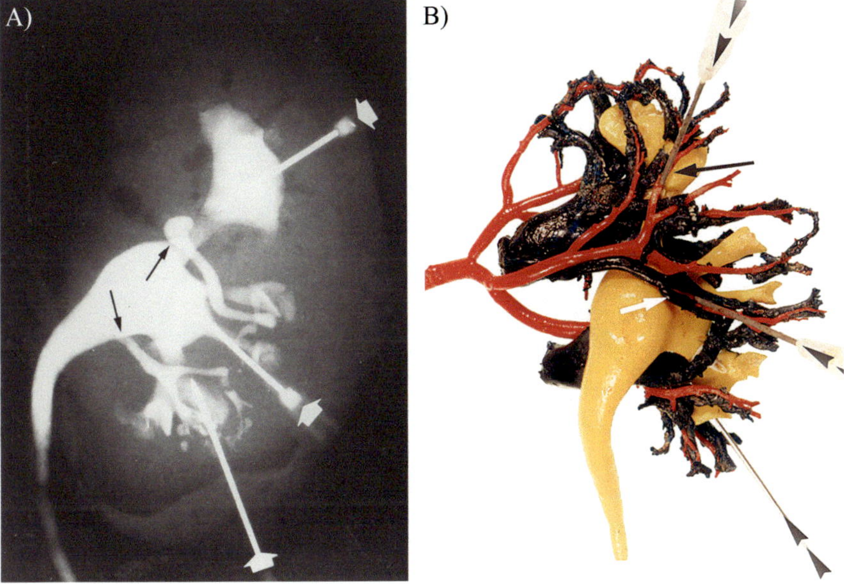

Fig. 6   A) Posterior view of a retrograde pyelogram from a right kidney reveals superior, middle, and inferior punctures (short arrows) and the contrast material in the superior and inferior infundibular arteries (black arrows). B) Posterior view of the corresponding endocast reveals injury to an upper infundibular artery (black arrow). The mid-kidney puncture (white arrow) was a through-and-through (two walls) puncture and injured an anterior segmental artery. The injured vessel furnished the postero-inferior branch filled with contrast on the pyelogram. The arrowheads point out the tracts of the needles

2.4   *Intrarenal Access Through the Renal Pelvis*

Direct puncture of the renal pelvis for endourologic surgery should be excluded. Besides the fact that the nephrostomy tube inserted at this site is easily dislodged and difficult to reintroduce during the operative maneuvers, renal pelvis puncture has a prohibitive and unnecessary risk of injuring a retropelvic vessel (artery and/or vein) (Clayman et al. 1984a; Sampaio and Aragao 1990a, b).

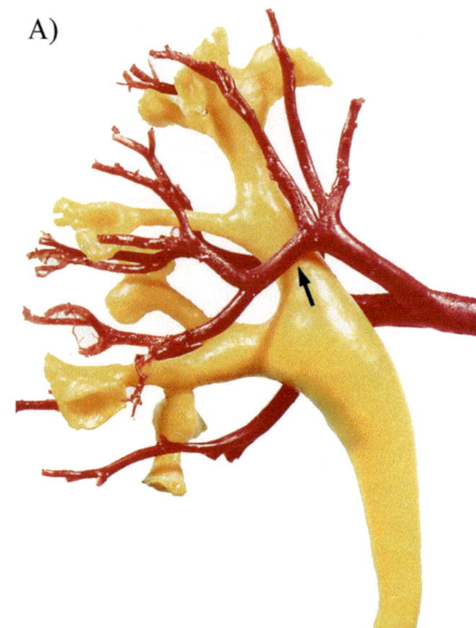
A)

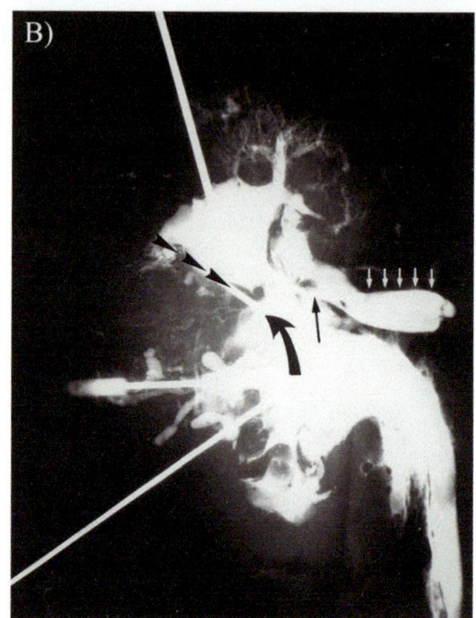
B)

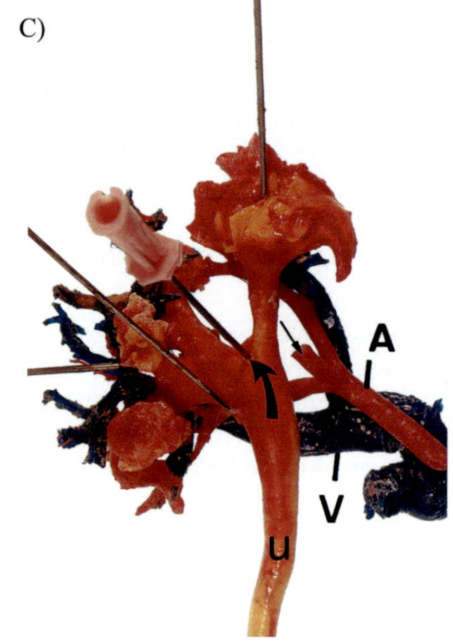
C)
A
V
u

◄**Fig. 7** (**A**) Posterior view of endocast (pelviocalyceal system and arteries) from a left kidney shows the posterior segmental artery (retropelvic artery) describing an arc and contacting the upper infundibulum (arrow). (**B**) Posterior view of a retrograde pyelogram from a left kidney shows contrast medium extravasation and contrast material in the arterial system and in the main trunk of the renal artery (short arrows). The retropelvic artery was injured by the needle pointed by the arrowheads. The curved arrow shows the lesion site. Straight arrow points the retropelvic artery filled with contrast medium extravasated from the collecting system. (**C**) Posterior view of the corresponding endocast reveals the retropelvic artery divided (straight arrow) and the needle responsible for the lesion (pink needle). The curved-arrow reveals the lesion site. A = renal artery; V = renal vein; u = ureter

2.5   *Intrarenal Access Through a Calyceal Fornix*

When we made a puncture through a fornix of a calyx, venous injury occurred in fewer than 8% of the kidneys. These injuries occurred indiscriminately, in the upper pole, mid-kidney and lower pole calices. We did not detect any arterial lesions as a consequence of a forniceal puncture (Sampaio et al. 1992).

In conclusion, the high rate of vascular injury and the possibility of associated complications mean that a nephrostomy tube should not be placed through an infundibulum of a calyx (Fig. 5). On the other hand, and regardless of the region of the kidney, puncture and placement of a nephrostomy tube through a fornix of a calyx is safe and must be the site chosen by the operator. Even in the superior pole, the intrarenal puncture through a calyceal fornix is harmless (Fig. 8A). In addition, when puncturing through a fornix of a calyx, in case of lesion, the injury was always to a periphery vessel, such as a small venous arcade (Figs. 8B).

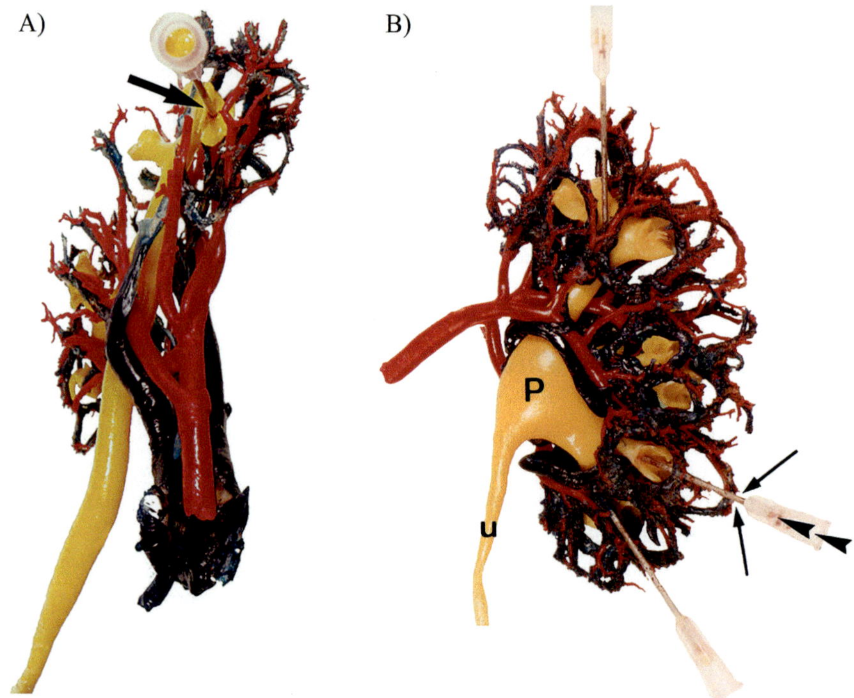

Fig. 8 (**A**) Superior view of an endocast from a left kidney shows that, even in the superior pole, a puncture through the fornix of a calyx (arrow) is safe. (**B**) Posterior view of an endocast from a right kidney and an inferior puncture performed through a fornix of a calyx. The arrows show a lesion to a small peripheric venous arcade. The arrowheads demonstrate the needle tract. P = renal pelvis; u = ureter

References

Clayman RV, Surya V, Hunter D, Castañeda-Zúñiga WR, Miller R, Coleman C, Amplatz K, Lange P. Renal vascular complications associated with the percutaneous removal of renal calculi. J Urol. 1984a;132:228–30.

Clayman RV, Hunter D, Surya V, Castañeda-Zúñiga WR, Amplatz K, Lange P. Percutaneous intrarenal electrosurgery. J Urol. 1984b;131:864–7.

Kaye KW, Goldberg ME. Applied anatomy of the kidney and ureter. Urol Clin N Amer. 1982;9:3–13.

Kaye KW, Reinke DB. Detailed caliceal anatomy for endourology. J Urol. 1984;132:1085–8.

Lee WJ, Smith AD, Cubelli V, Badlani GH, Lewin B, Vernace F, Cantos E. Complications of percutaneous nephro lithotomy. AJR. 1987;148:177–80.

Sampaio FJ. How to place a nephrostomy, safely. Contemp Urol. 1994;6:41–6.

Sampaio FJ. Renal anatomy: endourologic considerations. Urol Clin North Am. 2000;27:585–607.

Sampaio FJ. Renal collecting system anatomy: its possible role in the effectiveness of renal stone treatment. Curr Opin Urol. 2001;11:359–66.

Sampaio FJ, Aragao AH. Anatomical relationship between the intrarenal arteries and the kidney collecting system. J Urol. 1990a;143:679–81.

Sampaio FJ, Aragao AH. Anatomical relationship between the renal venous arrangement and the kidney collecting system. J Urol. 1990b;144:1089–93.

Sampaio FJ, Mandarim-de-Lacerda CA. 3-Dimensional and radiological pelviocalyceal anatomy for endourology. J Urol. 1988a;140:1352–5.

Sampaio FJ, Mandarim-de-Lacerda CA. Anatomic classification of the kidney collecting system for endourologic procedures. J Endourol. 1988b;2:247–51.

Sampaio FJ, Zanier JF, Aragao AH, Favorito LA. Intrarenal access: 3-dimensional anatomical study. J Urol. 1992;148:1769–73.

Sampaio FJ, Schiavini JL, Favorito LA. Proportional analysis of the kidney arterial segments. Urol Res. 1993;21:371–4.

Sampaio FJ. Basic Anatomic Features of the Kidney Collecting System. Three-dimensional and Radiologic Study. In Sampaio FJB, Uflacker R editors. Renal anatomy applied to urology, endourology, and interventional radiology. New York: Thieme Medical Publishers; 1993a. p. 7–15.

Sampaio FJ. Intrarenal access by puncture. Three-dimensional study. In Sampaio FJB, Uflacker R editors. Renal Anatomy Applied to Urology, Endourology, and Interventional Radiology. New York: Thieme Medical Publishers; 1993b. p. 68–76.

Sampaio FJ. Surgical Anatomy of the Kidney. In Smith's textbook of endourology, 2nd edition, chapter 12. Hamilton: BC Deker Inc.; 2007. p. 79–99.

Sampaio FJ, Aragao AH. Inferior pole collecting system anatomy. Its probable role in extracorporeal shock wave lithotripsy. J Urol. 1992;147:322–4.

Segura JW. The role of percutaneous surgery in renal and ureteral stone removal. J Urol, Part. 1989;2(141):780–1.

Weyman PJ. Air as a contrast agent during percutaneous nephrostomy. J Endourol. 1986;1:16–7.

Positioning in Percutaneous Renal Surgery

Jorge Gutierrez-Aceves, Louisa Ho, Silvia Proietti, Matheus Pupulin, Salvatore Di Pietro, and Guido Giusti

Abstract The most important aspect when planning a percutaneous access to treat kidney stones is the selection of the access site to the kidney. Since it was first described, PCNL was traditionally done with the patient in prone, with good success, few complications, and few limitations. As PCNL become more widely used, surgeons have developed alternate patient positions for PCNL, mainly the supine and supine-modified positions. Overall, both approaches have a number of advantages and drawbacks, but are both feasible and acceptable alternatives to access the kidney during percutaneous renal surgery with similar outcomes and rate of complications.

Keywords Percutaneous · Nephrolithotomy · Positioning · Prone · Supine · Urolithiasis · Endourology

1 Prone Position

Jorge Gutierrez-Aceves and Louisa Ho

The most important aspect when planning a percutaneous access to treat kidney stones with percutaneous nephrolithotomy (PCNL) is the selection of the access site to the kidney. Planning the access requires careful evaluation of the pre-operative CT scan in the three different planes, axial, coronal and sagittal, and the most important factors for the site selection are stone location and stone burden. Despite the widespread use of flexible nephroscopy, via either antegrade or retrograde approach, the access site should be selected to maximize access to the stone and stone removal via a rigid nephroscope.

J. Gutierrez-Aceves · L. Ho
Department of Urology, Glickman Urologic and Kidney Institute, Cleveland Clinic Foundation, Cleveland, OH, United States

S. Proietti · M. Pupulin · S. Di Pietro · G. Giusti (✉)
Department of Urology, San Raffaele Hospital, Milan, Italy
e-mail: drguidogiusti@gmail.com

© The Author(s), under exclusive license to Springer Nature Switzerland AG 2023   83
J. D. Denstedt and E. N. Liatsikos (eds.), *Percutaneous Renal Surgery*,
https://doi.org/10.1007/978-3-031-40542-6_6

The urologist should feel comfortable that the positioning of the patient will allow them to perform a lower, mid, or upper pole access, depending on the stone location and the patient anatomy. The position selected should not be a limitation to access any one of the renal calyceal groups.

2 Evolution of Patient Positioning

Several different patient positions have been described for obtaining percutaneous renal access. The classic prone position (Segura et al. 1985; Jones et al. 1990) that was described when PCNL was first introduced has been modified to a prone flex position (Ray et al. 2009), prone position with open split-legs (Grasso et al. 1993; Scarpa et al. 1997), and lateral flank decubitus (Karami et al. 2009). The supine position was initially described by Valdivia Uria in Zaragoza, Spain (Valdivia Uría et al. 1998), later modified to a lateral supine position by Gaspar Ibarluzea in Galdakao, Spain (Ibarluzea et al. 2007), and has since been further adapted with other minor modifications from several other authors (Sio et al. 2008; Papatsoris et al. 2008). Despite the increasing popularity of supine PCNL, prone is still the most commonly utilized position for performing percutaneous renal surgery worldwide. In the Global PCNL study from the Clinical Research Office of the Endourology Society CROES with 5803 patients worldwide, prone position was utilized in 80.3% (4637 patients) (Valdivia et al. 2011).

In the classic prone position (Fig. 1), the patient is placed in a prone decubitus position with both arms raised and slightly flexed at the elbows, with careful attention to prevent brachial plexus injury. The thorax is elevated to facilitate ventilation, and the superior abdomen is elevated to bring the kidney closer to the site of puncture and to decrease the movement of the kidney during ventilation. We typically use two rolls positioned in a horizontal manner with an elevation height of 15–20 cm depending on the weight of the patient. The first roll is positioned at the upper part of thorax, and a similar roll is placed just below the thoracic cage. The head is placed on a foam support to maintaining neck alignment while maintaining access to respiratory tubes, and all pressure points (knees, feet, forehead, eyes, elbows, fingers) are appropriately padded. Alternatively, the bolster may be positioned in a vertical manner extending from the shoulder to hip on each flank.

In the prone split-leg position, the patient's legs are appropriately padded and secured, and abducted at the hips without being flexed. The genitalia are positioned at the bottom of the operating table, providing room for retrograde access.

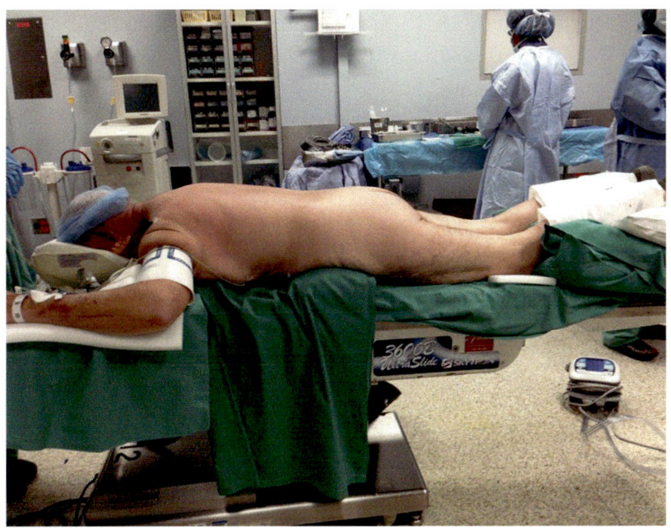

Fig. 1 Classic prone position for PCNL

3 Advantages and Drawbacks of Prone Position

3.1 Advantages

Easier access to all calyces

The main advantage of the prone position is that it completely exposes the lumbar area, providing a wide window to obtain access and space to maneuver the nephroscope and lithotripters. The access site is bordered by the 11th or 12th rib in the superiorly, the ileal crest inferiorly, the paravertebral medially, and the colon the laterally. These anatomical landmarks may vary from patient to patient, and adequate planning with the use of preoperative CT is necessary.

This broader surface area for an anatomical posterior puncture provides an easier access to posterior calyces. This broad window also facilitates access to all calyces, including upper pole and multiple calyceal access. In addition, the prone position allows for single-session bilateral PCNL in suitable cases without need for patient repositioning.

Shorter tract length

Prone position allows for a shorter tract length, which is a big advantage when treating obese patients, and facilitates a wider area for manipulation of instruments. Yazici et al. evaluated the renal anatomy with low-dose CT scan in a supine, prone, and 30° prone-flex position, and they reported that the mean tract lengths and the subcutaneous fat tissue lengths in the lower, middle, and upper poles of kidney were significantly longer in the supine position. The access field is also shorter and more limited in the supine (80.8–13.3 mm) compared to prone (86.3–15.0 mm) and prone-flex (86.7–18.4 mm) positions (p < 0.001) (Yazici et al. 2014).

3.2 Drawbacks

Need for patient repositioning

The classic prone position is a two-stage procedure. In the first part, patient is in the supine position for anesthesia induction and for obtaining retrograde access to the urinary tract with the placement of an externalized ureteral stent through cystoscopy. The patient is repositioned prone for the main part of the procedure.

A disadvantage of the classic prone position is a longer surgical time due to the need to reposition the patient. To this point, standardization of the patient repositioning is the most important factor for reducing surgical time. In our practice, once the patient is induced, we perform flexible cystoscopy and placement of an externalized ureteral stent with the patient supine on the stretcher. Alternatively, the flexible cystoscopy can be performed once the patient has been flipped to prone position, especially in a female patient. With either method, only one move is required, from supine on the stretcher, to prone on the surgical bed.

Limited endoscopic combined intrarenal surgery

Performing combined simultaneous flexible ureteroscopy and percutaneous nephrolithotomy is challenging in the classic prone position. However, this limitation is reduced with the use of a surgical bed that allows for a split-leg position. Several authors have reported routine endoscopic guided percutaneous access in the prone split-leg position with comparable outcomes to supine access. Battagelo et al., conducted a multicenter study comparing outcomes between endoscopic-guided prone split-leg PCNL and supine PCNL, and found no difference in rate of complications between groups. However, the endoscopic-guided prone split-leg PCNL group had a reduced operative time, radiation exposure, length of stay, and need for secondary procedures (Batagello et al. 2019).

Anesthetic challenges

Risk for ventilatory compromise and less airway control is frequently cited as a disadvantage of the prone position. Theoretically, it is more difficult for the anesthetist to manage any cardio-respiratory emergencies (Edgcombe et al. 2008). However, there is no evidence of increased anesthetic complications during prone PCNL. Moreover, recent studies have shown that prone positioning leads to more homogenous lung inflation and homogeneous distribution of alveolar ventilation, resulting in improved oxygenation and increased end-expiratory lung volume (Gattinoni and Caironi 2010). Similar effects were reported in awake patients with acute hypoxemic respiratory failure because of COVID-19 during spontaneous and assisted breathing, more than 20% improvement of oxygen pressure (pao_2) was documented with pronation of the patients (Telias et al. 2020), with a decrease in the pressure of carbon dioxide in arterial blood (paCo$_2$). In summary, general anesthesia in the prone position provides homogenous ventilation resulting in improved oxygenation and higher elimination of carbon dioxide (Tsaturyan et al. 2022).

Prone position in our opinion is not a contraindication for the treatment of the majority of obese patients. Overall, positioning and treating obese patients is a challenge with any of the potential positioning options. In patients who are considered severely morbidly obese, the only possible treatment option may be staged ureteroscopy. With respect to the prone position, the main determinant of whether it is safe to proceed with surgery once the patient has been placed in the prone position is adequate ventilation. It is of primary importance to have a good communication with the Anesthesiology team. We routinely evaluate with the Anesthesiology team the ventilation status, and decide to continue with the procedure if the patient is not having any ventilatory problems for the first 5 min after the patient has been placed in prone (Fig. 2A and B). The broader surface area providing an easy access to posterior calyces and the shorter length of the access tract are an even greater advantage of the prone position in obese patients (Yazici et al. 2014; Batagello et al. 2019).

4   Impact of Patient Position on Outcomes for PCNL

Overall, both prone and supine positioning, with or without various modifications, are feasible and acceptable alternatives to access the kidney during percutaneous renal surgery with similar outcomes and rate of complications.

The outcomes of supine and prone PCNL have been evaluated in a large number of retrospective and prospective randomized studies. The CROES report based on a global database in 5803 patients found that surgical time was significantly less in favor of prone position (82.7 versus 90.1 min), SFR was significantly better in favor of prone position (77.0% versus 70.2%), but the prone position presented a higher incidence of bleeding (6.1% versus 4.3%) and fever (11.1% versus 7.6%) (Valdivia et al. 2011). In a subsequent study from the same CROES database, Astroza et al., reported on outcomes of supine and prone position in PCNL for staghorn calculi. In this study, a total of 1079 PCNLs were performed in prone, and 232 PCNLs in supine, they found that a higher percentage of patients in the prone position had access through the upper pole (12.6% versus 3.6%). Surgical time was shorter (123 versus 103 min), stone free rate (SFR) was higher (59.2% versus 48.4%) and retreatment rate was lower (29.5% versus 36.1%) for patients in the prone position. There were no differences in complication rates (Astroza et al. 2013).

A multicenter retrospective study from a Europe based cooperation group evaluated outcomes in lower pole stones treated with prone versus supine PCNL. No differences were observed in terms of 1- and 3-month SFR (90.4% versus 87.7% and 92.3% versus 89.2%) and complication rates (7.6% versus 7.7%) when comparing prone versus supine PCNL, respectively (Sanguedolce et al. 2013).

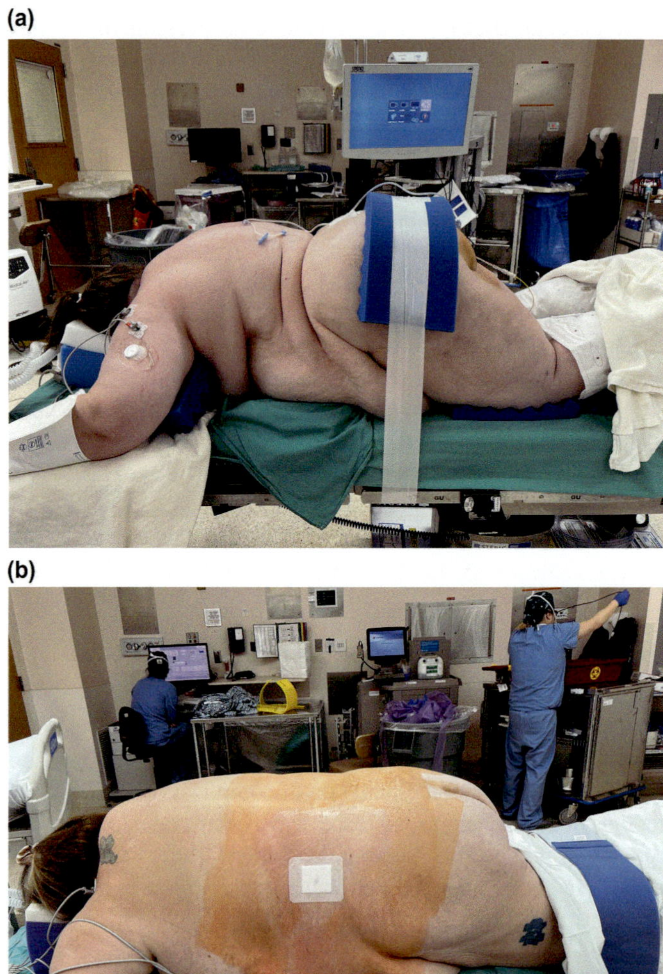

Fig. 2 Obese patient in prone position for PCNL, before (A) and after (B) treatment

Two recent meta-analyses have reported that SFR was higher in prone position compared to supine. Yun et al., reviewed 13 studies: 6 randomized, 7 retrospective studies with 6881 patients, prone position was associated with a higher rate of stone clearance (77.7% versus 74.3%), shorter mean operative time was observed in the supine groups (weighted mean difference [WMD]: -18.27; 95% CI: -35.77, -0.77; $p = 0.04$), with a lower incidence of blood transfusions in the supine group, and no difference was observed between the positions with regard to length of stay (LOS)

(Yuan et al. 2016). Zhang et al., reported on 6431 patients (4956 prone, 1457 supine), a shorter operative time (WMD 21.7) but lower SFR for supine (OR: 1.36) for supine, and no difference in LOS (WMD 0.05) or complication rate (OR: 1.1) (Zhang et al. 2014). Another recent meta-analysis by Li et al. which included 15 RCTs with 1474 patients showed no statistical difference in SFR, length of stay, or complication rate, although supine position had a shorter operative time (WMD -12.02) and lower rate of fever (RR 0.67) (Li et al. 2019).

Several prospective trials further support the findings from the retrospective studies reported above. Wang et al., presented a prospective randomized trial in 102 patients comparing prone versus modified supine position, they found that the rate of second PCNL was significantly higher (6 versus 0 patients) and the stone clearance rate (73.3% versus 88.7%) was significantly lower in the modified supine than in the prone position group. Mean operative time was significantly lower in the prone compared to the modified supine position group (78 versus 88 min). There were no significant differences in rates of rib and calyx puncture, numbers of punctures, estimated blood loss (EBL), and mean length of stay between the two groups (Wang et al. 2013). Most recently, Perrella et al., completed a multicenter randomized controlled trial in complex renal stones, and concluded that positioning during PCNL did not impact the success rates, however prone had a longer operative time (147.6 versus 117.9 min), and a higher rate of Clavien-Dindo $\geq$ III complications (14.3% versus 3.6%) (Perrella et al. 2022).

Results are similar when comparing miniaturized PCNL in the prone versus supine position. Zhan et al., completed a prospective trial and reported that SFR (90.1 versus 87.5%), EBL, number of access tracts, LOS (6 $\pm$ 1.1 versus 6 $\pm$ 1.5 days) and complications were similar. However, the operative time was significantly shortened in supine lithotomy position (56 $\pm$ 15 versus 86 $\pm$ 23 min) (Zhan et al. 2013).

5 Conclusion

In summary, prone position is still the most frequently utilized position globally to perform percutaneous renal surgery. There are very few limitations for using prone position during PCNL. Most contemporary series report a higher SFR in prone position compared to supine or supine modified position, with some studies reporting no statistical difference. All reports present comparable complications rate, and no significant difference in length of stay between the two approaches has been demonstrated, although the prone position was associated with an increase in the operative time. Ultimately, the decision of the patient position and surgical approach depends on preferences of the surgeon and the surgical team.

6 Supine Position

Silvia Proietti, Matheus Pupulin, Salvatore Di Pietro, Guido Giusti

Percutaneous nephrolithotomy (PCNL) was first described by Fernstrom and Johannson in 1976 in prone position (Fernström and Johansson 1976). Since then, this procedure has become the gold standard for treatment of large stones and it has improved over time resulting in decrease in invasiveness and morbidity with improvements in terms of results and ergonomics. Originally, PCNL was performed in the prone position due to concerns that other positions increased risk of inadvertent colon injury during percutaneous puncture of the kidney. Undoubtedly, at that time, the unavailability of both computed tomography (CT) scan or ultrasonography made the identification of interposed organs between the skin and the kidney impossible, thus largely justifying this intuitive approach.

Although the prone position was traditionally used to perform PCNL, anaesthetic concerns, especially in the morbidly obese or other high-risk patients and the need to reposition the patient during the procedure, were the reasons that initially induced urologists to consider alternative positions.

In 1987, Valdivia Uria introduced for the first time PCNL in the supine decubitus position using pre-operative CT scans for patient evaluation; he demonstrated similar outcomes and complications for PCNL performed in the supine position compared to the prone decubitus, with potential benefits in terms of ergonomics and the administration of anesthesia (Valdivia Uría et al. 1987; Valdivia 1990). In addition,

Hopper et al. back in 1987 demonstrated in an elegant study, performed with CT scan, that the colon becomes retrorenal in 1.8% and 10% of cases in supine and prone position respectively (Hopper et al. 1987), therefore definitely fading the idea of higher risk of puncturing the colon in supine than in prone.

Even though prone position remains the dominant position for PCNL, the use of supine PCNL is increasing—20% of all PCNLs entered into the Global PCNL study of the Clinical Research Office of the Endourological Society were performed in the supine position (Falahatkar et al. 2008). Herein we report different approaches to percutaneous renal access in the supine position, with a focus on variations in patient positioning.

7 Evolution of Patient Positioning

The original description of supine PCNL by Valdivia included the placement of a 3-L saline back under the patient's flank to improve exposure to the area where the percutaneous puncture is performed (Valdivia Uría et al. 1987). The patient is completely stretched out with extension of the ipsilateral leg. The ipsilateral arm is positioned across the thorax and soft pads are applied to pressure points (Fig. 3).

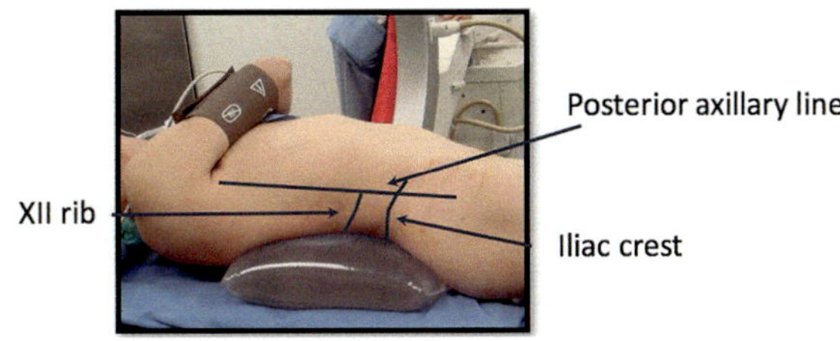

Fig. 3 Valdivia supine position

Since the supine position was initially introduced by Valdivia Uría et al. (1987), variations in the supine positions have been provided over time.

The most commonly used position is the Galdakao-modified Valdivia position (Ibarluzea et al. 2007) which is an evolution of the Valdivia's supine position, described by Ibarluzea et al. The supine Valdivia position is the same, the patient lies supine with a 3-L saline bag under the flank or by two separate jelly pillows placed under the thorax and the hip, but the patient's legs are placed in a modified lithotomy position with both legs in stirrups, the leg of the PCNL side is lengthened, while the contralateral one is abducted, in order to facilitate simultaneous percutaneous antegrade access and ureteroscopic and also retrograde transurethral access to the urinary system (Fig. 4).

Benefits from the Galdakao-modified Valdivia position include greater versatility upper urinary tract manipulation, given the increasing use of combined retrograde and percutaneous access to the urinary tract with both rigid and flexible instruments.

The Barts-modified Valdivia position provides a large surface area for percutaneous access with easy manipulation of the nephroscope, as the body is placed at 90° to the operating table (Papatsoris et al. 2008). The patient is positioned in the lithotomy position with the ipsilateral hemi-pelvis tilted by 45°. The ipsilateral lower limb is slightly flexed in a ventral direction and follows the lateral rotation of the trunk, while the contralateral lower limb remains fully abducted.

However, this position appears not ergonomic enough as such it cannot be used for every patient as it implies excessive flexibility of the spine. In addition, this position can generate some technical difficulties because of the overlap of the collecting system on the spine. For this reason, the Barts flank-free-modified supine position was introduced with good exposure of the flank but with less rotation of the trunk, with only 15° tilt of the ipsilateral flank (Bach et al. 2019).

Recently, another modification of the Galdakao-Valdivia position has been proposed, the Giusti's position, in order to overcome potential limitations in terms of nephroscope maneuverability resulting from the possible conflict between the nephroscope and the stirrup support (Proietti et al. 2019), especially when trying to reach the upper pole from a lower pole access. The patient is placed at the lateral edge of the table and the flank is elevated with a small bolster to obtain a mild rotation with an angle not exceeding 15°. The ipsilateral arm is placed lying over the thorax avoiding any stretch of the brachial plexus in order to allow for cephalad free tilting of C-arm during puncture. The leg of PCNL side is left straight on half of the operating bed without the stirrup and the contralateral leg is placed on a stirrup, so

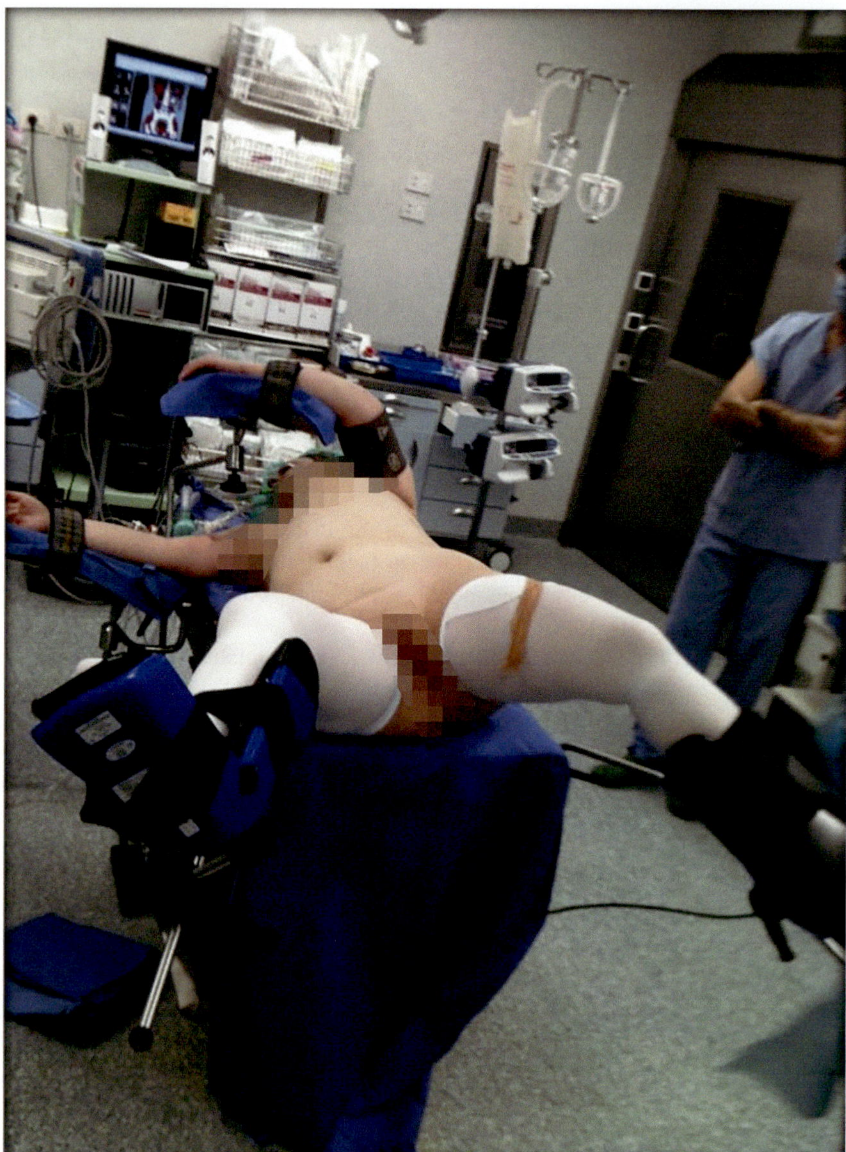

Fig. 4 Galdakao-modified Valdivia supine position

there is enough room for a second surgeon to perform retrograde manipulation of the upper urinary tract (Fig. 5).

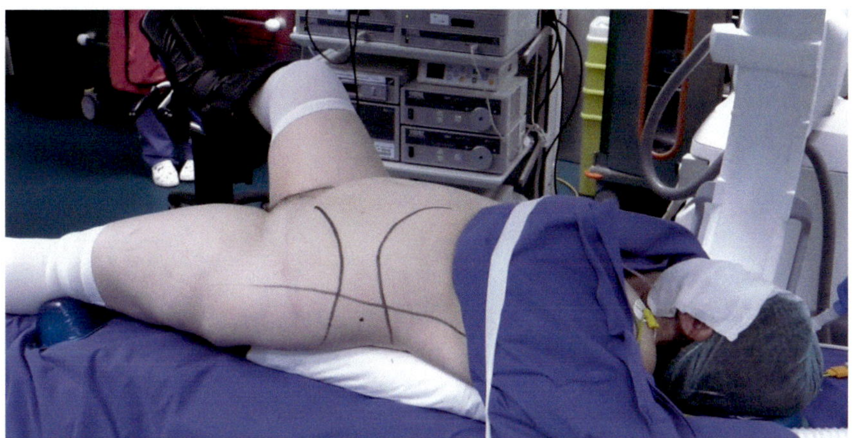

Fig. 5 Giusti's supine position

8   Benefits and Drawbacks of Supine Position

8.1   Benefits

Anesthesiologist advantages

Supine position for PCNL certainly offers some advantages over prone PCNL in terms of anesthesiologist management including the following: easier access to the patient for cardiovascular and pulmonary management, less risk of damage of central and peripheral nervous system (e.g. vascular, peripheral nerve and cervical spine injuries, tracheal compression and ocular damage) and better ventilator-associated parameters for obese patients (Manohar et al. 2007; Khoshrang et al. 2012). In addition, fluid absorption is also decreased in the supine position (Baard et al. 2014); this is of the utmost importance in patients with compromised cardiovascular status (Atkinson et al. 2011) as well as those at risk for systemic infection due to struvite or non-struvite stones colonized with bacteria.

Moreover, specific to issues with patient ventilation, the need to reposition the patients from the supine position to the prone position after intubation in patients undergoing prone PCNL increases the risk of single-lung ventilation because of the endotracheal tube displacement while the patient is rotated. Supine PCNL wipes out the risk of this pulmonary complication. Moreover, there is no need for extra anaesthesiologic armamentarium such as reinforced endotracheal tubes, stabilizing helmet, specialized paddings which may add additional cost to the procedure (Cracco and Scoffone 2011; Mazzucchi et al. 2012).

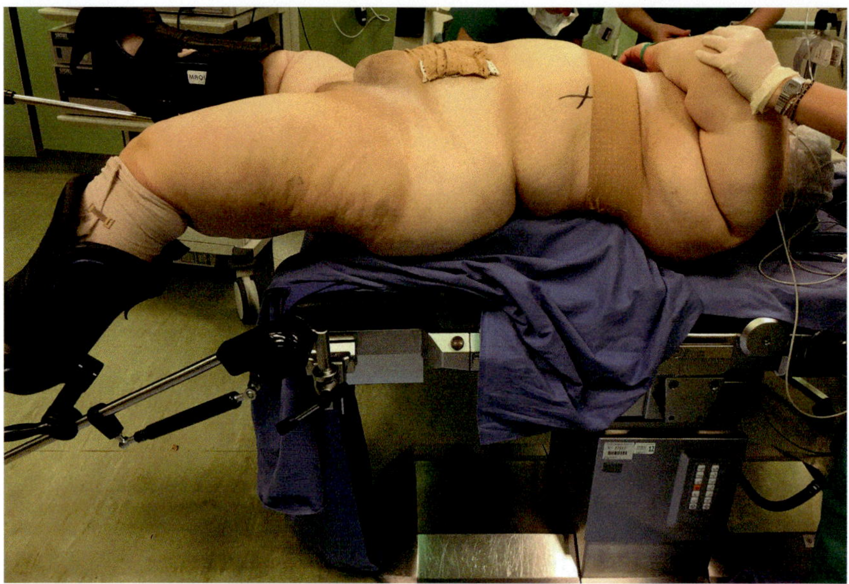

Fig. 6 Obese patient positioned for performing supine PCNL

Improvements in patient positioning and shorter operative time

Unquestionably, supine positioning is more ergonomic compared to prone decubitus with less labor for OR personnel and this advantage is even more evident in obese patients (De Sio et al. 2008) (Fig. 6). For supine PCNL a single draping and position is used throughout the entire procedure. The lack of this step of patients' repositioning result in a shorter overall operative time for supine PCNL compared with prone PCNL which has been demonstrated in several studies (Liu et al. 2010; Perrella et al. 2022; Scoffone et al. 2008).

Lower radiation exposure and improved ergonomics of fluoroscopy

Radiological exposure to the surgeon is decreased during supine PCNL because the surgeons' hands are not directly under the X-ray beam. Contrary, in prone PCNL, the surgeon's hands are inside the radiation field in particular when performing standard prone access techniques. Nevertheless, no comparison data have been published yet. Another advantage of supine position, is that due to the more lateral skin position for renal puncture in the supine position, there is typically the c-arm can be moved freely to evaluate the entire kidney during surgery without the risk displacing the nephroscope, which may happen more frequently in the prone position.

Easier endoscopic combined intrarenal surgery (ECIRS) or simultaneous bilateral endoscopic surgery (SBES)

The traditional Valdivia-Galdakao or in modified Valdivia position, can facilitate simultaneous manipulation antegrade and retrograde transurethral approaches to complex stone disease. Endoscopic Combined Intrarenal Surgery (ECIRS) was popularized by Scoffone in order to maintain high stone free rates of PCNL while decreasing the need for additional punctures to render patients stone free (Scoffone et al. 2008). ECIRS was also previously reported by Grasso et al. back in 1993 in prone position (Grasso et al. 1993), but, the lack of ergonomics of prone decubitus prevented the dissemination of this technique.

Single-session bilateral PCNL has been shown to be safe and feasible in the supine position. While one may argue that in the case of single-session bilateral PCNL the advantage of supine position (over prone position) in terms of operative time is outweighed by the necessity of changing position and draping between one side and the other, while in prone there is no need for that (Proietti et al. 2017). However, Proietti et al. showed that the total operative time (120 ± 45.4 min) for single-session bilateral PCNL was comparable to those reported in the literature for prone BPCNL (Giusti et al. 2018).

Recent publications have described the newest frontier in percutaneous stone surgery—simultaneous bilateral endoscopic surgery (SBES) combining supine PCNL and flexible ureteroscopy (fURS) in tandem fashion at the same time—that is, one surgeon performs supine PCNL while simultaneously another surgeon performs a contralateral fURS (Proietti et al. 2022). This technique was recently shown to be safe and feasible in a large prospective study and has advantages of reducing operative and anesthetic times in patients with bilateral urinary stone disease (Sofer et al. 2016).

Easier endoscopic access to the upper pole from lower pole puncture tract

Another aspect of PCNL that favors the supine position is that upper calyx endoscopic approachability through the lower calyx puncture tract is significantly higher in supine than in prone PCNL. Sofer et al. demonstrated that it is feasible to reach the upper calyx from the lower calyx puncture in 80% of cases for supine PCNL compared with only 20% of cases of prone PCNL (Altschuler et al. 2019) (Fig. 6). This may be justified by a thinner body wall, a thinner muscular layer, a lower muscle-to-fat thickness ratio and a wider angle between the lower and upper calyx axes afforded by the supine position. This is an important advantage of supine PCNL—access to the lower pole, renal pelvis, and upper pole can more effectively be accomplished through a lower pole puncture tract, which may, in turn decrease the need for upper calyx puncture and reduce the risks of thoracic complications associated with upper pole puncture in the prone position (Duty et al. 2012).

8.2 Drawbacks

Hypermobility of the kidney

One the most important drawbacks of supine position is the mobility of the kidney that is generally greater in the supine position than the prone position (Fig. 7).

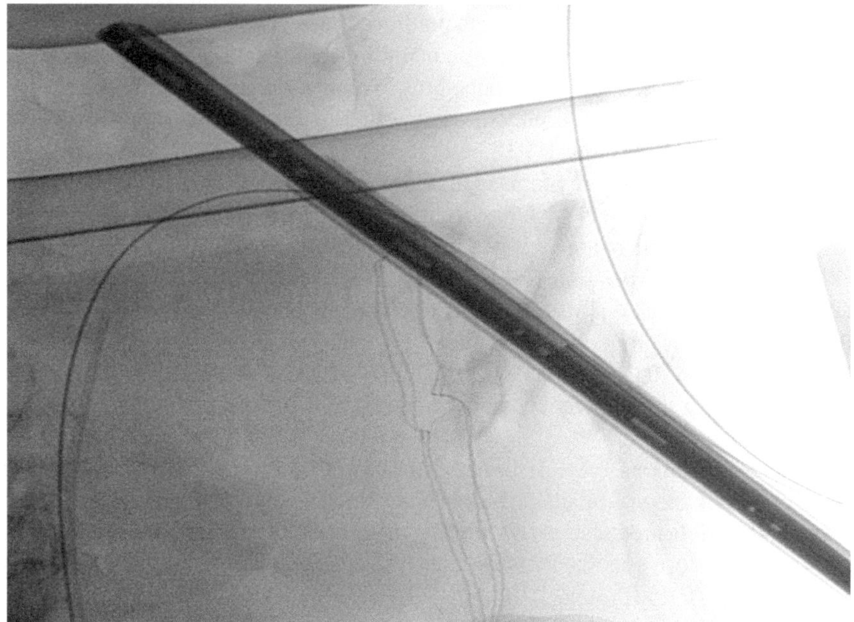

Fig. 7 Upper calyx approachability through the lower calyx in supine PCNL

In some patients, especially the thin ones, the mobility of the kidney is conspicuous during percutaneous puncture and tract dilation. This mobility is seen to a far lesser extent in the prone position where the kidney is fixed by the weight and rigidity of the posterior abdominal wall against the operating table.

Longer percutaneous tract

In the supine position, the tract length may be longer than in the prone position due to the fact that percutaneous puncture comes from a more lateral position on the patient's flank than in prone position. This comes also in part from the fact that the anterior abdominal wall is more bendable than the posterior abdominal wall. As a matter of facts, in the prone position, the more pliable anterior abdominal wall transmits pressure of the bed to the kidneys, limiting their mobility and shorterning the percutaneous tract (Proietti et al. 2019; Yazici et al. 2014).

In case of long access tract, the manoeuvrability within the collecting system could be challenging. As a consequence, the surgeon may need to adjust his or her technique to accommodate limitations in rigid nephroscopy or excessive torqueing in the supine position. These limitations may be overcome by routine use of a flexible nephroscope during supine PCNL. From a practical point of view, when planning to perform supine PCNL, it may be useful to have available longer length rigid nephroscopes and Amplatz sheaths, in particular in case of obese patients (Fig. 8).

In conclusion, the pros of supine PCNL compared with standard prone PCNL are as follows: (1) optimal cardiovascular and airway control, (2) better management in

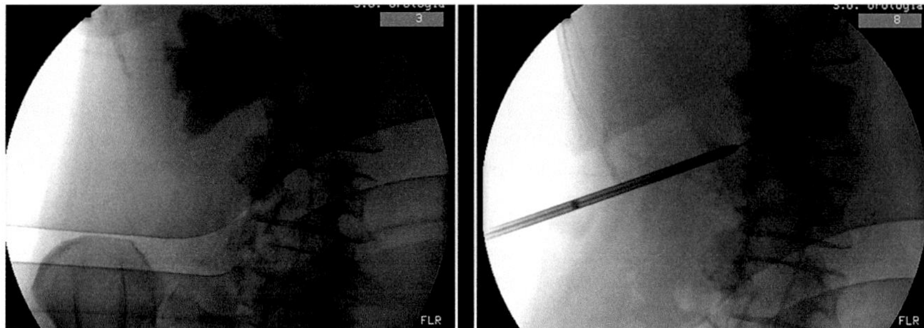

Fig. 8 Hypermobility of the kidney in supine PCNL

high-risk patients with heart failure or in obese patients, (3) easier, quicker and safer patient positioning with shorter operation time due to lack of need for repositioning, (4) possibility of a combined retrograde approach or simultaneous bilateral endoscopic surgery (5) better stone fragment washout due to the horizontal dorsal sheath angle (6) less radiation exposure to the surgeon' hands.

Nevertheless, supine PCNL also has some limitations, such as (1) limited area for renal puncture and nephroscope manoeuvrability; (2) upper pole calyx puncture could be more challenging; (3) potential difficulties in puncture and tract dilation due to kidney hypermobility; (4) decreased filling of the collecting system, which is constantly collapsed.

All of these issues are real, but supine percutaneous surgeons, by becoming more familiar with this position, have already developed tips and tricks to overcome them.

References

Altschuler J, Jain R, Ganesan V, Monga M. Supracostal upper pole endoscopic-guided prone tubeless "maxi-percutaneous nephrolithotomy": a contemporary evaluation of complications. J Endourol. 2019;33:274–8.

Astroza G, Lipkin M, Neisius A, Preminger G, De Sio M, Sodha H, Saussine C, de la Rosette J, CROES PNL Study Group. Effect of supine vs prone position on outcomes of percutaneous nephrolithotomy in staghorn calculi: results from the Clinical Research Office of the Endourology Society Study. Urology. 2013;82(6):1240–4.

Atkinson CJ, Turney BW, Noble JG, Reynard JM, Stoneham MD. Supine vs prone percutaneous nephrolithotomy: an anaesthetist's view. BJU Int. 2011;108:306–8.

Baard J, Kamphuis GM, Westendarp M, de la Rosette JJ. How well tolerated is supine percutaneous nephrolithotomy? Curr Opin Urol. 2014;24(2):184–8.

Bach C, Goyal A, Kumar P, Kachrilas S, Papatsoris AG, Buchholz N, Masood J. The Barts 'flank-free' modified supine position for percutaneous nephrolithotomy. Urol Int. 2012;89(3):365–8.

Batagello CA, Barone Dos Santos HD, Nguyen AH, Alshara L, Li J, Marchini GS, Vicentini FC, Torricelli FCM, Danilovic A, Pereira JG, Rose E, Srougi M, Nahas WC, Mazzucchi E, Monga M. Endoscopic guided PCNL in the prone split-leg position versus supine PCNL: a comparative analysis stratified by Guy's stone score. Can J Urol. 2019;26(1):9664–74.

Cracco CM, Scoffone CM. ECIRS (endoscopic combined intrarenal surgery) in the Galdakao-modified supine Valdivia position: a new life for percutaneous surgery? World J Urol. 2011;29:821–7.

De Sio M, Autorino R, Quarto G, Calabrò F, Damiano R, Giugliano F, Mordente S, D'Armiento M. Modified supine versus prone position in percutaneous nephrolithotomy for renal stones treatable with a single percutaneous access: a prospective randomized trial. Eur Urol. 2008;54(1):196–202.

Duty B, Waingankar N, Okhunov Z, Ben Levi E, Smith A, Okeke Z. Anatomical variation between the prone, supine, and supine oblique positions on computed tomography: implications for percutaneous nephrolithotomy access. Urology. 2012;79:67–71.

Edgcombe H, Carter K, Yarrow S. Anaesthesia in the prone position. Br J Anaesth. 2008;100(2):165–83.

Falahatkar S, Moghaddam AA, Salehi M, Nikpour S, Esmaili F, Khaki N. Complete supine percutaneous nephrolithotripsy comparison with the prone standard technique. J Endourol. 2008;22(11):2513–7.

Fernström I, Johansson B. Percutaneous pyelolithotomy. A new extraction technique. Scand J Urol Nephrol. 1976;10(3):257–9.

Gattinoni L, Caironi P. Prone positioning: beyond physiology. Anesthesiology. 2010;113(6):1262–4.

Giusti G, Proietti S, Rodríguez-Socarrás ME, Eisner BH, Saitta G, Mantica G, Villa L, Salonia A, Montorsi F, Gaboardi F. Simultaneous bilateral endoscopic surgery (SBES) for patients with bilateral upper tract urolithiasis: technique and outcomes. Eur Urol. 2018;74(6):810–5.

Grasso M, Nord R, Bagley DH. Prone split leg and flank roll positioning: simultaneous antegrade and retrograde access to the upper urinary tract. J Endourol. 1993;7(4):307–10.

Hopper KD, Sherman JL, Luethke JM, Ghaed N. The retrorenal colon in the supine and prone patient. Radiology. 1987;162(2):443–6.

Ibarluzea G, Scoffone CM, Cracco CM, Poggio M, Porpiglia F, Terrone C, Astobieta A, Camargo I, Gamarra M, Tempia A, Valdivia Uria JG, Scarpa RM. Supine Valdivia and modified lithotomy position for simultaneous anterograde and retrograde endourological access. BJU Int. 2007;100(1):233–6.

Jones DJ, Russell GL, Kellett MJ, Wickham JE. The changing practice of percutaneous stone surgery. Review of 1000 cases 1981–1988. Br J Urol. 1990;66(1):1–5.

Karami H, Arbab AH, Rezaei A, Mohammadhoseini M, Rezaei I. Percutaneous nephrolithotomy with ultrasonography-guided renal access in the lateral decubitus flank position. J Endourol. 2009;23(1):33–5. https://doi.org/10.1089/end.2008.0433.

Khoshrang H, Falahatkar S, Ilat S, Akbar MH, Shakiba M, Farzan A, Herfeh NR, Allahkhah A. Comparative study of hemodynamics electrolyte and metabolic changes during prone and complete supine percutaneous nephrolithotomy. Nephrourol Mon. 2012;4(4):622–8.

Li J, Gao L, Li Q, Zhang Y, Jiang Q. Supine versus prone position for percutaneous nephrolithotripsy: a meta-analysis of randomized controlled trials. Int J Surg. 2019;66:62–71.

Liu L, Zheng S, Xu Y, Wei Q. Systematic review and meta-analysis of percutaneous nephrolithotomy for patients in the supine versus prone position. J Endourol. 2010;24:1941–6.

Manohar T, Jain P, Desai M. Supine percutaneous nephrolithotomy: effective approach to high-risk and morbidly obese patients. J Endourol. 2007;21(1):44–9.

Mazzucchi E, Vicentini FC, Marchini GS, Danilovic A, Brito AH, Srougi M. Percutaneous nephrolithotomy in obese patients: comparison between the prone and total supine position. J Endourol. 2012;26:1437–42.

Papatsoris AG, Zaman F, Panah A, Masood J, El-Husseiny T, Buchholz N. Simultaneous anterograde and retrograde endourologic access: "the Barts technique." J Endourol. 2008;22(12):2665–6.

Perrella R, Vicentini FC, Paro ED, Torricelli FCM, Marchini GS, Danilovic A, Batagello CA, Mota PKV, Ferreira DB, Cohen DJ, Murta CB, Claro JFA, Giusti G, Monga M, Nahas WC, Srougi M, Mazzucchi E. Supine versus prone percutaneous nephrolithotomy for complex stones: a multicenter randomized controlled trial. J Urol. 2022;207(3):647–56.

Proietti S, de la Rosette J, Eisner B, Gaboardi F, Fiori C, Kinzikeeva E, Luciani L, Miano R, Porpiglia F, Rosso M, Sofer M, Traxer O, Giusti G. Bilateral endoscopic surgery for renal stones: a systematic review of the literature. Minerva Urol Nefrol. 2017;69(5):432–45.

Proietti S, Pavia MP, Rico L, Basulto-Martinez M, Yeow Y, Contreras P, Galosi A, Gaboardi F, Giusti G. Simultaneous bilateral endoscopic surgery: is it ready for prime time? J Endourol. 2022;36:1155–60.

Proietti S, Rodríguez-Socarrás ME, Eisner B, De Coninck V, Sofer M, Saitta G, Rodriguez-Monsalve M, D'Orta C, Bellinzoni P, Gaboardi F, Giusti G. Supine percutaneous nephrolithotomy: tips and tricks. Transl Androl Urol. 2019;8(Suppl 4):S381–8.

Proietti S, Sortino G, Giannantoni A, Sofer M, Peschechera R, Luciani LG, Morgia G, Giusti G. Single-session supine bilateral percutaneous nephrolithotomy. Urology. 2015;85(2):304–9.

Ray AA, Chung DG, Honey RJ. Percutaneous nephrolithotomy in the prone and prone-flexed positions: anatomic considerations. J Endourol. 2009;23(10):1607–14.

Sanguedolce F, Breda A, Millan F, Brehmer M, Knoll T, Liatsikos E, Osther P, Traxer O, Scoffone C. Lower pole stones: prone PCNL versus supine PCNL in the International Cooperation in Endourology (ICE) group experience. World J Urol. 2013;31(6):1575–80.

Scarpa RM, Cossu FM, De Lisa A, Porru D, Usai E. Severe recurrent ureteral stricture: the combined use of an anterograde and retrograde approach in the prone split-leg position without X-rays. Eur Urol. 1997;31(2):254–6.

Scoffone CM, Cracco CM, Cossu M, Grande S, Poggio M, Scarpa RM. Endoscopic combined intrarenal surgery in Galdakao-modified supine Valdivia position: a new standard for percutaneous nephrolithotomy? Eur Urol. 2008;54:1393–403.

Segura JW, Patterson DE, LeRoy AJ, Williams HJ Jr, Barrett DM, Benson RC Jr, May GR, Bender CE. Percutaneous removal of kidney stones: review of 1000 cases. J Urol. 1985;134(6):1077–81.

Sofer M, Giusti G, Proietti S, Mintz I, Kabha M, Matzkin H, Aviram G. Upper Calyx approachability through a lower calyx access for prone versus supine percutaneous nephrolithotomy. J Urol. 2016;195(2):377–82.

Telias I, Katira BH, Brochard L. Is the prone position helpful during spontaneous breathing in patients with COVID-19? JAMA. 2020;323(22):2265–7.

Tsaturyan A, Vrettos T, Ballesta Martinez B, Liourdi D, Lattarulo M, Liatsikos E, Kallidonis P. Position-related anesthesiologic considerations and surgical outcomes of prone percutaneous nephrolithotomy: a review of the current literature. Minerva Urol Nephrol. 2022;74(6):695–702.

Valdivia JG, Scarpa RM, Duvdevani M, Gross AJ, Nadler RB, Nutahara K, de la Rosette JJ, Croes PCNL Study Group. Supine versus prone position during percutaneous nephrolithotomy: a report from the clinical research office of the endourological society percutaneous nephrolithotomy global study. J Endourol. 2011;25(10):1619–25.

Valdivia JG, Valer J, Villarroya S, Lopez JA, Bayo A, Lanchares E, Rubio E. Why is percutaneous nephroscopy still performed with the patient prone? J Endourol. 1990;4(3):209–77.

Valdivia Uría JG, Lachares Santamaría E, Villarroya Rodríguez S, Taberner Llop J, Abril Baquero G, Aranda Lassa JM. Nefrolitectomía percutánea: técnica simplificada (nota previa) [Percutaneous nephrolithectomy: simplified technic (preliminary report)]. Arch Esp Urol. 1987;40(3):177–80.

Valdivia Uría JG, Valle Gerhold J, López López JA, Villarroya Rodriguez S, Ambroj Navarro C, Ramirez Fabián M, Rodriguez Bazalo JM, Sánchez Elipe MA. Technique and complications of percutaneous nephroscopy: experience with 557 patients in the supine position. J Urol. 1998;160(6 Pt 1):1975–8.

Wang Y, Wang Y, Yao Y, Xu N, Zhang H, Chen Q, Lu Z, Hu J, Wang X, Lu J, Hao Y, Jiang F, Hou Y, Wang C. Prone versus modified supine position in percutaneous nephrolithotomy: a prospective randomized study. Int J Med Sci. 2013;10(11):1518–23.

Yazici CM, Kayhan A, Dogan C. Supine or prone percutaneous nephrolithotomy: do anatomical changes make it worse? J Endourol. 2014;28(1):10–6.

Yuan D, Liu Y, Rao H, Cheng T, Sun Z, Wang Y, Liu J, Chen W, Zhong W, Zhu J. Supine versus prone position in percutaneous nephrolithotomy for kidney calculi: a meta-analysis. J Endourol. 2016;30(7):754–63.

Zhan HL, Li ZC, Zhou XF, Yang F, Huang JF, Lu MH. Supine lithotomy versus prone position in minimally invasive percutaneous nephrolithotomy for upper urinary tract calculi. Urol Int. 2013;91(3):320–5.

Zhang X, Xia L, Xu T, Wang X, Zhong S, Shen Z. Is the supine position superior to the prone position for percutaneous nephrolithotomy (PCNL)? Urolithiasis. 2014;42(1):87–93.

Ultrasound Guided Access

Wilson Sui, Jianxing Li, and Thomas Chi

Abstract Percutaneous nephrolithotomy is widely performed for treatment of large stones or stone burden. Historically, renal access is considered the most challenging step of the procedure with the greatest impact on the success of the case. Renal access is typically obtained under fluoroscopy by practicing urologists. There are however many disadvantages to fluoroscopic guidance, most prominently being the difficulty of learning this skill and radiation exposure to the patient, surgeon, and operating room staff. Advances in ultrasound technology have increased popularity of its use for renal access due to its many advantages including shortened learning curve, reduction or complete elimination of any ionizing radiation exposure, real time imaging of the renal anatomy and surrounding visceral organs, and improved operating room and surgeon ergonomics. Herein we review the history of ultrasonography and ultrasound-guided renal access in urology as well as the features of this modality and how it compared to fluoroscopy. In addition, we provide a practical overview of ultrasound fundamentals and technology and a step-by-step guide to performing ultrasound-guided renal access.

Keywords Nephrolithiasis · Nephrolithotomy · Percutaneous · Interventional ultrasonography · Radiation · Ionizing · Radiation exposure · Fluoroscopy · Learning curve

Abbreviations

CT   Computed tomography
ECIRS   Endoscopic combined intrarenal surgery
ESWL   Extracorporeal shockwave lithotripsy

W. Sui · T. Chi (✉)
Department of Urology, University of California, San Francisco, USA
e-mail: Tom.chi@ucsf.edu

J. Li
Department of Urology, Beijing Tsinghua Changgung Hospital, Beijing, China

© The Author(s), under exclusive license to Springer Nature Switzerland AG 2023   101
J. D. Denstedt and E. N. Liatsikos (eds.), *Percutaneous Renal Surgery*,
https://doi.org/10.1007/978-3-031-40542-6_7

OR   Operating room
PCNL   Percutaneous nephrolithotomy
TGC   Time-gain compensation

1 Introduction

Percutaneous nephrolithotomy (PCNL) is the recommended first line procedure for renal stones $\geq$ 20 mm, including staghorn calculi, due to its superior stone free rate and its limited morbidity when compared to extracorporeal shockwave lithotripsy (ESWL) or ureteroscopy (Turk et al. 2016; Assimos et al. 2016). The critical steps of a PCNL include obtaining renal access, dilation, lithotripsy and drainage. Obtaining renal access, the first step of this procedure, poses the most technical challenge to urologists, as demonstrated by survey data showing that only 11% of practicing urologists who routinely perform PCNL obtain their own access (Bird et al. 2003).

Fluoroscopy has been the preferred imaging modality for percutaneous access amongst urologists and is the most commonly used technique for PCNL access (Andonian et al. 2013). A Clinical Research Office of the Endourological Society report showed 86% of patients had fluoroscopic access versus just 14% with ultrasound guidance. Despite its popularity, fluoroscopy has many associated disadvantages including inability to identify surrounding organs or vasculature around the kidney, difficulty with assessing posterior calices and radiation exposure to the patient, surgeon, and operating room (OR) staff.

Considering these limitations to fluoroscopy, ultrasound technology has risen as a promising alternative, offering real time renal imaging with the potential to decrease the technical barriers to widespread use and improve patient outcomes. The objectives of this chapter are to review the evolution of ultrasound technology in urology, the benefits and learning curve of ultrasound guided access and the fundamentals of ultrasonography before describing a step-by-step approach to renal access.

2 History of Ultrasound Guided Access

In the 1950s, ultrasound technology was first applied in the medical field with early experiments used modified radar and sonar equipment in medical imaging (Wild 1950). The first use of ultrasound for nephrolithiasis was described in 1961 when Schlegel et al. reported on the use of intraoperative amplitude (A)-mode ultrasonography for renal stones. This was rudimentary however and the image generated was only a single spike representing a reflection from the stone (Schlegel et al. 1961). While these early images were crude and unusable for making medical diagnoses, they demonstrated the feasibility of applying this technology to medicine. It was not until the 1970s that innovations by Watanabe et al. and advancement of ultrasound technology made possible the first interpretable images of the prostate, bladder and kidney (Watanabe et al. 1976). At a time when most stones were identified by plain radiographs of the kidney, ureter and bladder or by intravenous pyeloureterograms, ultrasound imaging also showed promise in diagnosis of radiolucent matrix and uric acid stones (Pollack et al. 1978).

Subsequently in 1977, the first report of using intraoperative ultrasound to guide nephrolithotomy was published. Cook and Lytton used the brightness (B)-mode ultrasonography to localize a stones or stone fragments and access the collecting system (Cook and Lytton 1977). It was not until 1999 however that Desai and colleagues were the first to publish a large series of ultrasound-guided PCNLs with 45 procedures performed in pediatric patients (Desai et al. 1999). Next several randomized trials directly comparing ultrasound guided versus fluoroscopic PCNL were published demonstrating the safety and effectiveness of ultrasound guidance (Basiri et al. 2008; Karami et al. 2010; Agarwal et al. 2011; Jagtap et al. 2014).

3   Advantages of Ultrasound Guided Access

The advantages of ultrasound guided access include the reduction or complete elimination of any radiation exposure, real time imaging and improved ergonomics (Table 1). One in 11 people in the United States will suffer from a kidney stone over their lifetime, and 30% of these patients will develop a subsequent stone within 10 years (Turk et al. 2016; Assimos et al. 2016). Given the high recurrence of kidney stone disease, the cumulative exposure to radiation over a patient's lifetime from diagnostic imaging and treatment can be significant. For providers who routinely perform procedures to manage this disease, there is also a cumulative exposure to radiation which can lead to increased risk of cataracts, cancers, or other disease states that have been associated with radiation exposure for operators (Fulgham and Gilbert 2013). The decreased ionizing radiation exposure from utilizing ultrasound guidance can thus positively impact not only patients but providers as well. In populations especially vulnerable to the deleterious effects of ionizing radiation such as pediatric or pregnant patients, ultrasound is the preferred first line imaging modality for the diagnosis and treatment of kidney stones (Assimos et al. 2016).

The benefit of real time imaging of not only the kidney but also the surrounding viscera, pleura and vasculature allows the surgeon to minimize the risk of inadvertent injury during renal access (Andonian et al. 2013). In transplant and anomalous kidneys (ectopic, horseshoe) where the kidney is in an unfamiliar location, having the capability to identify surrounding organs in real time offers a distinct advantage. As no retrograde contrast is required to visualize the collecting system, ultrasound imaging can be utilized in cases even where retrograde access is not possible. Additionally, posterior calyces that are difficult to identify fluoroscopically are more straightforward to access using ultrasound guidance. Finally, examination of residual radiolucent stone fragments is not possible with fluoroscopy, but these fragments can be identified with ultrasonography.

Table 1 Advantages of ultrasound guided renal access

Radiation exposure
• Decreases or eliminates ionizing radiation exposure
• Visualization of radiolucent calculi
• Easy identification of posterior calyces
• Safer for use in the pediatric and pregnant populations
• Real time imaging
Real-time visualization of renal and stone configuration
• Visualization of surrounding visceral organs, pleura and vasculature, especially helpful in cases of transplant or anomalous kidneys
• Doppler flow imaging helps avoid vascular injury
Ergonomics
• Applicable to all patient positions
• Decreased operating room footprint
• Decreased physician and personnel fatigue and long-term orthopedic issues due to lack of lead aprons
• Lower cost of capital equipment
• Easier to teach and learn compared to fluoroscopic PCNL

Ultrasound guided access also offers advantages in ergonomics. This modality can be utilized for patients in a variety of positions and requires only minor adjustments to the OR set up or technique to obtain renal access compared to fluoroscopy. The smaller footprint of an ultrasound console as compared to a c-arm lends itself to use in tight-spaced ORs. Physicians and OR personnel also do not need to wear protective lead necessary for fluoroscopy use that can lead to orthopedic complaints and fatigue throughout the day.

4   Learning Curve

The steep learning curve for PCNL mastery is mostly related to achieving renal access. The importance of formal training in renal access was demonstrated in a survey that showed 92% of urologists trained in PCNL continued to perform PCNL in practice whereas only 33% of those untrained did ($p < 0.001$) (Lee et al. 2004). Furthermore, those trained in renal access performed a mean of 14 PCNLs per year versus 3.3 per year in the untrained. However only 27% of urologists trained in percutaneous access obtained their own access compared to 11% of those who were untrained ($p = 0.33$) highlighting again the difficultly with learning renal access. The major reported reasons included radiologists having better equipment or skills, access requiring extra time and surgeon comfort.

A critical review on renal access for PCNL recommended 24 PCNLs during residency to achieve basic proficiency, 60 to achieve competency and > 100 to reach excellence (Andonian et al. 2013). The studies this review was based on followed consecutive PCNL cases performed by novice surgeons or endourologists and found that operative/fluoroscopic time, renal access time, tract dilation time and complication rate improved over time and performance metrics approached that of expert surgeons within 60 to 100 cases (Allen et al. 2005; Tanriverdi et al. 2007). In transition from fluoroscopy to ultrasound guided PCNL access, one study reported the learning curve was as low as 20 cases for an experienced endourologist (Usawachintachit et al. 2016) Another study reported the learning curve for ultrasound guided access for a novice surgeon was 60 cases, similar to that of fluoroscopic PCNLs (Song et al. 2015). Overall, the learning curve for adopting ultrasound for renal access is shorter and more achievable by practicing urologists compared to fluoroscopy.

In obtaining ultrasound guided renal access, the urologist is faced with two technical challenges. First, one must be able to image the kidney and accurately interpret the displayed images. Second, one must be able to coordinate the needle and imaging hands when advancing the needle into the desired target. Early on in one's learning curve, failures may occur due to suboptimal imaging, misinterpretation of images or inaccurate needle placement. One consideration to improve the learning curve is to utilize a needle guide (Desai 2009). Needle guides fix the needle into a plane of imaging which can facilitate more accurate needle placement, especially when one is first starting to learn renal ultrasound, allowing the learner to focus on accuracy in imaging and reducing the need for accuracy of needle control. There are limitations however for needle guides in that the guides only allow for fixed angles of entry into the kidney. In addition, needle guide may limit one's ability to adjust to scenarios where a steeper or shallower trajectory to the skin is required to avoid bony structures. Ultimately, mastering both imaging and freehand needle control skills are important to applying ultrasound guidance for renal access.

5   Ultrasound Versus Fluoroscopy

Over the past decade, as PCNL technique and technology have progressed, ultrasound use has become more widespread. Given fluoroscopic guidance was heretofore the gold standard for access, randomized trials comparing this against fluoroscopic guidance were designed and published comparing them on several measures including time to puncture, radiation exposure, puncture attempts and complications.

The first randomized trial of fluoroscopy- versus ultrasound-guided access was published in 2008 and included 100 patients at a single center. The success rate for obtaining access was > 90% in either group with no differences in complications (Basiri et al. 2008). The ultrasound group had decreased radiation exposure and slightly longer access durations (p < 0.01). Another randomized trial of 60 patients in the flank position, 30 randomized to ultrasound guided access, showed similar operating and access times without any difference in complications or stone free rate

(Karami et al. 2010). In an additional randomized trial of 224 patients undergoing PCNL at a single center by a single provider, patients were randomized to fluoroscopic versus ultrasound guided access. Here the mean time to successful puncture was slower in the fluoroscopic group (3.2 min versus 1.8 min, p < 0.01), with increased radiation (28.6 s versus 14.4 s, p < 0.01) and with higher puncture attempts (3.3 versus 1.5, p < 0.01) and longer tract formation time with higher radiation exposure (p < 0.01) (Agarwal et al. 2011). There was no difference observed in complications.

While the aforementioned randomized trials all included experienced endourologists, there has been one trial that evaluated the trainee experience with ultrasound guidance. In a randomized trial of fluoroscopy versus ultrasound guided PCNL among trainees all with an experience of less < 25 PCNLs, there were no differences in operative time, post-operative complications, bleeding, analgesic requirement, length of stay or stone clearance (Jagtap et al. 2014). The authors noted however that while both methods of access were safe and effective, almost 20% of the ultrasound group required fluoroscopy as an adjunct for access due to lack of or mild hydronephrosis. This highlights an important point—while ultrasound and fluoroscopy have comparative different advantages and disadvantages, they are both excellent tools for facilitating renal access. The competent urologist should be familiar with both methods of access to be effective in all scenarios.

In most published trials, ultrasound guidance was used only in access and tract formation was performed under fluoroscopy, even if access was initially obtained using ultrasound. This is likely due to the level of provider comfort and familiarity with ultrasound imaging. This approach, however, only reduces and does not eliminate radiation exposure. Ultrasound-only PCNL, where ultrasound imaging is used to guide all portions of the case including tract dilation and placement of drainage tubes has been shown to be safe and efficient and of course completely avoids any radiation exposure (Yan et al. 2013). Applying ultrasound imaging guidance to renal tract dilation and drainage tube placement is outside the scope of this chapter, but achievable with a longer learning curve and stronger familiarity with the principles of excellent renal ultrasound imaging.

6 Ultrasound Guided Renal Access: Overview of Ultrasound Technology

Ultrasound guided renal access has been shown to provide safe and comparable access to fluoroscopically guided access with the advantages outlined above. Prior to our step-by-step description of ultrasound access, we recommend at least a superficial understanding of the basis of ultrasound technology to appreciate its strengths and limitations especially as it applies to imaging the kidney for renal access.

7   Fundamentals of Ultrasound Technology

Ultrasound waves are mechanical waves created by applying alternating electrical current to piezoelectric crystals housed in a transducer (Fulgham and Gilbert 2013). The piezoelectric effect (from Greek *piezein* meaning to squeeze or press) is the electric charge that accumulates in solid materials in response to mechanical stress (Katzir 2006). This alternating expansion and contraction of these crystals thus creates a mechanical wave that is transmitted via a coupling medium to the body. The waves produced are longitudinal, with particle motion in the same direction as the wave propagation. As the wave encounter tissue of different density and echogenic properties, they are reflected back towards the transducer with different characteristics depending on the tissue properties. In this way, the transducer works as both a receiver and transmitter of sound waves. The mechanical sound waves are then converted back into electrical energy and converted by the ultrasound machine into a displayed image.

8   Ultrasound Terminology

8.1   *Ultrasound Modes*

Gray-scale (Fig. 3A).

In gray scale imaging, a two-dimensional image is created where each pixel has a varying brightness. The image is created by measuring the time of travel for the soundwaves which determines the location of the pixel on the screen. The intensity on the other hand is reflected by the brightness of a given pixel. The image is typically refreshed at a rate of up to 40 frames per second giving the user a live image.

Doppler (Fig. 3B).

The doppler effect occurs when the frequency of sound waves are shifted after impacting a moving object based direction and velocity. Applied to medical imaging, color doppler ultrasound allows for evaluation of objects in motion in the human body such as blood flow. This is displayed with a color map, with greater velocities shown as brighter colors.

8.2   *Transducers*

Linear transducers are more commonly used for imaging superficial structures such as male genitalia and testes. Curved array transducers are more commonly used in abdominal imaging. This is because the curved probe allows for complete contact of the transducer with the skin after it is pressed onto the abdomen. In diagnostic renal ultrasonography, the ideal curved transducers are set to a frequency of 3.5 to 5.0 MHz. For special circumstances in renal imaging, a higher frequency transducer may be preferable. In pediatric patients, higher frequency transducers may be useful. Linear transducers of 6 to 10 MHz are utilized intraoperatively and laparoscopically for renal ultrasonography. The important principle guiding transducer selection to keep in mind is that higher frequency transducers offer greater detail and resolution of imaging while lower frequency transducers facilitate greater depth of penetration.

8.3   Contrast Agents

Nondilated systems, even with the use of retrograde saline or water injection, may be difficult to access due to poor collecting system visualization. To facilitate access, contrast agents containing gas microbubbles have been injected retrograde. Once struck by ultrasound waves, these bubbles oscillate and produce a return signal that can be more easily identified. One randomized trial demonstrated the use of contrast-enhanced ultrasound improves success rate for renal access while decreasing the number of access attempts and time to access in non-dilated collecting systems (Xia et al. 2021).

8.4   Echogenicity

Echogenicity refers to the capacity of a tissue or structure to reflect ultrasound waves compared to another structure. As echogenicity increases, so does the brightness of the target structure. An anechoic structure is one that reflect no sound waves and instead appears as black on the image. The most commonly encountered anechoic structures seen with genitourinary ultrasound imaging are fluid filled, including the bladder, blood vessels or collecting system, since fluid is generally anechoic (Fig. 1A). Hyperechoic structures are those who reflect more sound waves than surrounding structures and will appear bright on ultrasound imaging. This includes pleura, bones, and urinary stones (Fig. 2A). In contrast, hypoechoic structures reflect less than surrounding tissue and include subcutaneous fat and muscle (Fig. 1A). Notably some fat such as hilar fat or angiomyolipomas may be hyperechoic depending on the presence of connective tissue or other interfaces within the fat. Lastly isoechoic structures are those who reflect similar echoes. Typically, the liver, spleen and kidney are isoechoic.

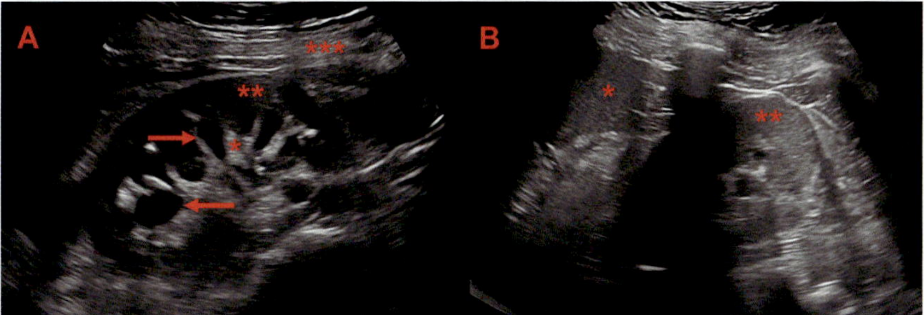

Fig. 1 Typical appearance of renal anatomy under ultrasound. A) Hypoechoeic dilated collecting system denoted by arrows with subcutaneous fat (***), renal parenchyma (**) and sinus fat (*) also visible. B) Isoechoic spleen (*) visualized next to renal parenchyma (**)

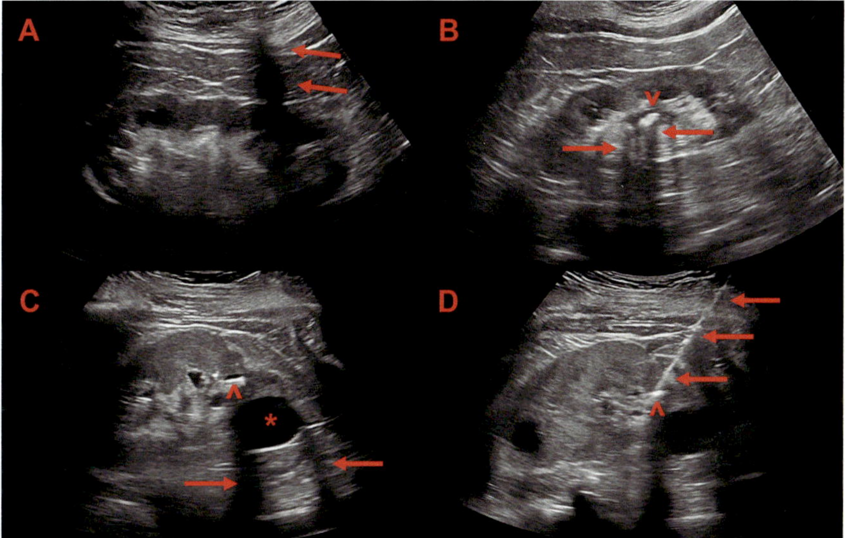

Fig. 2 Commonly encountered artifacts while performing ultrasound guided renal access. A) arrows denote rib shadowing due to acoustic shadowing B) post-acoustic shadowing denoted by arrows due to renal pelvis stone (v) C) Edging artifact denoted by arrows from rounded edges of a renal cyst (*) with peripherally located renal stone (^) with black rim denoting collecting system D) echogenic needle (denoted by arrows) traversing subcutaneous tissue and renal parenchyma, directly accessing a peripheral calyx containing a kidney stone (^)

8.5 *Attenuation*

Attenuation occurs when sound waves interact with tissues and fluid in the body resulting in a loss of kinetic energy (Fulgham and Gilbert 2013). Attenuation occurs via three major mechanisms: absorption, reflection and refraction. Absorption occurs

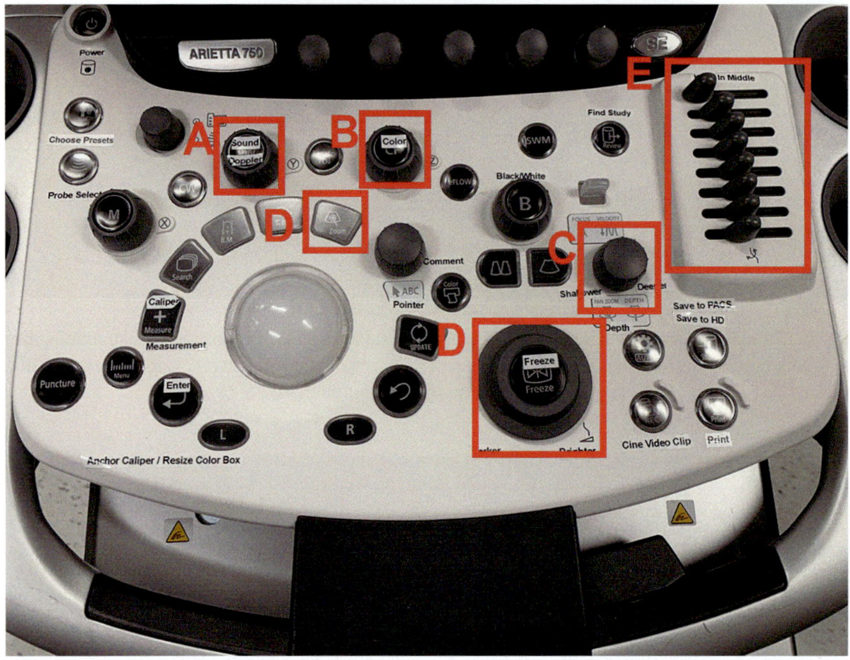

Fig. 3 Typical ultrasound machine setting controls including A) Gray scale mode, B) color doppler mode, C) frequency and depth, D) gain, E) time-gain compensation and F) field of view

when part of the kinetic energy of the sound wave is converted to heat after interacting with tissue. When a sound wave encounters an interface at an angle other than 90 degrees, refraction occurs which is when a portion of that sound wave is reflected while the other continues forward, leading to a loss of information. Finally, reflection occurs when sound waves interact with an interface between two unlike structures leading to scattering, especially if the interface is small or irregular, of the reflected wave. These interactions with tissue and interfaces within the body produce ultrasound artifacts that can interfere with accurate imaging.

8.6   Artifact

Ultrasound artifacts are commonly encountered during ultrasonography and may be due to scanning technique or intrinsic properties of the imaging modality. Understanding of ultrasound artifacts is important not only to improve image quality and avoid misdiagnosis but also some aid in the diagnosis of anatomy or pathology.

Acoustic shadowing occurs when there is a signal void behind a structure due to significant attenuation leading to loss of information distal to the interface. This occurs most often with solid structures, such as bone, where molecules are densely packed together. For the purposes of ultrasound guided renal access, the most commonly encountered shadowing is from the patient's ribs when attempting to visualize the kidney (Fig. 2A) or kidney stones within the collecting system (Fig. 2B). To avoid the former, the probe can be rotated on the body surface so that it is parallel to the ribs.

Edging artifact can be seen most often with rounded structures such as the upper or lower pole of the kidney, renal cyst walls, or testicles. This artifact occurs when sound waves impact a curved surface at a critical angle leading to refraction and loss of signal return to the transducer. Changing the angle of the ultrasound probe can help avoid this artifact.

The comet tail artifact occurs during gray scale ultrasonography due to reverberation of ultrasound signals between two closely spaced reflective surfaces. The bevel of an echogenic needle takes advantage of this artifact to give the tip of the needle more contrast compared to the surrounding tissue to make tracking the needle as it traverses to the target anatomy easier (Fig. 2D). Other foreign bodies may also cause this artifact such as catheter tips or surgical clips.

The twinkle artifact, also known as the color Doppler comet tail artifact, occurs in doppler mode due to reflection of sound waves from a strongly reflecting structure. This leads to machine noise and appears as a focus of alternating colors behind the structure mimicking turbulent blood flow. This is useful in identification of hyperechoic objects in the kidney such as kidney stones.

9 Patient Selection

For providers early in their learning curve for ultrasound access, we generally suggest choosing patients who have limited comorbidities and who are not morbidly obese. When imaging obese patients, the extra tissue between the initial needle puncture site and the kidney can make it difficult to image the kidney and track the needle through its subcutaneous trajectory. Choosing patients where retrograde access is possible can also facilitate greater renal access success. Retrograde instillation of fluid can facilitate induction of artificial hydronephrosis. Similarly, selecting patients in whom there is already moderate hydronephrosis can facilitate greater success with renal access as accessing a non-dilated system is challenging. In addition, the presence of staghorn stone configurations has been associated with greater renal access challenge. While there are no contraindications exclusive to ultrasound guided access when compared to fluoroscopic access, selecting patients with favorable anatomy can facilitate greater success for the operator, particularly when they have less experience in renal imaging.

10 Pre-operative Considerations and Patient Positioning

Prophylactic antibiotics are tailored the patients' pre-operative urine culture (or prior cultures if a recurrent stone former) and local antibiogram as recommended by American and European Urological Association guidelines (Turk et al. 2016; Assimos et al. 2016). Computed tomography imaging should be obtained in order to review renal anatomy in addition to surrounding vasculature and viscera in addition to stone characteristics. We typically prefer general anesthesia as this allows for minimization of movement leading to higher accuracy.

Patient positioning will depend on surgeon preference and comfort, patient body habitus, comorbidities, and renal anatomy. Options include supine, Galdakao-modified Valdivia or prone. Each position can provide different tradeoffs that can be advantageous depending on the clinical need. For example, the Galdakao-modified Valdivia preserves retrograde access with rigid instrumentation while allowing for adequate percutaneous access to the kidney and avoids the ventilatory issues sometimes associated with the prone position.

After positioning, there are several options to obtain upper urinary tract access. An externalized ureteral catheter can be placed via a flexible or rigid cystoscope. This is useful to induce hydronephrosis by retrograde injection of saline. Other options for upper tract access include placement of a ureteral access sheath both for instillation of saline and for the option to visualize the puncture site with a flexible ureteroscope and perform the dilation under direct vision, commonly referred to endoscopic combined intrarenal surgery, or ECIRS.

11 Procedural Steps

(1) Renal ultrasonography

The first step in obtaining access is adequately visualizing the kidney and its surrounding structures. Any portable ultrasound unit is viable. While the preferred option for a transducer is a curved array in the 3.5 MHz range, a linear transducer is also usable (Table 2). While ultrasound gel is typically utilized in ultrasound imaging as a coupling agent, we have found that this can result in slippery hands intraoperatively which is unfavorable for instrument handling. Instead, sterile water or saline is periodically applied to the patient's body as a reasonable alternative coupling agent.

11.1 Adjusting User Dependent Imaging Variables

Figure 3 Ultrasound machine settings

Frequency and depth (Fig. 3C).

Table 2 List of recommended equipment for ultrasound guided access

Reusable
• Ultrasound with transducer in the 3.5 MHz range
• Needle guide (optional)
• Nephroscope and lithotripter device
• C-arm with contrast (if preferred for tract dilation)
Disposable
• 18 to 24-gauge needle with an echogenic tip
• Fascial dilators (recommend 10Fr or 12Fr)
• Safety wire introducer (optional)
• Access tract dilation equipment (serial dilation kit or balloon set)
• Guidewire per surgeon preference (recommend J-tipped coaxial, hybrid or super stiff)
• Sterile ultrasound console cover
• Sterile ultrasound probe cover (if probe is not sterilized)
• Ultrasound contrast agent solution (optional, useful in non-dilated systems)

One should select the highest possible frequency that allows for adequate depth of penetration. Frequency and depth are inversely related. The higher the frequency, the better the quality of the image, however the lower the depth of penetration. Usually, renal imaging is done between 2.5 and 6 MHz to allow for adequate tissue penetration (in contrast for testicular imaging, a linear probe at 12 MHz is commonly used).

Setting the ultrasound to approximately 8–12 cm depth is usually adequate for the average patient however this should be adjusted to maximize the size of the kidney on the ultrasound screen.

Gain (Fig. 3D).

Gain determines how much a returning sound wave will be amplified when it strikes the transducer. When gain is increased, the image is brighter or hyperechoic. Too much gain leads to an image that appears "washed out." In contrast when gain is decreased, the image is darkened. With too little gain, it is difficult to distinguish between structures.

Gain should be adjusted so that the stone and renal parenchyma are clearly visible and there is adequate contrast between the access needle and the collecting system.

Time-gain compensation (Fig. 3E).

Unlike overall gain, time-gain compensation (TGC) adjusts imaging brightness for specific regions of the scanned field to be individually amplified. This function is used to increase amplification in regions where there is high attenuation or decrease amplification where attenuation is low. A common example in the kidney when TGC can be used to optimize imaging includes renal cysts. TGC for the region below the cyst can be decreased to accurately image this area.

Field of view (Fig. 3F).

Decreasing the field of view will limit the width of the image so that only a portion of ultrasound information is displayed. This may improve the refresh rate as it decreases the amount of data processing needed for returning ultrasound data. It can also be used to exclude distracting tissue or artifact for the surgeon to focus on the organ of interest.

(2)   Renal ultrasonography: identification of renal anatomy and vital structures

For patients undergoing PCNL, important landmarks include the midaxillary line, costal margin, the 11th and 12th ribs and the iliac crest. In the prone position, the paraspinous muscle is an important additional landmark. After identifying the 11th and 12th ribs, to optimize renal imaging, we recommend that the probe initially be placed along the midaxillary line just under the 11th rib. By convention, the probe should be oriented to the patient's body such that the cranial structures (i.e. the upper pole) should be to the left of the screen. Depending on the initial orientation, there will typically be post-acoustic shadowing by the ribs (Fig. 2A). This can be eliminated by rotating the probe to be parallel to the 11th rib (usually an adjustment of 30–45 degrees). The ideal initial view should be a longitudinal view that allows for identification of the renal cortex, collecting system and the target urinary stone(s).

Important surrounding structures that should be identified include bowel, pleura, vascular structures, and solid organs (Fig. 1B). Doppler flow can be used to facilitate vascular structure identification. To improve visualization of the collecting system, hydronephrosis may also be induced via manual or passive retrograde injection of saline via an externalized ureteral catheter, access sheath or flexible ureteroscope (Fig. 1A). Renal pyramids may be confused for calices so orienting to sinus fat and the collecting system and inducing hydronephrosis may help to differentiate these structures. In other cases where the stone occupies the collecting system or in minimally or mildly dilated systems, visualizing the stone post acoustic shadowing or a rim of darker black around the stone, representing urine next to the calyx, can confirm the target is in the collecting system (Fig. 2C).

(3)   Choosing the ideal calyx

When choosing the appropriate calyx under ultrasound guidance, identifying the calyx closest to the top of the screen will provide the shortest tract from the skin to the target and enable successful access. Ultrasound facilitates caliceal selection without the need to focus on the concept of posterior versus anterior caliceal positioning. In many cases, particularly with supine positioning, an anterior calyx may be the optimal target if it provides direct access to the target stone and collecting system. Ultrasound can also facilitate flexibility in selecting patient positioning. Compared to fluoroscopy, ultrasound guidance in renal access may lend itself to different skin entry points. For example, accessing horseshoe kidneys in the prone position will often result in a more medial skin entry compared to fluoroscopy due to the lie of the horseshoe kidney.

(4)   Renal puncture

The most technically challenging step to the case is the renal puncture. The surgeon must combine their kidney imaging interpretation with the technical skill of inserting the access needle. For needle insertion, we prefer to teach the renal puncture via the freehand approach which allows for more flexibility in needle adjustment. There are, however, several options for commercially available needle guides as described previously which attach to the ultrasound probe. These may facilitate learning as they decrease the challenge of coordinating the imaging with needle insertion and may be useful earlier in the surgeon's learning curve.

An 18-to-24-gauge needle with an echogenic tip should be used for access as these needles are more readily visible under ultrasound (Fig. 2D). We tend to favor the 18-gauge size for its stiffness, as the needle is less likely to deflect from its intended path during insertion. There are two options for needle insertion location in relationship to the probe, longitudinal and transverse. Both have their advantages. In the longitudinal approach, done by performing the puncture in line with the long axis of the probe, one can see the entire length of the needle as it traverses from the skin to the target calyx. In the transverse approach, the needle enters the skin from the side of the probe, providing a cross sectional view of the needle in any given imaging plane. This requires one to actively image the needle tip as it moves toward its target. While the transverse approach can allow one to navigate around ribs for example, we tend to favor the longitudinal approach for its safety profile.

Seeing the entire needle as it traverses the layers of body toward the target allows the operator confidence in avoiding peri-renal structures. For a lower pole puncture in the longitudinal approach, the needle is typically inserted approximately 1 cm from the caudal end of the probe and for an upper pole and mid kidney puncture, it enters the skin 1 cm from the cephalad end of the probe. Notably, if the probe is oriented correctly and the needle is inserted on the appropriate side of the probe, an upper pole and mid kidney puncture will be seen from the left of the screen whereas a lower pole puncture will be seen from the right. The needle should be visualized as it enters the skin and then passes the subcutaneous tissue including fat, fascia, and muscle (Fig. 2D). One critical principle is to visualize the target calyx, hold the image steady, and bring the needle into the target, rather than chase the needle.

For a transverse insertion, the access needle punctures the skin orthogonal to the long axis of the probe. Unlike the longitudinal approach where it is critical to hold the probe steady, with the transverse approach, the probe should be swept back and forth continuously to visualize the needle tip and trajectory to guide the needle to the calyx of interest. This active imaging movement with the ultrasound probe requires the operator to be moving both hands in concert with one another. The benefit of this approach however is that the needle can be inserted into the skin at any distance from the side of the ultrasound probe which allows for more flexibility in the angle and location of needle entry relative to the probe.

Learning to make real time adjustments to the needle can be challenging initially. If the needle tip is lost during insertion, two techniques can be of value. First, fanning the ultrasound probe back and forth to identify the needle location and adjusting the needle can bring it into the desired imaging plane. Second, with the ultrasound probe fixed in one position, the needle can be gently bounced in and out of the imaging plane to identify which direction it must be moved to enter the target imaging plane. One should be mindful not to enter the skin at too oblique of an angle which can not only make dilation more challenging but also cause the nephroscope to abut the patient's iliac crest. One advantage of ultrasound imaging is its live view imaging nature, compared to fluoroscopy that mostly entails spot imaging. The ability to monitor kidney movement during live imaging allows accurate coordination between the movement of the ultrasound probe and needle to ensure these remain in the same plane and approach the kidney as it moves. This can negate the need for temporary pause in ventilation commonly done with fluoroscopy to fix the kidney position in space during renal access.

(5)   Guidewire access, tract dilation and sheath placement

Once the access needle is successfully inserted into the target calyx, the inner stylet should be removed. If the collecting system is hydronephrotic (whether through natural or induced means) there is often brisk return of urine through the needle. Depending on surgeon preference and comfort, at this point, the rest of the procedure can be completed under ultrasound or fluoroscopic guidance. If a ureteroscope has been inserted retrograde, direct vision guidance for dilation is also another option. For the purposes of this chapter, we will describe the rest of the procedure under ultrasound guidance, though endoscopic direct vision guidance can bring surgeons to an X-ray free state for tract dilation with a potentially shorter learning curve compared to ultrasound guidance.

Under ultrasound guidance, any wrapped or lined guidewire should appear as linear and hyperechoic and can readily be seen traversing the renal parenchyma into the collection system. The exception are hydrophilic wires which may be so smooth that they are not visible under ultrasound. If there are issues with seeing the wire, a gentle in and out "jiggle" of the wire may facilitate identification.

After the wire has been inserted into the collecting system through the needle and the needle removed, a small skin incision is made to the size of the planned sheath. We commonly use fascial or serial dilators to facilitate tract dilation. Since these instruments in their disposable form are often made of polypropylene or other synthetic polymers, and while they are opaque and visible under fluoroscopic imaging, with ultrasound they are non-echogenic. As the dilator is advanced, the loss of signal of the wire signifies the tip of fascial dilator. Instead of looking for the dilator to appear, we look for the wire to disappear to know where the dilator tip is located. Critically when performing this step, it is important to first have a reliable ultrasound image of the wire. If there are concerns regarding depth of the fascial dilator, backing it out while keeping the wire in place should reveal the wire once more. Frequently active fanning of the ultrasound prob may be required to confirm visualization of the wire. When utilizing reusable serial dilators, such as Alken dilators, these metallic instruments can be seen as bright linear echos that cast a shadow.

In contrast, balloon dilation devices are more readily visible under ultrasound and most have a tip that is slightly more echogenic than the wire which facilitates locating them within the collecting system for accurate positioning. Again, with balloon dilation, it is important to keep a view of the wire to watch the balloon as it is advanced into the calyx. Once dilated, the contours of the balloon appear as a column of liquid and can be readily seen under ultrasound.

The percutaneous access sheath, whether advanced over a balloon or a serial dilator, is often difficult to visualize under ultrasound guidance thus it is often advanced keeping an eye on the back end of the sheath and stopping its advancement when it is matched with a known landmark of the dilator. For example, during balloon dilation, we typically advance this sheath until the back end of the balloon can just be seen through the sheath which approximates the correct depth matching the front of the sheath to the distal end of the balloon.

(6) After renal access and tract dilation are completed, nephroscopy and stone treatment is then performed. Please see detailed descriptions of these steps in the relevant chapters in this book
(7) Renal drainage

If an ultrasound-only procedure is sought, it is notable that nephrostomy tube placement can also be performed under ultrasound guidance. We routinely place 10 french cope pigtail nephrostomy tubes or 4.8/6 french internalized ureteral stents (in the supine position) under ultrasound guidance. While sometimes difficult to visualize, especially if there has been bleeding resulting in blood clot in the renal pelvis, the tube coils will appear as circular echogenic structures in the renal pelvis or bladder. To confirm accurate positioning of a stent, if the bladder cannot be visualized via ultrasound (such as in prone positioning) the proximal curl can be visualized using the nephroscope and the distal curl using a cystoscope or ureteroscope.

Complications with access

The most common reported complications of ultrasound guided access for nephrostomy tube placement by urologists includes urinary tract infection (1.1%), hemorrhage (1.9%), sepsis (0.76%), inferior vena cava injury (0.15%) and death (0.3%) (Fulgham and Gilbert 2013). Overall major complications have been reported in 3.3–6.7% of patients and minor complications in 5–38% of patients. Several meta-analyses have been performed comparing ultrasound versus fluoroscopic access percutaneous for PCNL. One found that the overall lower pooled odds ratio favored a significantly lower complication rate (OR 0.56, 95% CI 0.36–0.86) however the authors note that this was likely driven by impact of a single study of 8 that were included (Yang et al. 2019).

12 Summary

Ultrasound guided renal access has many different characteristics compared to fluoroscopic guided access including reduction or elimination of radiation exposure, real-time visualization of renal anatomy and surrounding structures and ergonomic improvements for the surgeon and OR staff. This is a safe method to access the kidney and has been shown in randomized data to have a comparable complication profile to fluoroscopic access. In obtaining renal access, the initial challenge lies in coordinating renal imaging with advancement of the access needle into the target calyx. Ultrasound can then be used to guide the remainder of the procedure including tract dilation and drainage tube placement effectively eliminating any radiation exposure.

References

Agarwal M, Agrawal MS, Jaiswal A, Kumar D, Yadav H, Lavania P. Safety and efficacy of ultrasonography as an adjunct to fluoroscopy for renal access in percutaneous nephrolithotomy (PCNL). BJU Int. 2011;108(8):1346–9.

Allen D, O'Brien T, Tiptaft R, Glass J. Defining the learning curve for percutaneous nephrolithotomy. J Endourol. 2005;19(3):279–82.

Andonian S, Scoffone CM, Louie MK, Gross AJ, Grabe M, Daels FP, et al. Does imaging modality used for percutaneous renal access make a difference? A matched case analysis. J Endourol. 2013;27(1):24–8.

Assimos D, Krambeck A, Miller NL, Monga M, Murad MH, Nelson CP, et al. Surgical management of stones: American urological association/endourological society guideline, Part I. J Urol. 2016;196(4):1153–60.

Basiri A, Ziaee AM, Kianian HR, Mehrabi S, Karami H, Moghaddam SMH. Ultrasonographic versus fluoroscopic access for percutaneous nephrolithotomy: a randomized clinical trial. J Endourol. 2008;22(2):281–4.

Bird VG, Fallon B, Winfield HN. Practice patterns in the treatment of large renal stones. J Endourol. 2003;17(6):355–63.

Cook JH, Lytton B. Intraoperative localization of renal calculi during nephrolithotomy by ultrasound scanning. J Urol. 1977;117(5):543–6. https://doi.org/10.1016/s0022-5347(17)58530-4.

Desai M. Ultrasonography-guided punctures—with and without puncture guide. J Endourol. 2009;23(10):1641–3.

Desai M, Ridhorkar V, Patel S, Bapat S, Desai M. Pediatric percutaneous nephrolithotomy: assessing impact of technical innovations on safety and efficacy. J Endourol. 1999;13(5):359–64.

Fulgham PF, Gilbert BR. Practical urological ultrasound. Springer; 2013.

Jagtap J, Mishra S, Bhattu A, Ganpule A, Sabnis R, Desai MR. Which is the preferred modality of renal access for a trainee urologist: ultrasonography or fluoroscopy? Results of a prospective randomized trial. J Endourol. 2014;28(12):1464–9.

Karami H, Rezaei A, Mohammadhosseini M, Javanmard B, Mazloomfard M, Lotfi B. Ultrasonography-guided percutaneous nephrolithotomy in the flank position versus fluoroscopy-guided percutaneous nephrolithotomy in the prone position: a comparative study. J Endourol. 2010;24(8):1357–61.

Katzir S. The discovery of the piezoelectric effect. In: The beginnings of piezoelectricity: a study in mundane physics; 2006. p. 15–64.

Lee CL, Anderson JK, Monga M. Residency training in percutaneous renal access: does it affect urological practice? J Urol. 2004;171(2):592–5.

Pollack HM, Arger PH, Goldberg BB, Grant MS. Ultrasonic detection of nonopaque renal calculi. Radiology. 1978;127(1):233–7.

Schlegel J, Diggdon P, Cuellar J. The use of ultrasound for localizing renal calculi. J Urol. 1961;86(4):367–9.

Song Y, Ma Y, Song Y, Fei X. Evaluating the learning curve for percutaneous nephrolithotomy under total ultrasound guidance. PLoS ONE. 2015;10(8): e0132986.

Tanriverdi O, Boylu U, Kendirci M, Kadihasanoglu M, Horasanli K, Miroglu C. The learning curve in the training of percutaneous nephrolithotomy. Eur Urol. 2007;52(1):206–12.

Turk C, Petrik A, Sarica K, Seitz C, Skolarikos A, Straub M, et al. EAU guidelines on interventional treatment for urolithiasis. Eur Urol. 2016;69(3):475–82. https://doi.org/10.1016/j.eururo.2015.07.041.

Usawachintachit M, Masic S, Allen IE, Li J, Chi T. Adopting ultrasound guidance for prone percutaneous nephrolithotomy: evaluating the learning curve for the experienced surgeon. J Endourol. 2016;30(8):856–63.

Watanabe H, Saitoh M, Igari D, Tanahashi Y, Harada K. Non-invasive detection of ultrasonic Doppler signals from renal vessels. Tohoku J Exp Med. 1976;118(4):393–4.

Wild JJ. The use of ultrasonic pulses for the measurement of biologic tissues and the detection of tissue density changes. Surgery. 1950;27(2):183–8.

Xia D, Peng E, Yu Y, Yang X, Liu H, Tong Y, et al. Comparison of contrast-enhanced ultrasound versus conventional ultrasound-guided percutaneous nephrolithotomy in patients with nondilated collecting system: a randomized controlled trial. Eur Radiol. 2021;31(9):6736–46. https://doi.org/10.1007/s00330-021-07804-1.

Yan S, Xiang F, Yongsheng S. Percutaneous nephrolithotomy guided solely by ultrasonography: a 5-year study of >700 cases. BJU Int. 2013;112(7):965–71.

Yang Y-H, Wen Y-C, Chen K-C, Chen C. Ultrasound-guided versus fluoroscopy-guided percutaneous nephrolithotomy: a systematic review and meta-analysis. World J Urol. 2019;37:777–88.

Radiation Hazards in Endourology

Ala'a Farkouh and D. Duane Baldwin

Abstract Patients with urinary stones are exposed to substantial amounts of radiation during diagnosis, treatment, and follow-up. Percutaneous nephrolithotomy (PCNL) is commonly performed for the management of large and complex renal stones and requires image-guided percutaneous access. This access is commonly done using fluoroscopy, exposing both patients and surgeons to radiation. The understanding of potential risks associated with radiation exposure has recently expanded from malignancy to include ischemic heart disease, cataracts, arthritis, and inflammation. This chapter will first review the hazards associated with radiation exposure, with emphasis on ionizing radiation used for medical imaging. Then, options for evaluation of patients that minimize radiation exposure will be discussed, including ultrasound and low and ultra-low dose CT scans. Next, intraoperative techniques designed to reduce radiation exposure during PCNL will be presented including ultrasound, pulsed fluoroscopy, shielding, distance, and other low dose techniques. In addition, follow-up strategies that minimize radiation exposure will be presented. Finally, after reading this chapter, the surgeon will be well-versed in the tenants of the ALARA principle (as low as reasonably achievable), and able to employ this principle in their practice to keep their patients and themselves safe from the harmful effects of excessive radiation exposure.

Keywords Radiation safety · Fluoroscopy · Computed tomography · Ultrasound · Percutaneous nephrolithotomy · Risk management

A. Farkouh · D. D. Baldwin (✉)
Department of Urology, Loma Linda University Health, Room A560, 11234 Anderson Street, Loma Linda, CA 92354, USA
e-mail: dbaldwin@llu.edu

A. Farkouh
e-mail: afarkouh@llu.edu

© The Author(s), under exclusive license to Springer Nature Switzerland AG 2023
J. D. Denstedt and E. N. Liatsikos (eds.), *Percutaneous Renal Surgery*,
https://doi.org/10.1007/978-3-031-40542-6_8

1   Introduction

The world around us is filled with potential dangers that intrude into our consciousness. These dangers include many visible and tangible threats, including poisonous spiders, venomous snakes, sharks, and lightning strikes. Although these tangible threats may arouse fear within us, the actual risks associated with many of these are quite low. In the United States, spider bites cause six deaths, rattlesnakes kill five people, shark attacks end the life of one, and lightning strikes kill eleven people on average per year.

In contrast, ionizing radiation cannot be felt, heard, or touched, and is completely invisible. For this reason, the risks associated with its use are easy to overlook. Despite being invisible, silent, and intangible, the effects of radiation pose a clear and present danger to the health and safety of kidney stone patients, urologic surgeons, and operating room staff. For patients with urinary stone disease specifically, radiation is used for diagnosis, during treatment, and for follow-up. Exposure to medical radiation from computed tomography (CT) scans, is projected to cause approximately 15,000 deaths per year in the USA alone (Berrington de Gonzalez et al. 2007).

Similarly, fluoroscopy employs ionizing radiation. The fluoroscopy machine was invented by Thomas Edison and much of the early work was done by his assistant Clarence Dally. Tragically, Mr. Dally developed severe non-healing skin burns on his hands requiring amputation, and ultimately became one of the first known casualties of medical radiation exposure when he died at the age of 39 from metastatic cancer. This had a profound effect upon Thomas Edison, who in 1903 said "Don't talk to me about x-rays; I am afraid of them" (Anon 1903). If the inventor of the fluoroscopy machine was afraid of its risks, perhaps we also should be afraid. Afraid enough that we do not use fluoroscopy indiscriminately and use it only when necessary and in accordance with the principles of ALARA (as low as reasonably achievable).

The aim of this chapter is to outline and review the health hazards associated with the ionizing radiation used in CT scans for the diagnosis and follow-up of stone disease, and fluoroscopy used to treat kidney stones. In addition, percutaneous nephrolithotomy (PCNL) techniques will be presented to facilitate diagnosis, treatment and follow-up of stones using the lowest possible dose of radiation.

2   Basic Principles of Medical Ionizing Radiation

Ionizing radiation has high frequency and energy, and is able to remove electrons from atoms, whether in living tissue or the surrounding environment. X-rays are ionizing radiation that have widespread use in medical imaging. In fact, diagnostic x-ray exposure is considered the largest source of all radiation exposure in the USA, accounting for over 40% of lifetime exposure (Donya et al. 2014). All radiographic studies including conventional plain films, CT scans, fluoroscopy, and nuclear medicine studies expose patients to ionizing radiation.

During medical imaging, sources of radiation include *primary beam radiation*, which travels directly from the source to the patient and constitutes the largest component of patient exposure, and *scatter radiation*, which are dispersed waves that are reflected when primary waves encounter the patient or some other object. Scatter radiation doses are lower than primary beam, but constitute the majority of radiation exposure to healthcare workers present during imaging or when performing radiation-guided procedures.

Different dose measurements can be used to quantify radiation exposure, which can create confusion among healthcare professionals. The three most commonly used doses are: absorbed dose, equivalent dose, and effective dose (Mitchell and Furey 2011).

Absorbed dose refers to the ionizing radiation deposited on and absorbed by tissue and is quantified by the unit Gray (Gy). *Equivalent dose* takes into account the properties of different types of ionizing radiation in causing harm and is calculated from the absorbed dose using radiation weighting factors. For x-rays, the radiation weighting factor is 1; therefore, both absorbed and equivalent doses are equal for medical radiation exposure. *Effective dose* is a calculated dose that further accounts for the susceptibility of different organs to radiation effects and is calculated from the equivalent dose using tissue weighting factors for a standard reference. Both equivalent dose and effective dose are reported in the unit Sievert (Sv). Effective dose is the radiation measure used in radiation protection practices, including setting annual exposure limits and measuring occupational exposures.

3 Health Risks of Ionizing Radiation

3.1 Radiation Effects—Defining the Terms

The harmful effects of radiation on cells and tissues can be classified into deterministic and stochastic effects. *Deterministic effects* refer to harms conferred to sensitive tissues as a result of radiation exposure that depends on the duration and dose. After a threshold is reached, any radiation exposure causes harm, and the severity is directly proportional to the dose. Common deterministic effects include dermatitis/burns, alopecia, infertility, cataracts, radiation sickness, and death (in cases of extensive exposure such as nuclear accidents).

Stochastic effects, on the other hand, occur by chance. No radiation threshold is needed for stochastic effects to occur and the severity of the effect is not related to the exposure dose. However, the risk of developing these stochastic effects is proportional to the radiation exposure, the greater the exposure, the more likely stochastic effects will take place. Stochastic effects include malignancy and genetic alterations.

3.2 Radiation Hazards

(A) Cancer

Evidence on the increased risk of malignancy associated with ionizing radiation exposure originates from epidemiological studies conducted on the atomic bomb survivors in Japan (Ozasa 2016). Shortly after the bombings, a high incidence of leukemia was noticed among survivors. For those exposed at a younger age (10 years), the risk of developing leukemia was 70 times higher. A decade after the bombings, an increased incidence of solid malignancies was also recorded and the risk of malignancy was dependent upon the individual dose exposure, such that the risk of developing a solid malignancy increased by 40–50% for each 1 Gy exposure (Ozasa 2016). These studies provided the evidence for the no threshold and linear dose–response relationship between radiation exposure and stochastic effects.

An increased risk of malignancy has also been reported after medical radiation exposure. This is largely based on cohort and case–control studies conducted on pediatric populations who underwent medical imaging. A meta-analysis conducted on these studies estimated the risk of malignancy associated with CT scan imaging in children and reported pooled excess relative risks of 26.9 per Gy for leukemia and 9.1 per Gy for brain tumors (Abalo et al. 2021). In fact, an increasing number of CT scans are being performed in both adults and children, such that up to 2% of malignancies in the United States may be attributable to the use of CT scans (Brenner and Hall 2007).

Similarly, physicians exposed to radiation and those performing radiation-guided interventions are at a higher risk of developing malignancies. In the United States, radiologists were found to have 38% higher all-cancer deaths compared to other specialists, and when analyzing leukemia specifically, the observed deaths were twice as many as expected (Yoshinaga et al. 2004). Radiation technologists were also found to have a higher incidence of leukemia, which was significantly associated with holding 50 or more patients during x-ray exams (relative risk 2.6) and working for five or more years before 1950 (relative risk 6.6) (Linet et al. 2005). The relationship between occupational radiation exposure among health professionals and the ensuing malignancy risk is further supported by the finding of a disproportionately high incidence of left-sided brain tumors among interventional radiologists. These right-handed interventionalists stand with the left side of the brain close to the source and subsequently receive much higher doses on that side (Roguin et al. 2013).

(B) DNA damage

Ionizing radiation can lead to DNA damage, including direct induction of double-strand DNA breaks. In fact, radiation-induced DNA damage leading to cell death forms the basis of radiation therapy for certain malignant neoplasms. However, not all radiation-induced DNA damage leads to cell death and if abnormal DNA accumulates or is inappropriately repaired, this may lead to consequences such as chromosomal abnormalities or malignancies.

One study measured the effects of acute radiation exposure on DNA among vascular surgeons and interventional radiologists after performing endovascular aortic repair (El-Sayed et al. 2017). In this study, all operators wore standard lead aprons and thyroid shields. After the procedure, blood samples from surgeons were collected. White blood cell markers of DNA damage and DNA repair were measured and were significantly elevated compared to baseline. A repeat test 24 hours later, revealed the markers had returned to baseline. During the same study, dosimeters placed on the surgeons' legs recorded significantly higher radiation exposures. A subset of surgeons was later asked to wear lower leg shields, and when doing so, there was no increase in DNA damage and repair markers after the procedure, suggesting that these leukocytes acquired DNA damage as they circulated in unshielded regions.

(C) *Cardiovascular disease*

Astronauts must be completely healthy with no medical comorbidities. Subsequently, it was not surprising that astronauts who have never flown or who flew low Earth orbital missions were significantly less likely to die of cardiovascular disease (CVD) compared to the age-matched general population. Conversely, the Apollo Lunar astronauts who flew into deep space had significantly higher CVD mortality compared to the other groups of astronauts (Delp et al. 2016). This may be attributed to the large amounts of cosmic radiation astronauts were exposed to when travelling beyond Earth's atmosphere.

Radiation can induce oxidative stress, increase inflammation, promote a profibrogenic state, and cause direct endothelial dysfunction (Meerman et al. 2021). This in turn may lead to accelerated atherosclerosis, ischemic heart disease, arrythmias, conduction defects, myocardial remodeling, cardiomyopathy, and heart failure.

Similarly, exposure to medical radiation can also increase the risk of CVD. Although medical imaging utilizes relatively less radiation than deep space travel, there is evidence of increased CVD with these smaller exposure levels, as demonstrated by a recent study on a large cohort of patients with tuberculosis who underwent repetitive fluoroscopy screenings (Tran et al. 2017). They reported approximately 25% higher excess relative risks per Gy for the development of all circulatory disease (p = 0.021) and for ischemic heart disease specifically (p = 0.048) among those exposed to cumulative radiation doses less than 0.5 Gy.

(D) *Thyroid disease*

Ionizing radiation is a known dose and age-related risk factor for developing thyroid cancer. Adults with low occupational radiation exposure have higher rates of thyroid cancer and a dose-related higher incidence of subclinical hypothyroidism (Luna-Sanchez et al. 2019).

(E) *Cataracts*

Occupational radiation exposure and its relationship to cataracts has been well documented. In one study, 52% of interventional cardiologists were found to have posterior lens opacities compared to 9% of controls, giving a significant relative risk of 5.7

(Ciraj-Bjelac et al. 2012). A similar high prevalence of 45% was also found among nurses working in interventional cardiology. A recent meta-analysis of 15 studies (n > 5,600), reported a 4.96 times greater risk of cataracts in the group with occupational radiation exposure (p < 0.00001) (Alhasan and Aalam 2022).

(F) *Skin Changes*

Patients receiving radiation therapy often experience radiation dermatitis, a common adverse effect due to the high amounts of exposure. Acute changes include desquamation, erythema, and hair loss, while chronic changes include atrophy, fibrosis, and pigmentation abnormalities (Hegedus et al. 2017). These skin changes are deterministic effects, which depend on the radiation dose received.

The exposures from medical imaging are unlikely to reach the threshold to cause radiation dermatitis similar to that seen in radiation therapy. However, recently more than 200 patients undergoing CT brain scans for the evaluation of stroke developed alopecia and skin burns in a single academic institution (Kuehn 2010). A subsequent FDA review found that the doses were increased to improve the image quality of the studies, with patient radiation exposure reaching up to 8 times greater than expected. Alarmingly, a review of regional hospitals found similar exposures in two other institutions. This led the US FDA to issue a white paper in 2010 specifically calling for a reduction in radiation exposure during CT scans, fluoroscopy, and nuclear medicine studies (United States Food and Drug Administration 2010).

In addition, surgeons who perform image-guided procedures with their hands under the direct radiation beam are exposed to relatively high doses for prolonged periods, leading to significant cumulative exposures. In fact, one study estimated that cumulative dose exposures to the dominant hand of urologists can reach levels up to 75 times higher than other regions (Park et al. 2021). In another study on orthopedic surgeons, high amounts of direct radiation exposure to the hands was associated with skin and nail pigmentation abnormalities (Fig. 1) (Asari et al. 2022).

(G) *Other Effects*

Ionizing radiation can affect any organ, however different organs have different susceptibilities and the effects depend on the dose and site of exposure. Radiation cystitis, radiation proctitis, and infertility are some effects of pelvic radiotherapy. Stomatitis, dysphagia, and alopecia are some effects of head and neck radiotherapy. Exposure to ionizing radiation may also trigger autoimmune diseases (Yahyapour et al. 2018), and chronic occupational exposure may lead to male infertility by causing damage to sperm DNA (Zhou et al. 2016). Surgeons with their hands in the direct radiation beam may experience hand joint pain and osteoarthritic changes (Willey et al. 2013).

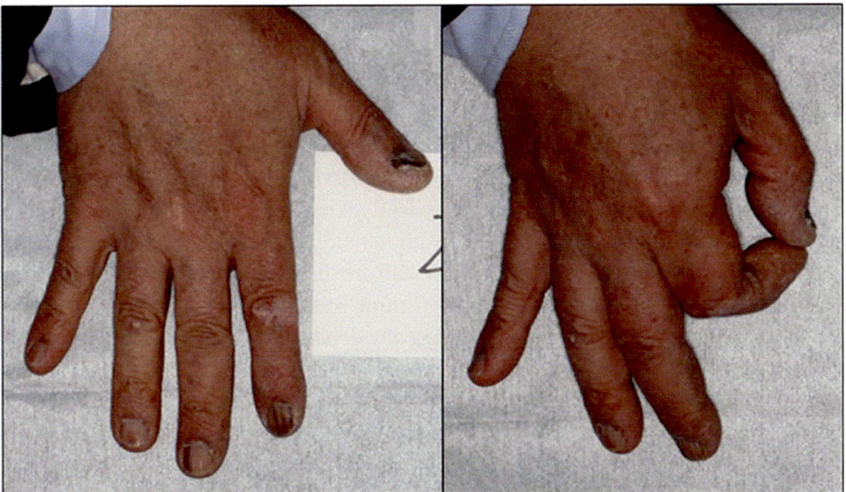

Fig. 1 Surgeon's hands demonstrating skin changes from occupational radiation exposure. These include nail discoloration, depigmentation, hyperkeratosis, and papules. Figure reproduced from Asari et al. (2022). With permission from Elsevier

3.3 Exposure Limits

To control radiation exposure and minimize harms, the International Commission on Radiological Protection (ICRP) has set occupational limits to an effective dose of 20 mSv per year, averaged over 5 years (no more than 100 mSv over 5 years) and also states the effective dose should not exceed 50 mSv annually (International Commission on Radiological Protection (ICRP) Guidance for Occupational Exposure 2023). The United States Nuclear Regulatory Commission (NRC) also sets whole body effective dose to 50 mSv per year (United States Nuclear Regulatory Commision Occupational Dose Limits 2023). These exposure limits are occupational upper limits. Furthermore, there are no guidelines regarding patient medical radiation exposure limits, but the goal should be to keep exposure as low as reasonably achievable (ALARA).

4 Radiation in Stone Disease—Diagnosis and Pre-operative Use

Patients with nephrolithiasis often undergo imaging to establish the diagnosis and plan for surgical intervention. The three most commonly used modalities are CT scan, kidney ureter bladder (KUB), and ultrasound (US).

The estimated radiation exposure to a patient from a single KUB is 0.7 mSv (Brisbane et al. 2016). However, a KUB film has low reported sensitivity (57%) in diagnosing nephrolithiasis and a specificity of 76% (Brisbane et al. 2016). A KUB is limited in that it only detects stones from a single angle and cannot visualize all stone types, including uric acid, cystine, and struvite stones.

US does not utilize ionizing radiation and is relatively inexpensive. There is marked variation in the reported sensitivity (45–84%) and specificity (53–94%) of US as a diagnostic modality (Brisbane et al. 2016). This may be attributed to the user-dependent nature of US imaging, as well as many factors which might affect image production including stone size, echogenicity, and patient body habitus.

CT scans have become widely available and are the most commonly used imaging modality for investigating urinary stones (Smith-Bindman et al. 2014). Up to three-quarters of patients presenting to the emergency department with flank pain or hematuria may receive CT imaging (Broder et al. 2007). CT has the highest sensitivity (95%) and specificity (98%) for detecting renal stones (Brisbane et al. 2016). It is able to detect almost all stone types, can provide multi-dimensional information regarding stone burden, and information regarding stone density. It also provides important anatomic information regarding the location of surrounding organs and the lungs, and detailed anatomic positions of the stones in three dimensions that can assist the surgeon in selecting the site of access prior to PCNL. Conversely, it is 10 times more expensive than a KUB and exposes patients to almost 15 times more radiation, at an average effective dose of 10–20 mSv per CT scan (Brisbane et al. 2016; Smith-Bindman et al. 2009). It is estimated that a single conventional non-contrast CT will lead to 1 in 1000 patients developing a fatal malignancy (Jellison et al. 2009).

Given the relative affordability of US and lack of radiation, the European Association of Urology (EAU) recommends US as the first diagnostic imaging modality for patients presenting with a picture suggestive of nephrolithiasis and recommends CT scan for confirmation of nephrolithiasis after the initial ultrasound (Skolarikos et al. 2022). The American Urological Association (AUA) guidelines for surgical management of stones recommend clinicians order a non-contrast CT scan prior to performing PCNL (Assimos et al. 2016). They also suggest clinicians order CT scans in stone patients to help determine the best management option when deciding between shock-wave lithotripsy (SWL) and ureteroscopy (URS).

Reducing radiation during evaluation of stone patients:

Safe radiation practices start from the time of patient presentation with a clinical picture suggestive of a urinary stone. Emergency care and primary care providers should be judicious in their selection of the appropriate diagnostic tests and imaging modality based on their clinical evaluation of the patient. In a multicenter prospective study (n = 2759), patients presenting to the emergency department with flank or abdominal pain were randomized to undergo either CT scan, formal US, or point-of-care US (Smith-Bindman et al. 2014). All three groups had similar adverse events and emergency department returns, but the two US groups had 40–46% lower radiation exposure compared to the CT group (p < 0.001).

If a CT scan is desired or indicated based on clinical judgement, the radiation exposure can be reduced by lowering the mAs or kVp. Low dose CT scans utilize settings to deliver < 3–4 mSv to the patient while maintaining diagnostic accuracy for urinary stones, with a meta-analysis including seven studies reporting pooled sensitivity and specificity of 97% and 95% respectively (Niemann et al. 2008). Ultra-low dose CT scans deliver doses less than 1–2 mSv and have also been reported to have satisfactory diagnostic ability for stones > 4 mm in size (Pooler et al. 2014). A cadaveric study, with blinded radiologists showed that reducing the mAs (140 to 7.5) resulted in no change in sensitivity and specificity in detecting calcium oxalate stones and resulted in a 95% reduction in radiation exposure (Fig. 2) (Jellison et al. 2009).

The main drawback of lowering the CT scan dose is a decline in the sensitivity and specificity for stone detection in patients who are overweight or underweight. The diagnostic accuracy of ultra-low dose CT scan ($\leq$ 7.5 mAs) was found to be significantly lower with high and low body weights compared to average weight, however when the mAs was increased to 15, the diagnostic accuracy was similar (Heldt et al. 2012). Reconstruction algorithms can also affect the image produced and alter the diagnostic ability of low dose CT scans. It has been reported that iterative image reconstruction is preferable for diagnosing stones in overweight patients using low dose CT scans (Chang et al. 2019). One exception to the performance of ultra-low dose CT would be a suspected infected obstructed stone, where the 20% mortality of urosepsis trumps the 0.1% risk of mortality from the conventional CT scan (Borofsky

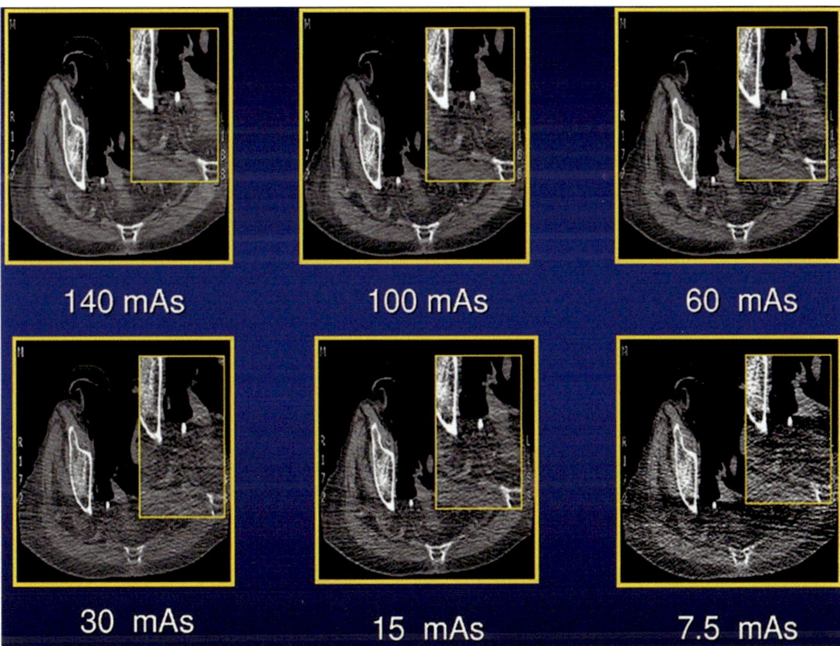

Fig. 2 Comparison of imaging between conventional 140 mAs CT with low and ultra-low dose CT settings. Figure reproduced from Jellison et al. (2009). With permission from Wolters Kluwer

et al. 2013). Also, patients with metal implants or hardware provide suboptimal picture quality with ultra-low dose CT due to the hardware-induced noise.

5 Radiation in Stone Disease—Intra-Operative Use

After diagnosing nephrolithiasis, surgical management may be indicated including SWL, URS, or PCNL. All of these approaches require image guidance, and fluoroscopy has commonly been used. Fluoroscopy is used to localize stones for SWL, and is used for stone localization and to guide insertion of wires and instruments in retrograde intrarenal surgery. For PCNL, image guidance is particularly crucial for establishing percutaneous access into the renal collecting system, which is also commonly performed under fluoroscopic guidance. During PCNL, fluoroscopy is also used to insert guidewires, for tract dilation, sheath insertion, identifying renal and surrounding anatomy, evaluating for residual stones, and stent or nephrostomy tube placement. One study reported a mean effective dose of 8.66 mSv from fluoroscopic radiation exposure during PCNL (Mancini et al. 2010). It is at this stage that surgeons may be exposed to both direct and scatter radiation. More recently, use of intraoperative CT scan as a surgical adjunct to confirm stone-free status has been reported (Patel et al. 2022). Use of conventional CT intraoperatively could substantially increase radiation exposure.

5.1 Fluoroscopy Settings and Doses

The radiation dose from fluoroscopy depends on: (1) the amount of radiation produced by the machine, measured in milliamperes (mA); and (2) the energy of the x-ray produced, reflecting its ability to penetrate objects, which is measured as the kilovoltage peak (kVp). The standard fluoroscopy machine setting is automatic exposure control (AEC), which automatically adjusts mA and kVp to optimize image quality.

5.2 Factors Affecting Radiation Dose During PCNL

Several studies have investigated factors which affect radiation doses during urologic procedures. Mancini et al. reported significantly higher effective dose during PCNL with increased BMI (p < 0.0001), greater stone burden (p = 0.04), and more access tracts (p = 0.024) (Mancini et al. 2010). Balaji et al. examined surgeon radiation exposure during PCNL and also reported significantly higher exposures with larger stone burden, multiple tracts, larger sheath size, and lower stone Hounsfield units (Balaji et al. 2019).

Although many of the above factors are beyond the control of the treating surgeon, it is important to consider their potential contribution to higher radiation exposure. In contrast, there are many factors which are directly under the control of the surgeon, including machine settings, shielding, collimation, positioning, and surgical technique.

5.3 Reducing Radiation During PCNL

(A) Fluoroscopy settings and use

The standard fluoroscopy mode is AEC, which uses continuous fluoroscopy at 30 pulses per second (pps), and continuously adjusts the mA and kVp to optimize image quality. However, many tasks during PCNL do not require optimal image quality, including confirming the position of guidewires, endoscopes, nephrostomies, and stents. For these tasks, where optimal image quality is not required, the surgeon can manually adjust the mA, kVp, pulse rate, and employ the "low dose" modality. Depression of the "low dose" button (Fig. 3) which is present on most modern c-arms has been shown to cut radiation exposure by more than half (Yecies et al. 2018).

Canales et al. compared radiation exposures and outcomes of PCNL between standard AEC (30 pps) and a protocol where the pulse rate was cut to 12 pps and the dose output was cut in half. They reduced the mean radiation exposure from 35.5 to 23.9 mGy (p < 0.001) (Canales et al. 2016). In their study, no patient required conversion from the reduced radiation protocol back to AEC, and the outcomes were similar.

In addition to altering the output dose and pulse rate, other settings on the fluoroscopy machine can also be employed to reduce radiation. Using a second screen with last image hold allows the surgeon to review the image without the use of live fluoroscopy (Mitchell and Furey 2011). Surgeon, instead of technician, fluoroscopy

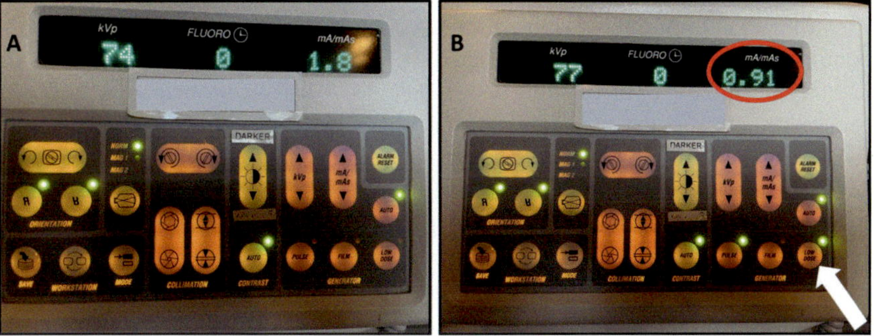

Fig. 3 (A) C-arm settings in standard automatic exposure control. (B) Depression of the low dose button (white arrow) results in reduction of dose output by half as reflected by the mA (red circle)

activation can also reduce radiation dose by eliminating unnecessary pedal activation. Another technique which significantly reduces radiation exposure is the use of collimation. In collimation, the x-ray beam leaving the source is narrowed to limit the field of exposure to only the areas of interest. Collimation is associated with improved image quality and reduced scatter radiation (Mitchell and Furey 2011).

(B) *Positioning and Set-Up*

C-arm positioning is crucial and can affect radiation dose (Mitchell and Furey 2011). Keeping the source underneath the patient reduces the scatter to staff members in the operating room (Harris 2018). When the x-ray source is close to the patient, the entrance dose will be higher. Subsequently, it is important to keep the x-ray source as far away from the patient as possible. In other words, the image intensifier or flat panel detector should be as close to the patient as possible. In addition, all staff should stand as far from the source as possible while completing their tasks. According to the inverse square law (dose $\propto$ 1/distance^2), if the distance from the source is doubled, the radiation dose is cut to a fourth (Le Heron et al. 2010). Non-essential personnel can step out of the room when fluoroscopy is in use.

Some c-arms come equipped with a laser pointer which will allow positioning of the c-arm without fluoroscopy activation. Markings on the drape can help with instrument location and depth, minimizing the need to use imaging to confirm placement. Markings on the drape or the floor can also be used to guide the technician in positioning the c-arm appropriately, minimizing "trial-and-error" in obtaining the desired image.

(C) *Surgical technique*

Modification of surgical techniques can further reduce the need for fluoroscopy. For example, in many steps of the procedure, relying on tactile feedback can decrease the need for imaging. Guidewires and the ureteroscope can be positioned using tactile feedback, reducing the need for fluoroscopy (Blair et al. 2013). Positioning of the surgeons' hands and equipment out of the primary beam can also reduce radiation exposure (Hajiha et al. 2019).

During PCNL, ancillary techniques have been developed that can reduce the requirement for fluoroscopy while obtaining percutaneous renal access. These modifications include use of ultrasound, endoscopic, laser, and electromagnetic guidance. US is extremely effective in locating the lung, pleura, and surrounding organs. US can also assess depth to the calyx of interest and aid in needle selection. Many authors have reported use of US to facilitate renal access and some have even performed PCNL completely under US guidance (Fig. 4A) (Emiliani et al. 2020).

Use of ureteroscopy in an endoscopic combined intrarenal approach (ECIRS) for access, can further reduce radiation as it will allow direct visual confirmation of needle position (Fig. 4B). Small corrections in needle position can be made under direct visualization. Similarly, balloon dilation and sheath insertion can be performed under direct vision to allow precise positioning that is not possible using fluoroscopy. A study comparing conventional fluoroscopic access to combined US and endoscopic

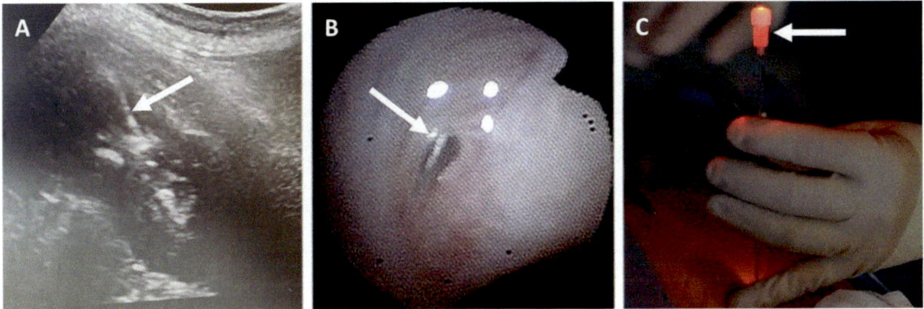

Fig. 4 (A) Ultrasound-guided access with needle seen entering kidney (arrow). (B) Endoscopic-guided access with tip of needle seen entering renal calyx (arrow). (C) Laser-guided access with laser glow seen at end of needle to maintain alignment (arrow)

access for PCNL reported 99% lower total fluoroscopy times, with similar outcomes in terms of complication and stone-free rates (Alsyouf et al. 2016).

The laser direct alignment radiation reduction technique (DARRT) is a hybrid technique which employs US and laser guidance. US is used to identify surrounding structures and the laser beam on the image intensifier is used to guide and maintain needle orientation during insertion (Fig. 4C), without the need for continuous fluoroscopic guidance. This has also been reported to significantly reduce fluoroscopy time (Khater et al. 2016).

Finally, a new robotic platform has recently become available which uses electromagnetic-guided percutaneous access. This device has just been approved by the FDA and may show promise for reducing radiation exposure to both patients and surgeons.

(D) *Shielding*

Use of lead shielding by medical personnel can significantly reduce their radiation exposure by more than 90% (Ong et al. 2021). These include aprons, vests and kilts, thyroid shields, and goggles. Given the availability of these personal protective equipment, it is expected that healthcare workers will take all necessary precautions to minimize harms to themselves, however a recent European study reported that although more than 99% wear aprons, only 52% wear thyroid shields, and only 7% wear lead glasses (Ong et al. 2021). In addition, maintaining the condition of these protective garments, with proper storage and periodic checks on their efficacy is also important to ensure maximal radiation protection. Other protective shields may also include under-table shields, table skirts, suspended shields, and portable rolling shields.

(E) *Awareness*

Awareness of radiation safety and reduction techniques has been demonstrated to cut fluoroscopy time in half (Weld et al. 2014). In one study, almost 44% of operating room staff working with radiation, reported receiving no training on radiation safety

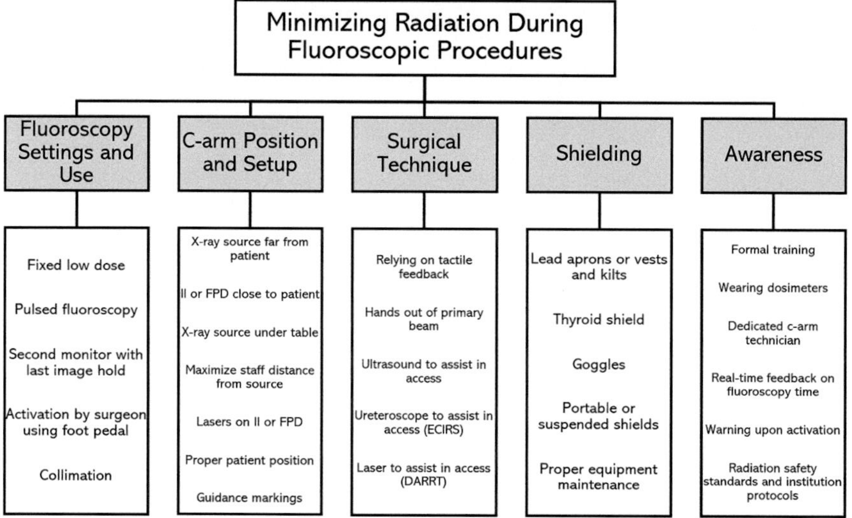

Fig. 5 Measures to reduce intraoperative radiation exposure. Abbreviations: DARRT: direct alignment radiation reduction technique; ECIRS: endoscopic combined intrarenal surgery; FPD: flat panel detector; II: image intensifier

(Ong et al. 2021). It is imperative that staff utilizing fluoroscopy are aware of its potential risks and strategies for reducing these risks. Surgeons and other staff, especially those who work in high volume centers, should also wear dosimeters to keep track of their cumulative exposures. Use of dedicated radiology technicians, who know how to calibrate, orient, and maneuver the c-arm, provides optimal images at the lowest radiation possible.

Keeping track of radiation during the procedure can help focus the surgeon's attention on reducing radiation exposure. This includes providing real time feedback to the surgeon on fluoroscopy time used, verbal warning by the surgeon to other personnel when fluoroscopy will be activated, and developing institutional protocols and standards to limit radiation. Figure 5 summarizes many different strategies that can be employed to reduce radiation during PCNL.

6 Radiation in Stone Disease—Follow-Up

After PCNL and other stone procedures, it is important to ensure there are no residual fragments which can subsequently lead to complications such as infection, dislodgement, obstruction, or growth and recurrence of stones. Post-operative imaging is also important to make sure there is no obstruction or hydronephrosis. There is no unanimous consensus on the appropriate imaging after PCNL, however similar to its use for diagnosis, CT scan has the highest sensitivity in detecting residual fragments, with a reported sensitivity of 100% compared to direct flexible nephroscopy (Pearle et al. 1999).

The AUA guidelines do not make explicit recommendations regarding follow-up of patients who underwent PCNL or other stone surgeries (Assimos et al. 2016). They do, however, recommend follow-up for stone patients managed by observation, but do not recommend a specific imaging modality or frequency. The EAU do make recommendations on follow-up after surgical treatment and give recommended durations and frequencies for imaging, depending on the presence of residual fragments post-operatively, the size of the residual fragments, and patient risk stratification (Skolarikos et al. 2022). The EAU also proposes KUB, US, or a combination of both as the imaging modality for follow-up, unless a patient becomes symptomatic, for which a CT scan should be ordered.

Reducing radiation for follow-up:

Ordering a low dose or ultra-low dose CT scan after PCNL to check for residual fragments or obstruction is an appropriate alternative to full dose CT scan. Similar to pre-operative and diagnostic use, deciding on the appropriate follow-up imaging should consider all patient factors and risks, while keeping radiation safety principles in mind. One should only order imaging studies with ionizing radiation that will affect management.

7 Special Populations

7.1 Children

Although the general approach to managing stone disease in children while maintaining radiation safety precautions is fairly similar to adults, clinicians should remember that because of their younger age and smaller body habitus, children are at a significantly higher risk for malignancy.

One recent study quantified the radiation dose for pediatric PCNL and reported a median fluoroscopy time of 11.7 minutes, with an estimated effective dose of 16.8 mSv (Ristau et al. 2015). One unique concern in children is the technical challenge in inserting the sheath, which may require additional fluoroscopy. This can be minimized by using retrograde ureteroscopic guidance for tract dilation and sheath insertion. Another study reported that the mean effective dose of an abdomen-pelvic CT scan in a child ranged from 10.6 to 14.8 mSv, with up to 25% of children receiving doses greater that 20 mSv (Miglioretti et al. 2013). When adding these numbers up, the exposure to a child undergoing preoperative CT scan, PCNL, and postoperative CT scan may surpass the annual occupational exposure limit for an adult.

With regards to guidelines on managing stones in the pediatric population, the AUA recommends obtaining a low dose CT scan if PCNL is planned (Assimos et al. 2016), while the EAU recommends US as the initial diagnostic test, followed by a KUB or a low dose CT if needed (Skolarikos et al. 2022).

7.2 Pregnancy

Developing fetuses are particularly susceptible to ionizing radiation. For diagnostic purposes, the EAU recommends US, followed by magnetic resonance imaging (MRI) if needed, with low dose CT scan being a last resort after careful consideration (Assimos et al. 2016). First-line management should be observation, with URS being a possible alternative should observation fail (Skolarikos et al. 2022). For pregnant women with stones, PCNL and SWL are contraindicated.

Pregnant surgeons and healthcare workers should be vigilant regarding the cumulative radiation dose they are exposed to and ensure all safety measures are in place, as the occupational exposure limit to the fetus during the entire pregnancy is set by the IRCP at 1 mGy (International Commission on Radiological Protection (ICRP) 2000).

8 Clinical Scenarios

Case A: Mr. Smith is a 55-year-old man who presented to the urgent care with right flank pain and hematuria. A conventional CT scan of the abdomen and pelvis was ordered and revealed a 3 cm right renal pelvic stone. Mr. Smith was referred to a urologist and PCNL was performed under fluoroscopy guidance with no radiation reduction protocols. The total fluoroscopy time was 9 minutes. A follow-up conventional CT scan was ordered on postoperative day 1 and revealed no residual fragments and a successful procedure. The total radiation doses received by Mr. Smith during the management of his stone were calculated and yielded: 16 mSv from preoperative CT scan, 6.3 mSv from intraoperative fluoroscopy, and 12 mSv from postoperative CT scan. Total radiation exposure was 34.3 mSv.

Case B: Mr. Jones is a 62-year-old man who presented to the urgent care with left flank pain. A renal ultrasound was ordered and revealed a large stone in the left kidney. Upon referral to a urologist trained in radiation safety, a low-dose CT scan was ordered for planning before PCNL. PCNL was then performed using a low-radiation protocol and combined access with ultrasound, laser, and endoscopic guidance, giving a total fluoroscopy time of 10 seconds. To ensure complete stone removal and no obstruction, an ultra-low dose CT scan confirmed the stone-free status. Mr. Jones received no radiation during ultrasound, 3.3 mSv from preoperative CT, 0.17 mSv from intraoperative fluoroscopy, and 1.1 mSv from postoperative CT scan. Total radiation exposure was 4.57 mSv.

When calculating the total radiation received during the stone episode, Mr. Smith received 7.5 times more ionizing radiation than Mr. Jones, yet both underwent similar procedures that resulted in similar favorable outcomes. Implementing radiation safety practices is essential, particularly in stone patients who may have recurrent episodes and may require repeat imaging and additional image-guided procedures. In one study, the radiation exposure received by stone patients over one year was quantified and was reported to be a median annual total effective dose of 29.7 mSv per patient, with one in five patients receiving radiation doses greater than the annual occupational limit (> 50 mSv) (Ferrandino et al. 2009). What is even more striking, is that these large values were calculated only from imaging studies and did not include radiation exposures from any operative procedures.

9 Summary of Key Points

- Radiation is important for diagnostic imaging and procedural guidance in endourology but can lead to high exposure levels to both patients and surgeons.
- High radiation exposure has been associated with an increased risk of malignancy, DNA damage, cardiovascular disease, thyroid disorders, cataracts, skin disease, and other health hazards.
- Use of low dose or ultra-low dose non-contrast CT scan is a suitable alternative to standard CT in most patients and minimizes radiation exposure without compromising sensitivity and specificity for diagnosis and follow-up of urolithiasis.
- Fluoroscopy settings and positioning that can lower radiation include pulsed mode, low dose settings, collimation, last image hold, surgeon foot pedal activation, x-ray source as far as possible from the patient, source below patient, and use of lasers and markings to guide c-arm positioning.
- Use of ultrasound, ECIRS, laser, or electromagnetic guidance during percutaneous renal access can significantly reduce the fluoroscopy needed, while ensuring safety and efficacy.
- Use of lead shielding, tracking radiation times, staff awareness and education are important to reduce radiation exposure.
- The concept of ALARA, as low as reasonably achievable, should be followed in everyday practice.

References

Abalo KD, Rage E, Leuraud K, Richardson DB, Le Pointe HD, Laurier D, et al. Early life ionizing radiation exposure and cancer risks: systematic review and meta-analysis. Pediatr Radiol. 2021;51(1):45–56. https://doi.org/10.1007/s00247-020-04803-0.

Alhasan AS, Aalam WA. Eye lens opacities and cataracts among physicians and healthcare workers occupationally exposed to radiation: a systematic review and meta-analysis. Saudi Med J. 2022;43(7):665–77. https://doi.org/10.15537/smj.2022.43.7.20220022.

Alsyouf M, Arenas JL, Smith JC, Myklak K, Faaborg D, Jang M, et al. Direct endoscopic visualization combined with ultrasound guided access during percutaneous nephrolithotomy: a feasibility study and comparison to a conventional cohort. J Urol. 2016;196(1):227–33. https://doi.org/10.1016/j.juro.2016.01.118.

Anon. Edison fears hidden perils of the X-Rays. New York World; 1903.

Asari T, Rokunohe D, Sasaki E, Kaneko T, Kumagai G, Wada K, et al. Occupational ionizing radiation-induced skin injury among orthopedic surgeons: A clinical survey. J Orthop Sci. 2022;27(1):266–71. https://doi.org/10.1016/j.jos.2020.11.008.

Assimos D, Krambeck A, Miller NL, Monga M, Murad MH, Nelson CP, et al. Surgical management of stones: American urological association/endourological society guideline. PART II J Urol. 2016;196(4):1161–9. https://doi.org/10.1016/j.juro.2016.05.091.

Balaji SS, Vijayakumar M, Singh AG, Ganpule AP, Sabnis RB, Desai MR. Analysis of factors affecting radiation exposure during percutaneous nephrolithotomy procedures. BJU Int. 2019;124(3):514–21. https://doi.org/10.1111/bju.14833.

Berrington de Gonzalez A, Mahesh M, Kim KP, Bhargavan M, Lewis R, Mettler F, et al. Projected cancer risks from computed tomographic scans performed in the United States in 2007. Arch Intern Med. 2009;169(22):2071–7. https://doi.org/10.1001/archinternmed.2009.440.

Blair B, Huang G, Arnold D, Li R, Schlaifer A, Anderson K, et al. Reduced fluoroscopy protocol for percutaneous nephrostolithotomy: feasibility, outcomes and effects on fluoroscopy time. J Urol. 2013;190(6):2112–6. https://doi.org/10.1016/j.juro.2013.05.114.

Borofsky MS, Walter D, Shah O, Goldfarb DS, Mues AC, Makarov DV. Surgical decompression is associated with decreased mortality in patients with sepsis and ureteral calculi. J Urol. 2013;189(3):946–51. https://doi.org/10.1016/j.juro.2012.09.088.

Brenner DJ, Hall EJ. Computed tomography–an increasing source of radiation exposure. N Engl J Med. 2007;357(22):2277–84. https://doi.org/10.1056/NEJMra072149.

Brisbane W, Bailey MR, Sorensen MD. An overview of kidney stone imaging techniques. Nat Rev Urol. 2016;13(11):654–62. https://doi.org/10.1038/nrurol.2016.154.

Broder J, Bowen J, Lohr J, Babcock A, Yoon J. Cumulative CT exposures in emergency department patients evaluated for suspected renal colic. J Emerg Med. 2007;33(2):161–8. https://doi.org/10.1016/j.jemermed.2006.12.035.

Canales BK, Sinclair L, Kang D, Mench AM, Arreola M, Bird VG. Changing default fluoroscopy equipment settings decreases entrance skin dose in patients. J Urol. 2016;195(4 Pt 1):992–7. https://doi.org/10.1016/j.juro.2015.10.088.

Chang DH, Slebocki K, Khristenko E, Herden J, Salem J, Grosse Hokamp N, et al. Low-dose computed tomography of urolithiasis in obese patients: a feasibility study to evaluate image reconstruction algorithms. Diabetes Metab Syndr Obes. 2019;12:439–45. https://doi.org/10.2147/DMSO.S198641.

Ciraj-Bjelac O, Rehani M, Minamoto A, Sim KH, Liew HB, Vano E. Radiation-induced eye lens changes and risk for cataract in interventional cardiology. Cardiology. 2012;123(3):168–71. https://doi.org/10.1159/000342458.

Delp MD, Charvat JM, Limoli CL, Globus RK, Ghosh P. Apollo lunar astronauts show higher cardiovascular disease mortality: possible deep space radiation effects on the vascular endothelium. Sci Rep. 2016;6:29901. https://doi.org/10.1038/srep29901.

Donya M, Radford M, ElGuindy A, Firmin D, Yacoub MH. Radiation in medicine: origins, risks and aspirations. Glob Cardiol Sci Pract. 2014;2014(4):437–48. https://doi.org/10.5339/gcsp.201 4.57.

El-Sayed T, Patel AS, Cho JS, Kelly JA, Ludwinski FE, Saha P, et al. Radiation-induced DNA damage in operators performing endovascular aortic repair. Circulation. 2017;136(25):2406–16. https://doi.org/10.1161/CIRCULATIONAHA.117.029550.

Emiliani E, Kanashiro A, Chi T, Perez-Fentes DA, Manzo BO, Angerri O, et al. Fluoroless endourological surgery for stone disease: a review of the literature-tips and tricks. Curr Urol Rep. 2020;21(7):27. https://doi.org/10.1007/s11934-020-00979-y.

Ferrandino MN, Bagrodia A, Pierre SA, Scales CD, Jr., Rampersaud E, Pearle MS, et al. Radiation exposure in the acute and short-term management of urolithiasis at 2 academic centers. J Urol. 2009;181(2):668–72; discussion 73. https://doi.org/10.1016/j.juro.2008.10.012.

Hajiha M, Smith J, Amasyali AS, Groegler J, Shah M, Alsyouf M, et al. The effect of operative field instrument clutter during intraoperative fluoroscopy on radiation exposure. J Endourol. 2019;33(8):626–33. https://doi.org/10.1089/end.2019.0285.

Harris AM. Radiation exposure to the urologist using an overcouch radiation source compared with an undercouch radiation source in contemporary urology practice. Urology. 2018;114:45–8. https://doi.org/10.1016/j.urology.2017.12.011.

Hegedus F, Mathew LM, Schwartz RA. Radiation dermatitis: an overview. Int J Dermatol. 2017;56(9):909–14. https://doi.org/10.1111/ijd.13371.

Heldt JP, Smith JC, Anderson KM, Richards GD, Agarwal G, Smith DL, et al. Ureteral calculi detection using low dose computerized tomography protocols is compromised in overweight and underweight patients. J Urol. 2012;188(1):124–9. https://doi.org/10.1016/j.juro.2012.02. 2568.

International Commission on Radiological Protection (ICRP) Guidance for Occupational Exposure. https://remm.hhs.gov/ICRP_guidelines.htm Accessed 15 Feb 2023.

International Commission on Radiological Protection (ICRP). Pregnancy and Medical Radiation; 2000.

Jellison FC, Smith JC, Heldt JP, Spengler NM, Nicolay LI, Ruckle HC, et al. Effect of low dose radiation computerized tomography protocols on distal ureteral calculus detection. J Urol. 2009;182(6):2762–7. https://doi.org/10.1016/j.juro.2009.08.042.

Khater N, Shen J, Arenas J, Keheila M, Alsyouf M, Martin JA, et al. Bench-top feasibility testing of a novel percutaneous renal access technique: the laser direct alignment radiation reduction technique (DARRT). J Endourol. 2016;30(11):1155–60. https://doi.org/10.1089/end.2016.0170.

Kuehn BM. FDA warning: CT scans exceeded proper doses. JAMA. 2010;303(2):124. https://doi. org/10.1001/jama.2009.1906.

Le Heron J, Padovani R, Smith I, Czarwinski R. Radiation protection of medical staff. Eur J Radiol. 2010;76(1):20–3. https://doi.org/10.1016/j.ejrad.2010.06.034.

Linet MS, Freedman DM, Mohan AK, Doody MM, Ron E, Mabuchi K, et al. Incidence of haematopoietic malignancies in US radiologic technologists. Occup Environ Med. 2005;62(12):861–7. https://doi.org/10.1136/oem.2005.020826.

Luna-Sanchez S, Del Campo MT, Moran JV, Fernandez IM, Checa FJS, de la Hoz RE. Thyroid function in health care workers exposed to ionizing radiation. Health Phys. 2019;117(4):403–7. https://doi.org/10.1097/HP.0000000000001071.

Mancini JG, Raymundo EM, Lipkin M, Zilberman D, Yong D, Banez LL, et al. Factors affecting patient radiation exposure during percutaneous nephrolithotomy. J Urol. 2010;184(6):2373–7. https://doi.org/10.1016/j.juro.2010.08.033.

Meerman M, Bracco Gartner TCL, Buikema JW, Wu SM, Siddiqi S, Bouten CVC, et al. Myocardial disease and long-distance space travel: solving the radiation problem. Front Cardiovasc Med. 2021;8: 631985. https://doi.org/10.3389/fcvm.2021.631985.

Miglioretti DL, Johnson E, Williams A, Greenlee RT, Weinmann S, Solberg LI, et al. The use of computed tomography in pediatrics and the associated radiation exposure and estimated cancer risk. JAMA Pediatr. 2013;167(8):700–7. https://doi.org/10.1001/jamapediatrics.2013.311.

Mitchell EL, Furey P. Prevention of radiation injury from medical imaging. J Vasc Surg. 2011;53(1 Suppl):22S-7Shttps://doi.org/10.1016/j.jvs.2010.05.139

Niemann T, Kollmann T, Bongartz G. Diagnostic performance of low-dose CT for the detection of urolithiasis: a meta-analysis. AJR Am J Roentgenol. 2008;191(2):396–401. https://doi.org/10.2214/AJR.07.3414.

Ong K, Warren H, Nalagatla S, Kmiotek E, Obasi C, Shanmugathas N, et al. Radiation safety knowledge and practice in urology theaters: a collaborative multicenter survey. J Endourol. 2021;35(7):1084–9. https://doi.org/10.1089/end.2020.0955.

Ozasa K. Epidemiological research on radiation-induced cancer in atomic bomb survivors. J Radiat Res. 2016;57 Suppl 1:i112-i7. https://doi.org/10.1093/jrr/rrw005

Park IW, Kim SJ, Shin D, Shim SR, Chang HK, Kim CH. Radiation exposure to the urology surgeon during retrograde intrarenal surgery. PLoS ONE. 2021;16(3): e0247833. https://doi.org/10.1371/journal.pone.0247833.

Patel PM, Kandabarow AM, Chuang E, McKenzie K, Druck A, Seffren C, et al. Using Intraoperative Portable CT Scan to Minimize Reintervention Rates in Percutaneous Nephrolithotomy: a Prospective Trial. J Endourol. 2022;36(10):1382–7. https://doi.org/10.1089/end.2022.0049.

Pearle MS, Watamull LM, Mullican MA. Sensitivity of noncontrast helical computerized tomography and plain film radiography compared to flexible nephroscopy for detecting residual fragments after percutaneous nephrostolithotomy. J Urol. 1999;162(1):23–6. https://doi.org/10.1097/00005392-199907000-00006.

Pooler BD, Lubner MG, Kim DH, Ryckman EM, Sivalingam S, Tang J, et al. Prospective trial of the detection of urolithiasis on ultralow dose (sub mSv) noncontrast computerized tomography: direct comparison against routine low dose reference standard. J Urol. 2014;192(5):1433–9. https://doi.org/10.1016/j.juro.2014.05.089.

Ristau BT, Dudley AG, Casella DP, Dwyer ME, Fox JA, Cannon GM, et al. Tracking of radiation exposure in pediatric stone patients: The time is now. J Pediatr Urol. 2015;11(6):339 e1–5. https://doi.org/10.1016/j.jpurol.2015.08.008.

Roguin A, Goldstein J, Bar O, Goldstein JA. Brain and neck tumors among physicians performing interventional procedures. Am J Cardiol. 2013;111(9):1368–72. https://doi.org/10.1016/j.amjcard.2012.12.060.

Skolarikos A, Neisius A, Petřík A, Somani B, Thomas K, Gambaro G. EAU guidelines on urolithiasis. EAU Guidelines Edn Presented at the EAU Annual Congress Amsterdam; 2022.

Smith-Bindman R, Lipson J, Marcus R, Kim KP, Mahesh M, Gould R, et al. Radiation dose associated with common computed tomography examinations and the associated lifetime attributable risk of cancer. Arch Intern Med. 2009;169(22):2078–86. https://doi.org/10.1001/archinternmed.2009.427.

Smith-Bindman R, Aubin C, Bailitz J, Bengiamin RN, Camargo CA Jr, Corbo J, et al. Ultrasonography versus computed tomography for suspected nephrolithiasis. N Engl J Med. 2014;371(12):1100–10. https://doi.org/10.1056/NEJMoa1404446.

Tran V, Zablotska LB, Brenner AV, Little MP. Radiation-associated circulatory disease mortality in a pooled analysis of 77,275 patients from the Massachusetts and Canadian tuberculosis fluoroscopy cohorts. Sci Rep. 2017;7:44147. https://doi.org/10.1038/srep44147.

United States Food and Drug Administration. Initiative to Reduce Unnecessary Radiation Exposure from Medical Imaging. 2010.

United States Nuclear Regulatory Commision Occupational Dose Limits. https://www.nrc.gov/reading-rm/doc collections/cfr/part020/part020-1201.html Accessed 15 Feb 2023

Weld LR, Nwoye UO, Knight RB, Baumgartner TS, Ebertowski JS, Stringer MT, et al. Safety, minimization, and awareness radiation training reduces fluoroscopy time during unilateral ureteroscopy. Urology. 2014;84(3):520–5. https://doi.org/10.1016/j.urology.2014.03.035.

Willey JS, Long DL, Vanderman KS, Loeser RF. Ionizing radiation causes active degradation and reduces matrix synthesis in articular cartilage. Int J Radiat Biol. 2013;89(4):268–77. https://doi.org/10.3109/09553002.2013.747015.

Yahyapour R, Amini P, Rezapour S, Cheki M, Rezaeyan A, Farhood B, et al. Radiation-induced inflammation and autoimmune diseases. Mil Med Res. 2018;5(1):9. https://doi.org/10.1186/s40779-018-0156-7.

Yecies T, Averch TD, Semins MJ. Identifying and managing the risks of medical ionizing radiation in endourology. Can J Urol. 2018;25(1):9154–60.

Yoshinaga S, Mabuchi K, Sigurdson AJ, Doody MM, Ron E. Cancer risks among radiologists and radiologic technologists: review of epidemiologic studies. Radiology. 2004;233(2):313–21. https://doi.org/10.1148/radiol.2332031119.

Zhou DD, Hao JL, Guo KM, Lu CW, Liu XD. Sperm quality and DNA damage in men from Jilin Province, China, who are occupationally exposed to ionizing radiation. Genet Mol Res. 2016;15(1). https://doi.org/10.4238/gmr.15018078.

Percutaneous Nephrolithotomy Access Under Fluoroscopic Control (Prone and Supine)

Maximiliano Lopez Silva, Pablo Contreras, and Norberto O. Bernardo

Abstract Percutaneous endourological procedures require an advanced level of skills and the techniques used should be understood by those treating patients with complex renal stone disease to improve their ability to manage these often challenging clinical problems. The bull's-eye and triangulation methods are the most commonly used approaches, but refinements in technique and applications of new technology offer the potential for improved access with reduced patient and surgeon morbidity. Percutaneous puncture, tract dilation, and antegrade nephrostomy sheath placement into the desired calyx can be achieved rapidly and with precision when fluoroscopy is adequately used. For this reason and for patient comfort access is best achieved in the operating room by the urologist even in special situations like staghorn stones requiring multiple or supracostal accesses, caliceal diverticulum and horseshoe kidneys.

Keywords Fluoroscopy · Guided · Percutaneous renal access · Nephrolithotomy · Kidney · Stones · Calyx

The last years of the 1970s and the early 1980s will probably be remembered by urologists as a time of tremendous changes, in particular the whole concept of minimally invasive surgery and the development of percutaneous surgery, which have shown spectacular clinical results and reduced the morbidity of open surgery (Smith et al. 1979a). Percutaneous stone extraction was first described more than 30 years ago and has become an increasingly common intervention for patients with stone disease (Lee et al. 2004), evolving into a safe and effective treatment for patients with large or otherwise complex stone disease. However, despite the increasing use of percutaneous renal surgery, Lee et al. reported that only a minority of urologists,

M. L. Silva · N. O. Bernardo (✉)
Hospital de Clínicas José de San Martín, University of Buenos Aires, Buenos Aires, Argentina
e-mail: nbernardo@hospitaldeclinicas.uba.ar

P. Contreras
Hospital Aleman, Buenos Aires, Argentina

J. D. Denstedt and E. N. Liatsikos (eds.), *Percutaneous Renal Surgery*,
https://doi.org/10.1007/978-3-031-40542-6_9

27% of who have trained in percutaneous access, actually gain their own access for percutaneous nephrolithotomy (PCNL) (Miller et al. 2007). One of the more common reasons given by respondents for not doing so was inadequate skills in the techniques of access.

The placement of percutaneous access into the intrarenal collecting system is one of the most critical aspects of percutaneous renal surgery. Image guidance is a critical factor for the performance of percutaneous minimally invasive procedures, which are being used with ever increasing frequency. Procedures such as PCNL are not performed without image guidance. The puncture of the kidney, insertion of guidewires, establishment of the percutaneous tract, and the disintegration and removal of stones are based on appropriate image guidance. For percutaneous renal surgery using fluoroscopy, access must be gained: different forms of access have been developed, all with the indispensable assistance of the image intensifier (Lee et al. 2004).

The first percutaneous nephrostomy to decompress an obstructed kidney was described by William Goodwin in 1955 (Lee et al. 2004). However, removal of a renal calculus via a percutaneous tract established specifically for that purpose was not performed until 1976, when Fernstrom and Johansson used the technique successfully in three patients (Lee et al. 2004). In their series, the tract was slowly dilated under fluoroscopic control over a 7-day period to a size sufficient for stone extraction. Similarly, Alken et al. in their experience with PCNL established access to the renal collecting system over the course of weeks (Alken et al. 1982). He subsequently developed the metal telescope dilators, which accelerates the procedure and allows stone removal in a single session. In 1982, Smith et al. described the rapid dilation of the nephrostomy tract in minutes with no untoward effects, which revolutionized the field of percutaneous stone surgery and contributed to the demise of open surgery (Smith et al. 1979b). Since that time the percutaneous approach has generated wide interest among the pioneers of endourology, and they developed and popularized most of the basic principles in this area in the late 1970s.

Fluoroscopy

Imaging equipment in percutaneous renal surgery typically uses radiation for image formation and guidance during access and tract dilation.

Fluoroscopy is useful during the advancement of guidewires, tract dilation, stone removal, and nephrostomy placement, providing realtime depiction of the collecting system and the stones therein. Percutaneous renal surgery is performed with a combination of fluoroscopic and endoscopic visualization of the collecting system. Fluoroscopy is a two-dimensional (2D) method and provides limited information regarding the surrounding soft tissue. Nevertheless, it has proven to be an invaluable tool for the performance of percutaneous procedures of the kidney and collecting system.

1   Radiation Exposure

All parameters of fluoroscopy affecting image quality, reproducibility, and radiation output from each radiographic unit must be evaluated routinely to ensure optimal image quality while minimizing the radiation dose (Chen et al. 2015). The endourologist can improve their imaging techniques and minimize both their and the patient's radiation exposure with no concurrent loss of image quality.

When attempting to obtain a diagnostic-quality image and the image is underpenetrated, and given the choice between increasing the total number of X-rays (mA) or the penetrability of the X-rays already present (kVp) to improve the image, the kVp should be increased initially as this will not increase the radiation output (Chen et al. 2015). Collimating the image to the minimum size necessary for performing the work will reduce the amount of unnecessary radiation.

The radiation output from the X-ray tube should have been evaluated within the past year by a radiologic physicist, who determines whether the unit's radiation output is within legal limits as well as optimal for each examination.

There have been various reports evaluating the typical radiation exposure from fluoroscopy during PNL, with an estimated effective dose (ED) between 7.63 and 8.66 mSv. Certain risk factors increase radiation exposure during PNL. These include high Body Mass Index (BMI), increased stone burden, and increased number of access tracts (Chen et al. 2015).

Radiation "spreads out" in a three-dimensional space with a discrete or fixed number of photons spreading out into successively larger spaces. As a result, the area geometrically increases as a function of distance from the source. Increasing the distance from the source is one of the least expensive and most dramatic ways to reduce the dose of radiation to which operating personnel are exposed. By doubling the distance from the source, the radiation is reduced to one-fourth of its original intensity because the same number of photons is in a space that is four times larger. Similarly, by tripling the distance, radiation is reduced to one-ninth. Moving 3 feet further away from an initial distance will reduce the dose by 89%.

The principle of radiation exposure As Low As Reasonably Achievable (ALARA) should be followed during procedures that require fluoroscopy. A drape placed over or under the patient helps reduce scatter radiation (Chen et al. 2015).

Shielding, whether provided by lead aprons or thyroid shields, is a method of last resort. They provide excellent protection and should always be worn by those who work near the fluoroscopy table to limit the dose of radiation to which they are exposed. When fluoroscopy is performed, the radiation dosimeter badge is worn on the collar, outside the apron. As a result of this technique, the actual effective whole-body exposure is up to 99% lower than the dose measured by the badge (Chen et al. 2015).

Component positioning on the C-arm can significantly influence scattered radiation fields. The image intensifier should be as close to the patient as possible and the image should be collimated as much as possible over the area of interest. When the image intensifier is placed above the patient, and the tube is shielded by the table, both leakage and scatter radiation are minimized. Foot control must be entrusted to the operator and not to a third party, allowing better coordination and audible alarms with fluoroscopy locking system are very useful.

The introduction of digital radiography has contributed to the reduction of radiation exposure as well as to the improvement of image quality (Spelic et al. 2010).

Radiation exposure can be a deleterious problem in percutaneous surgery, especially for the surgeon (Yang et al. 2002). There are two types of generalizable effects from radiation exposure: deterministic and stochastic effects. Deterministic effects are dose-related, and stochastic effects are characterized by the absence of a threshold dose. Risk of malignancy from radiation exposure is a stochastic effect. The National Council on Radiation Protection and Measurements has recommended an annual occupational limit of 50 mSv (United States Nuclear Regulatory Commission 1991). In medicine, there are no suggested limits for patient exposure. Instead, the risks from radiation must be balanced with the clinical necessity and benefit of the imaging study or procedure (Chen et al. 2015). The use of ultrasonography can eliminate or reduce the side effects of radiation exposure during fluoroscopy-guided PCNL.

2 Ultrasound Versus Fluoroscopy-Guided Access

The advantages of ultrasound over fluoroscopy-guided access into the collecting system include reduction of exposure to radiation for the urologist and operating room personnel. In pregnancy and in patients with transplanted, horseshoe, or ectopic kidneys, ultrasound represents the modality of choice (Evans and Wollin 2001; Francesca et al. 2002). Another advantage is proper localization of the adjacent organs for prevention of injury. The main disadvantage of this modality is the difficulty and the need for greater care when the collecting system is only mildly dilated.

Ultrasound has been used by several groups for the guidance of PCNL, especially during the puncture of the collecting system (Skolarikos et al. 2005). The performance of puncture with ultrasound guidance and without use of fluoroscopy has also been reported (Skolarikos et al. 2005). While ultrasound can be a useful complement to access the kidney, it should be emphasized that fluoroscopy is an indispensable component of safe percutaneous surgery.

Preoperative images

Conventional computed tomography (CT) has been used for diagnosis of urologic diseases for many years. Recently, unenhanced helical CT has become a serious alternative to intravenous urography (Thiruchelvam et al. 2005). For preoperative planning, helical CT depicts the extent, orientation, and location of renal calculi, which are useful for access selection in percutaneous procedures. In addition, the anatomic relationships of the collecting system with surrounding organs are delineated, and the performance of a safe puncture is possible (Thiruchelvam et al. 2005).

Nevertheless, the inability to provide realtime imaging capability has prevented wider application of CT in interventional procedures (Thiruchelvam et al. 2005).

The three-dimensional (3D) reconstruction of CT images for planning of percutaneous procedures has been reported to be feasible and accurate. With the use of 3D rendering software, the anatomic relationships of the collecting system are provided, and access selection is facilitated. The usefulness of 3D-reconstructed CT images, however, is not widely accepted (Park and Pearle 2006).

Systems as Uro Dyna-CT (Siemens Healthcare Solutions, Erlangen, Germany) installed in the endourologic operating suite provides not only standard X-ray and fluoroscopy but also interventional 3D imaging and cross-sectional image reconstructions. It also offers a 3D planning and laser-guiding puncture tool called the syngo iGuide. It may be an additional instrument that allows the urologist to handle complex punctures (Ritter et al. 2015).

Magnetic resonance imaging (MRI) provides better depiction of the soft tissue in comparison with fluoroscopy and CT, but remains unreliable for the identification of stones in the collecting system or ureter.

Each of these new technologies offers several potential advantages over the traditional percutaneous approach under fluoroscopic control. It should, however, be stated that all of these technologies are in a nascent stage of development. For that reason it is necessary to reinforce the basic concepts governing the realization of a conventional procedural approach to the kidney under fluoroscopic control. While this conventional approach is appealing, only a small percentage of urologists are familiar with it (Miller et al. 2007), and various training models are essential for consolidating the use of this surgery (Häcker et al. 2007).

Percutaneous renal access under fluoroscopic control

The information provided by preoperative helical CT is very valuable at the time of puncture under fluoroscopic control (El-Nahas et al. 2004), as it identifies the most suitable place to set the path of the needle from the skin to inside the calyx that has been chosen for tapping. A CT scan can assess the presence of adjacent organs brought into the path of the needle. In this case, there is the option to change that path at the time of puncture under fluoroscopic control or to decide that percutaneous access is contraindicated.

When deciding where to make the puncture, areas of parenchyma should be considered that are thick enough to maintain a stable needle path and prevent subsequent development of a fistula. Also, it is desirable to identify those calyces for which surrounding thickness of parenchyma will promote their spontaneous closure of the puncture. Areas of kidney with an extremely thin parenchyma should be avoided.

Also, the information provided by helical CT will allow paths to be planned that avoid simple cysts, which sometimes are present in the renal parenchyma and are frequently not picked up on fluoroscopy.

The collecting system is opacified with direct injection through the ureteral catheter of contrast. A posterolateral transparenchymal puncture minimizes the chance of injury to the major renal vessels. The chosen posterior calyx is visualized with the C-arm fluoroscopy unit in the posteroanterior direction initially.

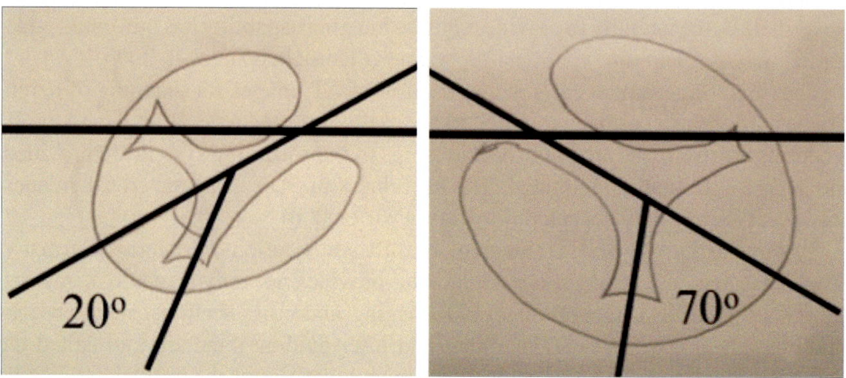

Fig. 1 Schematic view of both kidneys. Right kidney: posterior calyces positioned 20° posteriorly to the its own frontal plane. Left kidney: posterior calyces positioned 70° posterior to its frontal plane

The posterior calyces are positioned 20° posteriorly to the frontal plane of the kidney in most right kidneys, and 70° posterior to the frontal plane of the kidney in most left kidneys. In a normally rotated kidney, the frontal plane of the kidney is 30° posterior to the coronal plane of the body (Fig. 1).

In general, all patients undergoing any percutaneous renal procedure are given a general anesthetic.

2.1 PNL Position Variations

PNL may be performed in different positions, but some steps are common to the different techniques.

First step. A rigid cystoscope is used to place a 0.036-inch Teflon-coated guidewire into the upper collecting system. When a tortuous area blocks the progress of the guidewire, a wire with a hydrophilic guide-wire coating must be used. When the guidewire is in position, the 6F catheter is advanced over it to the renal pelvis, and the endoscope is removed.

To perform percutaneous access also some steps are common to every technique variations. The percutaneous access is created via an upper, middle, or lower calyx. Thorough evaluation of the renal collecting system anatomy is essential prior to definitive percutaneous puncture for access tract creation.

Percutaneous access to the upper urinary tract through a calyx must meet five conditions that guarantee safe access and avoid complications:

- Performed from a posterolateral position
- Performed through the renal parenchyma
- Toward the center of the calyx posterolaterally

- Toward the center of the renal pelvis
- As a result of these four conditions, the trajectory does not damage any major blood vessels.

2.2 PNL in Prone Position

The patient is placed in a lithotomy position for cystoscopy, with insertion of a 6F open-end ureteral catheter under fluoroscopy guidance.

A retrograde urogram then delineates the ureteral anatomy, as well as the exact stone location, degree of hydronephrosis, and the image of the selected calyx (Bernardo and Smith 2000).

After cystocopy, a 16F Foley catheter is inserted. Both catheters are tied with 2-0 silk to secure them in place. It is helpful to connect an empty syringe to the Luer lock adapter at the end of the ureteral catheter to prevent urine leakage.

The patient is positioned prone. The patient is moved slowly and gently to allow the body to adjust to the position change. A foam rubber pillow is placed under the head to prevent it from being angulated excessively in relation to the trunk. The endotracheal tube is placed in the side slot of the foam pillow, making sure that the tube is unobstructed and free from kinks. To reduce resistance to breathing, the chest and abdomen are elevated on two foam rubber rolls that extend from the shoulder to the hip. Knee donuts padded with sheepskin inside the ring are positioned between the knees and the operating table to protect the bony prominences. A foam rubber roll is placed anterior to the ankles. The arms are flexed and secured on padded arm boards, and the elbows are protected with sheepskin pads. At this time, the 2-0 silk tie securing the two catheters together is cut and discarded. The intravenous extension tubing is connected to a 60-mL syringe containing 25% diatrizoate (Hypaque) solution, and the tubing is primed and connected to the ureteral catheter.

Peercutaneous access. There are two primary methods used to gain fluoroscopy-guided percutaneous renal access: the "bullseye" technique and triangulation (Miller et al. 2007). Both techniques need a target, most commonly generated by opacification of the collecting system with iodinated contrast that is administered retrograde via a ureteral catheter. A calyceal entry point is selected to avoid the larger vascular structures that are found at the level of the infundibulum.

As with most percutaneous access techniques, the bullseye technique requires fluoroscopy to monitor and guide the procedure. To this end a ureteral catheter is placed and the patient is positioned as described above. With the C-arm in the 30° position, an 18G diamond tip access needle is positioned, so that the targeted calyx, needle tip, and needle hub are in line with the image intensifier, giving a bullseye effect on the monitor. In effect the surgeon is looking down the needle into the targeted calyx. The needle is advanced in 1–2-cm increments using a hemostat to minimize radiation exposure to the surgeon. Continuous fluoroscopic monitoring is performed to ensure that the needle maintains its proper trajectory. Needle depth is ascertained by rotating the C-arm to a vertical orientation. If the needle is aligned with the calyx in this view, the urologist should be able to aspirate urine from the collecting system, confirming proper positioning.

The triangulation technique is based on simple geometric principles and is guided by biplanar fluoroscopy; one plane is anteroposterior to the line of puncture and the other is oblique. The anteroposterior view may be considered to be in a plane parallel to the axis of puncture and is used to monitor mediolateral (left–right) adjustments. The oblique view gives information regarding depth to the site of puncture and is used to monitor needle adjustments in the cephalad–caudad (up–down) orientation.

The tip of the needle is oriented towards the calyx to be punctured in both the anteroposterior and oblique planes. Left–right adjustments are limited to the anteroposterior view only, and cephalad–caudad adjustments are limited to the oblique view. When making adjustments in the mediolateral axis, care should be taken not to inadvertently move the needle in the cephalad–caudad axis, and vice versa. In most cases, it is helpful for the surgeon to rest their arm on the patient during the access part of the procedure, as this minimizes unintended drifting of the needle away from the targeted axis and also provides additional needle stabilization.

To decrease the radiation exposure to the surgeon's hands, the C-arm should be oriented with the image intensifier angled toward the head of the patient. Whenever possible, the iris of the fluoroscope should be kept as small as possible, to further minimize stray radiation exposure. Once the needle is aligned with the targeted calyx in both the mediolateral and cephalad–caudad orientations, it is advanced with continuous fluoroscopy. The needle should always be advanced in the oblique view, which will allow for the assessment of the depth of the needle's penetration. It is helpful for the anesthesiologist to hold the patient's respirations while the needle is being advanced, to avoid having to "hit a moving target", as well as to minimize the risk of an inadvertent transthoracic puncture. After advancing the needle several centimeters in the oblique view, the anteroposterior view should be examined to confirm that the mediolateral trajectory of the needle is still properly aligned to the target. If necessary, the needle trajectory can be readjusted to maintain proper targeting. Again, it is critical not to alter the access needle's orientation in one plane while making adjustments in the other plane, particularly when advancing the needle.

Several groups have reported refinements in techniques, incorporating elements of the bullseye and triangulation methods, proposing new approaches, describing adjuncts, and using new technology. A geometric model was described to create a plane of coincidence between the C-arm and the needle, each at the same angle of 20–30° from the targeted calyx, but in opposite directions (Bernardo and Smith 2000). For lower pole access, the C-arm is rotated cranially 30° from the vertical plane, and a needle is advanced from a position distal to the calyx, rotated caudally 30° from the vertical plane. For mid-renal and upper pole calyceal access, the C-arm is rotated 20° away from the surgeon, and a needle is advanced from a position lateral to the calyx, at an angle of 20° toward the surgeon from the vertical plane. In either case, the C-arm remains fixed, and the needle is advanced until the point of coincidence between the calyx and the needle tip is reached. This technique purportedly eliminates the need for C-arm rotation, thus potentially reducing C-arm manipulation and fluoroscopic exposure time. This technique, however, requires a plumb, protractor, and ruler to calculate and confirm the necessary measurements.

Another recently proposed modification by Sharma and Sharma represents a hybrid of the bullseye and triangulation techniques (Sharma and Sharma 2009). The posterior calyx that provides the best access for stone clearance is selected. The initial puncture needle is held at this point. The needle with its overlying hub in the same line as the calyx creates a bullseye effect on the C-arm monitor. The site on the skin corresponding to the target calyx is thus determined, and its position is marked with a hemostat as point A. We place an intramuscular needle at this point instead of a hemostat. Then, under direct vision, the needle is placed vertically and the puncture is made at this point in the subcutaneous cellular tissue at a depth of about 1 cm (Fig. 2A). The visual control of the needle in the vertical position reduces fluoroscopic exposure to a few seconds. Subsequently, a brief fluoroscopic exposure is used to check the position of the needle and it is shown on the screen as a point. The trajectory of the line of puncture of the needle into the dorsal area represents an imaginary line through the selected calyx in the anteroposterior direction. However, this trajectory does not meet all five requirements for optimum puncture, described above, as the needle is not directed toward the center of the renal pelvis.

The C-arm is then angled toward the surgeon, 30° from the vertical in the axial plane. With the ventilation suspended in end expiration, the second puncture needle is held over the targeted calyx in such a way that the needle with its hub is in the same line with the calyx, which leads to a bullseye effect on the C-arm. This particular point on the skin is punctured with an intramuscular needle and is taken as point B (Fig. 2B). This position represents an imaginary line that is projected onto the center of the selected calyx. Again, all five requirements for safe renal puncture are not met because the trajectory is not toward the center of the renal pelvis. This position is checked in relation to the 12th rib. Visually observing the trajectory of the two small needles placed in the lumbar area, the intersection of two lines coincides with the desired calyx.

The distance between the two needles is measured (Fig. 3A). The C-arm is then brought back to its vertical position. Now the line of puncture is determined in alignment with the infundibulum from point A. Along this point line, the point B1 is marked. The distance between points A and B1 is equal to or greater than the distance between the intramuscular needles (points A and B) (Fig. 3B). The point B1 is the point where the skin is punctured for renal access. A small incision is then made at point B1 and the 18G needle is introduced for 1–1.5 cm (Fig. 4). Now, with the C-arm in the 90° vertical position (i.e. parallel to the line of puncture), the mediolateral (right to left) adjustments are made. Then the C-arm is tilted toward the head of the patient by 30° and adjustments are made in the cephalad and caudal orientation of the line of puncture. The needle orientation is maintained in one plane while making adjustments in the other plane. With the C-arm in the oblique orientation, the needle is advanced with ventilation suspended in full expiration. Under fluoroscopic control and from this position, the 18G needle is advanced towards the point of intersection of the two lines that project both intramuscular needles to reach the selected calyx.

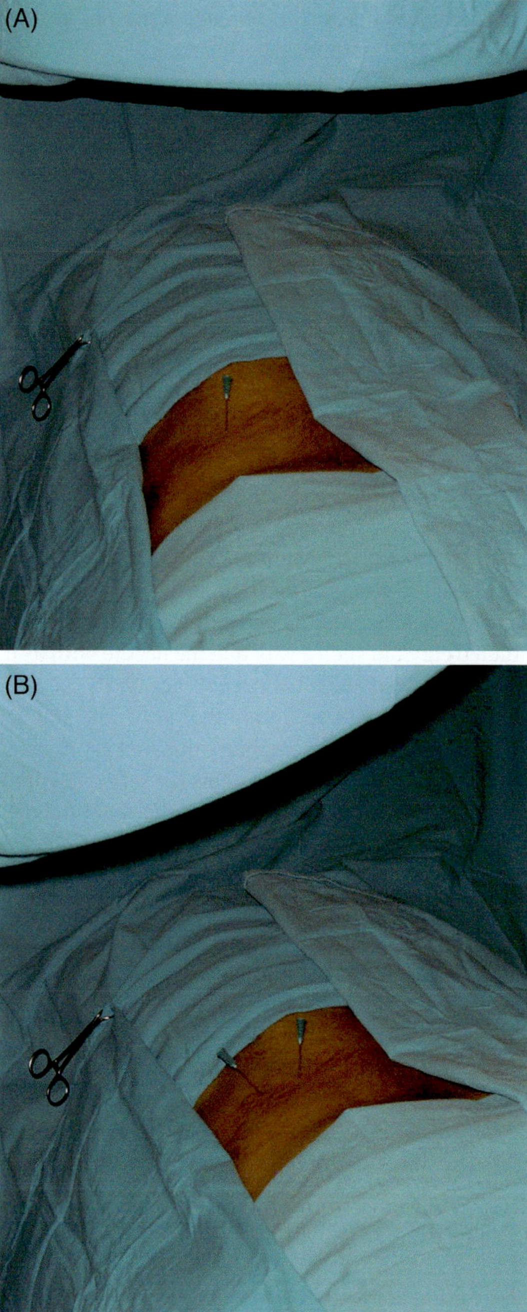

Fig. 2 (A) The intramuscular needle with its overlying hub in the same line as the calyx creates a bullseye effect on the C-arm monitor. The needle is placed upright and puncture is done at this point at a depth of about 1 cm in the subcutaneous cellular tissue. (B) The C-arm is angled 30° toward the surgeon. The second needle is held over the targeted calyx in such a way that the needle with its hub is in the same line with the calyx, which leads to a bullseye effect on the C-arm

This is the ideal path and the only one that meets the five requirements described above of a safe percutaneous renal puncture.

When the tip of the needle appears fluoroscopically to be within the collecting system, the needle trocar is removed, leaving only the needle cannula in place, and a small amount of urine is aspirated to confirm the needle's intraluminal position.

Definitive puncture of the renal collecting system with an 18G diamond needle permits the immediate introduction of a 0.038-inch guidewire into the collecting

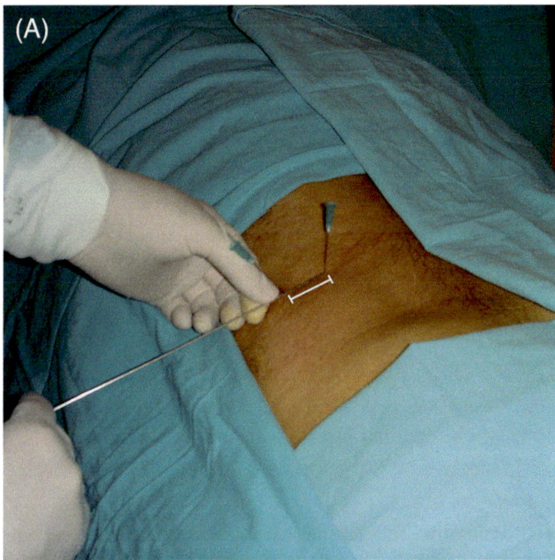
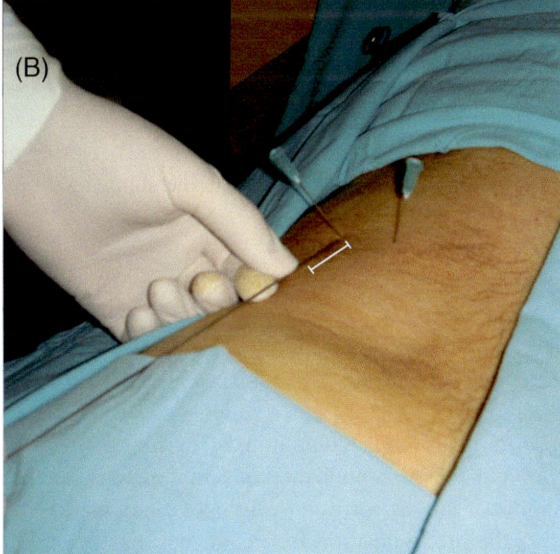

Fig. 3 (A) Distance between the two needles is measured (points A and B). (B) B1 is the point where the skin will be punctured for renal access. The distance between points A and B1 is equal to or greater than the distance between the intramuscular needles

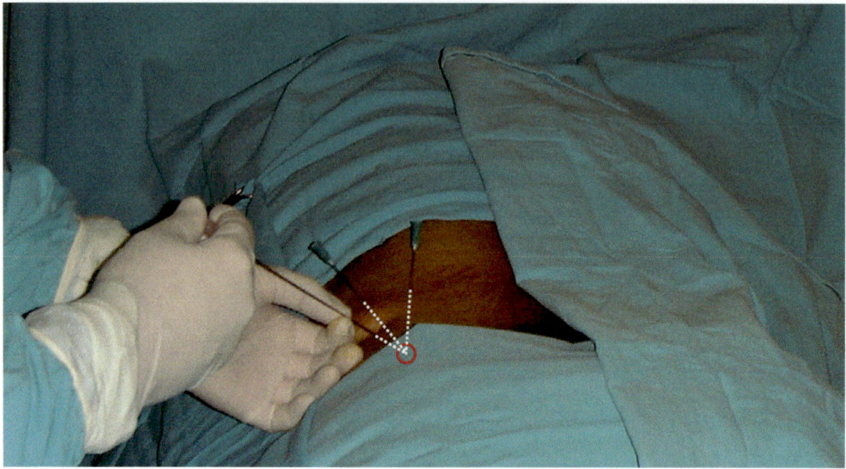

Fig. 4 The intersection of the two lines of small needles placed in the lumbar area coincides with the desired calyx. The 18G needle is advanced under fluoroscopic control towards the point of intersection of the lines that project both intramuscular needles in order to reach the selected calyx

system. The rigidity of this needle is advantageous for accurately directing the needle diamond tip as it is advanced through the fascial planes.

If at the point of withdrawing the trocar of the needle spontaneous output of urine has not been observed, it is advisable gently to try to introduce a hydrophilic guidewire, observing the advancement of the guidewire under fluoroscopy. Typically, it moves into the cavity of the calyx and progresses towards the renal pelvis. If for some reason the guidewire does not easily advance, it is advisable to inject an additional volume of contrast through the initially placed ureteral catheter with the intention of filling the calyx cavity and thereby facilitating the progression of the hydrophilic guidewire.

If no urine exits from the 18G needle, it is not advisable to inject contrast through the needle, since contrast can extravasate, creating a lake of radio-opaque material and making it difficult to visualize the shape of the kidney cavities.

2.3 PNL in Supine Position

Although PNL in prone position offers several advantages, as a larger surface area for the choice of puncture site, a wider space for instrument manipulation and a possibly a lower risk of splanchnic injury (Ibarluzea et al. 2007); in the last decades, several reports have been published of percutaneous renal surgery in the supine, modified supine or lateral position (Valdivia Uría et al. 1998). This has potential advantages over the prone position for PCNL and has been adopted by many urologists. The modified supine position preserves cardiovascular and ventilatory dynamics and allows better access to the respiratory tract. Additionally, the bowel slips away from the puncture area, lowering the risk of it being damaged. PCNL with the patient in a modified supine position may be considered for most patients, especially if concomitant ureteroscopy and Endoscopic Combined Intrrenal Surgery (ECIRS) is planned (Daels et al. 2009).

First descriptions of PNL in supine position were performed by Valdivia et al. in the late 80's (Ibarluzea et al. 2007). The key point in this surgery is to take time to locate the patient previous to initiate the surgery, instead of doing it at the time of position change (prone PNL). With the patient under general anesthesia, an inflated 3 L serum bag with water or air is placed under the patient's lumbar region of the side to be treated. This bag generates an intermediate lateral position. It is relevant to locate patient´s flank and the edge of the bag alongside the surgical table edge to allow a greater degree of movement to the nephroscope. The contralateral leg is flexed and located in a lower plane (this facilitates an eventual ureteroscopy access) on leg support 90 degrees, while the homolateral leg remains extended also on leg support. Ipsilateral arm is flexed and fixed. After locating the patient, simultaneous antisepsis to lumbar and genital regions are performed (Fig. 5A and B).

After cystoscopy (as descipted above), 6 Fr catheter is located and time to perform the access to the kidney has become.

With this technique it is possible to puncture the calyceal papilla without having to rotate the C-arm fluoroscope, fluoroscopic control is maintained perpendicular to the needle and renal access.

Initially a long metal instrument, as the nephroscope or Alken dilator, is overlaid on the patient's abdomen and under fluoroscopic control its distal tip is placed over the selected calyx. This point is marked on lumbar fossa of the patient and indicates the orientation of the needle. Entry point must be placed always behind the posterior axiallary line to avoid colonic damage.

Needle advances in an ascending direction in the search to the selected calyx papylla. Once kidney´s capsule is reached, calyx dilation with contrast is needed. At this point subjective perception of kidney movements is important. If backward kidney movement and/or calyceal distortion is perceived, the needle can advance and get into the selected calyx. If depth orientation is wrong, it is necessary to remove the needle from the kidney and retry to locate the calyx again in a higher or lower direction.

When the selected calyx has been reached and the first urine drops are obtained through the needle, the guidewire is introduced and the tract can be dilated (Valdivia Uría et al. 1998). After performing the needle access, procedure to check the correct location and to perform dilation are the same that were described above to PNL in prone position.

Many variation of the original supine position have been described. Some urologists prefer the "pure supine" position; to perform this technique, an special surgical table is needed (without metal bars) to locate the patient in the edge of the table and with no bag beneath the lumbar region. Other variant is to place two bags instead of one (in lumbar region and hip), what could allow more movement to the nephroscope. Finally, another variant of the way to locate the patient is to rotate the patient more

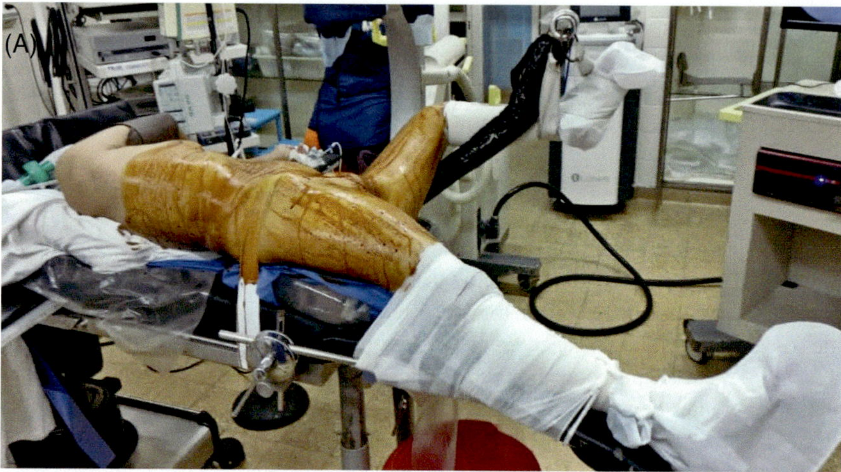

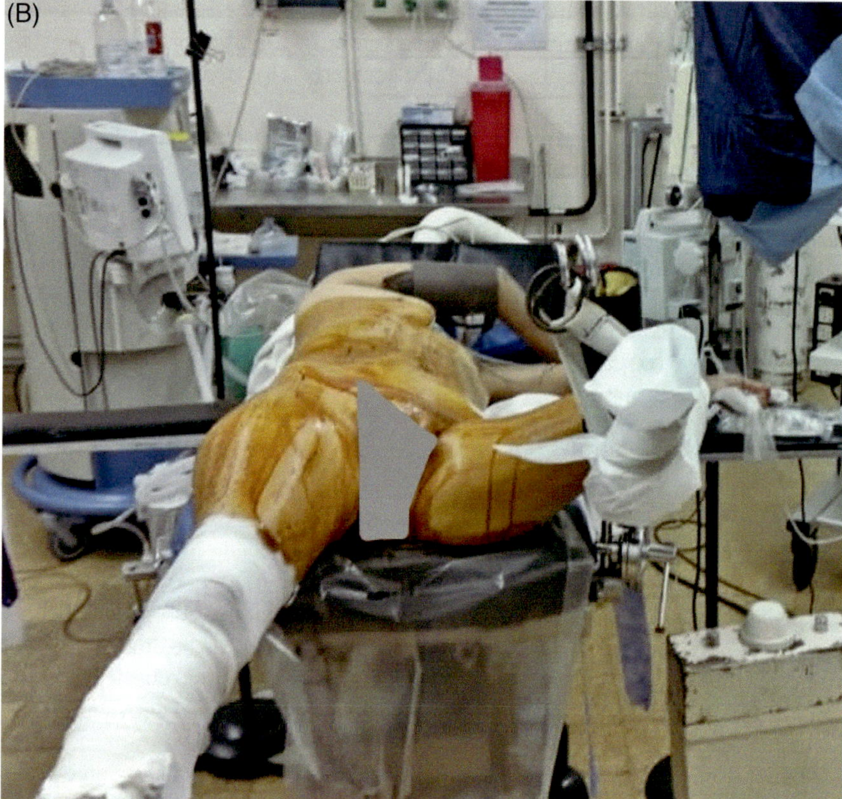

Fig. 5 View of patient in final position previous to initiate PNL in supine position. (A) punction view. (B) cystoscope view

than in original description; in this technique, the direction of the needle advance is more horizontal than ascending.

2.4 PNL in Lateral Position

When PNL is performed in lateral position it is important to consider the different degree of rotation presented by the posterior chalices of each kidney, as previously mentioned. In most right kidneys, the posterior calyces are positioned 20 degrees posteriorly to the frontal plane of the kidney, and in most left kidneys 70 degrees posterior to the frontal plane of the kidney (Fig. 1). This shows that in left stones the needle will be inserted in a direction almost parallel to the operating table, while, in right stones the needle will be inserted in downward position.

Triangulation technique is used, determining the cephalad-caudal axis with the C-arm in anteroposterior configuration, and determining the anteroposterior axis with the C-arm in oblique configurations (El-Husseiny et al. 2009).

Once reached the calyx, the wire is introduced and we can proceed to dilation.

2.5 Challenging Situations

In situations where the volume of the stone occupies the entire volume of the calyx selected to be punctured, the needle is advanced until there is the tactile sensation of the needle tip touching the hard surface of the stone. In this situation the tip of the trocar of the needle is in contact with the stone but the cannula of the needle is at a distance of 1–2 mm from the surface of the stone. It is advisable to then move the cannula on the trocar toward the stone until contact with the surface of the stone is felt. Then the trocar needle is removed and the hydrophilic guidewire is gently inserted into the narrow space between the urothelium of the calyx and the surface of the stone. Sometimes this allows the advancement of the guidewire to the renal pelvis, but in other situations it is only possible to locate the guidewire in the punctured calyx and attempting otherwise is risky because of the short length of the guidewire in the upper urinary tract. The guidewire is advanced carefully across the calyceal infundibulum.

2.6 Dilation

To perform the tracts dilation, 1-cm skin incision is made around the needle with a No. 10 blade, and the needle is removed. Then, in order to enlarge the defect in the lumbar fascia, a fascial incision needle can be used (No. 090070 Cook Urological). This instrument consists of an 18G needle fixed to a small, blunt, diamond-shaped blade that is passed over the puncture wire under fluoroscopic control, through the abdominal wall until it crosses the lumbar fascia. It is then withdrawn while gentle traction is placed on the puncture wire, and the tip of the blade is rotated 90° and then advanced again over the puncture wire in order to open the lumbar fascia more extensively. This action will facilitate the introduction of any of the available dilation systems.

Acute dilation of nephrostomy tracts can be performed with a variety of instruments. These instruments are inserted over a working guidewire. Because of the risk of perinephric guidewire kinking with loss of the nephrostomy tract and laceration of the renal parenchyma, all percutaneous dilator systems require fluoroscopic guidance (Falahatkar et al. 2009).

The nephrostomy tract is dilated to the desired width. In the serial dilation system, an 8F Teflon catheter is used as an obturator. Progressively larger dilators are then serially inserted over this guidewire. This additional obturator stiffness greatly reduces the risk of perinephric guidewire buckling.

With the access tract dilated, a working sheath is introduced into the collecting system. The renal pelvis is examined nephroscopically to identify the obstructed segment of the ureteropelvic junction (UPJ) and locate the previously placed ureteral catheter. If necessary, either the ultrasonic probe or the grasping forceps are passed into the renal pelvis to clean out clots.

The catheter is grasped and brought out through the nephrostomy tract. A 0.038-inch super-stiff wire, which is a fixed core guidewire with an extra-stiff shaft and a flexible tip, is advanced through the catheter. A surgical assistant removes the ureteral catheter, leaving the guidewire in place at the urethral meatus. This maneuver ensures the preservation of the nephrostomy tract, so that if the access route to the kidney is accidently lost, it is easily recovered by following the guidancedescribed above. Additionally, if for some reason the procedure has to be interrupted, placement of the nephroureteral stent will allow both drainage and subsequent easy access.

Special situations: multiple access

In the treatment of complex renal lithiasis with branches in multiple calyces, it is sometimes necessary to make multiple punctures through different calyces. The multiple punctures can all be made initially or after removing part of the stone burding.

If the planned multiple punctures are made at the beginning of surgery, the injection of contrast through the initially placed ureteral catheter facilitates visualization of all calyces and the most suitable for punctures can be chosen in accordance with the silhouette of the stone.

In contrast, if multiple punctures are made in addition to establishing a unique initial nephrostomy tract, the calyceal distention may be achieved by placing a Foley catheter and to inflate the balloon inside the Amplatz sheath to occlude its caliber. Thereafter it is possible to inject contrast either through the ureteral catheter placed at the beginning of surgery or the Foley catheter, and to place a clamp to prevent leakage of contrast from the distended renal cavity.

3 Conclusions

Percutaneous endourologic procedures require an advanced level of skill. The techniques used should be understood by those treating patients with complex renal stone disease to improve their ability to manage these often challenging clinical problems. The bullseye and triangulation methods are the most commonly used approaches, but refinements in technique and applications of new technology offer the potential for improved access with reduced patient and surgeon morbidity. Percutaneous puncture, tract dilation, and antegrade nephrostomy sheath placement into the desired calyx can be achieved rapidly and with precision when fluoroscopy is adequately used. For this reason and for patient comfort, access is best achieved in the operating room by the urologist, even in special situations like staghorn stones requiring multiple or supracostal accesses, calyceal diverticulum, and horseshoe kidneys.

References

Alken P, Hutschenreiter G, Günther R. Percutaneous kidney stone removal. Eur Urol. 1982;8:304–11.

Bernardo NO, Smith AD. Percutaneous endopyelotomy. Urology. 2000;56:322–7.

Chen T, Wang C, Ferrandino M, Scales C. Radiation exposure during the evaluation and management of nephrolithiasis. J Urol. 2015;194(4):878–85.

Daels F, González MS, Freire FG. Percutaneous lithotripsy in Valdivia-Galdakao decubitus position: our experience. J Endourol. 2009;23:1615–20.

El-Husseiny T, Moraitis K, Maan Z. Percutaneous endourologic procedures in high-risk patients in the lateral decubitus position under regional anesthesia. J Endourol. 2009;23:1603–6.

El-Nahas AR, Abou-El-Ghar M, Shoma AM. Role of multiphasic helical computed tomography in planning surgical treatment for pelvi-ureteric junction obstruction. BJU Int. 2004;94:582–7.

Evans HJ, Wollin TA. The management of urinary calculi in pregnancy. Curr Opin Urol. 2001;11:379–84.

Falahatkar S, Neiroomand H, Akbarpour M. One-shot versus metal telescopic dilation technique for tract creation in percutaneous nephrolithotomy: comparison of safety and efficacy. J Endourol. 2009;23:615–8.

Francesca F, Felipetto R, Mosca. Percutaneous nephrolithotomy of transplanted kidney. J Endourol. 2002;16:225–7.

Häcker A, Wendt-Nordahl G, Honeck P. A biological model to teach percutaneous nephrolithotomy technique with ultrasound and fluoroscopy-guided access. J Endourol. 2007;21:545–50.

Ibarluzea G, Scoffone C, Cracco C. Supine Valdivia and modified lithotomy position for simultaneous anterograde and retrograde endourological access. BJU Int. 2007;100(1):233–6.

Lee CL, Anderson JK, Monga M. Residency training in percutaneous renal access: does it affect urological practice? J Urol. 2004;171:592–5.

Miller NL, Matlaga BR, Lingeman JE. Techniques for fluoroscopic percutaneous renal access. J Urol. 2007;178:15–23.

Park S, Pearle MS. Imaging for percutaneous renal access and management of renal calculi. Urol Clin North Am. 2006;33:353–64.

Ritter M, Rassweiler MC, Michel M. The Uro Dyna-CT enables three-dimensional planned laser-guided complex punctures. Eur Urol. 2015;68:880–4.

Sharma G, Sharma A. Determining site of skin puncture for percutaneous renal access using fluoroscopy-guided triangulation technique. J Endourol. 2009;23:193–5.

Skolarikos A, Alivizatos G, de la Rosette. Percutaneous nephrolithotomy and its legacy. Eur Urol. 2005;47:22–8.

Smith AD, Lange PH, Fraley EE. Applications of percutaneous nephrostomy. New challenges and opportunities in endourology. J Urol. 1979a;121:382.

Smith AD, Reinke DB, Miller RP. Percutaneous nephrostomy in the management of ureteral and renal calculi. Radiology. 1979b;133:49–54.

Spelic DC, Kaczmarek RV, Hilohi. Nationwide surveys of chest, abdomen, lumbosacral spine radiography, and upper gastrointestinal fluoroscopy: a summary of findings. Health Phys. 2010;98:498–514.

Thiruchelvam N, Mostafid H, Ubhayakar G. Planning percutaneous nephrolithotomy using multi-detector computed tomography urography, multiplanar reconstruction and three-dimensional reformatting. BJU Int. 2005;95:1280–4.

United States Nuclear Regulatory Commission: 20.1201 Occupational dose limits for adults. 56 FR 23396. In: NRC regulations title 10, code of federal regulation. Washington, D.C.: U.S. Nuclear Regulatory Commission; 1991. Available at http://www.nrc.gov/reading-rm/doc-col lections/cfr/part020/full-text.html#part020-1201

Valdivia Uría JG, Valle Gerhold J, López López JA. Technique and complications of percutaneous nephroscopy: experience with 557 patients in the supine position. J Urol. 1998;160:1975–8.

Yang RM, Morgan T, Bellman GC. Radiation protection during percutaneous nephrolithotomy: a new urologic surgery radiation shield. J Endourol. 2002;16:727–31.

Endoscopic Combined IntraRenal Surgery (ECIRS)

S. Proietti, M. M. Oo, D. Santillan, C. Cristallo, S. Spagna, F. I. Tirapegui, G. Giusti, and M. S. Gonzalez

Abstract Endoscopic combined intrarenal surgery (ECIRS) is the simultaneous antegrade and retrograde approach to treating complex renal stone diseases by combining percutaneous nephrolithotomy (PCNL) with retrograde intrarenal surgery (RIRS). ECIRS has become popular over the last decade with the introduction of modified supine PCNL, as PCNL in this position makes retrograde approach to the kidney easily accessible without the need to reposition the patient. The goal of performing ECIRS is to achieve stone-free status for the operated renal unit in a one-stage surgery while minimizing the required percutaneous access to a single tract by taking advantage of the best of both PCNL and RIRS armamentarium.

Keywords Endoscopic Combined IntraRenal Surgery (ECIRS) · Kidney stone surgery · Endoscopic surgery · Minimally invasive surgery · Urolithiasis · Nephrolithiasis · Kidney stones · Stone removal · Renal calculi · Renal anatomy · Endourology · Flexible ureteroscopy · Percutaneous nephrolithotomy (PCNL) · Miniaturized percutaneous nephrolithotomy (mini-PCNL) · Retrograde intrarenal surgery (RIRS) · Holmium laser lithotripsy · Stone fragmentation · Renal access · Fluoroscopy · Postoperative care

S. Proietti (✉) · M. M. Oo · S. Spagna · G. Giusti
Department of Urology, European Training Center in Endourology, San Raffaele Hospital, IRCCS, Milan, Italy
e-mail: proiettisil@gmail.com

D. Santillan · C. Cristallo · F. I. Tirapegui · M. S. Gonzalez
Endourology, Stone Disease and Laser. Urology Department. Hospital Italiano de Buenos Aires, Aires, Argentina

J. D. Denstedt and E. N. Liatsikos (eds.), *Percutaneous Renal Surgery*,
https://doi.org/10.1007/978-3-031-40542-6_10

1   Introduction

Endoscopic combined intrarenal surgery (ECIRS) is the simultaneous antegrade and retrograde approach to treating complex renal stone diseases by combining percutaneous nephrolithotomy (PCNL) with retrograde intrarenal surgery (RIRS).

ECIRS has become popular over the last decade with the introduction of modified supine PCNL, as PCNL in this position makes retrograde approach to the kidney easily accessible without the need to reposition the patient.

After Valdivia-Urìa first demonstrated that PCNL can be done safely in the supine position with a 3L-saline bag under the flank in 1987 (Valdivia Uria et al. 1998), different variations in positioning have been reported in the literature—lateral, complete supine and modified supine positions (Kerbl et al. 1994; Falahatkar et al. 2008; Papatsoris et al. 2008; Bach et al. 2012). Yet none of these managed to replace the conventional prone positioning for PCNL until in 2001, when Professor Gaspar Ibarluzea from the Galdakao hospital shared his innovative concept of incorporating a modified lithotomy position to the supine Valdivia position (Ibarluzea González et al. 2001; Ibarluzea et al. 2007). This position is now known as Galdakao-modified supine Valdivia (GMSV) position and has led to supine PCNL gaining worldwide acceptance in the last decade as more urologists adopt this technique.

The term ECIRS was coined in 2008 by Scoffone et al. in the first report of the safety and efficacy of this combined approach (Scoffone et al. 2008). In their prospective study between 2004 and 2007, 127 patients underwent ECIRS, in which both PCNL and RIRS were simultaneously performed in the GMSV position, to treat large and/or complex urolithiasis. They reported high stone-free rates of 81.9% after the initial surgery and the mean operative time of 70 ± 28 min, including the time taken for positioning. Their reported complication rate of 38.6% for ECIRS was comparable to PCNL complication rates in the literature. Hence, they demonstrated that ECIRS could be performed efficiently and safely without the additional risk of complications from the combination of the two operations.

The goal of performing ECIRS is to achieve stone-free status for the operated renal unit in a one-stage surgery while minimizing the required percutaneous access to a single tract by taking advantage of the best of both PCNL and RIRS armamentarium.

ECIRS is particularly advantageous over PCNL or RIRS as monotherapy in treating complex renal stones such as staghorn or stones in multicalcyeal locations. In these challenging cases, PCNL as a single modality may lead to increased risk of renal parenchymal injury and resultant bleeding, either from the excessive swing of the nephroscope via a single access tract or from making multiple access tracts, in attempting to treat the stones located in difficult-to-reach calyces. On the other hand, RIRS alone on its own would result in high intrarenal pressures with resultant risk of sepsis, not to mention, prolonged operative time and its associated consequences.

In contrast, the dual approach enables a more effective lithotripsy, reduces operative time and increases surgical success for stone free rates while minimizing complications (Cracco et al. 2011, 2020; Hamamoto et al. 2014b; Nuño de la Rosa et al. 2014). In cases of large stones, simultaneous lithotripsy via antegrade and retrograde routes will fragment the stones more efficiently and reduce operative time. When there are multicalcyeal stones and the antegrade access via the percutaneous tract is unable to access the affected calyces (particularly if the stone is located in a calyx parallel to that of the access tract), retrograde flexible ureteroscope may be deployed to treat the stone, hence reducing the number of PCNL tracts or the need for staged surgery by improving stone clearance in a single operation.

Another example where ECIRS is indicated is in cases of ureteric strictures where retrograde access may be difficult or impossible—simultaneous antegrade and retrograde endoscopic assessment will delineate the extent of the disease accurately. The stricture may be treated by the antegrade approach if deemed suitable or planned for alternative appropriate intervention (Miyai et al. 2021; Scarpa et al. 1997). Similarly, in cases of reconstructed urinary systems such as ileal conduits, where retrograde approach may be complicated due to anastomotic stricture or obscure ureteric orifice, initial antegrade approach will allow the passage of wire down the ureter to identify the ureteric orifice for retrograde approach and thus, enabling assessment and potential treatment of the underlying pathology.

2 Patient Positioning

The same debate for patient positioning in PCNL exists for ECIRS. The choice of modified supine/lithotomy position versus prone position depends mostly on the familiarity of the approach by the surgeons.

2.1 *Galdakao-Modified Supine Valdivia (GMSV) Position and Giusti's Position*

These positions are commonly adopted for ECIRS due to their ease of positioning the patient without the need to turn the patient prone and because of the familiarity of urologists in doing RIRS in the lithotomy position rather than prone. Furthermore, there is an increasing shift from prone PCNL to supine PCNL with the use of ultrasound-guidance for access puncture over the last decade.

The details for these positions are discussed in the previous chapter on Supine PCNL.

2.2 Prone Split Leg Position

For urologists who are keen to maintain the prone approach for PCNL, ECIRS has also been reported to be successfully performed with the patient prone on an operating table that allows the legs to be placed in a split position in order to enable a second surgeon to perform retrograde ureterorenoscopy (Hamamoto et al. 2014a; Wang et al. 2022).

In this position, the ureteric orifice is first cannulated with the use of flexible cystoscopy and subsequent retrograde access is attained with flexible ureteroscopy. Antegrade access is established by traditional prone PCNL technique.

Those that advocate the prone position reported the advantages to be that of the availability of a wider surgical field for percutaneous access, an easier access to the upper pole calyces, less mobility of the kidney and shorter distance into the collecting system particularly in obese patients. Prone split leg position also enables the team to perform bilateral surgery without the need to reposition the patient (Hamamoto et al. 2014a; Wang et al. 2022; Duty et al. 2012).

Literature reports that there are no significant differences in outcomes in terms of stone-free rates and complications for the GMSV versus prone split leg position for ECIRS (Abouelgreed et al. 2022; Cracco and Scoffone 2020), though ECIRS became popular in the GMSV position and many have adopted this position in practice.

This is because ECIRS in GMSV position offer many anaesthesiologic advantages over prone positioning including easier access to the airway, less risk of endotracheal tube kinking or dislodgement, and improved cardiovascular and respiratory indexes (Ibarluzea et al. 2007; Khoshrang et al. 2012; Cracco and Scoffone 2011). It is also easier to position the patient in GMSV position as there is no need to turn over an anaesthetized patient, thus, decreasing need for manpower and lessening theatre occupancy time. More importantly, this avoids possible pressure injuries associated with the prone position, that can potentially lead to neurological or visual deficits. This is especially important in the challenging obese patients.

However, some disadvantages exist with modified supine positions. One of these is the limited access for puncture especially for the upper pole calyx where it may be associated with an increased risk of visceral injury. This risk may be decreased by the wide availability of pre-operative anatomical assessment with CT scans and the use of ultrasound to guide the needle puncture to ensure there is no intervening organ along the tract to the kidney. Hence, upper pole puncture is not necessarily excluded for ECIRS and may still be performed in selected cases. Furthermore, it is reported that access through lower pole in the supine position has a wider angle for manipulation to reach the upper pole (Proietti et al. 2019; Sofer et al. 2016). For cases where upper pole is not accessible through the percutaneous tract, this is precisely the indication for a combined approach surgery anyway.

Another critique for GMSV position is the difficulty with establishing antegrade access due to the increased mobility of the kidney in the supine position which makes percutaneous puncture and especially dilatation difficult, particularly so for patients of a thinner body habitus. In these cases, passing the guidewire down the ureter and out through the external urethral meatus in a through-and-through fashion (the "kebab" patient) can aid in stabilizing the kidney (Cracco and Scoffone 2020).

Lastly, in the GMSV position, as the antegrade access drains the irrigation fluid by gravity, it may be difficult to keep the calyces distended. However, with dual-access flow, endovision can be maintained well. In fact, keeping calyces less distended is advantageous in reducing intrarenal pressure, fluid reabsorption and its resultant risk of sepsis. The downward or horizontal position of the sheath also allows stone fragments to be flushed out (Nicklas et al. 2015), making fragment evacuation more efficient.

3 Equipment Positioning

Whether the surgeons prefer the GMSV or the prone split leg position, one of the main challenges for ECIRS is the arrangement of equipment in the confined space of the operating theatre. In ECIRS, two surgeries are being performed concurrently and therefore, two sets of equipment are needed including the bulky endoscopic video systems and lithotripsy machines. Also, fluoroscopy must be well-coordinated between the urologists and its imaging screen positioned to be easily seen by both the antegrade and retrograde teams.

Figure 1 suggests an example of how the equipment may be arranged in a theatre with two camera tower stacks—one for PCNL and one for RIRS. More commonly, not every hospital has the luxury of two sets of endoscopy camera towers for both the antegrade and retrograde surgeons. In these cases, the retrograde surgeon uses the camera system first for cystoscopy and semi-rigid ureteroscopy. Subsequently, the surgeon may switch to a disposable flexible ureteroscope as the disposable ureteroscopes come with their own monitor so that RIRS may be performed concurrently with the antegrade approach which will use the in-house endoscopic camera system.

Equipment positioning can be individualized based on the resources available. For example, if there are floating monitor screens available in the operating theatre, it will be better ergonomically for the surgeons to have the fluoroscopic imaging or the endoscopic video projected to these screens.

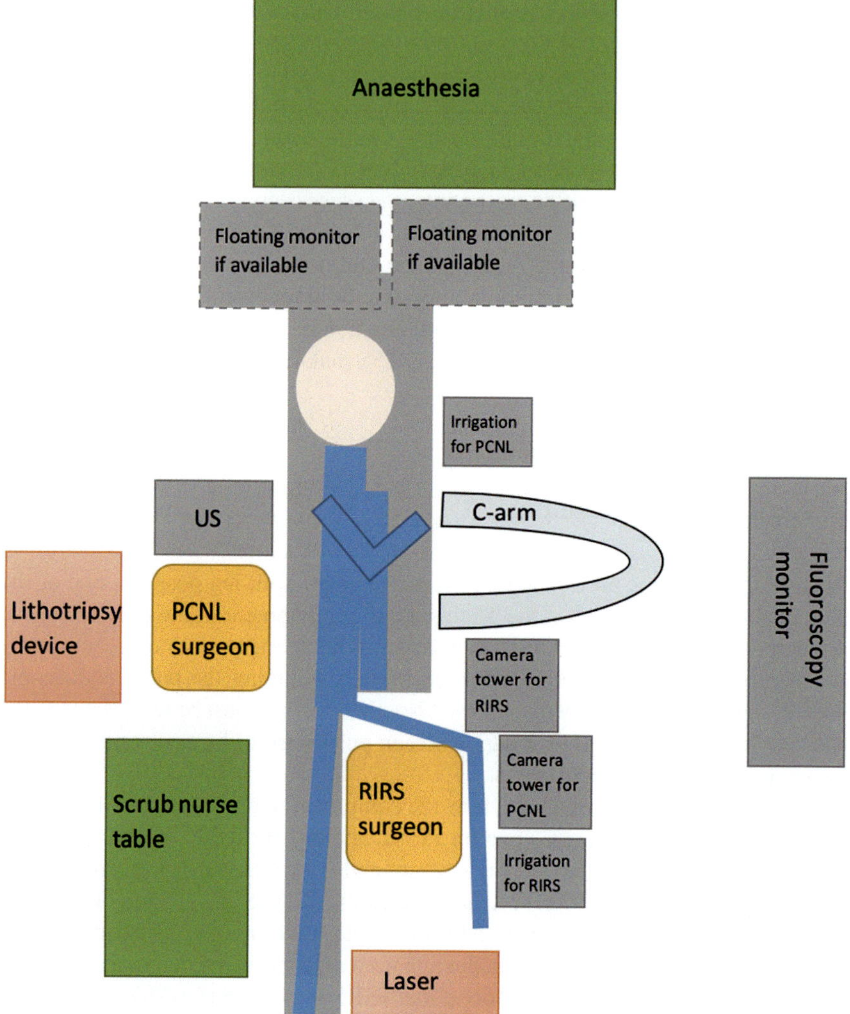

Fig. 1 Arrangement of ECIRS equipment in OR

4 Operative Steps

As with all surgeries, review of available radiological imaging is important for surgical planning by assessing the stone load and location as well as taking note of the presence of any aberrant anatomy such as retrorenal colon, liver ptosis, organomegaly or malrotated kidney.

After the patient is anaesthetized and prophylactic intravenous antibiotics are given, the patient is commonly placed in GMSV position with the equipment arranged as previously discussed. The surgeon then draws reference lines on the patient—the posterior axillary line, the iliac crest and the border of 12th rib—to mark the boundaries of the operative field.

The operative sites are cleaned and draped. One urologist starts off with cystoscopy and a safety guidewire is placed in the ureter on the side of the surgery. Ureteroscopy is then performed to assess for any abnormality of the lower tract and also for the presence of any ureteric stone or strictures and to gauge the caliber of the ureter to size for access with flexible ureteroscope.

Next, flexible ureteroscope is introduced in the retrograde fashion to survey the dynamic anatomy of the collecting system and the stone load and characteristics. This preliminary retrograde assessment is an important step as it provides the urologists with much valuable additional information but at the same time, is not time-consuming and poses little risk to the patient or the equipment. After the retrograde assessment, the surgeon also has the choice to not proceed with PCNL and may decide to perform only RIRS if the anatomy and stone burden are favourable.

If, however, the decision is made to proceed with ECIRS, a ureteric catheter is placed after withdrawal of the flexible ureteroscope for placement of contrast in the collecting system. A second urologist gains percutaneous access to the calyx of choice as per standard steps for PCNL. More urologists are now moving towards the use of ultrasound to gain access to the kidney, though fluoroscopy still plays an important role in establishing access. Ultrasound can aid to visualize surrounding organs during the puncture and avoid inadvertent injuries.

In suitable cases, instead of exchanging the flexible ureteroscopy to ureteric catheter, puncture may also be aided by flexible ureteroscopy under direct endoscopic vision. One of the pioneer teams of ECIRS from Cottolengo Hospital of Torino described their Turin Technique with this endovision-check percutaneous renal puncture for ECIRS (Cracco et al. 2022). Endovision minimizes bleeding as it checks the puncture and dilatation. It can also help to reduce the need for fluoroscopy and hence, decreasing radiation exposure for both the patient and healthcare staff.

Once the percutaneous access is established, lithotripsy is performed through the PCNL tract. Simultaneous laser lithotripsy via retrograde flexible ureteroscopy may also be performed. Ureteric access sheath may not always be necessary in cases of ECIRS, especially when combined with a standard size PCNL, as irrigation outflow through nephrostomy sheath will keep intrarenal pressures low. Also, stone fragments can be easily evacuated through the percutaneous tract, avoiding the need for multiple passage of the flexible ureteroscope up and down the ureter.

During lithotripsy, care must be taken by both surgeons not to damage the flexible ureteroscope by the antegrade lithotripsy energy device, in particular if a reusable ureteroscope is being used.

Stones in calyces that are not visible to the PCNL nephroscope can be retrieved with a basket via retrograde flexible ureteroscope and passed out through the antegrade tract (pass the ball technique Cracco and Scoffone 2020)] or repositioned for fragmentation in the part of the collecting system favourable to the PCNL access. Alternatively, the stones may be fragmented in-situ by laser via flexible ureteroscopy and the fragments then passed out through the PCNL tract for easier removal.

In addition to fluoroscopy, retrograde flexible ureterorenoscopy can aid in assessing stone clearance. Once stone clearance is established, a ureteric stent can be easily placed in the retrograde fashion and exit strategy as per surgeon's judgement.

5 Versatility of ECIRS

There can be variations to ECIRS by downsizing the PCNL tract to mini-PCNL or ultra-mini PCNL, provided two laser machines are available for both antegrade and retrograde lithotripsy.

Hamamoto et al. demonstrated in their 10-year retrospective study that ECIRS with mini-PCNL had superior outcomes when compared to conventional PCNL monotherapy or mini-PCNL monotherapy (Hamamoto et al. 2014b). For 161 patients with average renal stone size of 35–40 mm, they found operative time to be significantly shorter in mini-ECIRS arm (mini-ECIRS: 120.5 min vs. mini-PCNL: 181.9 min versus conventional-PCNL: 134.1 min, $P < 0.001$) with the best stone-free rates of 81.7% while mini-PCNL and conventional PCNL stone-free rates were 38.9% and 45.1% respectively.

Furthermore, although the aim of ECIRS is to reduce the number of PCNL tracts, in complex cases, it is still possible to perform multiple antegrade accesses to improve stone clearance. Figure 2 shows a patient with a conventional PCNL tract and an additional mini-PCNL tract for a stone in lower pole calyx at an angle that made it impossible to pass the retrograde flexible ureteroscopy.

Regardless of choice of positioning and size of percutaneous tract, systematic review of the available ECIRS literature in 2020 by Cracco and Scoffone (Cracco and Scoffone 2020) reported stone-free rates to be > 80% with a single percutaneous access in most cases with the overall range of 61–97%. The bigger the size of the percutaneous tract and the smaller the stone, expectedly, the higher was the stone free rate observed.

In their study, complication rates ranged from 5.8 to 44% and were associated with staghorn stones and longer operative time. Most complications classified under Clavien-Dindo grade 1 or 2 (Dindo et al. 2004). Bleeding risk was minimal regardless of the PCNL tract size. Infection and sepsis rates varied from 3 to 40%.

Notably, they found that most ECIRS were performed with single-access for PCNL, with only 1.6–10% of cases needing an additional access tract. Operative time was often found to be shorter compared to traditional PCNL monotherapy and was as fast as 70 minutes including the time taken for positioning. More importantly, ECIRS indicated a decreased need for additional procedures and was effective in achieving stone-free status even in cases of large and/or complex stones (Cracco and Scoffone 2020; Nuño de la Rosa et al. 2014).

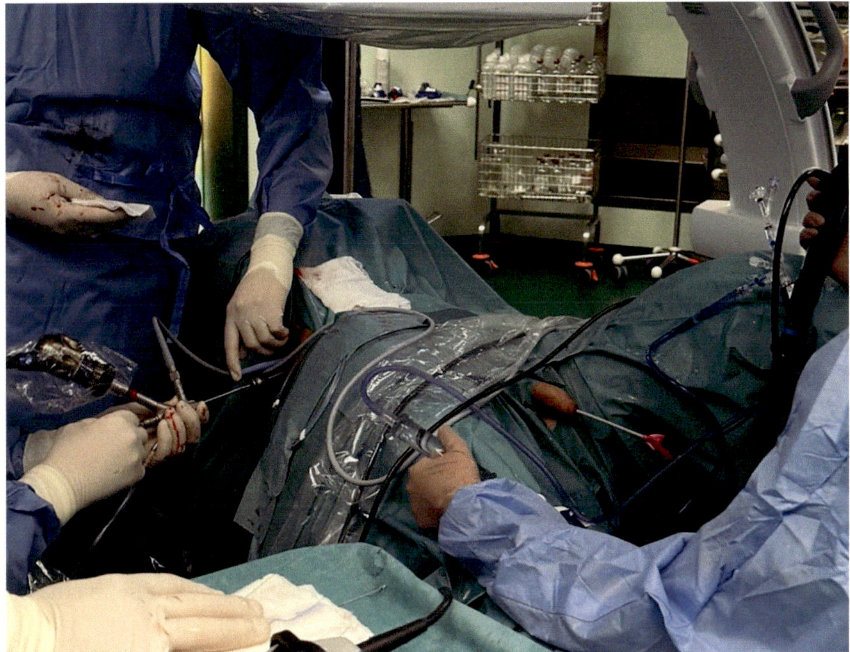

Fig. 2 ECIRS with standard and mini PCNL tracts

6 Disadvantages of ECIRS

While ECIRS has many merits, there are also some drawbacks. For a successful ECIRS, two operating teams and 2 sets of instruments are required simultaneously. This means additional manpower that may not always be available. Moreover, with the increase in the number of staff and extra equipment required, the operating theatre may be over-crowded. Well-trained and dedicated staff who are familiar with the set up and positioning of the equipment will increase efficiency.

In addition, there must also be synergy between the two urologists as well as between the surgeons and the scrub team and supporting theatre staff. Everyone should be familiar with the steps of the operation and the two surgeons need to communicate well in order to perform a successful ECIRS.

Lastly, since two operations are combined into one during ECIRS, the cost of each ECIRS will be more than that of either PCNL or RIRS alone due to additional instrument and consumables required for the combined surgery compared to PCNL or RIRS alone. However, since ECIRS reduces the need for ancillary procedures (Cracco and Scoffone 2020; Nuño de la Rosa et al. 2014), in the long run, it would be more cost effective. When patients can be rendered stone-free in a single step surgery rather than through repeated operations, there will be reduced need for operating theatre occupancy, hospitalization, repeated imaging and clinic visits, and this in turn will decrease overall healthcare costs. Nevertheless, one should be mindful of the indications for which ECIRS will be beneficial over PCNL/RIRS monotherapy and only perform ECIRS for cases that truly warrant it, rather than performing additional RIRS for all cases of PCNL, or vice versa, just because it is conveniently achievable. Avoiding unnecessary ECIRS will also reduce the amount of material waste so that we can be more environmentally-conscious.

7 Conclusion

ECIRS has revolutionized the management of complex renal stones. Its advantages for anaesthesia especially in the modified supine positions, and better results for one-step stone clearance with reduced need for ancillary procedures, make ECIRS the treatment of choice in cases of heavy stone burden or complex anatomy.

The debate on the best patient-positioning for ECIRS will continue based on the country of practice and personal preferences and familiarity of the performing urologists. In future, mini-PCNL paired with RIRS may replace standard-size antegrade access (Usui et al. 2020) as improvements in laser technology afford more efficient lithotripsy and the use of high powered lasers become more prevalent.

Besides its use in treatment of complex stones, ECIRS is also increasingly utilised in the treatment of other urological conditions. ECIRS has been reported to be successfully used for the treatment of ureteric strictures, encrusted stent removal, in paediatric population, in the transplanted kidney and even in a case of squamous cell carcinoma (Miyai et al. 2021; Scarpa et al. 1997; Juliebø-Jones et al. 2021; Mitome et al. 2018; Taguchi et al. 2015; Li et al. 2018; Santillán et al. 2021).

ECIRS with the maximal advantages of both PCNL and RIRS capabilities is no doubt fast-becoming the operation of choice for complex urolithiasis. As more urologists adopt this surgery for a variety of conditions, it will continue to result in improved outcomes and increased versatility.

References

Abouelgreed TA, Abdelaal MA, Amin MM, et al. Endoscopic combined intrarenal surgery in the prone split-leg position versus Galdakao-modified supine Valdivia position for the management of partial staghorn calculi. BMC Urol. 2022;22:163.

Bach C, Goyal A, Kumar P, et al. The Barts 'flank- free' modified supine position for percutaneous nephrolithotomy. Urol Int. 2012;89:365–8.

Cracco CM, Casablanca C, Peretti D, Scoffone CM. Endoscopic combined intrarenal surgery for complex stones—the Turin technique. Urol Video J. 2022;(16):100188. ISSN 2590-0897.

Cracco CM, Scoffone CM. ECIRS (Endoscopic Combined Intrarenal Surgery) in the Galdakao-modified supine Valdivia position: a new life for percutaneous surgery? World J Urol. 2011;29(6):821–7. https://doi.org/10.1007/s00345-011-0790-0. Epub 2011 Nov 6.

Cracco CM, Scoffone CM. Endoscopic combined intrarenal surgery (ECIRS)—tips and tricks to improve outcomes: a systematic review. Turk J Urol. 2020;46(Supp. 1):S46–57.

Dindo D, Demartines N, Clavien PA. Classification of surgical complications: a new proposal with evaluation in a cohort of 6336 patients and results of a survey. Ann Surg. 2004;240:205–13.

Duty B, Waingankar N, Okhunov Z, et al. Anatomical variation between the prone, supine, and supine oblique positions on computed tomography: implications for percutaneous nephrolithotomy access. Urology. 2012;79:67–71.

Falahatkar S, Moghaddam AA, Salehi M, et al. Complete supine percutaneous nephrolithotripsy comparison with the prone standard technique. J Endourol. 2008;22:2513–7.

Hamamoto S, Yasui T, Okada A, Takeuchi M, Taguchi K, Shibamoto Y, Iwase Y, Kawai N, Tozawa K, Kohri K. Developments in the technique of endoscopic combined intrarenal surgery in the prone split-leg position. Urology. 2014a;84(3):565–70.

Hamamoto S, Yasui T, Okada A, Taguchi K, Kawai N, Ando R, et al. Endoscopic combined intrarenal surgery for large calculi: simultaneous use of flexible ureteroscopy and mini-percutaneous nephrolithotomy overcomes the disadvantages of percutaneous nephrolithotomy monotherapy. J Endourol. 2014b;28:28–33.

Ibarluzea G, Scoffone CM, Cracco CM, et al. Supine Valdivia and modified lithotomy position for simultaneous anterograde and retrograde endourological access. BJU Int. 2007;100:233–6.

Ibarluzea González G, Gamarra Quintanilla M, Gallego Sánchez JA, Pereira Arias JG, Camargo Ibargaray I, Bernuy Malfaz C. Litotricia renal percutánea. Evolución, indicaciones y metodología actual en nuestra Unidad de Litotricia. Percutaneous kidney lithotripsy. Clinical course, indications, and current methodology in our Lithotripsy Unit. Arch Esp Urol. 2001;54(9):951–69.

Juliebø-Jones P, Pietropaolo A, Æsøy MS, Ulvik Ø, Beisland C, Bres-Niewada E, Somani BK. Endourological management of encrusted ureteral stents: an up-to-date guide and treatment algorithm on behalf of the European Association of Urology Young Academic Urology Urolithiasis Group. Cent European J Urol. 2021;74(4):571–8.

Kerbl K, Clayman RV, Chandhoke PS, et al. Percutaneous stone removal with the patient in a flank position. J Urol. 1994;151:686–8.

Khoshrang H, Falahatkar S, Ilat S, et al. Comparative study of hemodynamics electrolyte and metabolic changes during prone and complete supine percutaneous nephrolithotomy. Nephrourol Mon. 2012;4:622–8.

Li J, Wang W, Du Y, Tian Y. Combined use of flexible ureteroscopic lithotripsy with micro-percutaneous nephrolithotomy in pediatric multiple kidney stones. J Pediatr Urol. 2018;14(281):e1-6.

Mitome T, Tabei T, Tsuura Y, Kobayashi K. Squamous cell carcinoma in a calyceal diverticulum detected by percutaneous nephroscopic biopsy. Case Rep Oncol Med. 2018;24(2018):3508537.

Miyai T, Kawahara T, Kuroda S, Yasui M, Uemura H. Complete ureteral stenosis after ureteroscopic lithotripsy successfully managed using a simultaneous retrograde and antegrade flexible ureteroscopic approach. Clinical Case Reports. 2021;9(1):246–50.

Nicklas AP, Schilling D, Bader MJ, Herrmann TR, Nagele U. Training and research in urological surgery and technology (T.R.U.S.T.)-group. The vacuum cleaner effect in minimally invasive percutaneous nephrolitholapaxy. World J Urol. 2015;33(11):1847–53.

Nuño de la Rosa I, Palmero JL, Miralles J, Pastor JC, Benedicto A. A comparative study of percutaneous nephrolithotomy in supine position and endoscopic combined intrarenal surgery with flexible instrument. Actas Urol Esp. 2014;38:14–20.

Papatsoris AG, Zaman F, Panah A, et al. Simultaneous anterograde and retrograde endourologic access: "the Barts technique." J Endourol. 2008;22:2665–6.

Proietti S, Elias Rodríguez-Socarrás M, Eisner B, De Coninck V, Sofer M, Saitta G, Rodriguez-Monsalve M, D'Orta C, Bellinzoni P, Gaboardi F, Giusti G. Supine percutaneous nephrolithotomy: tips and tricks. Transl Androl Urol. 2019 Sep;8(Suppl 4):S381–8.

Santillán D, Schroh JCS, Gutierrez PA, Thomas F, Tirapegui FI, Moldes J, Cristallo C, González MS. Case report: mini-endoscopic combined intrarenal surgery in an en-bloc kidney transplant. Afr J Urol. 2021(27):147.

Scarpa RM, Cossu FM, De Lisa A, Porru D, Usai E. Severe recurrent ureteral stricture. the combined use of an anterograde and retrograde approach in the prone split-leg position without X- rays. Eur Urol. 1997; 31:254–6.

Scoffone CM, Cracco CM, Cossu M, Grande S, Poggio M, Scarpa RM. Endoscopic combined intrarenal surgery in Galdakao-modified supine Valdivia position: a new standard for percutaneous nephrolithotomy? Eur Urol. 2008;54:1393–403.

Sofer M, Giusti G, Proietti S, et al. Upper Calyx approachability through a lower calyx access for prone versus supine percutaneous nephrolithotomy. J Urol. 2016;195:377–82.

Taguchi K, Hamamoto S, Okada A, Mizuno K, Tozawa K, Hayashi Y, et al. First case report of staghorn calculi successfully removed by miniendoscopic combined intrarenal surgery in a 2year old boy. Int J Urol. 2015;22:978–80.

Usui K, Komeya M, Taguri M, Kataoka K, Asai T, Ogawa T, et al. Minimally invasive versus standard endoscopic combined intrarenal surgery for renal stones: a retrospective pilot study analysis. Int Urol Nephrol. 2020;52:1219–25.

Valdivia Uria JG, Valle GJ, Lopez Lopez JA, et al. Technique and complications of percutaneous nephroscopy: experience with 557 patients in the supine position. J Urol. 1998;160:1975–8.

Wang D, Sun H, Xie D, et al. Application of a new position in endoscopic combined intrarenal surgery: modified prone split-leg position. BMC Urol. 2022;22:38.

Papillary Versus Non-papillary Puncture for Percutaneous Nephrolithotomy

Panagiotis Kallidonis, Angelis Peteinaris, Vasileios Tatanis, and Wissam Kamal

Abstract Percutaneous nephrolithotomy (PCNL) constitutes the gold standard of treatment for large renal stones. Papillary access to the pelvicalyceal system (PCS) has been advocated as the safest approach to perform PCNL. The use of non-papillary access for PCNL has been proposed over the last few years. We herein review the current literature on the non-papillary approach for PCNL. Experimental and clinical studies are presented in detail. Two experimental studies investigating the feasibility of non-papillary access are included. Eleven cohort prospective and retrospective studies for non-papillary access and four comparative studies between papillary and non-papillary access are also discussed. Non-papillary access seems to be a safe and efficient solution in the latest endoscopic trends. A wider adaptation of this technical modification could be expected.

Keywords Papillary · Non-papillary · PCNL · Urolithiasis · Percutaneous · Access

1 Introduction

Percutaneous nephrolithotomy (PCNL) is reckoned to be the gold standard of the treatment for large renal calculi or smaller stones in specific locations (Geraghty et al. 2022). The puncture of the kidney and the access to the PCS constitute very important steps of PCNL, as they are associated with the approach to the stone and the maneuverability of the instruments. The access to the PCS through the fornix of the papilla (papillary puncture) was based on the anatomical studies of Sampaio et al. According to the aforementioned studies, a higher likelihood of complications was

P. Kallidonis (✉) · A. Peteinaris · V. Tatanis
Department of Urology, University Hospital of Rion, Patras, Greece
e-mail: pkallidonis@yahoo.com

W. Kamal
Department of Urology, King Fahad Hospital, Jeddah, Saudi Arabia

© The Author(s), under exclusive license to Springer Nature Switzerland AG 2023
J. D. Denstedt and E. N. Liatsikos (eds.), *Percutaneous Renal Surgery*,
https://doi.org/10.1007/978-3-031-40542-6_11

observed in the non-papillary access compared to the papillary one. Thus the "papillary dogma" dominated for many years (Sampaio and Aragao 1990). Recently this principle was questioned by some investigators who proposed non-papillary access to the PCS. Over the last years, non-papillary access has gained some popularity and is increasingly performed, proving its safety and advantages under various conditions.

2 The Papillary Dogma

The anatomical principles of PCNL have their background in the studies of Sampaio et al. The researchers conducted a detailed anatomical description of the internal renal branches and their relation to the PCS (Sampaio and Aragao 1990). According to their investigation, the more peripheral puncture was considered to be associated with safer access, proposing the fornix of the papilla as the ideal access location (Sampaio et al. 1992). Aiming the renal pelvis could lead to vascular trauma more commonly, due to the presence of the posterior branch of the renal artery (Sampaio and Aragao 1990). Additionally, the anatomical position of the arterial elements at an extremely short distance from the upper infundibulum and the pelvi-infundibular junction might increase the risk of injuries during access to the upper PCS (Sampaio 1992). Sampaio et al. evaluated the vascular injury risk of performing punctures to different locations of the PCS in cadaveric kidney models. The upper infundibular puncture was associated with a 67% risk for vascular injury, 26% of which were arterial branches. The puncture of the infundibulum of the middle calyceal groups was related to arterial injury in 23% of the cases. The lower infundibular access was associated with an incidence of 13% for arterial lesions in the studied kidney models (Sampaio et al. 1992; Sampaio 2000). The data presented by Sampaio et al. established the superiority of papillary access among endourologists, creating an unquestioned rule that affected the endourological practice for decades. On the other hand, the anatomical changes that occur at an obstructed or artificially dilated PCS were not evaluated and the incidence of vascular injury by the different access approaches have not been evaluated.

3 PCNL as a Surgical Technique

Numerous modifications of PCNL can be found in the literature, due to the variety in patient position, needle guidance and instrumentation (Yuan et al. 2016; Corrales et al. 2021). The location of access constitutes another controversial point resulting in the evolution of new different methods. The dispute of the 'papillary dogma' led to the emergence of the non-papillary PCNL. Over the last few years, various studies were conducted to investigate the safety and efficiency of this new surgical method under numerous conditions.

4   The Non-papillary Access

The main idea behind the papillary access is to achieve the entrance to the PCS as peripheral to the calyx as possible, entering by the fornix of the papilla. The non-papillary access is based on the idea of entering the PCS from any site that will be convenient for the management of the calculi. The following steps are conducted for the achievement of access to the PCS in non-papillary PCNL.

One of the widely used techniques of non-papillary access to PCS has been extensively described by Kyriazis et al. (2017). After the completion of artificial dilation of the PCS is achieved, if needed, a trocar needle (18G) is used to peak the entrance point, as the rotating C-arm device is turned 30° perpendicular to the long axis of the patient. The majority of the punctures are performed on the calyceal infundibulum or at the entrance of the calyces to the pelvis. The needle should be parallel to the axis of the C-arm as it is advanced for a few centimeters aiming at the selected entrance point (Bull's eye technique). Afterward, the distance between the needle and the PCS is estimated with fluoroscopy after the C-arm is rotated at 0°. After the entrance of the needle into the dilated system, a hydrophilic guidewire is advanced through the needle aiming to be inserted into the ureter (Fig. 1). Kallidonis et al. reported that when the infundibulum of the middle calyceal groups is the access point, the navigation in the PCS is easier and the manoeuvrability of the instruments is better in comparison to a papillary access (Kallidonis et al. 2022). The mentioned data constitute the advantages of non-papillary access.

A prospective clinical study including 40 patients with renal stones was conducted by Kallidonis et al. The authors investigated the anatomy for approaching the papilla and infundibulum of the calyx as well as the renal pelvis for PCNL. The vascularization of the sites which were related to the establishment of a PCNL access was evaluated (Kallidonis et al. 2017a). The enrolled patients underwent computed tomography perfusion (CTP) and 99mTc-dimercaptosuccinic acid (DMSA) single-photon emission computed tomography/computed tomography (SPECT/CT) aiming mainly at the level of the middle calyx. The design of the access was assessed in

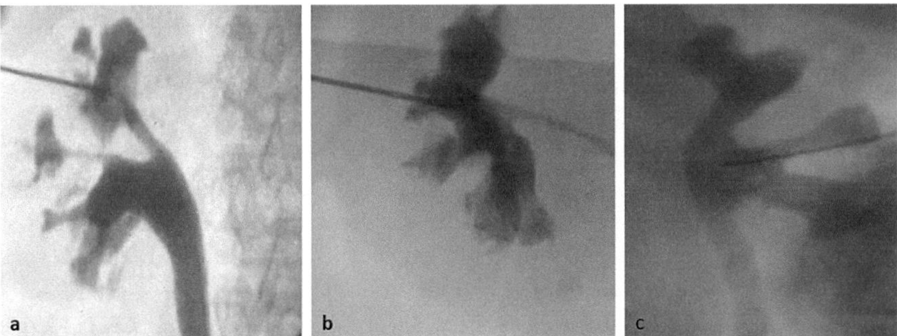

Fig. 1 Nonpapillary access to: a. The papilla of the upper calyx of a left kidney b. The infundibulum of the upper calyx of a left kidney c. The pelvis of a right kidney

the prone and supine positions. The subgroups created for a thorough investigation of the parameters were four. One group underwent DMSA SPECT/CT in the supine position and the second one in the prone position, while the same stratification happened with CTP. The angle of approach was calculated based on the Bull's eye technique access for prone and mirroring the procedure for supine access took place. The presented data revealed that the angles of approach are similar for the punctures to the papilla and infundibulum of the middle calyx as well as the renal pelvis. Additionally, the vascularization of the parenchyma at the potential entrance points was proved to be comparable. The tract dilation sites were overlapping for all three possible approaches.

An investigation of the renal anatomy and its relationship with vessels and calculi was also presented by Tsaturyan et al. (2021). The authors conducted a prospective pilot study, including 3 patients with renal stone who underwent a contrast CT with arterial, venous and excretory phase. After the appropriate 3D reconstruction of the images, an hyperaccuracy three-dimensional (HA3D™) model, including the collecting system, the stone and its surrounding vessels and tissues, was created. The patients underwent non-papillary PCNL one day after the CT scan and afterward, the reconstructive data were compared to the operative findings. The mean operative time was 39.4 min (range 35.2–44.0), while the median stone size was calculated to be 1170 mm^2 (range 830–1520). One of the patients underwent standard PCNL (dilation up to 30Fr), while the remaining two patients underwent mini PCNL (dilation up to 22Fr). One attempt was enough for the accumulation of access, and the cases were successfully completed with only one tract. A non-contrast CT was conducted on the 3rd postoperative day and all the patients were stone free. The authors concluded that a correlation between the 3D model and operative findings existed. They proposed that this model could minimize possible organ injuries and bleeding.

5 Experimental Data

Two experimental studies were conducted for the evaluation of the safety of papillary and non-papillary access. Adamou et al. performed an in vivo experimental study to investigate the possible effect of the dilation diameter on the renal parenchyma trauma during non-papillary access to the PCS (Adamou et al. 2022). Twenty-two non-papillary accesses with dilation ranging from 12 to 30Fr were performed in porcine model. No significant bleeding event was reported intra- or postoperatively. Kidney specimens for histopathological evaluation were retrieved immediately after the procedure and one month postoperatively. The researchers reported that the difference in renal function was not significant among different tract diameters, despite the larger kidney scar of the 30Fr dilatation.

Hou et al. conducted an in vitro experimental comparative study and concluded to a reduced likelihood of bleeding when a papillary access is performed in comparison to the non-papillary approach. The researchers used 70 porcine kidneys and performed punctures to different renal locations (papilla, infundibulum, renal column, minor calyceal neck). The arterial pressure of the kidney was maintained steady by continuous injection of natural saline. The authors observed that papillary access was associated with fewer bleeding events in comparison to the other possible puncture sites, suggesting it as the safest option (Hou et al. 2022).

6 Clinical Data

See Table 1.

Table 1 Clinical studies regarding papillary and non-papillary access and basic results presented

Author, year of publication	Type of surgery	Number of patients	Hemoglobin drop (gr/dL)	Operative time (min)	Stone free rate (SFR)
Güler et al. (2019)	Papillary Standard PCNL versus Papillary Mini-PCNL	97 in total, standard group:46 mini group:51	2.07 ± 1.59 (sg) 1.35 ± 1.11 (mg)	74.7 ± 44.5 (sg) 89.2 ± 40.4 (mg)	71.7% (sg) 76.5% (mg)
Kandemir et al. (2020)	Papillary Standard PCNL versus Papillary Mini-PCNL	148 in total, standard group:72 mini group:76	1.4 ± 1.5 (sg) 0.7 ± 1.3 (mg)	91.2 ± 33.2 (sg) 106.9 ± 38.8 (mg)	72.2% (sg) 75% (mg)
Kyriazis et al. (2017)	Non-papillary Standard PCNL	137	2.92 ($\pm$ N/A)	48.13 ± 14.8	84.6%
Kuzgunbay et al. (2011)	Papillary PCNL for Staghorn Calculi for young versus elederly patients	87 in total, Control group:45 Elderly group:37	145.8 ± 37.3 (cg) 132.6 ± 36 (eg)	1.70 ± 1.33 (cg) 1.46 ± 1.29 (eg)	92% (cg) 91.5%(eg)
Kallidonis et al. (2021a)	Non-papillary PCNL for Staghorn Calculi	53	$1,6 \pm 1,86$	54.57 ± 14.83	81.1%
Kallidonis et al. (2021b)	Non-papillary Mini-PCNL	32	1.23 ± 0.88	44.6 ± 13.44	96%
Tsaturyan et al. (2022)	Non-papillary Percutaneous Antegrade Ureterolithotripsy	72	1.02 ± 0.18	36.9 ± 14.8	95.8%

(continued)

Table 1 (continued)

Author, year of publication	Type of surgery	Number of patients	Hemoglobin drop (gr/dL)	Operative time (min)	Stone free rate (SFR)
Abouelgreed et al. (2022)	Papillary ECIRS Prone split-leg versus Galdakao-modified supine Valdivia (GMSV) position	66 (33–33)	N/A	118.87 ± 27.12 121.54 ± 26.73	87.87% 90.9%
Kallidonis et al. (2022)	Non-papillary ECIRS	33	1.2 (1.1–1.4)	47 (36–65)	90.9%

7 Standard PCNL

A randomized prospective study conducted by Güler et al. presents important data about the papillary access PCNL, including 97 patients (Güler et al. 2019). Fifty-one of the patients underwent mini-PCNL, while the rest of the participants was undergone a tract dilation of up to 30Fr. Flexible nephroscopy was performed in cases of high suspicion for residual lithiasis. In the standard PCNL group, the mean operative time was calculated to be 74.7 ± 44.5 min, varying from 56.1 ± 29.9 min for solitary stones to 79.2 ± 46.6 min for multiple stones. The authors reported that the mean stone size for this subgroup was 42.8 ± 22.5mm, while the mean hemoglobin drop was also estimated to be 2.07 ± 1.59 gr/dL postoperatively and the mean hospitalization time was 66.8 ± 43.2 h. The success rate was 88.8% and 67.6% for solitary and multiple stones, respectively. The overall success rate was 71.7%. Seven out of 46 patients (15.2%) needed a blood transfusion, while one of the patients underwent pleural effusion (2.2%). All the patients were followed up by Kidney-Ureter-Bladder (KUB) X-ray on the 1st post-operative day and by non-contrast computed tomography (CT) scan 4 weeks after the surgery for the stone-free rate (SFR) evaluation.

Kandemir et al. demonstrated data collected from a randomized control trial including 148 patients that underwent secondary papillary PCNL (Kandemir et al. 2020). All included patients had a prior history of PCNL and/or open renal procedures. Seventy-two of the patients underwent standard PCNL with tract dilation up to 30Fr. The mean stone size was calculated to be 33.1 ± 10.9mm and the stone-free rate was 72.2%. The mean operative time was 91.2 ± 33.2 min, while mean hospital stay was measured at 75.5 ± 34.0 h. Regarding complications, the authors reported a mean hemoglobin drop of 1.4 ± 1.5 gr/dL, while only 4 patients (5.6%) needed a blood transfusion. The encountered complications were 1 patient needed selective angioembolization (1.4%) and 2 patients underwent pleural effusion (2.8%). A KUB X-ray was conducted on the 1st postoperative day and a non-contrast CT 3 months after the surgery.

Kyriazis et al. were the first to present information about non-papillary PCNL, conducting a prospective study including 137 patients who underwent this type of access (Kyriazis et al. 2017). All the patients underwent standard PCNL with dilation up to 30Fr. Second access was needed in twenty-one participants in order to achieve a better SFR, while 4 patients needed 3 accesses. The mean operative time was 48.13 $\pm$ 14.8 min while the single stone subgroup required 47.87 $\pm$ 14.03 min, the multiple stones subgroup 54.18 $\pm$ 15.26 min, and staghorn calculi subgroup 78.26 $\pm$ 9.53 min. The time needed for the lithotripsy of staghorn calculi was prolonged in comparison with the other two subgroups. The primary stone-free rate was reported to be 84.6% and was defined as the presence of residual stones $\leq$ 1 mm or stone-free patient. The complication rate was in accordance with the literature, reaching 10.2%. The mean hemoglobin loss was estimated at 2.92 gr/dL and 2.9% of the patients needed a blood transfusion. One case of pseudoaneurysm was diagnosed 15 days after the surgery and was treated by angiographic embolization. Bleeding and transfusion rate was comparable to similar cohort studies of patients that underwent a papillary puncture (Kyriazis et al. 2015). The mean hospital stay was calculated to be 2.92 $\pm$ 1.13 days. The follow-up of the patients included a KUB X-ray and ultrasound evaluation 1 month after the surgery. The patients with radiolucent stones, abnormal findings or symptomatology were evaluated by non-contrast CT scan. This large prospective study suggested that non-papillary puncture for standard PCNL is a fast, safe and efficient technique in terms of perioperative complications and SFR.

8 Staghorn Calculi

The efficiency and safety of non-papillary access were evaluated in a series of patients with staghorn stones. A retrospective cohort study with 53 participants was conducted by Kallidonis et al. (2021a). The participants' average stone size was 60.1 $\pm$ 16.1 mm, and they were all treated with standard PCNL, which was performed with non-papillary access and two-step dilation up to 30Fr. In total, 64 accesses in 53 patients were performed with a mean number of 1.2 accesses per case. The authors reported that the mean operative time was 54.57 $\pm$ 14.83 min, which was shorter compared to similar studies of papillary puncture in the contemporary literature. The complication rate was found to be 20.7% with only one blood transfusion needed due to a bleeding pseudoaneurysm. The latter was treated by selective angiographic embolization. The mean hemoglobin loss was measured at 1.6 $\pm$ 1.86 gr/dL. The mean hospital stay was 3.9 $\pm$ 0.82 days. The SFR was calculated to be 81.1% at one month after the surgery. The follow-up consisted of a KUB X-ray and renal ultrasonography, while a CT scan was conducted in some cases that needed further evaluation. The reported data demonstrated that non-papillary PCNL for staghorn stones had comparable results to the literature in terms of safety and efficacy.

9   Mini PCNL

Non-papillary access for the performance of mini-PCNL has also been evaluated. Kallidonis et al. conducted a retrospective study with 32 patients who underwent one-step dilation to 22Fr (Kallidonis et al. 2021b). The mean stone size of the patients was 23.53 ± 6.6 mm, while the mean operative time was reported to be 44.6 ± 13.44 min. The mean operative time for the single access PCNL was calculated to be 44.66 ± 14.35 min, while for multiple accesses it was 44.6 ± 11.09 min. There is no significant difference regarding operative time between the single and multiple access groups. SFR was 96% for patients that underwent one access. Seven out of 32 patients needed multiple accesses and the SFR was calculated to be 85.7%. In addition, the complication rate did not exceed 9.37%. No severe bleeding was noticed and the mean hemoglobin drop was measured at 1.23 ± 0.88 gr/dL. The mean hospital stay was calculated to be 2.56 ± 0.98 days. The patients were evaluated 1 month postoperatively while the follow-up included KUB and ultrasound. CT scan was performed in case of abnormal radiological findings or persistent symptoms..

10   PAUL (Percutaneous Antegrade Ureterolithotripsy)

The evaluation of non-papillary medial puncture, which facilitates the ureteroscope insertion for the antegrade lithotripsy of ureteral stones has been proposed by a prospective cohort study from Tsaturyan et al. (2022). The authors presented the results of 72 cases. The patients underwent percutaneous access with 12Fr, 22Fr or 30Fr dilation based on the stone burden and the size of the PCS. The ureteral stones were treated using a high-power Holmium laser and the renal calculi were treated with one single-probe dual-energy lithotripter. Automated pump irrigation was used for the antegrade ureteroscopy since the continuous flow was useful for flushing the fragments to the bladder. The average cumulative stone size was measured at 24.2 ± 5.4 mm. The authors reported that the mean operative time was 36.9 ± 14.8 min, and included the treatment of renal and ureteral stones. The mean hospitalization time was 2.5 ± 0.5 days. The SFR rate at one month after the procedure was calculated to be 95.8%, while the perioperative and postoperative complication rate was 5.6%. No additional interventions were necessary. None of the patients needed a blood transfusion, while the mean hemoglobin drop was estimated to be 1.02 ± 0.18 gr/dL. Based on the data presented in the aforementioned study, non-papillary access could be used with safety for PAUL, as the more medial site of puncture is associated with easier insertion and more efficient manipulation of the flexible ureteroscope.

11   ECIRS (Endoscopic Combined Intrarenal Surgery)

Endoscopic combined intrarenal surgery (ECIRS) was introduced by Scoffone et al. in 2008.The safety and efficacy of ECIRS performed though a non-papillary access was evaluated by Kallidonis et al. (2022). A prospective cohort study was conducted including 33 patients. The indications for the endoscopic combined intrarenal surgery were the large and/or complex stone burden related to difficult renal anatomy. The authors reported 3 patients with horseshoe kidneys, 2 with complete duplicated systems and 2 cases of kidney malrotation, while 60% of the patients suffered from staghorn calculi (Fig. 2). The median stone size was calculated to be 35mm, ranging from 28.5 to 43.5 mm. The authors advocated the that high SFR from only one PCNL session with single access represented the main advantage of this technique. The median operative time was 47 min (ranging from 36 to 65 min) and most of the patients needed one access (78.8%), while 15.2% needed two and 6.1% needed three accesses. The complication rate was calculated to be 9.1% and blood transfusions were not needed. The SFR was estimated to be 90.9% at one month postoperatively. The mean hemoglobin drop was calculated be 1.2 gr/dL (with a range of 1.1 to 1.4 gr/dL) and the mean hospital stay was 3 days (ranging from 2 to 3 days). Considering the above evidence, ECIRS with a non-papillary approach should probably be considered as efficacious without compromising the safety.

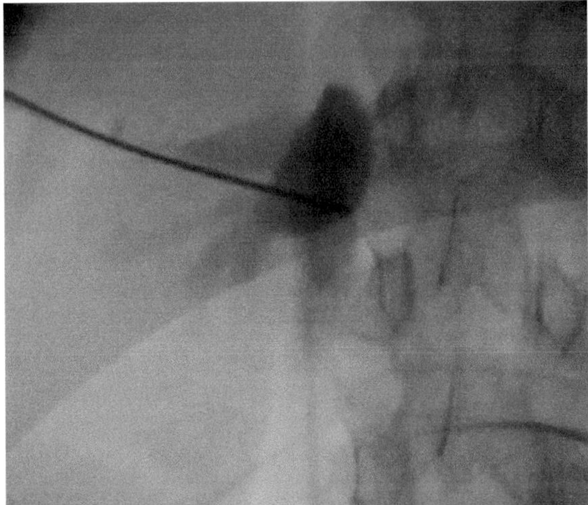

Fig. 2 Non-papillary access to the infundibulum of the lower calyx of a malrotated left kidney

12 The Comparison

Comparative cohort studies have been conducted to investigate the possible difference in the complication rate and SFR between the two access methods (Table 2).

Budak et al. conducted a retrospective comparison including 195 patients that underwent PCNL for the treatment of renal stones larger than 2 cm (Budak et al. 2018). The patients were divided into 2 groups based on the type of access that has been utilized. An infundibular approach ("Eye of the needle technique") was used in the first group of patients (91 patients), while the triangulation technique, aiming for the papilla of the calyx was used in the second group (104 patients). The complication rate of the infundibular group was 18.7% and of the papillary group was 26% without achieving statistical significance. The mean hemoglobin loss was 1.6 gr/dL (with a range from 0.8 to 8.7 gr/dL) and 1.8 gr/dL (with a range from 0.9 to 5.8 gr/dL) for the infundibular and the papillary group, respectively. The authors reported an operative time of 100 min (ranging from 45 to 200 min) and 102.5 min (ranging from 40 to 245 min) for the infundibular and the papillary group, respectively. Finally, the SFR was comparable between the two groups (73.6% and 71.2% for the first and the second group, respectively). The authors concluded that there are no significant differences between the two groups, regarding all the parameters that were investigated.

Kallidonis et al. conducted a prospective randomized study to investigate the hemoglobin drop and bleeding complications between 27 patients that underwent

Table 2 Comparative studies between papiilary and non-papillary PCNL

Author, year of publication	Number of patients	Hemoglobin drop (gr/dL)	Operative time (min)	Stone free rate (SFR)
Budak et al. (2018)	195 in total Non-papillary acces:91 Papillary access:104	NPA: 1.6 (0.8–8.7) PA: 1.8 (0.9–5.8)	NPA: 100 (45–200) PA: 102.5 (40–245)	NPA: 73.6% PA: 71.2%
Kallidonis et al. (2017b)	55 in total Non-papillary acces:91 Papillary access:104	NPA: 1.35 ± 0.79 gr/dL PA: 1.54 ± 1.29	NPA: 43.21 ± 12.38 PA: 51.97 ± 16.1	N/A
Tahra et al. (2020)	276 in total Non-papillary acces:207 Papillary access:69	N/A	NPA: 56.8 ± 15.3 PA: 58.3 ± 14.3	NPA: 85.5% PA: 86.4%
Kashi et al. (2022)	134 in total Non-papillary acces:67 Papillary access:67	NPA: 1.873 ± 1.126 PA: 1.978 ± 1.292 (1st postoperative day)	NPA: 87.58 ± 25.80 PA: 90.22 ± 22.52	NPA:76% PA:82%

papillary PCNL and 28 patients that underwent non-papillary PCNL (Kallidonis et al. 2017b). The comparison of the operative time between the infundibular and the papillary puncture group revealed that the mean operative time of the non-papillary group was 43.21 ± 12.38 min and 51.97 ± 16.1 min for the papillary group. The hemoglobin loss was 1.35 ± 0.79 gr/dL and 1.54 ± 1.29 gr/dL for the infundibular and the papillary group, respectively. The mean hospitalization time for the former group was 5.8 ± 2.56 days and for the latter group 5.57 ± 1.7 days. In terms of complications, the infundibular group was associated with a complication rate of 7.14%, while complications occurred in 7.4% of the cases in the papillary group. Based on the presented data, it is suggested that no significant difference in terms of hemoglobin drop and bleeding complications was found between the two groups.

The above-mentioned results are in accordance with the findings of Tahra et al. (2020) The authors conducted a retrospective, match-paired case–control study including 207 patients who underwent PCNL with non-papillary access and 69 who underwent PCNL with papillary access. The mean operative time of the non-papillary group was calculated to be 56.8 ± 15.3 min and of the papillary group 58.3 ± 14.3 min. The hemoglobin level drop was similar and the mean hospitalization time was calculated to be 4.51 ± 1.8 and 4.45 ± 1.9 days for the papillary and the non-papillary groups, respectively. The authors reported a similar SFR between the two groups (85.5% for the non-papillary group and 86.4% for the papillary group), while the complication rate was also comparable (7.2% for the non-papillary and 7.1% for the papillary group).

In addition, Kashi et al., compared papillary and non-papillary PCNL, including 134 patients in a prospective cohort study (Kashi et al. 2022). The authors reported that the mean hemoglobin drops, on the first postoperative day, were 1.873 ± 1.126 and 1.978 ± 1.292 gr/dL for the non-papillary and the papillary group, respectively. No significant difference was also noticed on the second postoperative day. The mean operative time was 87.58 ± 25.80 min, and 90.22 ± 22.52 min for the non-papillary and papillary groups, respectively. The SFR was calculated to be 76% for the former and 82% for the latter group. Considering the above comparative studies, it is clear that different investigating groups conclude to the clinical safety of the non-papillary approach.

13 Conclusion

Non-papillary access seems to be safe and efficient alternative for the papillary approach. It can be performed in different clinical scenarios such as standard and mini PCNL, ECIRS, antegrade ureteroscopy and staghorn stones. The complication rate does not differ between different puncture sites. The available evidence suggests that short operative times are related to an easy navigation and lithotripsy in the PCS constituting the main advantage of this type of access. Nevertheless, the surgical habits of each department and the techniques that any surgeon has been trained to use, play an important role in their preferred practice. It could be proposed that these two techniques complement each other.

References

Abouelgreed TA, Abdelaal MA, Amin MM, Elatreisy A, Shalkamy O, Abdrabuh AM, et al. Endoscopic combined intrarenal surgery in the prone split-leg position versus Galdakao-modified supine Valdivia position for the management of partial staghorn calculi. BMC Urol. 2022;22(1):163. https://doi.org/10.1186/s12894-022-01115-3.

Adamou C, Tsaturyan A, Kalogeropoulou C, Tzelepi V, Apostolopoulos D, Vretos T, et al. Comparison of renal parenchymal trauma after standard, mini and ultra-mini percutaneous tract dilation in porcine models. World J Urol. 2022;40(8):2083–9. https://doi.org/10.1007/s00345-022-040 69-1.

Budak S, Yucel C, Kisa E, Kozacioglu Z. Comparison of two different renal access techniques in one-stage percutaneous nephrolithotomy: triangulation versus eye of the needle. Ann Saudi Med. 2018;38(3):189–93. https://doi.org/10.5144/0256-4947.2018.189.

Corrales M, Doizi S, Barghouthy Y, Kamkoum H, Somani B, Traxer O. Ultrasound or fluoroscopy for percutaneous nephrolithotomy access, is there really a difference? A review of literature. J Endourol. 2021;35(3):241–8. https://doi.org/10.1089/end.2020.0672.

Geraghty RM, Davis NF, Tzelves L, Lombardo R, Yuan C, Thomas K, et al. Best practice in interventional management of urolithiasis: an update from the European Association of urology guidelines panel for urolithiasis 2022. Eur Urol Focus. 2022. https://doi.org/10.1016/j.euf.2022. 06.014.

Güler A, Erbin A, Ucpinar B, Savun M, Sarilar O, Akbulut MF. Comparison of miniaturized percutaneous nephrolithotomy and standard percutaneous nephrolithotomy for the treatment of large kidney stones: a randomized prospective study. Urolithiasis. 2019;47(3):289–95. https:// doi.org/10.1007/s00240-018-1061-y.

Hou B, Wang M, Song Z, He Q, Hao Z. Renal puncture access via a nonpapillary track in percutaneous nephrolithotomy: an in vitro porcine kidney experience. Urolithiasis. 2022;50(3):357–60. https://doi.org/10.1007/s00240-022-01302-9.

Kallidonis P, Kalogeropoulou C, Kyriazis I, Apostolopoulos D, Kitrou P, Kotsiris D, et al. Percutaneous nephrolithotomy puncture and tract dilation: evidence on the safety of approaches to the infundibulum of the middle renal calyx. Urology. 2017a;107:43–8. https://doi.org/10.1016/ j.urology.2017.05.038.

Kallidonis P, Kyriazis I, Kotsiris D, Koutava A, Kamal W, Liatsikos E. Papillary versus nonpapillary puncture in percutaneous nephrolithotomy: a prospective randomized trial. J Endourol. 2017b;31(S1):S4-s9. https://doi.org/10.1089/end.2016.0571.

Kallidonis P, Vagionis A, Lattarulo M, Adamou C, Tsaturyan A, Liourdi D, et al. Non-papillary percutaneous nephrolithotomy for treatment of staghorn stones. Minerva Urol Nephrol. 2021a;73(5):649–54. https://doi.org/10.23736/s2724-6051.20.04124-7.

Kallidonis P, Vagionis A, Vrettos T, Adamou K, Pagonis K, Ntasiotis P, et al. Non papillary mini-percutaneous nephrolithotomy: early experience. World J Urol. 2021b;39(4):1241–6. https:// doi.org/10.1007/s00345-020-03267-z.

Kallidonis P, Tsaturyan A, Faria-Costa G, Ballesta Martinez B, Peteinaris A, Adamou C, et al. Nonpapillary prone endoscopic combined intrarenal surgery: effectiveness, safety and tips, and tricks. World J Urol. 2022. https://doi.org/10.1007/s00345-022-04178-x.

Kandemir E, Savun M, Sezer A, Erbin A, Akbulut MF, Sarılar Ö. Comparison of miniaturized percutaneous nephrolithotomy and standard percutaneous nephrolithotomy in secondary patients: a randomized prospective study. J Endourol. 2020;34(1):26–32. https://doi.org/10.1089/end.2019.0538.

Kashi AH, Basiri A, Voshtasbi A, Ghead MA, Dadpour M, Nazempour F, et al. Comparing the outcomes of papillary and non-papillary access in percutaneous nephrolithotomy. World J Urol. 2022. https://doi.org/10.1007/s00345-022-04256-0.

Kuzgunbay B, Turunc T, Yaycioglu O, Kayis AA, Gul U, Egilmez T, et al. Percutaneous nephrolithotomy for staghorn kidney stones in elderly patients. Int Urol Nephrol. 2011;43(3):639–43. https://doi.org/10.1007/s11255-010-9885-6.

Kyriazis I, Panagopoulos V, Kallidonis P, Özsoy M, Vasilas M, Liatsikos E. Complications in percutaneous nephrolithotomy. World J Urol. 2015;33(8):1069–77. https://doi.org/10.1007/s00345-014-1400-8.

Kyriazis I, Kallidonis P, Vasilas M, Panagopoulos V, Kamal W, Liatsikos E. Challenging the wisdom of puncture at the calyceal fornix in percutaneous nephrolithotripsy: feasibility and safety study with 137 patients operated via a non-calyceal percutaneous track. World J Urol. 2017;35(5):795–801. https://doi.org/10.1007/s00345-016-1919-y.

Sampaio FJ. Anatomical background for nephron-sparing surgery in renal cell carcinoma. J Urol. 1992;147(4):999–1005. https://doi.org/10.1016/s0022-5347(17)37445-1.

Sampaio FJ. Renal anatomy. Endourologic considerations. Urol Clin North Am. 2000;27(4):585–607. https://doi.org/10.1016/s0094-0143(05)70109-9.

Sampaio FJ, Aragao AH. Anatomical relationship between the intrarenal arteries and the kidney collecting system. J Urol. 1990;143(4):679–81. https://doi.org/10.1016/s0022-5347(17)40056-5.

Sampaio FJ, Zanier JF, Aragão AH, Favorito LA. Intrarenal access: 3-dimensional anatomical study. J Urol. 1992;148(6):1769–73. https://doi.org/10.1016/s0022-5347(17)37024-6.

Tahra A, Sobay R, Bindayi A, Suceken FY, Kucuk EV. Papillary vs non-papillary access during percutaneous nephrolithotomy: retrospective, match-paired case-control study. Archivio italiano di urologia, andrologia: organo ufficiale [di] Societa italiana di ecografia urologica e nefrologica. 2020;92(1):50–2. https://doi.org/10.4081/aiua.2020.1.50.

Tsaturyan A, Bellin A, Barbuto S, Zampakis P, Ntzanis E, Lattarulo M, et al. Technical aspects to maximize the hyperaccuracy three-dimensional (HA3D(™)) computed tomography reconstruction for kidney stones surgery: a pilot study. Urolithiasis. 2021;49(6):559–66. https://doi.org/10.1007/s00240-021-01262-6.

Tsaturyan A, Boviatsis V, Peteinaris A, Adamou C, Pagonis K, Natsos A, et al. Non-papillary access for the percutaneous antegrade treatment of renal and ureteral stones. Urology. 2022. https://doi.org/10.1016/j.urology.2022.08.037.

Yuan D, Liu Y, Rao H, Cheng T, Sun Z, Wang Y, et al. Supine versus prone position in percutaneous nephrolithotomy for kidney calculi: a meta-analysis. J Endourol. 2016;30(7):754–63. https://doi.org/10.1089/end.2015.0402.

Tract Dilation for PCNL

Lazaros Tzelves, Nariman Gadzhiev, Titos Markopoulos,
Bhaskar Somani, and Andreas Skolarikos

Abstract Percutaneous nephrolithotomy success and safety largely depend on two steps: renal puncture and percutaneous tract dilation. The tract dilation can be performed using several techniques like Alken or Amplatz dilators, balloon single-use dilator, or the most recently developed one-shot technique. All the methods were initially dependent on the use of fluoroscopy for guidance, but recent expertise on the use of ultrasound permitted tract dilation under complete ultrasound guidance, eliminating the harmful effects of radiation exposure.

Keywords PCNL · Tract dilation · Amplatz · Alken · Balloon dilation · One-shot dilation

1　Introduction

Since its introduction in 1976 by Fernstrom and Johansson, percutaneous nephrolithotripsy (PCNL) has revolutionized the management of urolithiasis. It is the minimally invasive nature of this procedure that leads to high stone-free rates (SFRs), while at the same time permitting surgeons to offer excellent clinical outcomes avoiding the complications related to copious open surgery for removal of complex and/or large stone volumes (Skolarikos et al. 2022). It is nowadays considered the

L. Tzelves
Department of Urology, University College London Hospital, London, UK

N. Gadzhiev
Department of Urology, Pavlov First Saint Petersburg State Medical University, Saint Petersburg, Russia

T. Markopoulos · A. Skolarikos (✉)
Department of Urology, School of Medicine, Sismanoglio Hospital, National and Kapodistrian University of Athens, Athens, Greece
e-mail: andskol@yahoo.com

B. Somani
University Hospital Southampton NHS Trust, Southampton, UK

gold-standard option for stones >2 cm in maximum diameter (Skolarikos et al. 2022). To master the fundamental principles of this procedure, endourologists have to reach and surpass the learning curve which is steep. Along with puncture of the renal parenchyma, percutaneous tract dilation is one of the most critical steps of PCNL. It is the success of these two steps that greatly affect the duration of operation, total fluoroscopic time, rate of bleeding complications, perforation of the renal collecting system, urine leakage, and injury to adjacent organs (Geraghty et al. 2022).

2   Tract Dilation Under Fluoroscopic Guidance

Fluoroscopy has been utilized for many years during endourological procedures and PCNL to guide stone localization, needle entry into collecting systems, insertion of guidewires and access sheaths, as well as creation and dilation of the percutaneous tract. The size of the tract to be created during standard PCNL is supposed to accommodate the insertion of a sheath with an inner diameter of 30Fr and outer diameter of 34Fr, while during mini-PCNL usually sheaths less than 20–24Fr are inserted.

There are several methods for dilation of the tract: use of metallic, sequential, co-axial Alken dilators (Alken et al. 1981), use of polyurethane, serial, Amplatz dilators (Castaneda-Zuniga et al. 1982), use of the single step balloon dilators (Clayman et al. 1983) and creation of the tract by one-stage dilation using a single 25–30Fr Amplatz dilator (Frattini et al. 2001) (Fig. 1). Each of these techniques has its advantages and disadvantages which will be analyzed further but is imperative to understand that the dilator should not be advanced further than the calyx because otherwise the collecting system or ureteropelvic junction and even surrounding organs and vessels may be perforated (Fig. 2). The desired point of entry of the distal end of the dilator is just into the calyx and proper positioning should be confirmed with the nephroscope and adjustments should be made over the guidewire if needed (Figs. 3 and 4). Another important technical detail is that skin incision should extend to an adequate depth into underlying fascial layers so that dilators can be easily advanced without kinking and bending.

Alken metallic dilators are serial rigid dilators advanced over the guidewire in a coaxial manner without the need to remove the previous dilator before the next one is advanced (Alken et al. 1981) (Fig. 5). After the guidewire is properly inserted into the pelvicalyceal system or ideally down to the ureter/bladder, an 8Fr guide rod is advanced initially, and its distal end is recognized with a ball at its tip so that it is easy to confirm position under fluoroscopic guidance (Alken et al. 1981). Subsequently, dilation continues up to 30Fr. They are reusable and considered to lead to less blood loss due to the tamponade effect of the dilators on small vessels of the renal parenchyma. A major advantage is that metallic dilators can override dense and fibrotic tissue, encountered after previous renal surgeries, making them ideal for these cases. The main disadvantage is the increased fluoroscopy and procedural time needed until dilators of all sizes are inserted sequentially, while at the same time due to repeated manipulations over the guidewire, there is an increased chance of displacement or kinking due to the force applied.

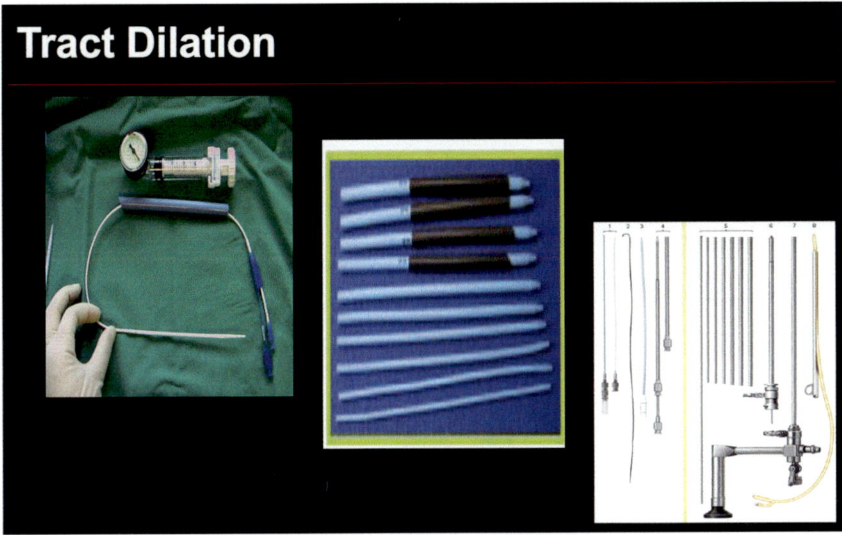

Fig. 1 Tract Dilation—Balloon Dilation, Amplatz dilators, Metallic Dilators

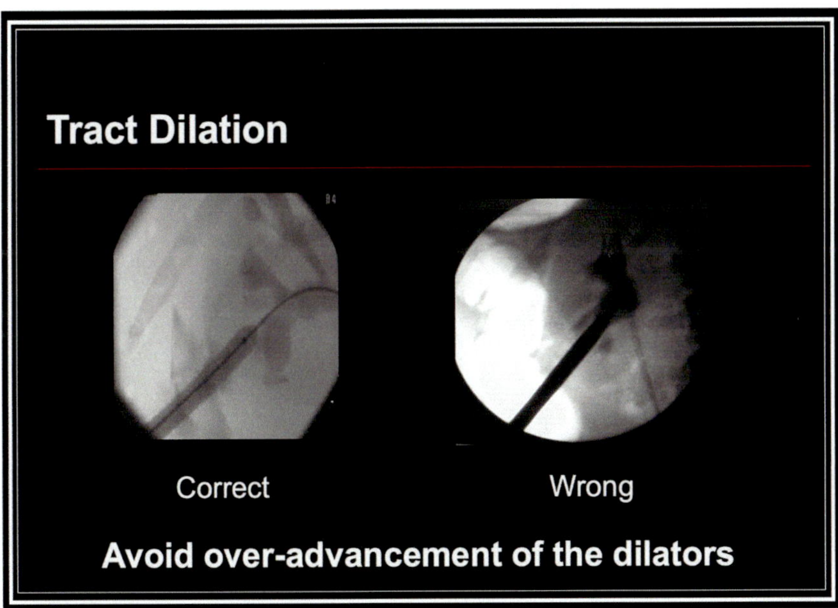

Fig. 2 Correct advancement of the dilator

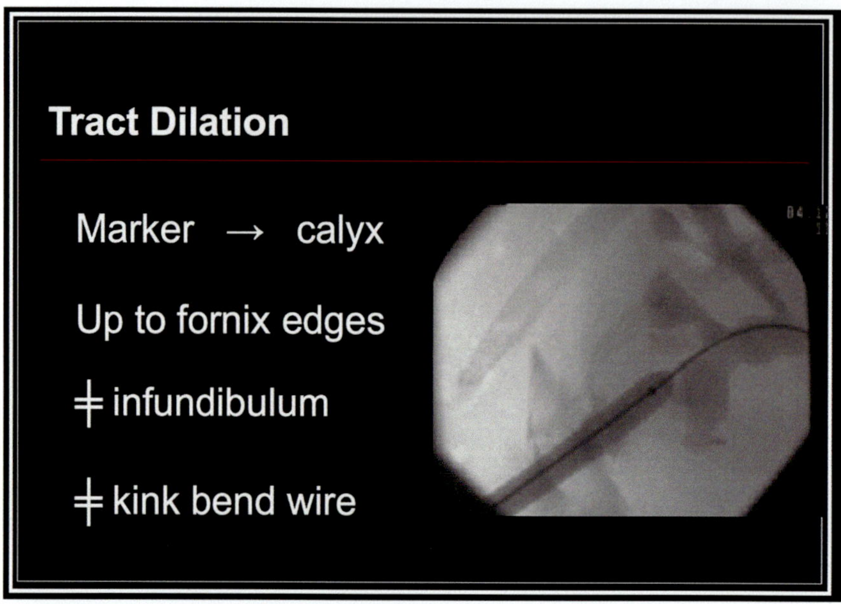

Fig. 3 Balloon dilation of the PCNL tract—Landmarks

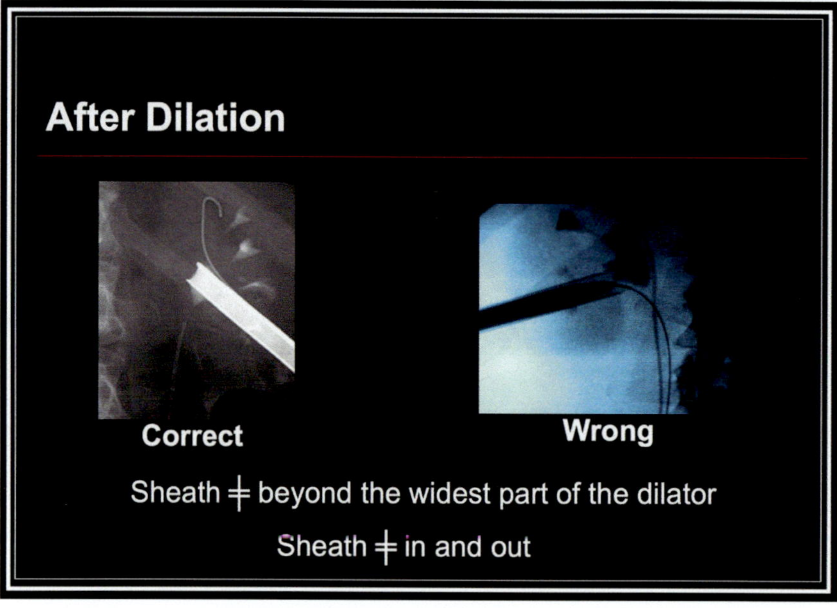

Fig. 4 Proper advancement of the sheath after tract dilation

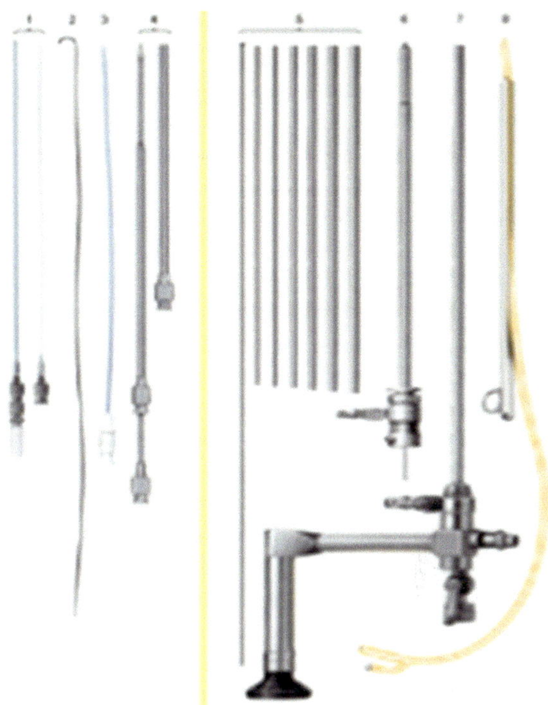

Fig. 5 Peter Alken's metallic dilators

In a similar manner, Amplatz semi-rigid dilators are sequential dilators that are progressively advanced over an initial 8Fr guiding catheter, but in contrast with Alken dilators, they are not inserted coaxially since the smaller diameter dilator should be removed before the next one is advanced at increments of 2Fr (Castaneda-Zuniga et al. 1982). Since they are composed of softer material, they are considered to be less traumatic for tissue than metallic dilators. Drawbacks of this technique are increased use of fluoroscopy and time needed to create access and increased chance of tract loss or guidewire kinking during the sequential exchange of dilators. Amplatz dilators are used once, therefore increasing procedural costs, while the tamponade effect is lost due to the removal of smaller-size dilators before the next one is advanced leading to hemorrhage.

Single-step balloon dilator overpasses the need for repetitive dilation of Alken and Amplatz dilators leading to decreased use of fluoroscopy and quicker creation of the percutaneous tract (Clayman et al. 1983). Before the balloon dilator is advanced over the guidewire, the working sheath is loaded on the balloon catheter and then the dilator is advanced over the working guidewire into the pelvicalyceal system (Clayman et al. 1983). The balloon is inflated with contrast up to 30 atm and this pressure is maintained for 30–60 s. The atm applied is guided from the "waist" that appears during balloon dilation, which signifies the area of maximum resistance.

The indication of adequate dilation is when the "waist" disappears (Clayman et al. 1983). At the point of maximum balloon dilation, the working sheath is advanced under continuous fluoroscopic guidance just distally to the end of the maximum balloon dilation and not further beyond this point (Clayman et al. 1983). Although this is considered one of the safest techniques, the literature contains some controversial data regarding bleeding complications. Most studies suggest that the use of balloon leads to reduced bleeding, but results from the Clinical Research Office of the Endourological Society Percutaneous Nephrolithotomy Global Study over 5537 patients, indicate that compared to telescopic/serial dilation, single-step balloon dilation led to increased rates of bleeding (9.4% versus 6.7%, $p < 0.001$), more transfusions (7.0% versus 4.9%, $p = 0.001$) and greater drop in mean hematocrit levels (4.5% versus 2.5%) (Lopes et al. 2011). These findings were mainly attributed to the heterogeneity of technique among the centers recruiting patients (Lopes et al. 2011). Although the main disadvantage is the increased costs since it is single use, it can decrease the use of fluoroscopy and procedural time devoted to tract dilation but literature has shown increased failure rates, especially if there is a history of renal surgery, reaching up to 25% (Joel et al. 2005).

The one-stage dilation method was introduced by Frattini et al. in 2001 who proposed that after successful puncture and guidewire insertion, a single 25–30Fr dilator to be loaded on the Alken guide rod or an 8Fr polyurethane dilator and subsequently a 34Fr sheath to be advanced (Frattini et al. 2001). Fahmy et al. assessed the use of single-step tract dilation in 70 children with stone burden 2–4 cm using a 20Fr Amplatz working sheath after tract dilation (Fahmy et al. 2011). In this randomized controlled trial (RCT), in the first group, Alken dilators were used, while in the second group a single step 20Fr Amplatz dilator was advanced (Fahmy et al. 2011). Authors reported that dilation was successful in all cases and there were no significant differences between the groups regarding operative time, total fluoroscopy time, length of stay (LOS), and SFRs (Fahmy et al. 2011). The overall complication rate was higher in the group of Alken dilators (28.5% versus 14.2%, $p = 0.018$), the need for intraoperative transfusion was lower in the single-step dilation (2.8% versus 11.4%, $p = 0.045$), fluoroscopy time during dilation favored single step dilation (8.8 versus 23.3 s, $p = 0.042$), while hemoglobin drop was greater in cases where Alken dilators were used (1.5 versus 0.6 gr/dl, $p = 0.026$) (Fahmy et al. 2011). Ghoneima et al. performed an RCT to assess the feasibility and safety of one-shot dilation compared to sequential dilation in a tubeless PCNL (Ghoneima et al. 2022). In the group where only one 30Fr Amplatz dilator was used, authors reported decreased dilation time (34.4 versus 166.2 s, $p < 0.001$), decreased fluoroscopy time during dilation (15.6 versus 98.5 s, $p < 0.001$), decreased total operative time (73.2 versus 97.9 min, $p < 0.001$), decreased need for transfusion (4.2% versus 17.2%, $p = 0.015$), decreased urine leakage (1.4% versus 15.5%, $p = 0.003$), but similar SFRs and rest complication rates were observed (Ghoneima et al. 2022). Although most studies indicate the advantageous effects of single-step dilation, Aminsharifi et al. in their study suggested that this technique may lead to more parenchymal damage than gradual dilation (Aminsharifi et al. 2011). Authors quantified the decrease in renal function and renal scar formation using 99m-Tc DMSA scan one month after PCNL in two distinct groups: one where single-step dilation was performed and the second where Alken dilators were inserted (Aminsharifi et al. 2011). Although their findings complied with literature regarding shorter access time and radiation exposure in the single-stage dilation group, they detected a significant drop in 99m-Tc uptake in this group one month postoperatively ($-2.4 \pm 0.3\%$, p = 0.001), while in the group of Alken dilators, no significant drop was noted (Aminsharifi et al. 2011).

The main advantages and disadvantages of each technique are shown in Table 1.

Several meta-analyses tried to address the differences between these techniques and provide a clear insight into the pros and cons of each one of them. Peng et al. in their study included 7 RCTs with 697 patients in total, comparing one-shot versus serial dilation (Peng et al. 2019). In their pooled analysis they found that although SFRs, success in dilation, LOS, and complication rates were similar between groups, the one-shot technique offered 110 s decreased access time, 0.23 gr/dl decreased blood loss but similar transfusion rates, and shorter fluoroscopy time in all included studies, although a pooled analysis was not performed for this outcome due to extreme heterogeneity in definition (Peng et al. 2019). In a more recent analysis, Peng et al. (2020) compared balloon with Amplatz dilation using data from 6 RCTs and 1317 patients in total. They reported similar overall complication rates, transfusion rates, SFRs, LOS, operative time, fluoroscopy time, and success rates among the two groups, but less hemoglobin drop by 0.21 gr/dl and shorter access time by 2.6 min when balloon dilation was used (Peng et al. 2020). Finally, Wu et al. in their

Table 1 Advantages/disadvantages of percutaneous tract dilation techniques

Alken metallic dilators	Amplatz semi-rigid plastic dilators	Single-step balloon dilator	One-stage dilation method
Less blood loss due to tamponade effect	Softer material causing less tissue trauma	Tamponade effect of the dilated balloon	Reduced cost
Reusable	Single use	Single use	No need to use a whole set of dilators
Rigid material able to be advanced through fibrotic tissue	Increased time needed to create tract	Less time consuming	Less time consuming
Increased time needed to create tract	Increased use of fluoroscopy	Decreased use of fluoroscopy	Decreased use of fluoroscopy
Increased use of fluoroscopy	Increased chance of tract loss or guidewire kinking due to force applied repetitively	8–25% failure rate, especially in cases with dense fibrotic tissue from previous surgery	Less successful in patients with previous renal surgery
Increased chance of tract loss or guidewire kinking due to force applied repetitively			

analysis compared all 4 methods between them by pooling data from 11 studies and 1415 patients (Wu et al. 2020). They found that the fluoroscopy time was decreased by 30.7 s in one-shot dilation compared to Alken dilators and by 26.4 s in balloon versus Alken dilators, but was similar between the balloon and one-shot dilation (Wu et al. 2020). Access time was shorted by 2.15 min for one-shot versus Alken dilators, while hemoglobin drop was less in one-shot dilation compared to Alken dilators (-0.19 gr/dl), less in balloon versus Amplatz dilation (-0.65 gr/dl), but similar between balloon versus one-shot dilation and Amplatz versus Alken dilators (Wu et al. 2020). Finally, overall SFRs, LOS, transfusion rates, and success rates were similar between the groups (Wu et al. 2020).

3 Creation of Percutaneous Tract in a Modified or Supine Position

Creation of a percutaneous tract in a supine or modified position can prove challenging due to existing anatomic structures through the course of dilators compared to the prone position; however, it is important for endourologists to be familiar with this technique, since supine PCNL reduces cardiopulmonary complications in high-risk patients and also permits simultaneous retrograde access for performing endoscopic combined intrarenal surgery (Mourmouris et al. 2018). In their study, Chung et al. proposed a modified tract dilation technique in patients undergoing PNCL in a prone or modified position, which compared to the standard technique led to reduced fluoroscopy time (68.9 versus 212.1 s, $p < 0.05$), decreased LOS (5.9 versus 6.7 days, $p < 0.05$) and increased success rate (77.2% versus 63.6%, $p < 0.05$), although total operative time, complication and transfusion rates were similar (Chung et al. 2021). The authors proposed steps in order to decrease the mobility of the kidney during advancing the dilators in a supine position by applying traction to the guidewires at two points: one at its exit from the dilator towards the kidney and the other from the urethra since the guidewire was advanced into the bladder and grabbed with a cystoscopic forceps (Chung et al. 2021). Although there is the theoretical risk of damaging the pelvicalyceal system from the excessive force over the guidewire, in this study no such event was noted, implying that the use of a hydrophilic guidewire instead of a more rigid shows a protective effect (Chung et al. 2021).

4 Tract Dilation Under Ultrasonographic Guidance

Exposure to ionizing radiation leads to tissue damage either when a certain threshold is acutely surpassed (deterministic effect) which is not that common or even with repeated low doses which gradually accumulate and can lead to mutations and carcinogenesis (stochastic effect). Both patients and operating room staff are exposed to harmful doses of radiation during endourological procedures (Vassileva et al. 2020, 2021) but also during their diagnosis and follow-up leading to an accountable burden (Tzelves et al. 2022a). One of the most effective ways to reduce radiation exposure is the use of ultrasound, which not only eliminates radiation but also facilitates the detection of radiolucent stones and better visualization of renal calyx anatomy (anterior versus posterior) and recognition of surrounding structures and vessels (when using Doppler function). Nowadays, there are centers performing PCNL entirely under ultrasonographic guidance which has stood the test of time and proven its effectiveness and safety (Tzelves et al. 2022b).

To perform a completely fluoroscopy-free PCNL, tract dilation should be performed under ultrasonographic guidance as well. The main obstacle in this is that Amplatz and Alken dilators have low echogenicity in contrast to the high echogenicity of the guidewire. Therefore, a method to observe the course of dilators is to detect the point where the guidewire signal is lost and thereby estimate the position of the dilator tip. However, this method can be obscured by adipose tissue and is not applicable to patients with increased body mass index. In obese patients, the estimated depth can be measured by the needle length that was inserted to enter the calyx, therefore providing a metric.

Another method to perform the tract dilation under ultrasonographic guidance, the two-step technique, was proposed by Li et al., who advanced 8–16Fr fascial dilators over the guidewire to a pre-determined depth according to needle length used for puncture (Li et al. 2014). Subsequently, a 16Fr peel-away sheath was placed and a ureteroscope was inserted through the sheath to confirm proper positioning (Li et al. 2014). In case of short dilation, the 16Fr sheath was advanced over the ureteroscope (Li et al. 2014). Following this, a 15Fr metallic dilator was placed and the tract was dilated up to 24Fr (Li et al. 2014).

Finally, balloon dilation can also be applied to dilate the tract under ultrasonographic guidance. Jin et al. compared this technique against serial metallic dilators (Jin et al. 2020). The balloon was inflated up to 30 atm for 60 s, while the course and final position of the balloon was monitored and confirmed only by ultrasound (Jin et al. 2020) In the comparator group, the two-step technique was used as described above (Jin et al. 2020). Authors reported that SFRs need for ancillary procedures, transfusion, and infection rates were similar between the two groups, while the time needed for tract dilation was less for the balloon group (3.4 versus 4.3 min, p < 0.001) and similarly a reduced total operative time was observed (62.2 versus 70.2 min, p = 0.024) (Jin et al. 2020). The only RCT existing is the study by Pakmanesh et al. who compared Amplatz dilators to balloon dilation in ultrasound-guided PCNL (Pakmanesh et al. 2019). In the Amplatz group, a single 28–30Fr dilation was used with the desired depth estimated according to the length of the inserted needle to perform a successful puncture, while in the balloon group, a 28–30Fr balloon dilator was used and monitored by ultrasound (Pakmanesh et al. 2019). Authors reported that short dilation was more frequent in the Amplatz group (57.6% versus 36.4%), although not reaching statistical significance, while the time needed for tract dilation, SFRs, and complications were similar (Pakmanesh et al. 2019). Importantly, the cost of the balloon was higher than Amplatz dilators (603 versus 718 US dollars, $p = 0.0001$) (Pakmanesh et al. 2019). They also observed that lower pole access led to significantly more short dilations compared to middle or lower pole access (61% versus 18% versus 40% respectively, $p = 0.01$) (Pakmanesh et al. 2019). Not only the location of the punctured calyx seems to affect tract dilation success when using the balloon under ultrasound guidance. Li et al. suggested that the degree of hydronephrosis is important since in patients with moderate or severe pelvicalyceal system dilation, balloon insertion was nearly 100% successful, in contrast with non-dilated systems (Li et al. 2014). Other factors leading to the reduced success of balloon dilation are obesity, previous open surgery, and staghorn stones (Usawach-intachit et al. 2016), therefore It is advisable that novice surgeons may use fluoroscopy under these circumstances.

5　Conclusion

Percutaneous tract dilation in PCNL is of similar importance as renal puncture, as operation success and bleeding complications are mostly affected by these two steps of the procedure. For many years, tract dilation was performed solely under fluoroscopic guidance with the main methods being Alken metallic or Amplatz polyurethane sequential dilators, single-step balloon dilation, or one-shot dilation. Each technique offers specific pros and cons, although in cases with previous renal surgeries and the existence of fibrotic tissue along the tract, the use of metallic dilators is advisable. Gaining expertise in the use of ultrasound led to PCNL being completely performed under ultrasound guidance in several centers and tract dilation can also be performed using either Amplatz/Alken or balloon dilators without the need for fluoroscopic guidance. The familiarity of the surgeon with each of these methods should be taken into serious consideration before choosing the technique (Fig. 6).

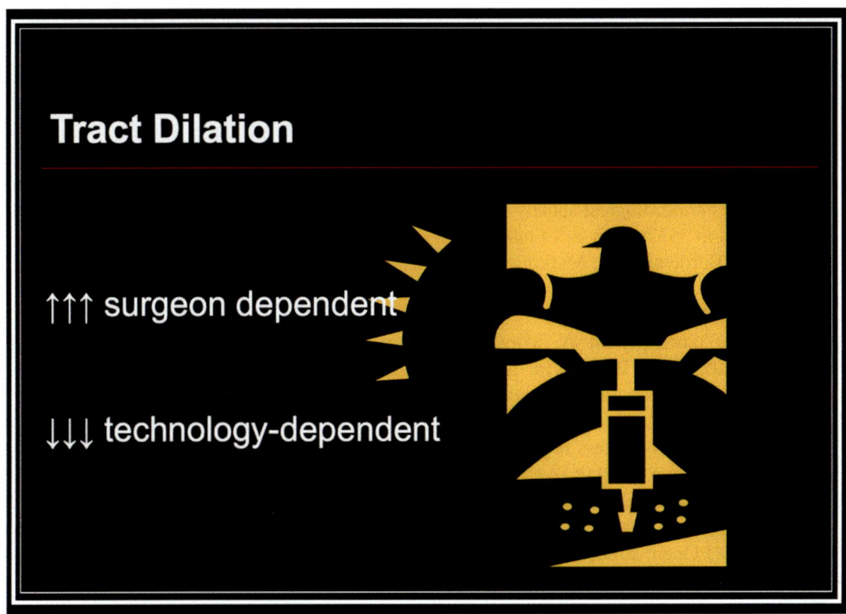

Fig. 6 Track dilation is surgeon dependent

References

Alken P, Hutschenreiter G, Günther R, Marberger M. Percutaneous stone manipulation. J Urol. 1981;125(4):463–6.

Aminsharifi A, Alavi M, Sadeghi G, Shakeri S, Afsar F. Renal parenchymal damage after percutaneous nephrolithotomy with one-stage tract dilation technique: a randomized clinical trial. J Endourol. 2011;25(6):927–31.

Castaneda-Zuniga WR, Clayman R, Smith A, Rusnak B, Herrera M, Amplatz K. Nephrostolithotomy: percutaneous techniques for urinary calculus removal. 1982. J Urol. 2002;167(2 Pt 2):849–53; discussion 54.

Chung JW, Ha H, Park DJ, Ha YS, Lee JN, Chun SY, et al. Efficacy and safety of modified tract dilation technique using simultaneous pulling of proximal and distal ends of a guidewire for percutaneous nephrolithotomy in modified supine position. Investig Clin Urol. 2021;62(2):186–94.

Clayman RV, Castaneda-Zuniga WR, Hunter DW, Miller RP, Lange PH, Amplatz K. Rapid balloon dilatation of the nephrostomy track for nephrostolithotomy. Radiology. 1983;147(3):884–5.

Fahmy AMW, Elbadry M, Moussa A. Single step track dilatation for percutaneous nephrolithotomy in children. Int Urol Nephrol. 2011;54(11):2789–95.

Frattini A, Barbieri A, Salsi P, Sebastio N, Ferretti S, Bergamaschi E, et al. One shot: a novel method to dilate the nephrostomy access for percutaneous lithotripsy. J Endourol. 2001;15(9):919–23.

Geraghty RM, Davis NF, Tzelves L, Lombardo R, Yuan C, Thomas K, et al. Best practice in interventional management of urolithiasis: an update from the European Association of Urology Guidelines Panel for Urolithiasis 2022. Eur Urol Focus. 2022.

Ghoneima W, Makki M, Lotfi MA, Mostafa A, Elkady A, Rammah AM. The feasibility and safety of one-shot dilatation compared to conventional sequential dilatation in tubeless percutaneous nephrolithotomy: a prospective randomized controlled study. Urolithiasis. 2022;51(1):3.

Jin W, Song Y, Fei X. The Pros and cons of balloon dilation in totally ultrasound-guided percutaneous Nephrolithotomy. BMC Urol. 2020;20(1):82.

Joel AB, Rubenstein JN, Hsieh MH, Chi T, Meng MV, Stoller ML. Failed percutaneous balloon dilation for renal access: incidence and risk factors. Urology. 2005;66(1):29–32.

Li J, Xiao B, Hu W, Yang B, Chen L, Hu H, et al. Complication and safety of ultrasound guided percutaneous nephrolithotomy in 8025 cases in China. Chin Med J (engl). 2014;127(24):4184–9.

Lopes T, Sangam K, Alken P, Barroilhet BS, Saussine C, Shi L, et al. The clinical research office of the endourological society percutaneous nephrolithotomy global study: tract dilation comparisons in 5537 patients. J Endourol. 2011;25(5):755–62.

Mourmouris P, Berdempes M, Markopoulos T, Lazarou L, Tzelves L, Skolarikos A. Patient positioning during percutaneous nephrolithotomy: what is the current best practice? Res Rep Urol. 2018;10:189–93.

Pakmanesh H, Daneshpajooh A, Mirzaei M, Shahesmaeili A, Hashemian M, Alinejad M, et al. Amplatz versus Balloon for tract dilation in ultrasonographically guided percutaneous nephrolithotomy: a randomized clinical trial. Biomed Res Int. 2019;2019:3428123.

Peng P-x, Lai S-c, Ding Z-s, He Y-h, Zhou L-h, Wang X-m, et al. One-shot dilation versus serial dilation technique for access in percutaneous nephrolithotomy: a systematic review and meta-analysis. BMJ Open. 2019;9(4): e025871.

Peng PX, Lai SC, Seery S, He YH, Zhao H, Wang XM, et al. Balloon versus Amplatz for tract dilation in fluoroscopically guided percutaneous nephrolithotomy: a systematic review and meta-analysis. BMJ Open. 2020;10(7): e035943.

Skolarikos ANA, Petrik A, Somani B, Thomas K, Gambaro G, et al. EAU guidelines on urolithiasis; 2022.

Tzelves L, Geraghty R, Lombardo R, Davis NF, Petřík A, Neisius A, et al. Duration of follow-up and timing of discharge from imaging follow-up, in adult patients with urolithiasis after surgical or medical intervention: a systematic review and meta-analysis from the European Association of Urology Guideline Panel on Urolithiasis. Eur Urol Focus. 2022a.

Tzelves L, Juliebø-Jones P, Manolitsis I, Bellos T, Mykoniatis I, Berdempes M, et al. Radiation protection measures during endourological therapies. Asian J Urol. 2022b.

Usawachintachit M, Masic S, Chang HC, Allen IE, Chi T. Ultrasound guidance to assist percutaneous nephrolithotomy reduces radiation exposure in obese patients. Urology. 2016;98:32–8.

Vassileva J, Zagorska A, Basic D, Karagiannis A, Petkova K, Sabuncu K, et al. Radiation exposure of patients during endourological procedures: IAEA-SEGUR study. J Radiol Prot. 2020;40(4).

Vassileva J, Zagorska A, Karagiannis A, Petkova K, Sabuncu K, Saltirov I, et al. Radiation exposure of surgical team during endourological procedures: international atomic energy agency-southeastern European group for urolithiasis research study. J Endourol. 2021;35(5):574–82.

Wu Y, Xun Y, Lu Y, Hu H, Qin B, Wang S. Effectiveness and safety of four tract dilation methods of percutaneous nephrolithotomy: a meta-analysis. Exp Ther Med. 2020;19(4):2661–71.

Mini Percutaneous Nephrolithotomy

Oriol Angerri, Matthias Boeykens, and Thomas Tailly

Abstract While percutaneous nephrolithotomy is the most efficient of endourologic procedures to treat large stone burdens, it is also the most prone to severe complications. Miniaturization of equipment is therefore an appealing approach to reduce complications while maintaining efficacy of the procedure. Although reducing the tract size is not the only change that is achieved or needed by miniaturization of the technique. Mini-PCNL comes with a different armamentarium of scopes, a different strategy for stone fragmentation, fragment extraction as well as an evolution in exit strategy. This chapter is intended to cover all these topics and emphasize the main advantages of mini-PCNL.

Keywords Percutaneous nephrolithotomy · Laser · Tubeless · Lithotripter · Miniaturization · Stent · Nephrostomy · Ambulatory · Vacuum

1 Percutaneous Access

"Mini-PCNL" means the use of nephroscope and Amplatz sheaths of smaller caliber as compared to the conventional PCNL. It utilizes a nephroscope of 12 F size with an Amplatz sheath size of 15–18 F., or under 22 Fr. The technique of initial puncture remains the same.

Access is obtained to the desired calyx with either USG or fluoroscopic guidance and a Terumo or extra-stiff guidewire is inserted in the pelvicalyceal system. It is important to place a good length of the wire in the pelvicalyceal system, preferably

O. Angerri
Department of Urology, Fundacio Puigvert, Barcelona, Spain

M. Boeykens
Department of Urology, General Hospital Delta, Roeselare, Belgium

T. Tailly (✉)
Department of Urology, University Hospital Ghent, Corneel Heymanslaan 10, 9000 Gent, Belgium
e-mail: Thomas.tailly@uzgent.be

   199
J. D. Denstedt and E. N. Liatsikos (eds.), *Percutaneous Renal Surgery*,
https://doi.org/10.1007/978-3-031-40542-6_13

in the upper ureter, to avoid slippage of the wire. The puncture should be in line with the infundibulum through which access is intended, to minimize the torque effect on the parenchyma. If multiple tracts are needed in a given case, it is advisable to obtain all accesses at the beginning itself, with separate guidewires for each access. These tracts can be dilated later on a preferential basis as needed.

1.1 *Metal Telescopic Dilatation (Alken Dilatation)*

This was the first described method for percutaneous tract dilatation, proposed by Alken (Alken et al. 1981) (1) An Alken's cannula is introduced over the guidewire under fluoroscopic control which is followed by a guide rod. This is followed by an introduction of serial telescopic metal dilators which slide one over the other till the required diameter of Amplatz sheath to be placed is reached. The advantage of this system is that a central rod is always there to guide the dilator, and if the initial angle and depth are maintained, there is minimal chance of under or over dilatation. The equipment, being metallic, is reusable and thus cost effective, and remains a popular approach in conventional PCNL. In mini-PCNL dilatation is faster because you are using less metal dilators. However, it has largely been replaced by the simpler single-step dilatation in mini-PCNL.

1.2 *Single-Step Dilatation*

This system was proposed by Frattini et al. in (2001). Herein the desired tract size is created in a single step with the dilator of appropriate size without resorting to multiple steps (Fig. 1). After initial puncture and guidewire placement, the desired sized dilator is passed over the guidewire followed by the access sheath. This takes considerably less time and the amount of radiation exposure is also less with this technique (Wu et al. 2020). In mini-PCNL, this approach is often the preferred form of dilatation, thanks to the smaller tract size.

An alternative, is to use a single-step screw dilator. The dilator is made of PTFE and is flexible to allow easy passage through the muscles and fascia (Abdelwahab et al. 2022). This has a considerable advantage over conventional dilators, as this screw dilator can be passed straight over the initial guidewire. The dilator is advanced in a screwing motion till it reaches the desired position. The access sheath can be backloaded over the dilator and can be slid in all the way once the dilator is in place. The entire process is over quickly, saving on time as well as radiation exposure (Abdelwahab et al. 2022).

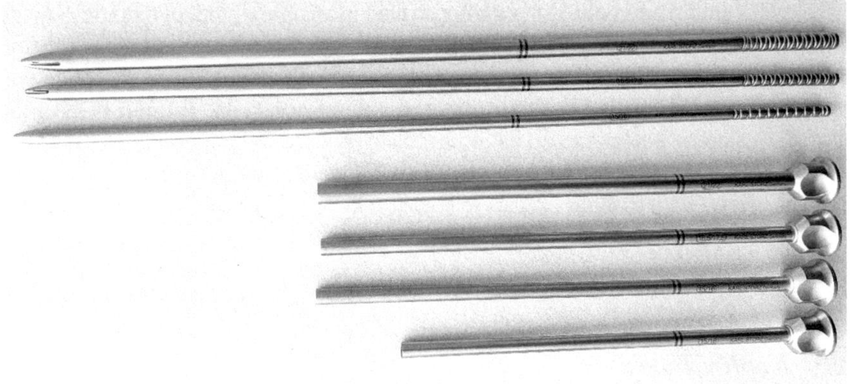

Fig. 1 One step dilators and accompanying Amplatz sheaths sizes 15/16 (short and long), 16.5/ 17.5 and 21/22, from Storz (Karl Storz, Tuttlingen, Germany)

1.3 Balloon Dilatation

The use of a balloon dilator for tract dilatation was proposed by Clayman et al. in (1983). This involved passing a balloon over the guidewire into the pelvicalyceal system over which the desired access sheath can be passed. This has been a popular approach in conventional PCNL where a tract size of 30 Fr was used. The balloon dilates the tract in one shot;. The smallest currently available balloon dilator is 18F in size (Cook Medical, Bloomington, IN) and is as such suitable for mini-PCNL.

The procedure involves passing a 0.035- or 0.038-inch guidewire into the pelvicalyceal system through the puncture needle once an appropriate puncture is made. As an initial step, a 6F, 8F or 10F fascial dilator can be advanced over the guidewire. After these steps, tract dilatation is performed with a balloon dilator which is inflated to 20 atmospheres with diluted or non-diluted contrast dye. Balloon dilatation is usually performed under fluoroscopic guidance. A fluoroscopic image will inform the user of the correct position of the balloon dilator that has two radio-opaque markers identifying the distal and proximal end of the balloon, the completeness of the inflation and any potential indentations in the balloon due to for instance a stiff renal capsule. The Amplatz sheath is then passed over the balloon into the collecting system (Gönen et al. 2008).

1.4 Sequential Amplatz Dilatation

This method of tract dilatation is comparable to telescopic metal dilatation. In standard PCNL, serial passage of Amplatz dilators is done, progressing from 8 to 30 F, followed by placement of the Amplatz sheath over the last dilator (Al-Kandari et al.

2007). Al-Kandari and colleagues demonstrated in an animal model that the damage to the renal parenchyma was similar to the damage caused by balloon dilatation (Al-Kandari et al. 2007). The disadvantage is that when one dilator is withdrawn, it allows bleeding in the tract until the next dilator comes in. In mini-PCNL, the number of steps is less as the dilatation needs to proceed only up to 15–18 Fr, which also provides an opportunity to use one-step dilatation in these cases.

2 Equipment Available for Mini-PCNL

2.1 Nephroscopy

Nephroscopy refers to the introduction of a nephroscope through the access sheath placed in the tract created, to inspect the collecting system and remove the stone. In the case of mini-PCNL, the tract size is < 22Fr, so only miniaturized nephroscopes are available for use in these settings. Mini-nephroscopes are supplied by several manufacturers, and the most popular size is 12 Fr. Smaller sizes including 7.5 Fr, called by several names including "ultra- mini" PCNL and "MIP XS" are also available (Fig. 2).

With the initial introduction of the nephroscope, we must assess the adequacy of dilatation and any trauma to the collecting system. The Amplatz sheath must be

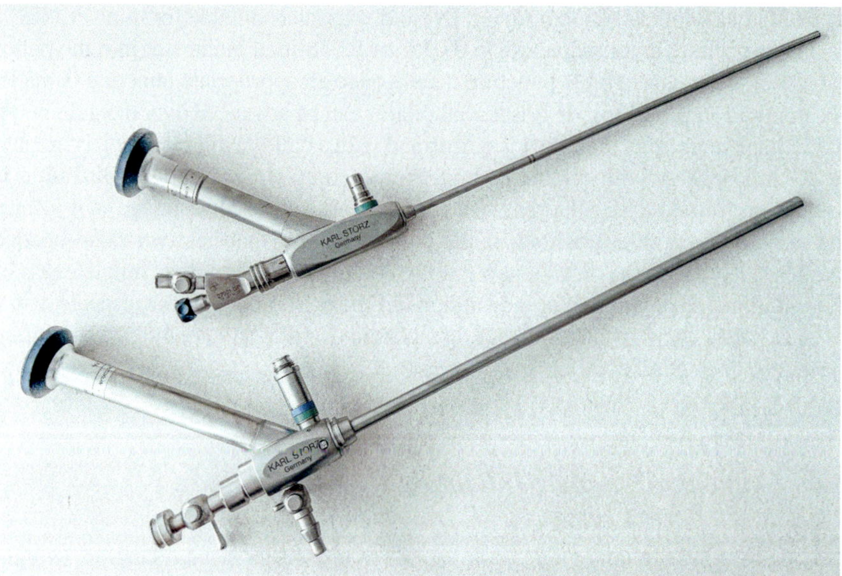

Fig. 2 Top: 12F nephroscope that fits through a 15/16 Amplatz sheath; bottom: 18F nephroscope that fits through a 21/22 Amplatz sheath, both from Storz (Karl Storz, Tuttlingen, Germany)

advanced or retracted as required under vision to get a clear view of the collecting system and the stone burden. It should be our endeavor to have a direct access to the stone without much torque on the renal parenchyma. Any clot if present should be either washed out or removed with appropriate grasping forceps. Once the collecting system is clear of clots and debris, stone fragmentation should be started.

Working with an Amplatz sheath of 15–18 Fr and a 12 Fr nephroscope leaves adequate space between the telescope and sheath for the outflow of irrigation fluid during nephroscopy. This helps in keeping the intrarenal pressures low and also allows outflow of any stone dust and fragments, clots, and infected urine and debris (Tokas et al. 2021).

The nephroscope is also useful to pass a guidewire across the Pelvi-Ureteric Junction (PUJ) for placement of a DJ stent at completion. Stenting is optional in mini-PCNL but is often required in the case of upper ureteric stones, edematous PUJ, or in presence of bleeding or significant trauma to the mucosa.

Ideally, a flexible nephroscopy should be performed at the end of a PCNL procedure to evaluate procedural success. One of the pitfalls of mini-PCNL is the difficulty of passing a flexible cystoscope antegradely through the tract. A flexible cystoscope of 16Fr outer diameter size, should however be able to fit through an 18Fr mini percutaneous access sheath and easily passes through a 22 F tract. It allows you to check all different calyces with a flexible scope, and to remove or treat any stones in different parts of the kidney with laser lithotripsy.

2.2 Lithotripsy

Lithotripters

Various lithotripsy devices are available for stone fragmentation, ranging from pneumatic and ultrasonic lithotripters which work very well for larger stone bulk, to lasers that can do effortless lithotripsy for any stone type. Combination of ballistic and ultrasonic devices are a really good option to increase efficiency during surgery. The type of lithotripter chosen is decided by the stone burden, type of stone and surgeon's preference.

Lasers

Laser energy devices are the most versatile lithotripters available, since they can be used with flexible and rigid scopes. Holmium: YAG laser is the most commonly used laser for lithotripsy and is the current gold standard for laser intracorporeal lithotripsy (Emiliani et al. 2023). Lasers providing pulsed mode are best suited for lithotripsy as compared to continuous mode lasers, which are better suited for soft tissue ablation (Pal et al. 2016).

The major advantages offered by lasers are smooth operation, smaller fragments and limited retropulsion. Holmium is the most popular laser for stone fragmentation, as being a pulsed laser, it is highly efficient in stone fragmentation. There are various settings available for stone fragmentation or dusting during laser lithotripsy. In mini-PCNL, fragmentation may be chosen as the primary modality to clear the stone completely and rapidly. The usual laser settings are frequency ranging from 10 to 30 Hz with the energy of 1.5–3 J with power outputs ranging from 15 to 50 Watts (Emiliani et al. 2023). One can work with 550 μm fiber, which passes easily through the working channel of the nephroscope. High-power settings in Holmium YAG laser, beyond 50 watts, can be very useful for large and hard stones but should be used with caution (Bujons et al. 2016).

A new addition to the laser armamentarium is the Thulium Fiber Laser (TFL). TFL has been found to be effective for soft tissue application as well as lithotripsy. Due to its continuous-wave form and high-frequency format, it has been found to have a special benefit for stone dusting and is believed to produce less retropulsion as compared to conventional holmium laser (Korolev et al. 2021).

Optimal use of laser fiber is extremely important to obtain the optimal outcome at the same time preventing damage to scopes.

Mechanical or Ballistic Lithotripters

These lithotripters work similarly to a jackhammer where the projectile inside the hand piece is accelerated either using electromagnetic energy or pneumatic energy (compressed air). Pneumatic lithotripters are the most commonly used mechanical lithotripter device for breaking renal stones. Using compressed air, ballistic energy is generated which gets transferred onto a metallic probe which further breaks the stone like a hammer and chisel effect. It breaks all types of stones irrespective of their composition but stone fragments generated are larger which have to be manually retrieved. The probe vibrates longitudinally either in single or multiple pulses (Hemal et al. 2003). The Swiss Lithoclast® (EMS, Electro medical systems SA, Nyon, Switzerland) was first introduced in 1991 which was further improved in 2005, Swiss Lithoclast® 2 (EMS, Electro medical systems SA, Nyon, Switzerland) with better fragmentation and less pushback effect. The lithoclast probes come in various sizes and lengths for use in standard PCNL, mini-PCNL, and semirigid ureteroscopic surgery. Probes specifically designed for use in mini-PCNL are smaller in size ranging from 0.8 to 2 mm. Recently, flexible pneumatic probes of size 0.89 mm and length 600–940 mm were also introduced for use in retrograde intra-renal surgery (RIRS). During PCNL both the frequency and the air pressure can be adjusted according to the hardness of the stone for optimal fragmentation. The major disadvantage of pneumatic lithotripters is a significant amount of retropulsion and also bleeding due to friction between the stone and the pelvicalyceal mucosa while breaking the stones.

Ultrasonic Lithotripters

These lithotripters convert electrical energy into mechanical energy with the help of piezo-ceramic elements. A very high frequency of 20,000 Hz will be transmitted to the probe which helps in breaking the stone into smaller fragments and also generation of fine dust. This high-frequency oscillations can lead to generation of heat, which might risk damaging the scopes. Hence continuous cooling of the generator is achieved by continuous saline irrigation and also suctioning. Simultaneous suctioning helps in the clearance of stone fragments and stone dust at a faster speed leading to decreased operation times. Isolated ultrasonic lithotripters are currently not commonly used in day-to-day practice. Retropulsion is significantly less with ultrasonic lithotripters. Lithotripters with both pneumatic and ultrasonic energy capabilities have entered the market two decades ago and have been shown to have superior efficiency than lithotripters with either energy used alone in stone fragmentation (Auge et al. 2002). Examples of such lithotripters include Swiss Lithoclast® Master/ Ultra (EMS, Electro medical systems SA, Nyon, Switzerland), Swiss Lithoclast® Select TM (EMS, Electro medical systems SA, Nyon, Switzerland), and Calcuson Lithotripter® (Karl Storz, Tuttlingen, Germany). Swiss Lithoclast® Master has a facility for both pneumatic and ultrasonic lithotripters. Recently ultrasound probes of size less than 2 mm have been introduced for use in mini-PCNL. Xiong et al. have designed a Micro Ultrasonic probe (HuifuKang Co. Ltd., China) of size 2 mm, which combines the high efficiency of ultrasonic lithotripsy while retaining the ability to pass through mini nephroscopes as well (Xiong et al. 2020).

New Generation Dual Lithotripters

Lithotripters like Swiss Lithoclast® Master or CyberWand™ have double probes (inner and outer probes) for providing both pneumatic and ultrasonic energies for fragmenting and suctioning of stone fragments. Newer generation dual energy lithotripters with single probes were developed with better fragmentation/dusting and faster stone clearance rates (Bader et al. 2020). These include ShockPulse Stone Eliminator™ (Olympus, Tokio, Japan) and Swiss Lithoclast® Trilogy (EMS). They have single lumen probes with larger inner lumen compared to dual-probe lithotripters leading to better suctioning of even larger stone fragments without the need for active removal of stone fragments. Both these lithotripters have plug and play facility and have a handpiece to which single lumen probes of various sizes are attached for use in standard or mini-PCNL and ureteroscopic surgery (URS). Effective and variable suction facility with these lithotripters greatly reduces the operating times (Chew et al. 2017).

Single and reusable probes are available with this equipment. For use in mini-PCNL, a single or reusable 1.83 mm probe of length 418 mm is available (Fig. 3) (Carlos et al. 2018; Sabnis et al. 2020).

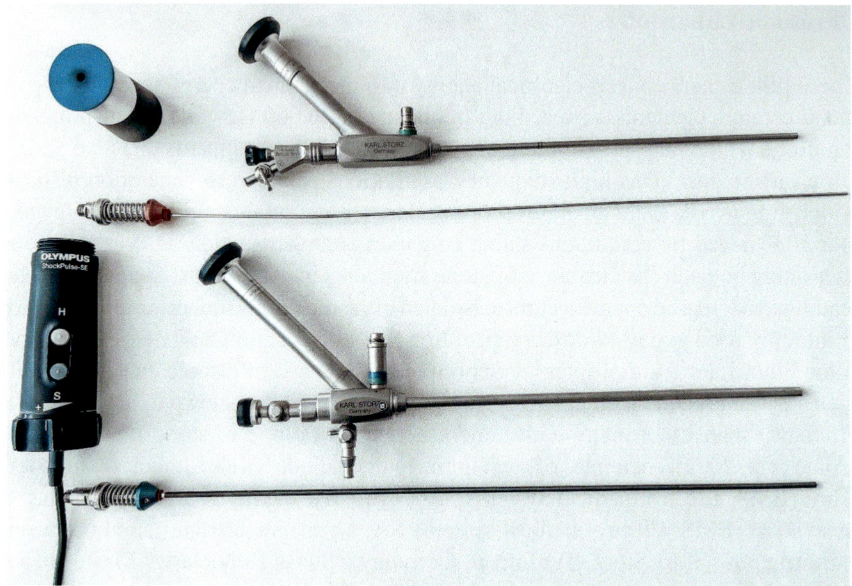

Fig. 3 Left: Shockpulse SE Handpiece with nose cone (Olympus, Tokio, Japan); From top to bottom: 12F Nephroscope from Storz, 1.83 mm diameter Shockpulse probe (Red) that fits the working channel of the 12F nephroscope, 18F nephroscope from Storz, 3.4 mm diameter Shockpulse probe (Blue) that fits the working channel of the 18F nephroscope

Electro Hydraulic Lithotripters (EHL)

These were the first intracorporeal lithotripters introduced in 1955 for treating bladder stones that were subsequently extended to breaking ureteric and renal stones as well. They work by the generation of a spark between two electrodes leading to the formation of a cavitation bubble. Collapse of this bubble generates a shock wave that helps in fragmentation of the stones. Significant retropulsion of the stone and tissue perforation are the drawbacks of this modality. Because of this, use of EHL is hardly ever practiced in modern-day practice for treating renal stones (Vorreuther et al. 1995).

3   Extraction of Fragments in Mini-PCNL

As mini-PCNL is performed through smaller tracts than standard PCNL, fragments need to be smaller before extraction can be achieved. This has always been the Achilles' heel of mini-PCNL, causing the procedure to need slightly more time to achieve similar stone free results as standard PCNL (Sharma et al. 2022). Several methods however do exists to efficiently clear the kidney from stone fragments, specific to mini-PCNL.

3.1 Hydrodynamic Evacuation of Fragments

Purging, washing out and the vacuum cleaner effect are all hydrodynamic strategies for fragment extraction that can be used during mini-PCNL without the use of additional disposable equipment.

Washout of fragments can be achieved in one of two ways. Smaller fragments and dust may evacuate next to the scope outside of the percutaneous tract with the continuous backflow of irrigation fluid. Alternatively, when the scope is suddenly removed from the tract after filling the collecting system, fragments can wash out with the irrigation fluid that flows out of the tract, relieving the intrarenal pressure (Nagele and Nicklas 2016). The **purging** effect consists of antegrade or retrograde fragment evacuation by increased irrigation. Antegradely, this can be achieved by providing inflow through the percutaneous tract and outflow through a ureteric catheter or better yet an ureteral access sheath. Retrogradely, the inflow comes from the ureteric catheter or a flexible ureteroscope, purging out fragments through the percutaneous tract (Nagele and Nicklas 2016).

The **vacuum cleaner effect** was first described in 2008 by Nagele et al. and has since proven to be one of the unique features of mPCNL (Nagele and Schilling et al. 2008). The physics of the vacuum cleaner effect are based on Bernoulli's principle, the Venturi effect and the de Laval nozzle (Nicklas et al. 2015; Mager et al. 2016). Depending on the size of the percutaneous tract, the shape and size of the nephroscope and the irrigation flow, a reversal of irrigation flow and a turbulence occur a short distance in front of the nephroscope that can act as a hydrodynamic trap for stone fragments that are smaller than the inner diameter of the sheath (Nicklas et al. 2015; Mager et al. 2016). This effect decreases with an increasing tract-to-scope ratio and appears to be optimal when a 12F nephroscope is used with a 15F ID (inner diameter) Amplatz sheath (Nicklas et al. 2015; Mager et al. 2016). Practically, the Amplatz sheath should be placed over or in front of the stone with the nephroscope retracted in the tract. Then the scope is advanced towards the stone with running irrigation fluid. At a certain distance from the stone, depending on the irrigation pressure, and the scope-to-tract ratio, the stone will be drawn inside of the tract, towards the scope. By gently extracting the scope, the stone, captured in the turbulence in front of the scope, will follow outside of the tract. Once the scope exits the tract, the turbulence in front of the scope suddenly disappears and the stone can be dropped outside of the tract. Although this can be achieved in both prone and supine position, this effect may be more efficient in supine position (Gadzhiev et al. 2017).

3.2 Active Evacuation by Suction

Suction devices for mPCNL have been developed to improve visualization, to efficiently evacuate fragments, and to reduce intra-renal pressure (IRP), thereby reducing pyelo-venous reflux and presumably reducing the rate of infectious complications (Li et al. 2022).

Vacuum Suction Sheath

A fairly recent addition to the armamentarium in mini-PCNL, vacuum suction sheaths are similar in shape to conventional PCNL sheaths but have a sidearm that can be connected to negative pressure to apply suction. Several designs have been developed and the most commonly known and commercially available suction sheath is the disposable ClearPetra sheath (WellLead Medical, Guangdong, China). A meta-analysis of the three randomized controlled trials (RCTs) that have been published to date comparing vacuum-assisted sheaths with conventional sheaths in mPCNL concluded that a vacuum-assisted sheath improves the stone free rate (SFR), while decreasing the operative time and risk of post-operative urinary tract infection (Zhu et al. 2021). As can be expected with a vacuum assisted sheath, the intrarenal pressures are lower than when using a regular mini-PCNL tract, which may be a factor influencing post-operative fever rate (Croghan et al. 2023).

Lithotriptors with Suction

As mentioned previously, several lithotripters that can be used through a miniaturized nephroscope have additional suctioning capabilities, such as the ShockPulse (Olympus, Tokio, Japan), Lithoclast Master (EMS, Electro medical systems SA, Nyon, Switzerland) or Trilogy (EMS, Electro medical systems SA, Nyon, Switzerland) devices. These devices allow for aspiration of fragments as they are created during lithotripsy. While this suction is continuous with the Trilogy® (EMS, Electro medical systems SA, Nyon, Switzerland) device, it is manually operated with the ShockPulse™ (Olympus, Tokio, Japan) device, which can add a level of control. A benchtop study comparing the efficacy of Shockpulse™ and Trilogy® probes suited for mini-PCNL demonstrated the 1.9 mm Trilogy® probe to have superior results in comparison to the 1.5 mm Trilogy® probe and the 1.83 mm ShockPulse™ probe (Tabib et al. 2022).

As aspiration of fragments is an appealing idea to clear fragments while keeping the pressure in the kidney lower, this concept has also been applied to laser fragmentation with the development of laser suctioning handpieces (Dauw et al. 2016). In a retrospective study, Singh et al. compared the efficacy of laser lithotripsy with a suctioning handpiece by EMS (EMS, Electro medical systems SA, Nyon, Switzerland) to laser lithotripsy without additional suctioning, used trough a 12F nephroscope (Singh et al. 2022). They could only identify a benefit in stone clearance rate in a subgroup of patients with stone burden >18 mm. When the Trilogy™ (EMS, Electro medical systems SA, Nyon, Switzerland) was compared to the TFL laser with a vacuum assisted sheath, they both achieved complete stone free status in all patients at one month postoperatively, although the trilogy achieved higher stone fragmentation rates (Patil et al. 2022).

3.3 Baskets and Graspers

Mini-nephroscopes between 12 and 15F from different manufacturers usually have a 6F working channel, accommodating a wide array of reusable or disposable graspers and baskets. Slightly larger nephroscopes, such as the 18F slender scope from Storz (Karl Storz, Tuttlingen, Germany) have a larger working channel, up to 13.7F, allowing larger and more rigid graspers and baskets to be inserted, such as the disposable Perc N-Circle or Perc N-Gage from Cook (Cook, Bloomington, U.S.A.). Which basket to use is at the urologist's discretion, although a systematic evaluation of stone baskets favored tipless baskets with linear opening for faster stone extraction combined with less mucosal trauma (Monga et al. 2004).

4   Exit Strategies in Mini-PCNL

Historically, the standard PCNL exit strategy was to leave a nephrostomy tube (NT) with or without a double-J (DJ) stent. The rationale of a NT was threefold: to tamponade the PCNL tract to prevent bleeding, post-operative urinary drainage, and maintaining the tract for easy re-entry in case of necessity for a second-look procedure (Ghani et al. 2016; Veser et al. 2020).

Several modifications have been proposed, most notably 'tubeless' (leaving a DJ stent without a NT) and 'totally tubeless' (leaving neither a NT nor a DJ stent) PCNL. The reduced tract size of mini-PCNL has motivated more and more surgeons to adapt and adopt a (totally) tubeless approach (DiBianco and Ghani 2021).

4.1 Tubeless Mini-PCNL

In the past two decades multiple RCTs have been published comparing a standard to a tubeless or totally tubeless procedure. The meta-analyses that evaluated these studies all concur that a tubeless procedure allows for a shorter operative time and reduced length of stay without influencing the SFR or complication rate of the procedure (Gauhar et al. 2022; Chen et al. 2020; Xun et al. 2017). It should be nuanced however that although between 14 and 26 studies were included in the meta-analyses, only three of the included RCTs reported on mini-PCNL and no subgroup analysis was performed (Sebaey et al. 2016; Liu et al. 2017; Lu et al. 2013). All three tubeless mini-PCNL RCTs reported that the tubeless procedure was associated with reduced pain level whereas Lu et al. and Liu et al. agreed that a tubeless approach allowed for a shorter length of stay (Sebaey et al. 2016; Liu et al. 2017; Lu et al. 2013). As there was no significant difference for operative time, SFR or complication rate, a tubeless approach can be supported in mini-PCNL.

Although reduced length of stay and post-operative pain are definitely important outcomes, the patient reported outcome of Quality of Life (QoL) should be taken into account as well. Whereas a nephrostomy tube may be removed shortly after the procedure and prior to the patient's discharge home, a DJ stent will most often stay in place for a week or longer and another procedure, albeit a stent extraction with flexible cystoscopy in the outpatient clinic, is needed for its removal. Zhao and colleagues demonstrated in an RCT that in fact patients identified the DJ stent as more bothersome than a nephrostomy tube and had a worse QoL according to the Wisconsin QoL questionnaire, despite the nephrostomy tube causing more post-operative pain (Zhao et al. 2016). These results were corroborated by both Jiang and Zhang, who additionally demonstrated that a post-operative ureteric catheter for a few days was tolerated far better than a DJ stent (Jiang et al. 2017; Zhang et al. 2019). The benefits of reduced post-operative pain and length of stay should thus be weighed against the potential decreased QoL and the need for an additional procedure in patients that are eligible for a tubeless procedure.

4.2 Totally Tubeless Mini-PCNL

In select patients, a totally tubeless procedure can be considered, leaving no drainage whatsoever. A meta-analysis including 14 studies concluded that a totally tubeless procedure resulted in a shorter operative time and a shorter length of stay, with no significant difference in SFR or complication rate (Li et al. 2020). Although it is often hinted that mini-PCNL may increase the opportunity for totally tubeless PCNL, all the studies included in this meta-analyses reported on standard PCNL with tract sizes of 28–30F (Li et al. 2020; Zeng et al. 2018).

The same exit strategy cannot always be applied to all patients and selection criteria are useful to identify patients in whom a tubeless or totally tubeless procedure can be considered. If a second-look procedure is anticipated, leaving a nephrostomy tube provides an easy re-entry.

In the absence of any residual fragments, any perforations to the collecting system, damage to the ureter, significant bleeding, a history of infections or anatomical abnormalities that would necessitate leaving a stent such as a solitary kidney, a totally tubeless procedure can be considered (Ghani et al. 2016; Veser et al. 2020).

4.3 Tract Sealing

To prevent post-operative bleeding or leakage from the percutaneous tract after PCNL, a variety of hemostatic agents have been explored for direct application in the tract (Veser et al. 2020; Misra and Gkentzis 2020).

A systematic review including 9 RCTs comprising a total of 694 patients, could not demonstrate any beneficial effects from the use of hemostatic agents after PCNL.

Importantly, all these patients underwent a standard PCNL with tract sizes of 28–34F. As mini-PCNL has already been demonstrated to have a lower risk of post-operative bleeding in comparison to standard PCNL and considering the significant cost of these hemostatic agents, the use of these agents after mini-PCNL cannot be supported based on currently available data (Sharma et al. 2022; Veser et al. 2020; Misra and Gkentzis 2020).

5 Outpatient Mini-PCNL

In 2010, Beiko and Shahroer almost simultaneously reported on their initial series of highly selected patients undergoing outpatient tubeless PCNL demonstrating this to be safe and effective considering certain selection criteria (Beiko and Lee 2010; Shahrour and Andonian 2010).

Over the years, the body of literature on outpatient PCNL grew and Gao and associates performed a systematic review and meta-analysis in 2020 including 6 studies, comprising only one RCT and two studies covering mini-PCNL (Gao et al. 2020). The analysis showed a lower complication rate and shorter operative time for outpatient procedures, which of course needs to be interpreted with caution as the mainly retrospective data is highly subject to selection bias. No other significant differences were noted from the analysis. They emphasized that patient selection is key to identify patients eligible for an outpatient procedure, with criteria including adequate counseling, a Body Mass Index (BMI) < 30, American Society of Anesthesiologists (ASA) score of $\leq$ 2, absence of intraoperative complications and living within 30 min of the hospital (Gao et al. 2020).

Most recently, these criteria have been extended to include virtually all patients undergoing an uncomplicated PCNL procedure, regardless of the ASA score, BMI, stone burden or number of tracts used (Bechis et al. 2018; Hosier et al. 2021; Chong et al. 2021). As the outcomes appear quite similar to inpatient PCNL with a fairly low rate of unplanned admission or readmissions, there is an increased support for routine outpatient PCNL in high-volume centers with experienced surgeons (Bechis et al. 2018; Hosier et al. 2021; Chong et al. 2021).

Interestingly, this shift towards more outpatient PCNL procedures has already been identified from IBM® Marketscan® data by Johnston et al. who demonstrated that 85.3% of patients in that database had underwent an outpatient procedure in 2019 (Johnston et al. 2023). Although the database unfortunately did not allow to specify if there was also a proportionate increase in mini-PCNL, Thakker and colleagues suggested that mini-PCNL most likely played a role in their own transition to outpatient PCNL (Johnston et al. 2023; Thakker et al. 2023). Additionally and importantly, both Thakker et al. and Lee et al. proved that outpatient PCNL comes with a significant cost saving in comparison to inpatient PCNL (Thakker et al. 2023; Lee et al. 2022). Considering all the above, the road seems to be paved for ambulatory PCNL to be adopted by more and more surgeons worldwide.

6 Mini-PCNL Versus Other Stone Treatments

Now that the technique with all its specificities has been outlined, the question remains whether this technique is worth adopting by urologists who prefer standard PCNL or who prefer retrograde intrarenal surgery for larger stone burdens in the kidney.

The most recent systematic review and meta-analysis by Sharma et al. included 16 RCTs on mini- versus standard PCNL with a total of 3961 patients (Sharma et al. 2022). When evaluating the included studies, it becomes clear that there's a large degree of heterogeneity between the studies. Not only regarding tract sizes and stone burden treated, but also for the definition of SFR and the imaging modality used to assess this. Additionally, there are some serious concerns regarding the risk of bias, mainly due to unclear concealment of allocation (Sharma et al. 2022). Despite these important limitations, the meta-analysis demonstrated that the SFR was not different between mini- or standard PCNL, even in subgroup analyses for different stone sizes and access sheath tract sizes (Sharma et al. 2022). The use of a miniaturized tract did significantly reduce the need for transfusions by 56% (95%CI RR [0.37,0.78], p = 0.001) (Sharma et al. 2022). As the stone burden needs to be reduced to smaller fragments for extraction, it is not surprising that a standard PCNL is statistically significantly faster with a mean difference in operative time of 8.28 min, (95% CI [3.96,12.59], p = 0.000) (Sharma et al. 2022). Then again, the hospitalization time is considerably shorter after mini-PCNL with a mean difference of −0.59 days (approximately 14 h) (95% CI [−0.81,−0.37], p = 0.000) (Sharma et al. 2022). Although the patients undergoing mini-PCNL had fewer minor complications, there was no statistically significant difference in major complications or fever rate between the two procedures (Sharma et al. 2022).

As mini-PCNL can often be performed tubeless and even an outpatient procedure is feasible, it ventures into the realm of patients undergoing RIRS regarding post-operative complications and length of stay. Dorantes-Carrillo and colleagues performed a systematic review and identified 8 RCTs totaling a mere 891 patients for analysis (Dorantes-Carrillo et al. 2022). They concluded that the SFR was significantly in favor of mini-PCNL (RR: 1.06 [95%CI: 1.01–1.10], p = 0.008), accepting however a longer hospitalization time (MD 1.11 days [95%CI: 0.06–2.16], p = 0.04) and slightly more blood loss (mean difference 0.35 g/dL [95%CI: 0.05–0.65], p = 0.02) without an increased transfusion rate (Dorantes-Carrillo et al. 2022). The results should be interpreted with caution as a large proportion of the stones were located in the lower pole and five of the included studies even reported solely on the treatment of lower pole stones (Dorantes-Carrillo et al. 2022). As such, these results may not be generalizable to all renal stones. Kallidonis et al., evaluating the results of mini-PCNL and RIRS only for lower pole stones of less than 2 cm, reached the same conclusions as Dorantes-Carrillo (Kallidonis et al. 2022).

It appears from these meta-analyses that mini-PCNL is quite the contender for both standard PCNL and retrograde intrarenal surgery. With an increasing body of evidence in the published literature, strong advocates of the technique and the simple fact that seeing is believing, we would expect this approach to gain momentum in the near future and be adopted by more and more colleagues in the field.

References

Abdelwahab K, El-Babouly IM, Mahmoud MM, Elderey MS. Comparative study between a new screwed Amplatz sheath and the ordinary one in percutaneous nephrolithotomy. World J Urol. 2022;40:213–9.

Al-Kandari AM, Jabbour M, Anderson A, Shokeir AA, Smith AD. Comparative study of degree of renal trauma between Amplatz sequential fascial dilation and balloon dilation during percutaneous renal surgery in an animal model. Urology. 2007;69:586–9.

Alken P, Hutschenreiter G, Günther R, Marberger M. Percutaneous stone manipulation. J Urol. 1981;125:463–6.

Auge BK, Lallas CD, Pietrow PK, Zhong P, Preminger GM. In vitro comparison of standard ultrasound and pneumatic lithotrites with a new combination intracorporeal lithotripsy device. Urology. 2002;60:28–32.

Bader MJ, Eisel M, Strittmatter F, Nagele U, Stief CG, Pongratz T, Sroka R, Training and research in urological surgery and technology (T.R.U.S.T.)-group. Comparison of stone elimination capacity and drilling speed of endoscopic clearance lithotripsy devices. World J Urol. 2020. https://doi.org/10.1007/s00345-020-03184-1

Bechis SK, Han DS, Abbott JE, Holst DD, Alagh A, Dipina T, Sur RL. Outpatient percutaneous nephrolithotomy: the UC San Diego health experience. 2018;32:394–401. https://home.liebertpub.com/end

Beiko D, Lee L. Outpatient tubeless percutaneous nephrolithotomy: the initial case series. J Canadian Urol Assoc. 2010;4:86–90.

Bujons A, Millán F, Centeno C, Emiliani E, Sánchez Martín F, Angerri O, Caffaratti J, Villavicencio H. Mini-percutaneous nephrolithotomy with high-power holmium YAG laser in pediatric patients with staghorn and complex calculi. J Pediatr Urol. 2016;12:253.e1-253.e5.

Carlos EC, Wollin DA, Winship BB, et al. In Vitro comparison of a novel single probe dual-energy lithotripter to current devices. J Endourol. 2018;32:534–40.

Chen ZJ, Yan YJ, Zhou JJ. Comparison of tubeless percutaneous nephrolithotomy and standard percutaneous nephrolithotomy for kidney stones: a meta-analysis of randomized trials. Asian J Surg. 2020;43:60–8.

Chew BH, Matteliano AA, De Los RT, Lipkin ME, Paterson RF, Lange D. Benchtop and initial clinical evaluation of the shockpulse stone eliminator in percutaneous nephrolithotomy. J Endourol. 2017;31:191–7.

Chong JT, Dunne M, Magnan B, Abbott J, Davalos JG. Ambulatory percutaneous nephrolithotomy in a free-standing surgery center: an analysis of 500 consecutive cases. 2021;35:1738–1742. https://home.liebertpub.com/end

Clayman RV, Castaneda-Zuniga WR, Hunter DW, Miller RP, Lange PH, Amplatz K. Rapid balloon dilatation of the nephrostomy track for nephrostolithotomy. Radiology. 1983;147:884–5.

Croghan SM, Skolarikos A, Jack GS, Manecksha RP, Walsh MT, O'Brien FJ, Davis NF. Upper urinary tract pressures in endourology: a systematic review of range, variables and implications. BJU Int. 2023;131:267–79.

Dauw CA, Borofsky MS, York N, Lingeman JE. A usability comparison of laser suction handpieces for percutaneous nephrolithotomy. J Endourol. 2016;30:1165–8.

DiBianco JM, Ghani KR. Precision stone surgery: current status of miniaturized percutaneous nephrolithotomy. Curr Urol Rep. 2021. https://doi.org/10.1007/s11934-021-01042-0.

Dorantes-Carrillo LA, Basulto-Martínez M, Suárez-Ibarrola R, Heinze A, Proietti S, Flores-Tapia JP, Esqueda-Mendoza A, Giusti G. Retrograde Intrarenal surgery versus miniaturized percutaneous nephrolithotomy for kidney stones >1 cm: a systematic review and meta-analysis of randomized trials. Eur Urol Focus. 2022;8:259–70.

Emiliani E, Kanashiro A, Angerri O. Lasers for stone lithotripsy: advantages/disadvantages of each laser source. Curr Opin Urol. 2023. https://doi.org/10.1097/MOU.0000000000001092.

Frattini A, Barbieri A, Salsi P, Sebastio N, Ferretti S, Bergamaschi E, Cortellini P. One shot: a novel method to dilate the nephrostomy access for percutaneous lithotripsy. J Endourol/endourol Soc. 2001;15:919–23.

Gadzhiev N, Sergei B, Grigoryev V, Okhunov Z, Ganpule A, Pisarev A, Iskakov Y, Petrov S. Evaluation of the effect of Bernoulli maneuver on operative time during mini-percutaneous nephrolithotomy: a prospective randomized study. Investig Clin Urol. 2017;58:179–85.

Gao M, Zeng F, Zhu Z, et al. Day care surgery versus inpatient percutaneous nephrolithotomy: a systematic review and meta-analysis. Int J Surg. 2020;81:132–9.

Gauhar V, Traxer O, García Rojo E, et al. Complications and outcomes of tubeless versus nephrostomy tube in percutaneous nephrolithotomy: a systematic review and meta-analysis of randomized clinical trials. Urolithiasis 2022;50:511–522.

Ghani KR, Andonian S, Bultitude M, Desai M, Giusti G, Okhunov Z, Preminger GM, de la Rosette J. Percutaneous nephrolithotomy: update, trends, and future directions. Eur Urol. 2016;70:382–96.

Gönen M, Istanbulluoglu OM, Cicek T, Ozturk B, Ozkardes H. Balloon dilatation versus Amplatz dilatation for nephrostomy tract dilatation. J Endourol. 2008;22:901–4.

Hemal AK, Goel A, Aron M, Seth A, Dogra PN, Gupta NP. Evaluation of fragmentation with single or multiple pulse setting of Lithoclast for renal calculi during percutaneous nephrolithotripsy and its impact on clearance. Urol Int. 2003;70:265–8.

Hosier GW, Visram K, McGregor T, Steele S, Touma N, Beiko D. Ambulatory percutaneous nephrolithotomy is safe and effective in patients with extended selection criteria. Can Urol Assoc J. 2021. https://doi.org/10.5489/cuaj.7527.

Jiang H, Huang D, Yao S, Liu S. Improving drainage after percutaneous nephrolithotomy based on health-related quality of life: a prospective randomized study. J Endourol. 2017;31:1131–8.

Johnston SS, Johnson BH, Rai P, Grange P, Tony A, Ghosh S, Buchholz N, Amos T, Buchholz N. Trends and patterns of initial percutaneous nephrolithotomy and subsequent procedures among commercially-insured US adults with urinary system stone disease: a 10-year population-based study. World J Urol. 2023;41:235–240.

Kallidonis P, Adamou C, Ntasiotis P, Pietropaolo A, Somani B, Özsoy M, Liourdi D, Sarica K, Liatsikos E, Tailly T. The best treatment approach for lower calyceal stones ≤20 mm in maximal diameter: mini percutaneous nephrolithotripsy, retrograde intrarenal surgery or shock wave lithotripsy a systematic review and meta-analysis of the literature conducted by the European section of Uro-technology and young academic urologists. Minerva Urol and Nephrol. 2022;73:711–23.

Korolev D, Akopyan G, Tsarichenko D, Shpikina A, Ali S, Chinenov D, Corrales M, Taratkin M, Traxer O, Enikeev D. Minimally invasive percutaneous nephrolithotomy with SuperPulsed thulium-fiber laser. Urolithiasis. 2021;49:485–91.

Lee MS, Assmus MA, Agarwal DK, Rivera ME, Large T, Krambeck AE. Ambulatory percutaneous nephrolithotomy may be cost-effective compared to standard percutaneous nephrolithotomy. J Endourol. 2022;36:176–82.

Li Q, Gao L, Li J, Zhang Y, Jiang Q. Total tubeless versus standard percutaneous nephrolithotomy: a meta-analysis. Minim Invasive Ther Allied Technol. 2020;29:61–9.

Li P, Huang Z, Sun X, Yang T, Wang G, Jiang Y, Ke C, Li J. Comparison of vacuum suction sheath and non-vacuum suction sheath in minimally invasive percutaneous nephrolithotomy: a meta-analysis. J Invest Surg. 2022;35:1145–52.

Liu M, Huang J, Lu J, Hu L, Wang Z, Ma W, Zhang J, Zhao X, Chen X, Su B. Selective tubeless minimally invasive percutaneous nephrolithotomy for upper urinary calculi. Minerva Urol Nefrol. 2017;69:366–71.

Lu Y, Gen PJ, Jun ZX, Kun HL, Xian PJ. Randomized prospective trial of tubeless versus conventional minimally invasive percutaneous nephrolithotomy. World J Urol. 2013;31:1303–1307.

Mager R, Balzereit C, Gust K, Hüsch T, Herrmann T, Nagele U, Haferkamp A, Schilling D. The hydrodynamic basis of the vacuum cleaner effect in continuous-flow PCNL instruments: an empiric approach and mathematical model. World J Urol. 2016;34:717–24.

Misra V, Gkentzis A. The use of haemostatic agents in percutaneous nephrolithotomy: a systematic review. SN Compr Clin Med. 2020;2:192–202.

Monga M, Hendlin K, Lee C, Anderson JK. Systematic evaluation of stone basket dimensions. Urology. 2004;63:1042–4.

Nagele U, Schilling D, Anastasiadis AG, Walcher U, Sievert KD, Merseburger AS, Kuczyk M, Stenzl A. Minimal-invasive perkutane Nephrolitholapaxie (MIP). Urologe 2008;47:1066–1073.

Nagele U, Nicklas A. Vacuum cleaner effect, purging effect, active and passive wash out: a new terminology in hydrodynamic stone retrival is arising–Does it affect our endourologic routine? World J Urol. 2016;34:143–4.

Nicklas AP, Schilling D, Bader MJ, Herrmann TRW, Nagele U. The vacuum cleaner effect in minimally invasive percutaneous nephrolitholapaxy. World J Urol. 2015;33:1847–53.

Pal D, Ghosh A, Sen R, Pal A. Continuous-wave and quasi-continuous wave thulium-doped all-fiber laser: implementation on kidney stone fragmentations. Appl Opt. 2016;55:6151.

Patil A, Sharma R, Shah D, Gupta A, Singh A, Ganpule A, Sabnis R, Desai M. A prospective comparative study of mini-PCNL using Trilogy^{TM} or thulium fibre laser with suction. World J Urol. 2022;40:539–43.

Sabnis RB, Balaji SS, Sonawane PL, Sharma R, Vijayakumar M, Singh AG, Ganpule AP, Desai MR. EMS Lithoclast Trilogy^{TM}: an effective single-probe dual-energy lithotripter for mini and standard PCNL. World J Urol. 2020;38:1043–50.

Sebaey A, Khalil MM, Soliman T, Mohey A, Elshaer W, Kandil W, Omar R. Standard versus tubeless mini-percutaneous nephrolithotomy: a randomised controlled trial production and hosting by Elsevier. Arab J Urol (Official J Arab Assoc Urol 2016;14:18–23.

Shahrour W, Andonian S. Ambulatory percutaneous nephrolithotomy: initial series. Urology. 2010;76:1288–92.

Sharma G, Sharma A, Devana SK, Singh SK. Mini versus standard percutaneous nephrolithotomy for the management of renal stone disease: systematic review and meta-analysis of randomized controlled trials. Eur Urol Focus. 2022;8:1376–85.

Singh AG, Palaniappan S, Jai S, Tak G, Ganpule A, Sabnis R, Desai M. The clinical outcomes of laser with suction device in mini-percutaneous nephrolithotomy. Asian J Urol. 2022;9:63–8.

Tabib C, Whelan P, Kim C, Dionise Z, Soto-Palou F, Terry R, Antonelli J, Preminger G, Lipkin M. Benchtop evaluation of miniature percutaneous nephrolithotomy lithotrites. J Endourol. 2022;36:1483–8.

Thakker PU, Mithal P, Dutta R, Carreno G, Gutierrez-Aceves J. Comparative outcomes and cost of ambulatory PCNL in select kidney stone patients. Urolithiasis. 2023;51:1–6.

Tokas T, Tzanaki E, Nagele U, Somani BK. Role of intrarenal pressure in modern day endourology (Mini-PCNL and Flexible URS): a systematic review of literature. Curr Urol Rep. 2021;22:1–8.

Veser J, Fajkovic H, Seitz C. Tubeless percutaneous nephrolithotomy: evaluation of minimal invasive exit strategies after percutaneous stone treatment. Curr Opin Urol. 2020;30:679–83.

Vorreuther R, Corleis R, Klotz T, Bernards P, Engelmann U. Impact of shock wave pattern and cavitation bubble size on tissue damage during ureteroscopic electrohydraulic lithotripsy. J Urol. 1995;153:849–53.

Wu Y, Xun Y, Lu Y, Hu H, Qin B, Wang S. Effectiveness and safety of four tract dilation methods of percutaneous nephrolithotomy: a meta-analysis. Exp Ther Med. 2020;2661–2671.

Xiong LL, Huang XB, Ye XJ, Chen L, Ma K, Liu J, Hong Y, Xu QQ, Wang X. Microultrasonic probe combined with ultrasound-guided minipercutaneous nephrolithotomy in the treatment of upper ureteral and renal stones: a consecutive cohort study. J Endourol. 2020;34:429–33.

Xun Y, Wang Q, Hu H, Lu Y, Zhang J, Qin B, Geng Y, Wang S. Tubeless versus standard percutaneous nephrolithotomy: an update meta-analysis. BMC Urol. 2017;17:1–17.

Zeng G, Zhu W, Lam W. Miniaturised percutaneous nephrolithotomy: its role in the treatment of urolithiasis and our experience. Asian J Urol. 2018;5:295–302.

Zhang Y, Wei C, Pokhrel G, Liu X, Ouyang W, Gan J, Ding B, Liu Z, Peng E, Chen Z. Mini-percutaneous nephrolithotomy with ureter catheter: a safe and effective form of mPCNL offers better quality of life. Urol Int. 2019;102:167–74.

Zhao PT, Hoenig DM, Smith AD, Okeke Z. A randomized controlled comparison of nephrostomy drainage versus ureteral stent following percutaneous nephrolithotomy using the Wisconsin stone QOL. J Endourol. 2016;30:1275–84.

Zhu L, Wang Z, Zhou Y, Gou L, Huang Y, Zheng X. Comparison of vacuum-assisted sheaths and normal sheaths in minimally invasive percutaneous nephrolithotomy: a systematic review and meta-analysis. BMC Urol. 2021. https://doi.org/10.1186/S12894-021-00925-1.

Ultra Mini PCNL

Satyendra Persaud, Ramandeep Chalokia, and Janak Desai

Abstract Mini percutaneous nephrolithotomy (mini-PCNL) has emerged as a promising technique in the field of kidney stone surgery, offering a minimally invasive approach for the management of renal calculi.Mini-PCNL involves the use of a smaller-caliber nephroscope compared to traditional percutaneous nephrolithotomy (PCNL). The miniaturized instruments allow for a less invasive procedure, resulting in reduced morbidity, shorter hospital stays, and faster recovery for patients with kidney stones. This technique combines the advantages of both PCNL and flexible ureteroscopy, enabling efficient stone fragmentation and removal.Procedural details of mini-PCNL, include patient selection criteria, renal access techniques, and the utilization of holmium laser lithotripsy for effective stone fragmentation. The advantages and limitations of mini-PCNL are discussed, providing valuable insights for urologists considering this approach for their patients.Mini-PCNL has demonstrated excellent stone clearance rates, particularly for medium-sized renal calculi and staghorn stones. The reduced risk of bleeding and potential for outpatient management further enhance its appeal in the management of urolithiasis.Mini percutaneous nephrolithotomy is a safe and effective alternative to conventional PCNL.

Keywords Mini percutaneous nephrolithotomy (mini-PCNL) · Kidney stone surgery · Urolithiasis · Nephrolithiasis · Percutaneous nephrolithotomy · Minimally invasive surgery · Renal calculi · Stone removal · Renal access · Small-caliber nephroscope · Flexible ureteroscopy · Renal anatomy · Stone fragmentation · Holmium laser lithotripsy · Endourology · Retrograde intrarenal surgery (RIRS) · Fluoroscopy · Postoperative care · Nephrostomy tube · Outpatient procedure

---

S. Persaud
Division of Clinical Surgical Sciences, University of the West Indies, West Indies, Trinidad and Tobago
e-mail: satyendra.persaud@sta.uwi.edu

R. Chalokia
Warrington and Halton Teaching Hospitals, NHS Foundation Trust, Warrington, UK

J. Desai (✉)
Samved Hospital, Ahmedabad, Gujarat, India
e-mail: drjanakddesai@gmail.com

© The Author(s), under exclusive license to Springer Nature Switzerland AG 2023   217
J. D. Denstedt and E. N. Liatsikos (eds.), *Percutaneous Renal Surgery*,
https://doi.org/10.1007/978-3-031-40542-6_14

In 1941 Rupel and Brown removed a stone whole from an obstructed the kidney via a previously placed nephrostomy and percutaneous nephrolithotomy (PCNL) was born (Patel and Nakada 2015). Fernstrom and Johannson subsequently described the creation of a percutaneous access specifically to remove stones using a cystoscope and rigid graspers to remove the stone (Fernstrom 1976). In 1977, Alken would help create the percutaneous nephroscope and eventually Arthur Smith along with Kurt Amplatz created the 30Fr Amplatz sheath (Desai 2021). Eventually, 30Fr was described as the standard for PCNL at the time, being limited to this size by the availability of appropriately sized fibreoptic and lithotripsy devices. In the decades since, the procedure has evolved tremendously.

PCNL is now the procedure of choice for large kidney stones with stone free rates superior to shockwave lithotripsy or ureteroscopy (Assimos et al. 2016). The procedure has seen numerous innovations in instrumentation, radiology as well positioning and has entered an era of miniaturization. This was initially driven by the need to treat stones in the pediatric population and initially vascular access sheaths were repurposed and modified for this purpose, with Jackman and colleagues coining the term "mini-perc" in 1998 (Desai 2021). Subsequently, a number of minimally invasive PCNLs were developed, accompanied by purpose-built instruments. This has been possible with the concomitant development of fiberoptics and lasers which permitted lithotripsy through small calibre endoscopes.

One should be familiar with the terms describing the various categories of PCNL—these are described based on the outer diameter of the sheath and are as follows (Miernik 2019):

24–32Fr—Standard PCNL
14–22Fr—Mini PCNL
11–13Fr—Ultra-Mini PCNL
4.8–11Fr—Micro PCNL

1 Benefits of Miniaturization and the Development of Ultra-Mini PCNL

One dreaded complication of PCNL is bleeding and the risk of bleeding is directly related to tract size. In an analysis of over 5000 procedures in the Clinical Research Office of the Endourological Society (CROES) Global PCNL database, it was noted that transfusion risk varied between 1.1% with an 18fr tract to as high as 12.1% among patients whose tracts were over 30Fr (Yamaguchi et al. 2011) Table 1. Dr Desai and team in Ahmedabad similarly noted that bleeding seemed to increase significantly with tracts dilated beyond 14 to 16fr. They postulated that the elasticity of the kidney may be able to tolerate dilation up to this point, tearing once the tracts were dilated beyond this. This led the team to the development of the ultra-mini PCNL (UMP) with dilation to a maximum of 13Fr (Desai and Solanki 2013). This was first described in 2013 and since then has become an established option for the treatment of stones up

Table 1 Transfusion rate in relation to PCNL sheath size

	No of patients	% Blood transfusion
Small (18Fr or less)	271	1.1%
Medium (24Fr–26Fr)	1039	4.8%
Large (27Fr–30Fr)	3533	5.9%
Larger (>30Fr)	371	12.1%

Table 2 Comparisons of various miniaturized versions of PCNL

	Mini-PCNL	UMP	Micro-perc
Size of Sheath	18–22Fr	11Fr and 13Fr	4.8Fr
Stone removal	Forceps and ultrasonic disintegration with suction	Creating a fluid vortex	Leave for natural expulsion
Telescope size	3 mm	1 mm	0.9 mm
Resolution of telescope	30,000 pixels	17,000 pixels	10,000 pixels

to 2 cm. UMP falls on the miniaturization spectrum between traditional PCNL and micro-PCNL with several options lying in between (Table 2) (Smith et al. 2018)—the choice of procedure will depend on patient and stone characteristics as well as surgeon experience and comfort as well as availability of equipment. The technique, while it requires some experience, has proven to reproducible with authors reporting stone free rates as high as 99% with few or no complications (Agrawal et al. 2016).

2 Instruments and Technique

Instruments were specially created including a 3.5Fr 0-degree telescope (17,000 pixels) which fits into a 6Fr inner sheath with the latter having two ports, one for irrigation and the other permitting passage of a laser fiber. There is also an outer sheath, 11 or 13Fr in diameter with a small inner tube, 3fr in diameter, running along its length and connected to a side port (Figs. 1 and 2). The latter is a special feature—injection of fluid via this port creates a vortex within the collecting system with fluid moving from the high pressure renal pelvis into the outer sheath and allows evacuation of stone fragments.

The procedure is carried out under general anesthesia. Puncture is done in standard prone fashion following the cystoscopic placement of a ureteric catheter. This facilitates dilation of the tract under fluoroscopy using small Teflon dilators. The outer sheath, over an obturator, is inserted into the collecting system followed by the inner sheath with the attached camera. Under direct vision, stone disintegration is carried out via a 365-um laser fibre and fragments, which are less than 2mm. Following disintegration, the inner sheath is removed and saline is injected via the

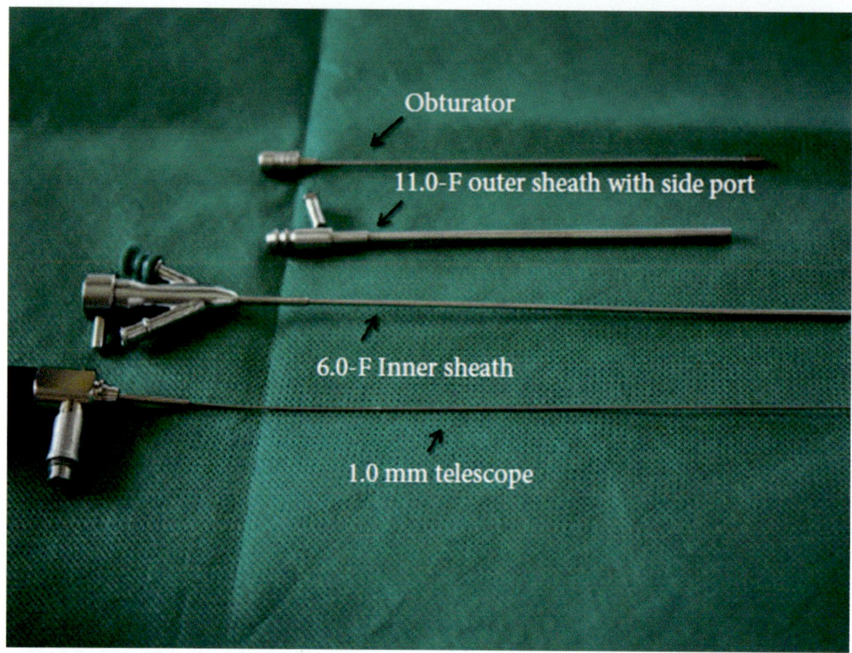

Fig. 1 UMP Instruments including telescope, inner sheath, and specially designed outer sheath (with obturator) which may be 11 or 13 Fr

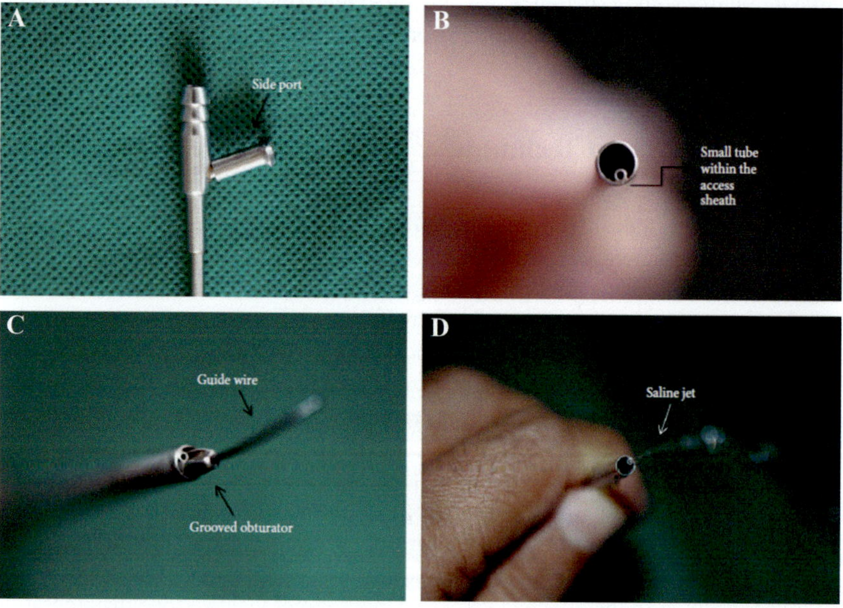

Fig. 2 (A) Outer sheath with side port for irrigation via water tube on the sheath (B). (C) Grooved obturator sliding over a guidewire. (D) Demonstration of waterjet function of the outer sheath

port on the outer sheath. The tiny fragments are agitated and are washed out via the vortex described above. This effect can also be created by flushing the ureteric catheter. Following this, the instruments are removed, and firm pressure is applied to the tract for a few moments. The ureteric catheter is kept for a few hours following surgery and barring no complications, this and the urinary catheter is removed and the patient is typically discharged within 24 h (Desai and Solanki 2013).

3 When Is UMP Appropriate?

UMP forms an important part of the stone treatment arsenal and falls along the spectrum of miniaturization between traditional PCNL and micro-PCNL—it is an option for stones up to 2 cm. One primary advantage of tract miniaturization is a decrease in blood loss. In an analysis of factors leading to bleeding during PCNL the authors noted that blood loss may be minimized via the utilization of smaller tracts in pediatric patients, those non hydronephrotic kidneys or narrow narrow infundibula as well as mopping up of smaller calyceal stones as part of a multi-puncture procedure (Kukreja et al. 2004). In the case of the latter, UMP is used as an adjunct to remove stones in a calyx which cannot be accessed by the primary PCNL tract—this avoids having to make larger secondary punctures. Apart from the blood loss related advantages, UMP offers a stent and nephrostomy-free option meaning that patient comfort is maximized, and hospital stay is minimized.

One of the key advantages in UMP over fURS (Flexible ureterorenoscopy) lies in the management of stones in lower pole calyces. In these cases, it is easier to access stones via UMP rather than fURS. This is well illustrated in a RCT by Datta and colleagues—almost a quarter of the patients had stones in their low poles with 100% clearance being achieved via UMP. This is contrasted with the fURS group where almost half of those with residual stones had lower pole stones pre intervention (Datta et al. 2016).

4 How Does Ultra Mini PCNL Compare to Ureteroscopy and Standard PCNL?

In a recent randomized trial, 98 patients with stones 10–30 mm were randomized to UMP and 46 to flexible ureteroscopy (fURS). Both mean laser time (41.17 min versus 73.58 min) and consumable costs ($45.73 versus 423.11) were significantly less in the UMP group. Additionally the stone free rate at 1 month of follow-up was 100% for UMP group and 73% for the fURS group. Grades I and II complications were 10% in the UMP group and 35% in the fURS group (Datta et al. 2016). In this study laser and evacuation times were significantly less for UMP and this may be due to quicker fragmentation and retrieval due to the vortex effect described above.

Schoenthaler and colleagues found similar stone free and complication rates between both procedures but cost of consumables was much less among patients undergoing UMP (Schoenthaler et al. 2015). In a Meta-Analysis, Jung found higher stone free rates, but similar complication rates, with UMP compared to fURS (Do et al. 2022).

Zhong and colleagues compared minimally invasive PCNL (16Fr) versus standard PCNL (26Fr) noting that miPCNL was associated with a higher stone clearance rate—89.7 versus 68%. There were similar complication rates between the two procedures but less chance of needing an adjunctive procedure with miPCNL (Zhong et al. 2011). The authors also noted that multiple mini tracts led to improved stone clearance for staghorn stones. While this study didn't use the kit as described by Desai, the data are nonetheless helpful. Adamou et al. compared standard, mini and ultra-mini PCNLs for single renal stones among 84 patients. They noted that while stone free rates were similar among different PCNL types, ultra-mini PCNL was associated with a shorter hospitalization and a smaller haemoglobin drop. They did note that operative time was longer in the ultra-mini group (Adamou et al. 2022).

5   Synopsis

In the era of miniaturization, there are several minimally invasive options to standard PCNL. The primary driver of the development of these options has been a reduction in blood loss that follows a smaller tract. One such option is the Ultra-mini PCNL. This has proven to be safe and efficacious and is an option for stones 2 cm or less. For these stones UMP may be used as the sole treatment modality and has the advantages of lower cost, faster operation times and being truly tube/stent free when compared to ureteroscopy. Additionally, for larger stones, UMP may be used as an adjunct to traditional PCNL for smaller stones which cannot be accessed with the primary tract and in this way avoids the bleeding risk that follows multiple large tracts. UMP also outperforms fURS when it comes to clearance of lower pole stones. One final advantage of UMP over fURS is the reduction in the cost of disposables. The financial and environmental benefits of this cannot be understated.

References

Adamou C, Evangelia Goulimi E, Pagonis K, Peteinari A, Tsaturyan A, Vagionis A, Lattarulo M, Giannitsas K Liatsikos EKP. Comparison between standard, mini and ultra-mini percutaneous nephrolithotomy for single renal stones: a prospective study. World J Urol. 2022;40(10):2543–8.

Agrawal M, Agarwal K, Jindal T, Sharma M. Ultra-mini-percutaneous nephrolithotomy: a minimally-invasive option for percutaneous stone removal. Indian J Urol [Internet]. 2016;32(2):132. Available from: http://www.indianjurol.com/text.asp?2016/32/2/132/174778

Assimos D, Krambeck A, Miller N. Kidney stones: surgical management guideline—American Urological Association. American Urological Association; 2016.

Datta SN, Solanki R, Desai J. Prospective outcomes of ultra mini percutaneous nephrolithotomy: a consecutive cohort study. J Urol. 2016;195(3):741–6.

Desai JSH. Mini percutaneous kidney stone removal applicable technologies. Urol Clin N Am. 2021.

Desai J, Solanki R. Ultra-mini percutaneous nephrolithotomy (UMP): one more armamentarium. BJU Int. 2013;n/a.

Fernstrom IJB. Percutaneous pyelolithotomy. A new extraction technique. Scand J Urol Nephrol. 1976.

Jung HDo, Chung DY, Kim DK, Lee MH, Lee SW, Paick S, et al. Comparison of ultra-mini percutaneous nephrolithotomy and retrograde intrarenal surgery for renal stones: a systematic review and meta-analysis from the KSER update series. J Clin Med [Internet]. 2022;11(6):1529. Available from: https://www.mdpi.com/2077-0383/11/6/1529

Kukreja R, Desai M, Patel S, Bapat S, Desai M. Factors affecting blood loss during percutaneous nephrolithotomy: prospective study. J Endourol. 2004;18(8):715–22.

Miernik ADJ. Small-caliber percutaneous nephrolithotomy: mini, UMP, and micro-perc. In: Smith A, Badlani G, Preminger GKL, editor. 4th ed. John Wiley and Sons; 2019. p. 301–309.

Patel SR, Nakada SY. The modern history and evolution of percutaneous nephrolithotomy. J Endourol. 2015.

Schoenthaler M, Wilhelm K, Hein S, Adams F, Schlager D, Wetterauer U, et al. Ultra-mini PCNL versus flexible ureteroscopy: a matched analysis of treatment costs (endoscopes and disposables) in patients with renal stones 10–20 mm. World J Urol [Internet]. 2015;33(10):1601–5. Available from: https://doi.org/10.1007/s00345-015-1489-4

Smith AD, Preminger G, Kavoussi L, Badlani GRA. Smith's textbook of endourology. 4th ed. Wiley; 2018.

Yamaguchi A, Skolarikos A, Buchholz N-PN, Chomón GB, Grasso M, Saba P, et al. Operating times and bleeding complications in percutaneous nephrolithotomy: a comparison of tract dilation methods in 5537 patients in the clinical research office of the endourological society percutaneous nephrolithotomy global study. J Endourol. 2011;25(6):933–9.

Zhong W, Zeng G, Wu W, Chen WWK. Minimally invasive percutaneous nephrolithotomy with multiple mini tracts in a single session in treating staghorn calculi. Urol Res. 2011;39(2):117–22.

Super-Mini-PCNL (SMP)

Guohua Zeng and Wei Zhu

Abstract Super-mini-PCNL (SMP) is an innovative endoscopic system that comprises an 8.0 F super-mini nephroscope and a specially designed irrigation-suction sheath available in either 12 or 14 Fr. The irrigation-suction sheath is a unique feature of SMP that allows for both irrigation and suction, leading to improved efficiency in stone clearance and irrigation, despite using instruments with smaller dimensions. Clinical studies have confirmed that the SMP technique is a safe, feasible, and effective method for managing moderate-sized renal calculi. This technique has several advantages, including a small percutaneous tract, minimal blood loss, high efficacy in stone clearance, improved visual field, high totally tubeless rate, short operation duration, and ease of use.

Keywords PCNL · SMP · Miniaturization · Irrigation-suction sheath · Renal calculi

According to the latest guidelines from the European Association of Urology (EAU), PCNL is recommended as the primary treatment for large renal calculi (>20 mm) and also for smaller stones (10–20 mm) located in the lower pole of the kidney when unfavorable factors for SWL are present (Professionals S-O Urolithiasis 2019). Compared to open surgery, PCNL offers high stone-free rates and is less invasive. However, PCNL is a challenging surgical technique associated with the possibility of significant complications that may affect its efficacy. These complications include bleeding, as well as injuries to the kidney, adjacent visceral structures, or vascular structures. The accuracy of the nephrostomy tract placement and its size are factors that can impact the incidence of PCNL complications. To reduce the morbidity associated with conventional-sized PCNL instruments, several modifications have been developed to miniaturize standard PCNL. These modifications include the use of miniature endoscopes via small percutaneous tracts (14–20 F), generally referred

G. Zeng (✉) · W. Zhu
Department of Urology and Guangdong Key Laboratory of Urology, The First Affiliated Hospital of Guangzhou Medical University, Guangzhou, China
e-mail: gzgyzgh@vip.tom.com

  225
J. D. Denstedt and E. N. Liatsikos (eds.), *Percutaneous Renal Surgery*,
https://doi.org/10.1007/978-3-031-40542-6_15

to as minimally invasive PCNL, mini-PCNL, or min-perc. In addition, Desai et al. (2013) have reported their ultra-mini PCNL (UMP), and micro-PCNL has also been introduced for clinical use (Desai and Mishra 2012). Developing miniature endo-scopes and access sheaths is necessary to reduce the size of nephrostomy tracts. However, using smaller nephrostomy tracts may compromise visual fields and make stone extraction more difficult. Increasing the irrigation pressure using a pressure pump can improve the visualization and passive egress of stone fragments, but it may also increase intra-luminal pressure.

The super-mini-PCNL (SMP) technique was developed to address the limitations of miniaturized PCNLs (Zeng et al. 2016, 2017). SMP is a recent addition to the miniaturized PCNL techniques, using an access sheath size of 10–14 F. Its design has been shown to prevent excessive intrarenal pressure while providing excellent endoscopic visual quality for stone fragmentation and extraction.

1   Materials

The SMP system comprises two essential components: an 8.0 Fr miniaturized nephroscope and a newly designed irrigation-suction sheath (Zeng et al. 2018a).

Miniaturized nephroscope

The SMP nephroscope has an outer diameter of 8.0 F and an inner diameter of 7.5 F, with a dismountable sheath. The telescope is made up of a 1.4-mm (4.2 F) fibre-optic bundle, providing a 120° angle of view and a resolution of up to 40,000 pixels. Once the telescope is inserted into the sheath during the procedure, a 3.3 F space is left in the bottom half of the sheath, which serves as the working channel (as shown in Fig. 1). The working channel can accommodate a laser fibre up to 550 μm in size for stone fragmentation. Alternatively, a 0.8 mm pneumatic lithotripter probe, or a 3.0 F stone basket or forceps, can also pass through the working channel during the procedure. The working length of the scope is 25.2 cm.

Irrigation-suction sheath

The irrigation-suction sheath is a crucial component of the SMP system, enabling efficient irrigation and stone clearance within a miniaturized setup. It comprises two parts: a straight sheath and a handle.

The straight sheath is a two-layered metallic tube, with a diameter ranging from 12 to 14F, and can provide a working length of either 8 or 14 cm. The space between the two layers functions as a channel for irrigation, while the central lumen of the sheath serves as a conduit for continuous suction. Additionally, the distal tip of the sheath has side holes that allow for the egress of irrigant through the irrigation channel.

The "handle" component of the SMP system allows for the control of irrigation and suction during the procedure. The oblique bifurcated tube is used for continuous suction of the irrigation fluid and the stone fragments, while the irrigation port with integral stopcock is used for regulating the flow rate of the irrigant. The straight tube, which is contiguous with the suction conduit of the straight sheath, has a receptacle for inserting lithotripsy instruments or endoscopic baskets. The negative aspiration pressure can be controlled and adjusted by opening or occluding the pressure vent located in the axis of the oblique tube (Fig. 2). The use of a specimen collection bottle between the handle and the aspirator facilitates efficient collection of stone fragments.

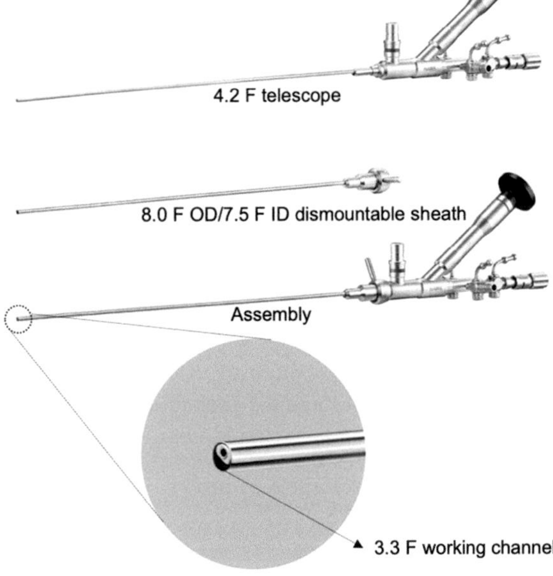

Fig. 1 Detailed structure of the miniaturized nephroscope (OD = outer diameter; ID = inner diameter)

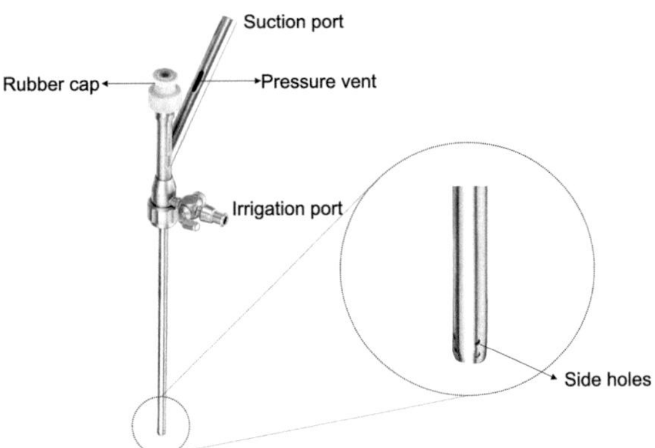

Fig. 2 Irrigation-suction sheath

2 Indications and Contraindications

Indications

- Adult patients with kidney stones between 1.5–3.0 cm in size, including those who have previously undergone unsuccessful stone clearance with shock wave lithotripsy (SWL) or ureteroscopic lithotripsy (URS), patients with cystine calculi, or those with anatomical abnormalities that prevent retrograde access or distal passage of stones.
- Patients with unfavorable renal anatomy for retrograde intrarenal surgery (RIRS), such as those with narrow (<5 mm) or long (>30 mm) infundibulum.
- Pediatric patients with stones < 2.5 cm in size that have not been effectively treated with SWL.

Contraindications

- Patients who are currently on anticoagulant therapy must discontinue it before the procedure. For instance, patients taking aspirin should discontinue use 7 days prior to the procedure, while those taking warfarin should stop 5 days beforehand.
- Patients with untreated urinary tract infections (UTIs), pregnant patients, patients with atypical interposition of visceral organs (such as bowel, spleen or liver), patients with tumors in the probable access tract area, or patients with potential malignant renal tumors should not undergo the procedure.

3 Technique

Routine preoperative preparations should be carried out, as with any percutaneous surgery. This should involve a thorough evaluation of available imaging, such as CT and IVU, to help determine the primary calyx of the puncture site, through which the majority of the stone bulk can be safely cleared. In cases where the patient has a complex stone burden or unfavorable renal anatomy, stones located in separate calyces that are unlikely to be removed through the primary tract should also be identified. Pre-operative planning for the creation of secondary tracts to safely access these calyces may be necessary.

Traditionally, SMP has been performed with the patient in the prone position, which provides direct access to the posterior calyx. However, SMP can also be performed with the patient in the supine position. This allows the use of endoscopic combined intrarenal surgery (ECIRS), which provides simultaneous antegrade and retrograde access to facilitate stone clearance. Supine SMP also enables easier switching from regional to general anesthesia, if necessary, and may be advantageous for patients with co-morbidities that make it difficult to anesthetize them in the prone position. However, establishing multiple percutaneous tracks can be challenging due to space limitations in the supine position.

During the SMP procedure, a retrograde 5 Fureteral catheter is inserted into the target kidney, followed by percutaneous access using an 18-gauge coaxial needle. A flexible tip guidewire is then inserted, and access track dilatation is performed using 10 F fascial dilators. The irrigation-suction straight sheath, along with an obturator, is then advanced over the guidewire and into the pelvicalyceal system. The handle component of SMP is connected to the sheath, and the irrigation port is connected to the irrigation unit of the pump, while the oblique tube is connected to the aspirator unit via a specimen collection bottle. The irrigation fluid pressure is set between 200 to 250 mmHg, and the suction pressure between 100 to 150 mmHg. The miniaturized endoscope is inserted into the sheath through the cap to visualize targeted renal stones for lithotripsy using a holmium-YAG laser or pneumatic lithotripter. Suction is continuously applied to evacuate tiny stone fragments through the oblique sluice. If stone fragments are too large to pass around the scope inside the sheath, the scope can be withdrawn slowly to create an unobstructed channel for larger fragments evacuation. Multiple tracks may be required for patients with a large stone burden. Fluoroscopic imaging is used to assess stone-free status, and antegrade insertion of a double-J stent may be considered in certain cases. Finally, the sheath is removed, and the wound is sutured or sealed with absorbable gelatin.

It is important to note that the decision to perform a tubeless or totally tubeless procedure should be made on an individual patient basis, taking into consideration the size and location of the stone, the complexity of the procedure, and the patient's overall health status. In addition, close postoperative monitoring is necessary to detect any potential complications early, such as bleeding or obstruction, which may require prompt intervention.

Nephrostomy tubes can provide effective drainage of urine and debris from the kidney, and may be necessary in certain cases to prevent obstruction or infection. The decision to place a nephrostomy tube should also be based on individual patient factors, and the potential benefits and risks should be carefully weighed. Close monitoring and follow-up is important in all cases to ensure the best possible outcome for the patient.

4 Advantages Over Other Miniaturized PCNLs

1. *Active removal of stone fragments and maintaining low renal pelvic pressure (RPP)*

SMP is a highly efficient miniaturized PCNL technique that removes most stone fragments through the negative pressure aspiration system. It offers several advantages over other miniaturized PCNL techniques, including the ability to extract stones using both fragmentation and dusting techniques, promoting efficient lithotripsy and removal of stone fragments, and maintaining a continuous irrigation system that reduces the occurrence of a "dust storm" caused by stone pulverization and improves the visual field. The use of a miniaturized access track also reduces access-related bleeding and improves vision. Additionally, negative pressure aspiration facilitates irrigation drainage and maintains a low average RPP throughout the procedure (Alsmadi et al. 2018).

2. *Improved irrigation*

The two-layered irrigation-suction sheath used in the SMP system offers a unique advantage over other miniaturized PCNL systems. In most miniaturized PCNL systems, the main irrigation is delivered through the same channel as the working instruments, leading to reduced irrigation efficiency once the laser fiber or pneumatic lithotripter probe is inserted. However, with the SMP system, the space between the two layers of the sheath acts as an independent irrigation channel. This frees up the working channel space of the nephroscope, allowing larger instruments such as 550 um laser fibers or 1.0 mm lithotripters to be used without compromising irrigation efficacy.

3. *A more efficient hydrodynamic mechanism for retrieval of fragments*

Other miniaturized PCNL systems often use irrigation systems that require both inflow and outflow of irrigation through the same lumen of the sheath. However, this can partially offset the effect of outflow and push stone fragments back into the collecting system. This decreases stone clearance efficiency and may even lead to stone migration, resulting in increased operation time. In contrast, the irrigation-suction sheath in the SMP system allows for separate channels for inflow and outflow, following a one-way flow system. The inflow enters the collecting system through the irrigation channel and is then aspirated out of the system through the suction conduit of the sheath (as shown in Fig. 3). This system ensures efficient stone removal and reduces operative time.

5 Enhanced SMP (eSMP)

The eSMP technology was developed to address the limitations of treating large burden kidney stones with SMP, which is only suitable for small to moderate-sized stones. The eSMP system includes an 11 Fr miniaturized nephroscope and an 18 Fr single-layer suction sheath. The sheath for eSMP is larger than that used in SMP, which allows for better performance.

One concern with small tract PCNL for large burden stones is the potential risk due to prolonged operation time. However, the use of the suction sheath in eSMP has significantly accelerated the lithotripsy procedure. In a retrospective study, the stone size in eSMP was 3.27 ± 0.85 cm, while the operation time was only 51.7 ± 14.4 min, demonstrating high efficiency in stone extraction. The safety of eSMP was supported by a postoperative fever rate of 4.34% and a transfusion rate of 2.17%. Therefore, in experienced hands, eSMP is a safe and effective option for managing 2–5 cm renal stones (Zhong et al. 2021).

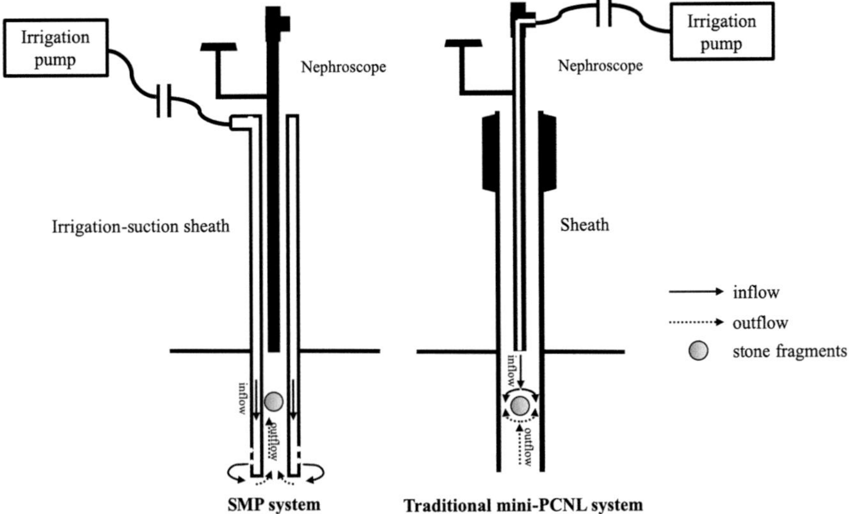

Fig. 3 The hydrodynamic mechanisms for retrieval fragments in SMP system and traditional miniPCNL system

6 Comment

Despite being introduced several years ago, SMP has not yet gained widespread popularity in the field of urology. However, both the safety and efficacy of SMP have been investigated in both adult and pediatric populations (Liu et al. 2018; Sarica et al. 2017). In fact, a multicenter, prospective, randomized controlled trial has demonstrated that SMP is more effective than RIRS for treating lower calyceal calculi, with higher stone-free rates and lower auxiliary rates (Zeng et al. 2018b). Additionally, SMP appears to be an excellent alternative for patients with small to medium-sized stones, and a previous study has demonstrated higher totally tubeless rates associated with this technique (Liu et al. 2018). In certain medical units, SMP has been commonly used to manage moderate-sized renal calculi. For patients with multiple or staghorn stones with a larger stone burden, eSMP with a larger size suction sheath may be a better choice.

References

Alsmadi J, Fan J, Zhu W, Wen Z, Zeng G. The influence of super-mini percutaneous nephrolithotomy on renal pelvic pressure in vivo. J Endourol. 2018;32:819–23.

Desai M, Mishra S. "Microperc" micro percutaneous nephrolithotomy: evidence to practice. Curr Opin Urol. 2012;22:134–8.

Desai J, Zeng G, Zhao Z, Zhong W, Chen W, Wu W. A novel technique of ultra-mini-percutaneous nephrolithotomy: introduction and an initial experience for treatment of upper urinary calculi less than 2 cm. Biomed Res Int. 2013;490793.

Liu Y, AlSmadi J, Zhu W, Liu Y, Wu W, Fan J, Lan Y, Lam W, Zhong W, Zeng G. Comparison of super-mini PCNL (SMP) versus Miniperc for stones larger than 2 cm: a propensity score-matching study. World J Urol. 2018. https://doi.org/10.1007/s00345-018-2197-7.

Professionals S-O Urolithiasis (2019). In: Uroweb. https://uroweb.org/guideline/urolithiasis/. Accessed 13 Apr 2019

Sarica K, Eryildirim B, Tuerxun A, Batuer A, Kavukoglu O, Buz A, Zeng G. Super-mini percutaneous nephrolithotomy for renal stone less than 25mm in pediatric patients: could it be an alternative to shockwave lithotripsy? Actas Urol Esp. 2017. https://doi.org/10.1016/j.acuro.2017.08.005.

Zeng G, Wan S, Zhao Z, et al. Super-mini percutaneous nephrolithotomy (SMP): a new concept in technique and instrumentation. BJU Int. 2016;117:655–61.

Zeng G, Zhu W, Liu Y, Fan J, Zhao Z, Cai C. The new generation super-mini percutaneous nephrolithotomy (SMP) system: a step-by-step guide. BJU Int. 2017. https://doi.org/10.1111/bju.13955.

Zeng G, Zhu W, Lam W. Miniaturised percutaneous nephrolithotomy: its role in the treatment of urolithiasis and our experience. Asian J Urol. 2018;5:295–302.

Zeng G, Zhang T, Agrawal M, et al. Super-mini percutaneous nephrolithotomy (SMP) vs retrograde intrarenal surgery for the treatment of 1–2 cm lower-pole renal calculi: an international multicentre randomised controlled trial. BJU Int. 2018;122:1034–40.

Zhong W, Wen J, Peng L, Zeng G. Enhanced super-mini-PCNL (eSMP): low renal pelvic pressure and high stone removal efficiency in a prospective randomized controlled trial. World J Urol. 2021;39:929–34.

Micro PCNL

Abhishek Singh, Rohan Batra, and Mahesh Desai

Abstract Microperc is a technique of miniaturised PCNL which does not require tract dilatation. It is the smallest available armamentarium to access the pelvi-calyceal system for therapeutic dusting and fragmentation of renal stones. Bader et al. in 2010 demonstrated an all-seeing needle to visualize the entire tract during standard PCNL. Extending the concept of this, Desai et al. demonstrated the feasibility and efficacy of this needle which helped in performing single-step miniaturised tract PCNL of 4.85-Fr. The visualising needle helps in confirming the puncture of selected desired calyx and correct papilla. It consists of a 0.9 mm flexible fibre optic telescope over a 4.85 Fr needle. The three- way connector helps in utilisation of irrigation and laser together thus dusting and fragmentation of renal stones. The microperc is indicated in paediatric stones, small renal stones less than 1.5 cm, calyceal diverticular stones, stones in calyces with infundibular stenosis, ectopic and horseshoe kidneys, paediatric urolithiasis and as adjunct to standard PCNL. Modification of microPCNL in the form of mini-micro PCNL using 8 Fr metal sheath gives better manoeuvrability and stability. Microperc has emerged as a complement armamentarium to PCNL and an alternative procedure to RIRS. It is safe and feasible for carefully selected cases of renal calculi with a very important role in paediatric renal calculi.

Keywords PCNL · Microperc · Mini-microperc · microPCNL · Laser

1 Introduction

Since the advent of PCNL in 1976, it has become the standard technique for treatment of renal stones (Fernstrom and Johansson 1976). The ideal procedure for the treatment of renal stone should be such that it provides a complete clearance of stone without injuring kidney or ureter. However, at present, we have not reached the goal of ideal treatment yet. In last few decades, by the year 2010, the size of the PCNL has kept on decreasing with the advent of miniPCNL to size of 16–18

A. Singh · R. Batra · M. Desai (✉)
Department of Urology, MPUH, Nadiad, India
e-mail: mrdesai@mpuh.org

© The Author(s), under exclusive license to Springer Nature Switzerland AG 2023   233
J. D. Denstedt and E. N. Liatsikos (eds.), *Percutaneous Renal Surgery*,
https://doi.org/10.1007/978-3-031-40542-6_16

Fr with the expectation of decreasing PCNL access related complications. The main reason for the miniaturization of PCNL is due to a major morbidity of PCNL which is bleeding complications. Although most bleeding associated with PCNL is managed conservatively and does not cause any consequences, 0.6–1.4% of patients require angioembolization. In a study by Kukreja et al., it was observed that as the tract size of PCNL decreases, the bleeding complications decreases (Kukreja et al. 2004).

Additionally, other complications of PCNL tract dilatation include increased fluoroscopic time, increased radiation to patient as well as surgeon. Sometimes infundibular tears can occur due to tract dilatation. So, a simple solution to decrease these complications was to reduce the tract size as low as possible. MiniPCNL has given answers to these issues to some extent but the problems still persist and not have been eliminated fully. Microperc is the smallest tract size instrument available today which can treat renal stones percutaneously.

2 Development of Armamentarium

Markus Bader et al. presented the all-seeing needle at the AUA 2010 in USA. The purpose of this needle was to permit the visualization of the entire tract during the percutaneous access up to the pelvi-calyceal system. The authors used this needle prior to the standard PCNL in 15 patients in 2010 (Bader et al. 2010).

Additionally, during peritoneal access in laparoscopic surgeries, optical trocars help in visualization of entry of trocar into the peritoneal cavity.

Standing on the shoulders of these concepts, Desai et al. moved ahead and extended the use of this 'all seeing needle' for a single step PCNL through a small tract as small as 4.85 Fr. Thus, the term 'Microperc' was defined for this technique. It is a one-step PCNL without the need for any tract dilatation (Desai et al. 2011). This technique was performed on 10 patients as initial technical feasibility and safety study. There were no tract related complications in these patients and stone free rate on 88.9% was reported.

3 Armamentarium

The parts of a Microperc assembly include:

(1) 3-part needle of 16 G (4.85 Fr). Needle includes the shaft, with outer diameter of 1.6 mm (4.85 Fr) and needle with bevelled edge (1.3 mm) (Figs. 1, and 2)
(2) Fiber-optic telescope (0.9 mm). It contains 10,000 fiber-optic bundles (10,000-pixel resolution) and is flexible (Fig. 1) with light cable and camera attachment head
(3) 3-part plastic adaptor
(4) Irrigation tubing (which can be connected to irrigation pressure pump) (Fig. 3).

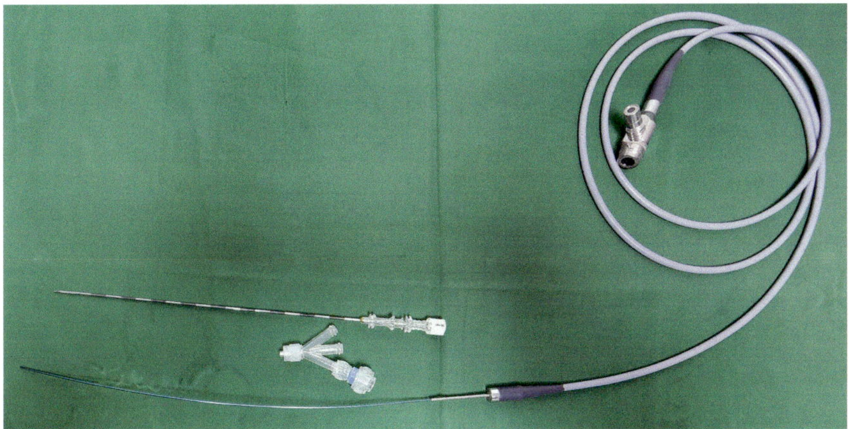

Fig. 1 Three-part needle with telescope

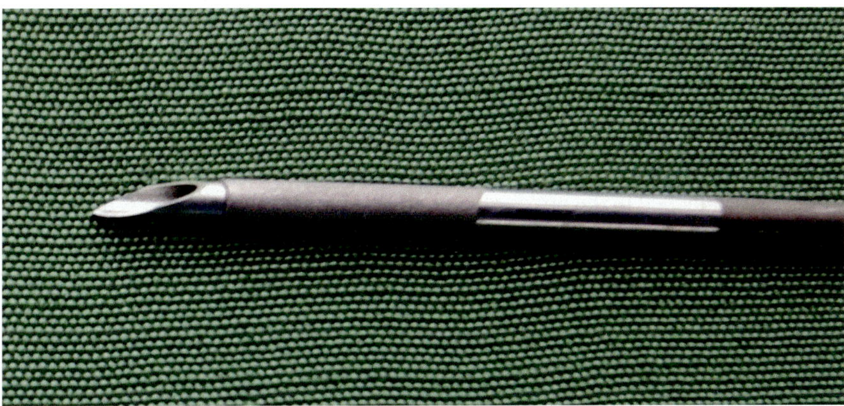

Fig. 2 Bevelled needle with sheath

The fiber optic telescope is connected to the standard endoscopic camera system and a light source. The three-way adapter(connector) allows simultaneous irrigation, laser fiber insertion and telescope to work simultaneously.

4 Technique of the Procedure

The patient is in general anaesthesia and in lithotomy position. A 6 Fr or 7 Fr open ended ureteral catheter is placed transurethrally with a cystoscopy. Multiple side holes can be made in the ureteric catheter to improve drainage of fluid as the tip may get clogged due to small stone fragments or small clots. After inserting the

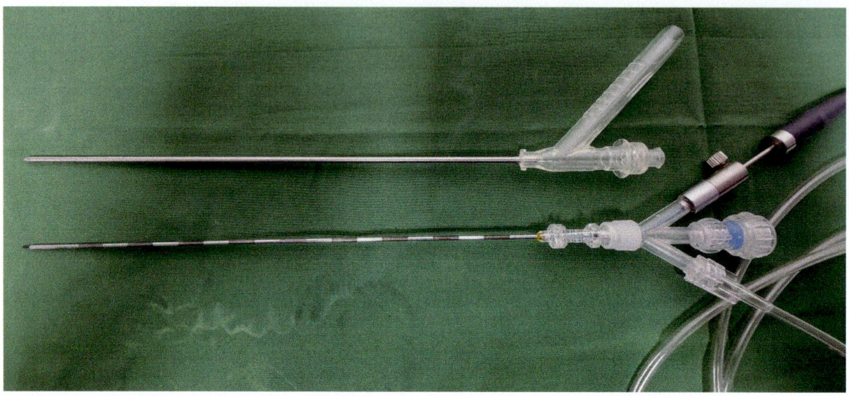

Fig. 3 Assembled needle and telescope with irrigation port

ureteric catheter and a foley's catheter, the patient is turned into prone position. The procedure can also be performed in supine position.

A targeted calyceal puncture is made under USG or fluoroscopic guidance with a 16-gauge all-seeing needle under optical vision. The optical vision may or may not be used during the initial puncture. USG guidance using a puncture attachment aids in the puncture of desired targeted stone containing calyx. After the access is confirmed with efflux of urine from PCS, the bevelled inner needle is removed and then a 3-way connector is attached to the proximal end of the sheath. The telescope is then passed through the side port and the other side port has to be used for irrigation purpose. The optic is relayed through a multi-joint mounting arm with attached camera and light cable. The central port is used to pass the laser fiber. The stone can be fragmented by a holmium laser or a thulium fiber laser (TFL). The vision is controlled in such a way that the stones are clearly seen in the PCS. Irrigation pump can be used as required and is controlled by a foot pedal by the operating surgeon. The ureteric catheter helps in continuous drainage of the system.

At the end of the procedure dusting, fragmentation of stones and clearance are assessed by fluoroscopy. If the need to keep DJ stent is felt, it has to be kept retrogradely. The patient is monitored for postoperative complications. The foley catheter and ureteric catheter is removed on postoperative day 1 and the patient is subsequently discharged home. CT KUB can be done to assess the stone free rate in patients at 1-month follow up.

5   Salient Features of Microperc

16 G needle has to accommodate 0.9 mm telescope as well as laser fiber. So due to lack of space, a pressure irrigation pump is required. The laser fiber of more than 272 microns is not desirable. The camera head and light cable are away and held with articulating arms mounted away from the assembly.

6   Modification of Microperc

Since microperc is single step insertion in PCS and with a needle, it can bend in pelvicalyceal system if a lot of manipulation is done. To overcome this situation, an 8 fr metallic sheath is developed. This is called 'Mini-microperc-sheath'. It allows the same three-way connector as in microperc. It consists 3.5 Fr telescope which is mounted inside a 6 Fr sheath. The inner telescope sheath has two side ports. One is used for irrigation and the other one for passing laser fiber. A thin lithotripter can also be used with this system. The sheath of this mini-microperc allows intra renal manipulation of scope without risking of bending of needle or damage to the scope (Sabnis et al. 2012) (Figs. 4 and 5).

Fig. 4 Mini-microperc sheath

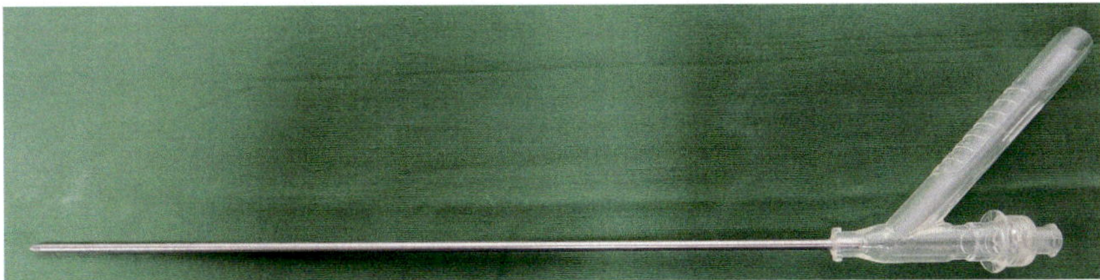

Fig. 5 Mini-microPCNL sheath with suction port

7 Advantages of Microperc

The Microperc is of immense benefit in Lower polar calculi which are not amenable to flexible ureteroscopy due to awkward calyxes. Microperc is also advantageous in patients with stones in calyceal diverticulum and pediatric stone patients, lower polar stones, narrow infundibular width, malrotated kidneys, ectopic kidney stones, horse shoe kidney isthmus stone, failed RIRS cases. It can be used as an adjunct to standard PCNL or miniPCNL without increasing the morbidity of the procedure.

8 Disadvantages of Microperc

There is a chance of elevated intrarenal pressures that can cause intravasation of irrigation fluid and resultant sepsis. So, irrigation should be kept in such a way that vision is optimum. If the stone fragments migrate to other calyces, it is difficult to manoeuvre the microperc in different calyces. So, a conversion to miniperc may be required in such cases. Fragment retrieval is not possible in microperc. So, if DJ stenting is to be done, then the DJ stent has to be placed in a retrograde manner. Since microperc is a very delicate instrument, wear and tear of the instrument is higher than miniperc or standard PCNL instruments.

9 Role of Microperc in the Era of RIRS

A prospective randomised trial was done by Sabnis et al. in 2013 between microperc and RIRS for renal stone < 1.5 cm. The authors determined the safety and stone free rate of microperc as similar to that of RIRS. However, microperc was associated with higher haemoglobin drop and more pain. RIRS had higher incidence of DJ stenting (Sabnis et al. 2013). Tepeler et al. in 2013 (Tepeler et al. 2013) reported a stone free rate of 85.7% using microperc in 21 patients with lower calyceal stones. Microperc has a high stone clearance rate that can offset its invasive nature. The surgeon discomfort score was higher in the RIRS group and RIRS has an initial learning curve.

Armagan et al. in 2015 compared microperc and RIRS in a retrospective manner for stones less than 2 cm in lower pole. They concluded that microperc is feasible, safe and efficacious with significantly higher SFR (Armagan et al. 2015). Baş O et al. in 2016 compared microperc vs RIRS for paediatric renal stones of 10–20 mm. retrospectively. Both RIRS and microperc were comparable and had similar complication rates. However, hospital stay and radiation exposure were lower in the RIRS patients (Baş et al. 2016). Li MM et al. in 2018 performed a meta-analysis of nine studies (842 patients) which compared microperc with RIRS. Microperc had higher stone-free rate, longer hospital stays, longer fluoroscopy time, and higher decrease in haemoglobin in comparison to RIRS. The operative time, stone free rate, complication rate, or auxiliary procedures were similar in both the groups (Li et al. 2018). Zhang B et al. did a systematic review and meta-analysis of comparison of microperc and RIRS. He concluded that microperc has lesser DJ stent insertions and higher SFR but drop in haemoglobin and hospital stay are higher. However, the operative time for RIRS and Microperc for lower pole stones was not statistically significant and it was comparable (Zhang et al. 2020).

In RIRS, if the ureters are tight, it leads to DJ stenting for 10–14 days and the procedure has to be postponed. Whereas in microperc, the stone clearance can be achieved in a single sitting.

10 Comparison of Microperc with SWL

SWL usually needs a multiple sessions and auxiliary procedures to achieve stone clearance. In contrast, microperc is associated with high stone clearance in a short hospital stay. In Indian context, majority (75%) of renal calculi are composed of calcium oxalate monohydrate (Srisubat et al. 2009). Thus, SWL is not very effective in these patients. Hatipoglu et al. compared microperc with SWL and found that retreatment rates are lower with microperc in comparison to SWL (Hatipoglu et al. 2013).

11 Comparison of Microperc with Miniperc

Miniperc is a similar to standard PCNL, except that the tract size is smaller, but still, it has to be dilated stepwise. On the contrary, microperc is a single step renal access.

Karatag T et al. in 2015 retrospectively compared both these procedures for pediatric renal stones of size between 10 to 20 mm in 119 patients. They concluded that microperc has similar stone clearance and complications rates as that of miniperc. The stone-free rate at 1 month was 92.8% versus 93.6% for Microperc and Miniperc respectively (Karatag et al. 2015). In 2016, Tok A et al. compared outcomes of 98 patients for treatment of lower polar stones of 10–20 mm. The results were comparable in both arms (Tok et al. 2016). Dundar G et al. in 2016 compared Miniperc and Microperc in 43 paediatric patients for low volume stones ls size less than 2 cm after unsuccessful SWL. The stone clearance rate for Microperc was 93.8% and for Miniperc was 92.6% (Dundar et al. 2016).

12 Microperc in Today's Scenario

In today's scenario, microperc is an adjunct and complimentary to other modalities like miniPCNL and RIRS. There are definite indications and advantages for microperc in carefully selected patients.

13 Conclusion

Microperc has a unique place in today's era of miniperc and RIRS. It gives all advantages of RIRS without disturbing the ureter and gives stone free rates equivalent to RIRS. It does not have the complications of PCNL. Also, we fragment and dust all the stones under vision. Thus, it has the best of both the procedures. The indications have to be very diligently selected to get optimum outcomes with microperc. It is a very handy armamentarium in specific situations like pediatric renal stones, calyceal diverticulum stones and lower polar stones.

References

Armagan A, Karatag T, Buldu I, Tosun M, Basibuyuk I, Istanbulluoglu MO, et al. Comparison of flexible ureterorenoscopy and micropercutaneous nephrolithotomy in the treatment for moderately size lowerpole stones. World J Urol. 2015;33(11):1827–31.

Bader M, Gratzke C, Schlenker B, Tilki D, Reich O, Gozzi C, et al. 1890 The "all-seeing needle"–an optical puncture system confirming percutaneous access in Pcnl. J Urol. 2010;183(4s):E734–5.

Baş O, Dede O, Aydogmus Y, Utangaç M, Yikilmaz TN, Damar E, et al. Comparison of retrograde intrarenal surgery and micro-percutaneous nephrolithotomy in moderately sized pediatric kidney stones. J Endourol. 2016;30(7):765–70.

Desai MR, Sharma R, Mishra S, Sabnis RB, Stief C, Bader M. Single-step percutaneous nephrolithotomy (microperc): the initial clinical report. J Urol. 2011;186(1):140–5.

Dundar G, Gokce G, Gokcen K, Korgali E, Asdemir A, Kaygusuz K. Microperc versus miniperc for treatment of renal stones smaller than 2 cm in paediatric patients. Urol J. 2016;13(5):2829–32.

Fernstrom I, Johansson B. Percutaneous pyelolithotomy. A new extraction technique. Scand J Urol Nephrol. 1976;10:257–9.

Hatipoglu NK, Sancaktutar AA, Tepeler A, Bodakci MN, Penbegul N, Atar M, et al. Comparison of shockwave lithotripsy and microperc for treatment of kidney stones in children. J Endourol. 2013;27(9):1141–6.

Karatag T, Tepeler A, Silay MS, Bodakci MN, Buldu I, Daggulli M, et al. A comparison of 2 percutaneous nephrolithotomy techniques for the treatment of Pediatric kidney stones of sizes 10–20 mm: microperc versus miniperc. Urology. 2015;85(5):1015–8.

Kukreja R, Desai M, Patel S, et al. Factors affecting blood loss during percutaneous nephrolithotomy: prospective study. J Endourol. 2004;18:715.

Li M-M, Yang H-M, Liu X-M, Qi H-G, Weng G-B. Retrograde intrarenal surgery versus miniaturized percutaneous nephrolithotomy to treat lower pole renal stones 1.5–2.5 cm in diameter. World J Clin Cases 2018;6(15):931.

Sabnis RB, Ganesamoni R, Sarpal R. Miniperc: what is its current status? Curr Opin Urol. 2012;22:129–33.

Sabnis RB, Ganesamoni R, Doshi A, Ganpule AP, Jagtap J, Desai MR. Micropercutaneous nephrolithotomy (microperc) versus retrograde intrarenal surgery for the management of small renal calculi: a randomized controlled trial. BJU Int. 2013;112(3):355–61.

Srisubat A, Potisat S, Lojanapiwat B, Setthawong V, Laopaiboon M. Extracorporeal shock wave lithotripsy (ESWL) versus percutaneous nephrolithotomy (PCNL) or retrograde intrarenal surgery (RIRS) for kidney stones. Cochrane Database Syst Rev. 2009;4:CD007044.

Tepeler A, Armagan A, Sancaktutar AA, Silay MS, Penbegul N, Akman T, et al. The role of microperc in the treatment of symptomatic lower pole renal calculi. J Endourol. 2013;27(1):13–8.

Tok A, Akbulut F, Buldu I, Karatag T, Kucuktopcu O, Gurbuz G, et al. Comparison of microperc and mini-percutaneous nephrolithotomy for medium-sized lower calyx stones. Urolithiasis. 2016;44(2):155–9.

Zhang B, Hu Y, Gao J, Zhuo D. Micropercutaneous versus retrograde intrarenal surgery for the management of moderately sized kidney stones: a systematic review and meta-analysis. Urol Int. 2020;104(1–2):94–105.

Percutaneous Nephrolithotomy in Patients with Medullary Sponge Kidney

Ravindra B. Sabnis and Pawan Survase Jain

Abstract Medullary sponge kidney (MSK) aka Lenarduzzi–Cacchi–Ricci disease is characterized by dilatation of medullary and papillary parts of the collecting ducts due to cystic damage to the distal nephron. MSK derives its name from the classical cysts found within the nephron which can grow from 1 to 8 mm and appear as "sponges" upon cross-sectional examination. Prevalence in the general population is estimated to be around 0.5–1% in few studies, but the disease is commonly observed among recurrent stone formers. The increased stone forming tendency in MSK patients is due to morphological anomalies (cystic dilations favouring urinary stasis) and functional disorders. The diagnosis of MSK is radiographic, and intravenous urography is the gold standard technique. Treatment of MSK patients with symptomatic stones requires either extracorporeal shock-wave lithotripsy (SWL) for stones less than 2 cm in diameter or a percutaneous nephrolithotomy (PCNL) for stones > 2 cm. PCNL is very challenging in anomalous kidneys and may be associated with difficulty in achieving an optimal access. Minimally invasive PCNL has been proven to be safe and effective for patients with large stone burden or complex stones. Endoscopic combined intrarenal surgery (ECIRS) is a new and adaptable concept for the treatment of large and/or complex urolithiasis in MSK.

Keywords Medullary sponge kidney · Nephrocalcinosis · PCNL · ECIRS

1 Background

Medullary sponge kidney (MSK) is a rare sporadic renal malformation recognized by Lendarduzzi in 1939. Although it was first recognized by G Lenarduzzi in 1939, its thorough description was done by a multidisciplinary team of a radiologist (Lenarduzzi), a urologist (Cacchi), and a pathologist (Ricci) hence referred to as Lenarduzzi–Cacchi–Ricci disease.

R. B. Sabnis (✉) · P. Survase Jain
Muljibhai Patel Urological Hospital, Nadiad, Gujarat 287001, India
e-mail: rbsabnis@mpuh.org

J. D. Denstedt and E. N. Liatsikos (eds.), *Percutaneous Renal Surgery*,
https://doi.org/10.1007/978-3-031-40542-6_17

MSK is generally considered a sporadic disorder. Despite its sporadic nature, MSK rarely presents with familial inheritance in an autosomal dominant fashion (Fabris et al. 2013). The exact prevalence of the disease is unknown. In a series published by Palubinskas et al. (1963), features demonstrating definite to weak radiological signs of MSK were detected in 0.5–1% of cases. The prevalence of MSK among recurrent renal calcium stone formers has been observed as high as 20% (Thomas et al. 2000). MSK is characterized by the dilatation of the medullary and papillary parts of the collecting ducts due to cystic damage to the distal nephron. MSK derives its name from the classical cysts found within the nephron which can grow from 1 to 8 mm and appear as "sponges" upon cross-sectional examination. This disorder usually affects the medulla where the cortical structures are almost always spared.

2 Pathophysiology

The disease is considered congenital because of its frequent association with other developmental disorders like congenital hemihypertrophy and Beckwith-Wiedemann syndrome, horseshoe kidney, unilateral renal aplasia, and contralateral congenital small kidney.

As MSK is a rare disease, there is a paucity of literature at present. The congenital disease involving abnormal epigenetic mechanisms and the acquired disease secondary to calcium accumulation or hyperparathyroidism are the main explanations for the occurrence of MSK (Pisani, et al. 2020; Fabris et al. 2010). Existing knowledge does not reveal the apparent heritability of MSK. Mutations in glial cell–derived neurotrophic factor (GDNF) in 12% of MSK cases (Torregrossa et al. 2010).

A growing literature demonstrates that mutations and variants of GDNF and RET (RET proto-oncogene) have been noted in fetuses with renal agenesis and renal tract malformations (Skinner et al. 2008). Although GDNF and RET does not justify for most cases of MSK, variants of these might act as predisposition genes interrelating with other genes and anonymous factors. This condition may also be amplified by a defective expression of other key regulators of renal development including hepatocyte nuclear factor 1β (HNF1B) (Desgrange et al. 2017 Dec 15), a transcription factor that regulates endoderm development (Kolatsi-Joannou et al. 2001). Molecular analysis confirmed that HNF1B might act both upstream and downstream of RET signalling by directly regulating GDNF family receptor alpha 1 and ETS variant transcription factor 5. Eventually, HNF1B deletion may lead grossly mis patterned ureteric tree network, faulty collecting duct differentiation, and disrupted tissue architecture, which can induce cystogenesis (Desgrange et al. 2017).

3   Clinical Presentation

MSK usually manifests with nephrocalcinosis and recurrent renal stones; other signs may also be renal acidification and concentration defects, pre-calyceal duct ectasias (erroneously diagnosed as cysts), and neglected proximal tubular defects. The most common presenting clinical sign of MSK is recurrent calcium oxalate and/or phosphate nephrolithiasis. The increased stone-forming tendency in MSK patients is not yet fully explained, as the majority of authors consider that the association of morphological anomalies (cystic dilations favoring urinary stasis) and functional disorders (hypercalciuria, hypocitraturia, distal renal tubes acidosis, and defective acidification) create the environment for stone formation (calcium phosphate and oxalate) (Katabathina et al. 2010) (Fig. 1). Macro- and micro-haematuria, renal failure, and hyperparathyroidism (Maschio et al. 1982) can be the presenting features in a small number of patients. However, in many patients, hypercalciuria, nephrocalcinosis, and renal stones precede the onset of hyperparathyroidism over many years. It has also been suggested that hypercalciuria can stimulate secondary hyperparathyroidism (Dlabal et al. 1979). The disease doesn't exhibit gender preponderance and is generally diagnosed in adulthood, because of recurrent calcium nephrolithiasis and nephrocalcinosis. It rarely manifests in children, but when this happens, the disease is rather severe and the bone-related consequences of distal renal tubular acidosis dominate the clinical picture, with failure to thrive, short stature, and rickets-like symptoms (Sluysmans et al. 1987; Kasap et al. 2006).

4   Management

The diagnosis of MSK is radiographic, and intravenous urography is the gold standard technique. Radiographs reveal collections of contrast medium in ectatic papillary ducts, giving the appearance of a blush (in the mildest cases) or linear striations, or bouquets of papillae, whereas cystic dilation of the collecting ducts are seen in the full-blown cases. Medullary nephrocalcinosis is a common feature. Distinctive cases involve all renal papillae bilaterally, but involvement may also be unilateral or affect only a few papillae, the latter cases pose more challenges in diagnosis. A medullary sponge kidney lacking calcifications appear on the sonogram as a kidney with prominent hypoechoic calyces thereby posing a challenge to diagnose. On the contrary, MSK with nephrocalcinosis has a classic appearance of highly echogenic renal pyramids.

Treatment of MSK patients with symptomatic stones requires the correction of the metabolic disorders, eradication of infection, and removal of the offending stones. Extracorporeal shock-wave lithotripsy (SWL) is the preferred treatment modality for stones less than 2 cm in diameter. Percutaneous nephrolithotomy (PCNL) remains the accepted standard for stones > 2 cm and for stones that are refractory to SWL.

Most recently retrograde intra- renal surgery (RIRS) has also been advocated for the treatment of medium-sized stones.

With regards to the treatments for medullary sponge kidney, the primary focus is to prevent the possible development of stones, next in line is to treat the complications. The points of highlight in the management of medullary sponge kidneys are.

- Patients should be provided an insight about their nutritional intake, especially with regards to higher fluid intake, to keep their urine output at more than 3 L per day as this will help to reduce the risk of some stones and the development of UTIs. Dietary modifications like avoidance and reduction of dairy products and vitamin D supplements reduce calcium intake thereby reducing the risk of stone production (Pak 1998). Avoiding foods rich in oxalate, like tea, chocolate, nuts, strawberries, rhubarb, spinach, and beetroot, will reduce the production of oxalate stones (Brinkley et al. 1990). In general diet deficient in protein or sodium, will also have a positive influence on reducing stone production (Heilberg 2000).
- UTI or evolving pyelonephritis should be addressed with antibiotics as quickly as possible.
- If a medullary sponge kidney patient presents with pain and haematuria, they should receive a full battery of investigation to stay vigilant regarding the sequel of the disease.
- In medullary sponge kidney, regular urinalysis, and plain abdominal X-ray can help to detect infection and renal tract calcification and should be a made a protocol. Renal function can be monitored using urea, electrolytes, creatinine, and eGFR. Children have to be screened for Wilms' and other abdominal tumors (Beetz et al. 1991).

Treatment with potassium citrate is generally recommended for patients with MSK with at least one stone risk factor (SRF; hypercalciuria, hypocitraturia, hyper-uricosuria, hyperoxaluria). The initial dosage of potassium citrate is 20 mEq (2 g)/d of citrate; if tolerated, the dosage is titrated for patients initially failing to achieve a citraturia level > 450 mg/24 h, adding 10 mEq (1 g) citrate at a time until the desired level is reached, provided the urine pH in a 24-h collection is < 7.5. Patients are followed up once a month until the treatment dose is fixed and thereafter once every 6 months. Long-term treatment with potassium corrects incomplete dRTA leading to a reduced calcium mobilization from bone buffering of acids, thus reducing calci-uria. The reduction in hypercalciuria and the increase in hypocitraturia prevents lithogenesis (Zerwekh et al. 2002; Pak 1994).

PCNL is one of the most efficient treatment modes for large (larger than 300 mm2) and complex stones in anomalous kidneys with a higher SFR (>90%).

However, PCNL is very challenging in anomalous kidneys and may be associated with difficulty in achieving optimal access due to abnormality in renal position and relation of the calyces to the renal pelvis and upper ureter; or may lead to increased frequency of visceral and vascular injuries caused by the altered relationship of the kidney to the surrounding structures and the presence of aberrant vasculature (Binbay et al. 2011; Al-Otaibi and Hosking 1999). Osther et al. (2011), reported that access failure for PCNL was significantly more in patients with renal anomalies (5%) when compared to normal kidneys (1.7%).

In order to combat these unfavorable facts of PCNL, minimally invasive PCNL (MPCNL) is a modified PCNL using a miniaturized endoscope through a smaller size of nephrostomy tract (14–20 Fr.) was tried. It has been proven to be safe and effective for patients with large stone burdens or complex stones and has fewer perioperative complications than the conventional PCNL. In the study published by Sun et al. (Sun et al. 2016) titled "Safety and efficacy of minimally invasive percutaneous nephrolithotomy in the treatment of patients with medullary sponge kidney" minimally invasive percutaneous nephrolithotomy was performed in 15 medullary sponge kidneys. All the patients included in this study had complex renal stones including 14 multiple stones and 3 partial staghorn calculi. The mean stone surface area was 779.5 ± 421.1 mm^2. The total operative time was 87.3 ± 32.3 min. An initial stone-free rate of 60% was achieved after the MPCNL, and the final stone-free rate was 86.6% after the auxiliary second look and/or shock-wave lithotripsy. SFR after primary MPCNL was 60%. It was appreciably low when compared to the patients without MSK. This was owing to the abnormal tubular etiology of stone formation. Two patients included in this study had a failed procedure. Clavien grade I and II complications occurred in 3 (21.4%) patients including one (7.1%) patient who required a transfusion. All the complications were managed conservatively. No major complications were recorded. This retrospective analysis confirmed that MPCNL was a safe alternative for medullary sponge kidney patients with complex renal calculi.

A high incidence of UTI had been documented in MSK patients with renal calculi and especially after the intervention. UTI can result in sepsis or even septic shock, and it is one of the most dreaded and life-threatening conditions in endourological surgery. In order to avoid septic complications, it is critical to effectively treat the UTI preoperatively. Hemorrhage and the need for blood transfusions are major concerns in PCNL. MPCNL has been proven to be a safe and effective treatment option for complex or staghorn stones. It had less blood loss and a lower incidence of blood transfusion than the conventional PCNL.

Currently, PNL is the preferred first-line, minimally invasive treatment but the need for two or more access sites and greater blood loss especially in anomalous kidneys like MSK makes it less favorable. The use of single-tract PCNL with adjuvant procedures such as flexible ureteroscopy/nephroscopy may reduce the challenges faced with PCNL without compromising on stone-free rates. Endoscopic combined intrarenal surgery (ECIRS) is a new and adaptable concept for the treatment of large and/or complex urolithiasis. Combining the anterograde and retrograde approach to the renal cavities, ECIRS allows the use of all the rigid and flexible endourological instruments, optimal end vision percutaneous renal puncture, preliminary evaluation of renal stones features, the negligible need for multiple percutaneous accesses, immediate treatment of concomitant ureteral calculi and final visual control of the stone-free status.

The most important drawback of PCNL is the inability to reach all the papillae through a single access. In MSK with repeated recurrences of symptomatic stones,

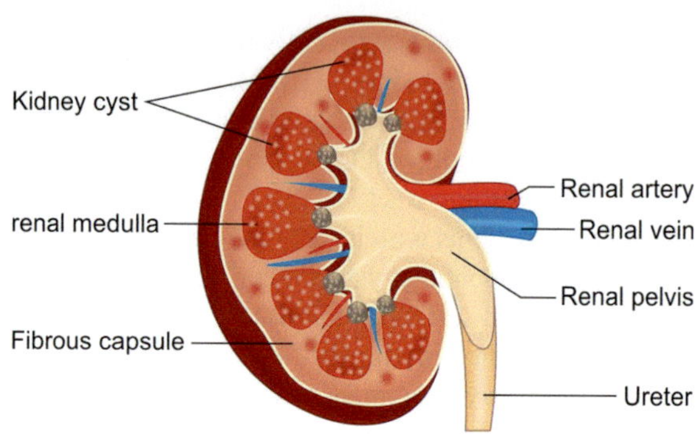

Fig. 1 Kidney showing the classical cysts found within the nephron which can grow from 1 to 8 mm and appear as "sponges" with nephrocalcinosis and multiple calyceal stones

ureteroscopic laser papillotomy (Xu et al. 2015) is a viable option for radiographically visible intraductal papillary calculi. With the consortium of treatment options available, the best treatment to prevent the stone passage, avoid renal function damage, improve life quality, and also relieve pain, hematuria, and urinary infection associated with MSK has to be offered to the patient (Fig. 1).

References

Al-Otaibi K, Hosking DH. Percutaneous stone removal in horseshoe kidneys. J Urol. 1999;162:674–7.

Beetz R, Schofer O, Riedmiller H, Schumacher R, Gutjahr P. Medullary sponge kidneys and unilateral Wilms tumour in a child with Beckwith-Wiedemann syndrome. Eur J Pediatr. 1991;150:489–92.

Binbay M, Istanbulluoglu O, Sofikerim M, et al. Effect of simple malrotation on percutaneous nephrolithotomy: a matched pair multicenter analysis. J Urol. 2011;185(5):1737–41.

Brinkley LJ, Gregory J, Pak CY. A further study of oxalate bioavailability in foods. J Urol. 1990;144(1):94–6.

Desgrange A, Heliot C, Skovorodkin I, Akram SU, Heikkila J, Ronkainen VP, et al. HNF1B controls epithelial organization and cell polarityduring ureteric bud branching and collecting duct morphogenesis. Development. 2017;144(24):4704–19.

Dlabal PW, Jordan RM and Dorfman SG. Medullary sponge kidney and renal-leak hypercalciuria. A link to the development of parathyroid adenoma? JAMA 1979;241:1490–1491.

Fabris A, Lupo A, Bernich P, et al. Long-term treatment with potassium citrate and renal stones in medullary sponge kidney. Clin J Am Soc Nephrol. 2010;5(9):1663–8.

Fabris A, Anglani F, Lupo A, Gambaro G. Medullary sponge kidney: state of the art. Nephrol Dial Transplant. 2013;28(5):1111–9.

Heilberg IP. Update on dietary recommendations and medical treatment of renal stone disease. Nephrol Dial Transplant. 2000;15(1):117–23.

Kasap B, Soylu A, Oren O, et al. Medullary sponge kidney associated with distal renal tubular acidosis in a 5-year-old girl. Eur J Pediatr. 2006;165:648–51.

Katabathina VS, Kota G, Dasyam AK, Shanbhogue AKP, Prasa SR. Adult renal cystic disease: a genetic, biological, and developmental primer. Radiographics. 2010;30:1509–23.

Kolatsi-Joannou M, Bingham C, Ellard S, Bulman MP, Allen LIS, Hattersley AT, et al. Hepatocyte nuclear factor-1beta: a new kindred with renal cysts and diabetes and gene expression in normal human development. J Am Soc Nephrol. 2001;12(10):2175–80.

Maschio G, Tessitore N, D'Angelo A, et al. Medullary sponge kidney and hyperparathyroidism–a puzzling association. Am J Nephrol. 1982;2:77–84.

Osther PJ, Razvi H, Liatsikos E, Averch T, Crisci A, Garcia JL, Mandal A, de la Rosette. on behalf of the CROES PCNL Study Group J. Percutaneous nephrolithotomy among patients with renal anomalies: patient characteristics and outcomes; a subgroup analysis of the clinical research office of the endourological society global percutaneous nephrolithotomy study. J Endourol. 2011;25(10):1627–32.

Pak CY. Citrate and renal calculi: an update. Miner Electrolyte Metab. 1994;20:371–7.

Pak CY. Kidney stones. The Lancet. 1998;351(9118):1797–801.

Palubinskas AJ. Renal pyramidal structure opacification in excretory urography and its relation to medullary sponge kidney. Radiology. 1963;81:963–70.

Pisani R, Giacosa S, Giuliotti et al. Ultrasound to address medullary sponge kidney: a retrospective study. BMC Nephrol. 2020;21(1):430.

Skinner MA, Safford SD, Reeves JG, et al. Renal aplasia in humans is associated with RET mutations. Am J Hum Genet. 2008;82:344–51.

Sluysmans T, Vanoverschelde JP, Malvaux P. Growth failure associated with medullary sponge kidney, due to incomplete renal tubular acidosis type 1. Eur J Pediatr. 1987;146:78–80.

Sun H, Zhang Z, Yuan J, Liu Y, Lei M, Luo J, Wan SP, Zeng G. Safety and efficacy of minimally invasive percutaneous nephrolithotomy in the treatment of patients with medullary sponge kidney. Urolithiasis. 2016;44:421–6.

Thomas E, Witte Y, Thomas J, et al. Maladie de Cacchi et Ricci: remarques radiologiques, epidémiologiques et biologiques. Prog Urol. 2000;10:29–35.

Torregrossa R. Anglani F. Fabris A, et al. Identification of GDNF gene sequence variations in patients with medullary sponge kidney disease. Clin J Am Soc Nephrol. 2010;5:1205–1210.

Xu G, Wen J, Wang B, Li Z, Du C. The clinical efficacy and safety of ureteroscopic laser papillotomy to treat intraductal papillary calculi associated with medullary sponge kidney. Urology. 2015;86(3):472–6.

Zerwekh JE, Reed-Gitomer BY, Pak CY. Pathogenesis of hypercalciuric nephrolithiasis. Endocrinol Metab Clin North Am. 2002;31:869–84.

PCNL for Calyceal Diverticula

Raymond Khargi, Ryan M. Blake, Samuel M. Yim, and Mantu Gupta

Abstract Calyceal diverticula are a unique urologic pathology that occasionally cause bothersome symptoms for patients. Diagnosis is challenging and is accomplished only with appropriate imaging and experienced clinicians. A variety of treatment options exist for calyceal diverticula. Percutaneous nephrolithotomy (PCNL) is a valuable treatment for calyceal diverticula as it can be used in majority of patients and has excellent success rates. This chapter will review the topic of calyceal diverticula and provide an in depth discussion of the role of PCNL in their treatment.

Keywords Calyceal diverticulum · Percutaneous nephrolithotomy · Nephrolithiasis · Endourology · Minimally invasive

1 Introduction

Calyceal diverticula are congenital non-secretory outpouchings that communicate with the renal collecting system. Embryologically, calyceal diverticula are thought to arise from the persistence of small ureteral buds, which fail to undergo normal regression and instead aberrantly connect to the renal collecting system. The phenomenon was first described by Rayer in 1841 and later the nomenclature "calyceal diverticula" was coined by Prather in 1941 (York et al. 2019). The incidence of calyceal diverticula is estimated to be less than 1%, ranging from 2.1 to 6.0 per 1000 individuals, with 3% presenting bilaterally (Gross and Herrmann 2007).

The diverticular cavities are lined with urothelium and passively receive urine from the collecting system via a narrow diverticular neck. This can result in various symptoms related to urinary stasis, including hematuria and recurrent urinary tract infections (UTIs). The most common presenting complaint, however, is flank

R. Khargi · R. M. Blake · M. Gupta (✉)
Icahn School of Medicine at Mount Sinai, New York City, USA
e-mail: mantu.gupta@mountsinai.org

S. M. Yim
SUNY Downstate Health Sciences University, Brooklyn, USA

© The Author(s), under exclusive license to Springer Nature Switzerland AG 2023   251
J. D. Denstedt and E. N. Liatsikos (eds.), *Percutaneous Renal Surgery*,
https://doi.org/10.1007/978-3-031-40542-6_18

pain. Stone formation has been observed in 9.5–50% of patients (Middleton and Pfister 1974). However, in a reported pooled series by Waingankar et al., 96% of symptomatic patients presented with stones in the diverticulum that required treatment (Waingankar et al. 2014). The presence of calyceal diverticula can thus have significant clinical implications and may require intervention to manage associated complications.

In this chapter we will review the presentation, diagnosis, and management of calyceal diverticular stones.

2 Presentation

The majority of patients with calyceal diverticula are asymptomatic, and the diagnosis is made incidentally on imaging performed for other indications. When symptomatic, patients can present with flank pain, recurrent urinary tract infection, and/or hematuria. Additionally, if the diverticular neck proves to be patent enough, passage of multiple tiny smooth stones can also be observed within this patient population.

In children, calyceal diverticula commonly present with UTIs and association between the calyceal diverticulum and vesicoureteral reflux should be ruled out (Estrada et al. 2009).

Due to the similarity of symptoms with other renal pathologies such as renal or parapelvic cysts, hydrocalycosis secondary to an obstructed infundibulum, cystic tumors, and renal abscess, imaging studies such as computed tomography (CT) and ultrasound (US) are typically employed to differentiate between these conditions.

3 Diagnostic Workup

The diagnostic workup for calyceal diverticula typically includes a comprehensive medical history, physical examination, urinalysis, urine culture, complete blood count, and a basic metabolic panel. Additionally, imaging studies of the abdomen are usually performed to confirm the diagnosis. Renal ultrasound or non-contrast computed tomography scans are the most common imaging modalities employed in the diagnosis of this condition.

3.1 KUB

Although plain abdominal radiographs cannot make a definitive diagnosis of a calyceal diverticulum, there are often subtle clues that suggest the diagnosis. This is important because recognizing these clues can then lead to an appropriate imaging study to make the correct diagnosis, usually a CT urogram. If not recognized, it

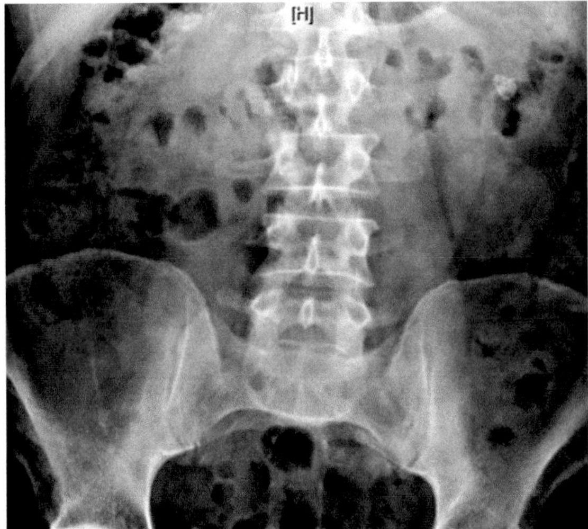

Fig. 1 Mulberry appearance of calyceal diverticular stones on KUB. This patient had over 100 stones in his diverticulum cavity. The peripheral location is due to the fact that diverticula are peripheral to a calyx, so they are not as centrally located except in the less common scenario when a diverticulum comes off of the renal pelvis directly (type II calyceal diverticulum). The ground glass appearance is due to the fact that most diverticula contain numerous tiny stones, that due to their close proximity give off a bland, homogenous appearance on KUB as opposed to the typical stone that has sharp, sometimes irregular border

can lead to the stone being treated just like any other stone, and lead to a failed ureteroscopy or ESWL procedure. The tell-tale signs of a calyceal diverticulum on KUB are a peripheral location, closer to the renal capsule than would be expected for a collecting system stone, or a mulberry or ground glass appearance (see Fig. 1).

3.2 Ultrasound

Renal ultrasound will accurately diagnose calyceal diverticulum in 80% of cases (Rathaus et al. 2001). A 3.5–5 MHz curvilinear transducer is typically used to scan the kidney. When devoid of calculi, calyceal diverticula on ultrasonography appear to have a similar appearance and echotexture to renal cysts. When stones are present, they appear as hyperechoic, mobile, position-dependent structures and can have acoustic shadowing coming from within the juxtaposing radiolucent cavities (see Fig. 2). A classic ultrasound finding is a cyst containing "milk of calcium", a colloidal suspension of precipitated calcium crystals (Patriquin et al. 1985). The milk of calcium will appear as a meniscus-like, semilunar calcification that changes position on upright and lateral decubitus radiography. The major drawback to ultrasound is that its accuracy is operator dependent.

                                                                                R. Khargi et al.

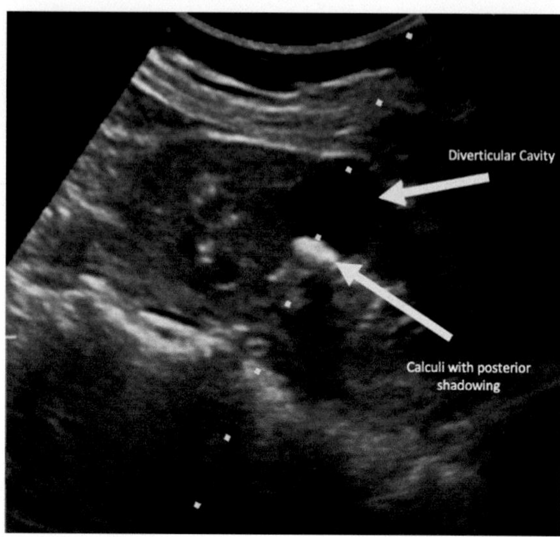

Fig. 2 Renal ultrasound showing a meniscus-like, semilunar calcification

3.3 Computed Tomography

Calyceal diverticula are typically identified in noncontrast CT as a dilated stone-containing collecting system outpouchings (see Fig. 3). When a calyceal diverticulum is suspected, imaging of the renal collecting system should be done to determine where the diverticulum is located and how it communicates with other components of the collecting system. The best imaging technique to characterize the diverticulum is a CT urogram. If there is sufficient diverticular neck patency, the diverticulum will fill passively in retrograde fashion from the connected calyx or renal pelvis leading to opacification of the cavity in the delayed phase. The cavity may not opacify if the neck or accompanying infundibulum are both blocked, which could affect surgical access.

In 1980, Wulfsohn et al. proposed a classification system for calyceal diverticula (Wulfsohn 1980). They are classified into two main types based on their location within the renal collecting system. Type I diverticula communicate with a minor calyx or an infundibulum, while type II diverticula emanate from the renal pelvis or a major calyx. Type II diverticula, although quite rare, tend to be larger, symptomatic, and located centrally within the kidney (see Figs. 4 and 5). This is because they are in closer proximity to the renal pelvis and therefore more likely to become obstructed, leading to hydronephrosis, infections, and stone formation.

The optimal treatment strategy for each type of calyceal diverticulum depends on several factors, including the size and location of the diverticulum, the presence of associated stones or infection, and the patient's overall health status. In 1992, another classification system was proposed by Dretler which takes into account not only the location of the diverticulum but also the characteristics of its neck and mouth, as well as the optimal treatment strategy for each type (Dretler 1992). Type I diverticula have

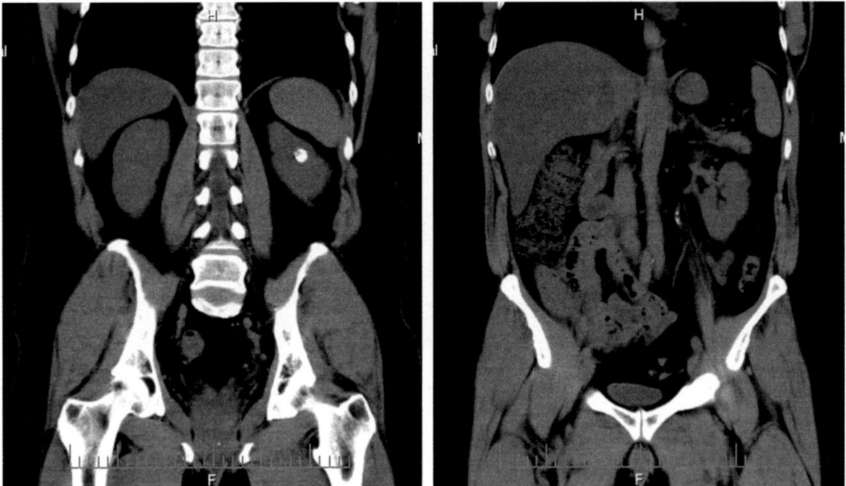

Fig. 3 Coronal images of patient with numerous stones in a diverticular cavity with passage of stones causing symptoms

Fig. 4 Type I diverticulum. *Note* Peripheral location

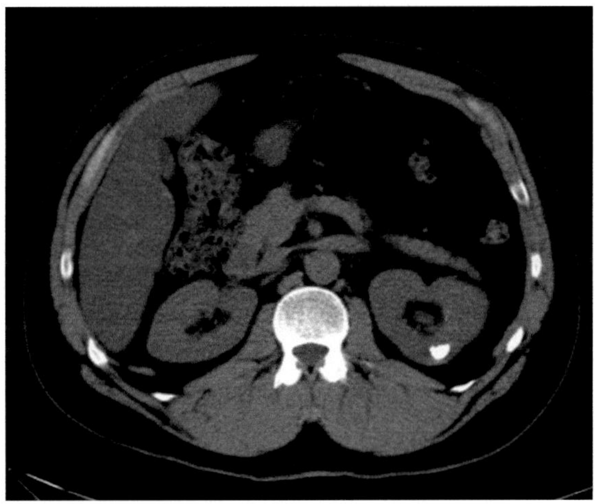

an open mouth and short neck, type II has a closed mouth and short neck, type III has a closed mouth and long neck, and type IV has an obliterated neck. Shock-wave lithotripsy (SWL) can on occasion be recommended for type I diverticula, as they are more likely to pass stone fragments through the wide neck and the neck does not necessarily need to be treated surgically. Ureteroscopic management can be recommended for some type II diverticula that are not in the lower pole and that do not have a large stone burden. The closed mouth and short neck can be treated endoscopically. Percutaneous treatment is often recommended for types III and IV,

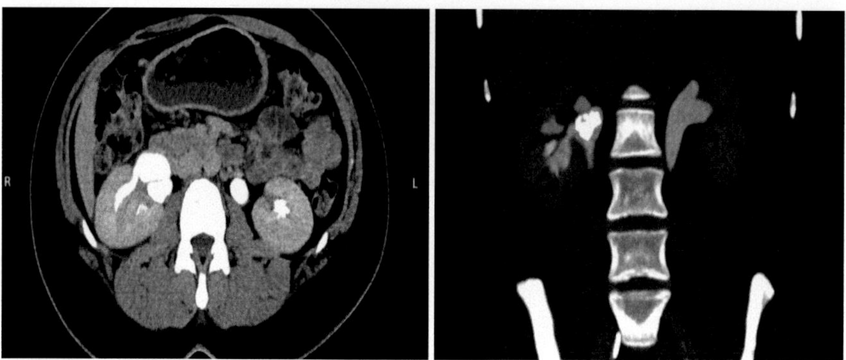

Fig. 5 Type II diverticulum, axial and coronal images

as they have a closed mouth and long neck or an obliterated neck, which may require more invasive treatment.

4 Treatment Strategies

The treatment of calyceal diverticula is typically reserved for symptomatic patients. In milder cases, medical management with antibiotics and analgesics may suffice, while surgical intervention may be necessary for more severe symptoms. Historically, open marsupialization and fulguration of the diverticular cavity or partial nephrectomy were performed. However, with the advancement of endoscopic technology, minimally invasive options including extracorporeal shock wave lithotripsy (ESWL), ureteroscopy, percutaneous nephrolithotomy (PCNL), and laparoscopy/robotic surgery have become more widely utilized. The choice of treatment modality depends on various factors such as the location and size of the diverticulum, the severity of symptoms, and the risk of complications associated with each treatment approach.

4.1 *Extracorporeal Shock Wave Lithotripsy*

Extracorporeal Shock Wave Lithotripsy (ESWL) has been used as a primary yet controversial treatment approach for stone-bearing calyceal diverticula, primarily for smaller stones in the middle and upper pole of the kidney. For successful passage of stone fragments following ESWL, it is required for the diverticulum to have a patent neck in order to clear the fragments. One benefit of ESWL is that it is the least invasive treatment available because it does not require an incision or endoscopic equipment. Nevertheless, stone-free rates are poor and stone particles may not be able to pass through a narrow diverticular neck. In short-term follow-up, 36–70% of patients may experience success in the form of pain reduction (Jones et al. 1991). Some claim that ESWL has minimal usefulness in the treatment of calyceal diverticula and should only be used in individuals who are ineligible for more effective treatments because of the reported stone-free rates of 0–58% (Monga et al. 2000). ESWL can only address the stone component of the issue, unlike other treatment methods that allow for ablation of the calyceal diverticulum.

4.2 Ureteroscopy

URS has been shown to be an effective alternative option with greater efficacy than ESWL alone. During ureteroscopy, a retrograde pyelogram is used to aid in potentially identifying the ostium to the diverticular neck, followed by laser incision of the neck to allow for stone extraction. Following the removal of the stones, either laser or electrocautery ablation of the lining is performed. This technique is most suited for upper- to mid-pole diverticular stones with mild to moderate stone burden. Ito et al. conducted a comprehensive evaluation of 153 patients who underwent flexible ureteroscopy/retrograde intrarenal surgery and observed a stone-free rate of 61.4%, a symptom-free rate of 67.9%, and a complication rate of 3.3% (Ito et al. 2018). Due to the acute angle deflection required for access, URS has traditionally not been recommended for lower pole calyceal diverticula. Nevertheless, if technology progresses and flexible ureteroscopes become more miniaturized, the indication may evolve in the future.

One of the major disadvantages of ureteroscopy is the moderately high rate of failure to detect diverticular ostia. Reportedly, up to 30% of patients undergoing ureteroscopic management fail treatment due unsuccessful identification of the ostium (Batter and Dretler 1997). Furthermore, this has been proposed as a potential explanation for prolonged operative times in ureteroscopy in some series, and if completely unidentifiable, subsequent percutaneous or laparoscopic surgeries may be required. One adjunctive diagnostic method that can be useful is to fill the collecting system with dilute indigo carmine or methylene blue solution. The fluid is then aspirated and irrigation with saline is resumed at a very slow rate. Often efflux of tinted fluid from the ostium can then be noted.

4.3 Laparoscopic/Robotic Approach

Open surgery was an early approach for the management of calyceal diverticula; however, advances in minimally invasive techniques, including laparoscopic and robotic surgery, have reduced its utilization. Laparoscopic or robotic surgery is considered suitable for anteriorly located calyceal diverticula with an undetectable ostium precluding endoscopic management, those with a large stone burden, and those with a thin overlying parenchyma. Nevertheless, due to the invasiveness of the laparoscopic/robotic surgery compared to alternative modalities, such as ESWL, percutaneous, and ureteroscopic techniques, this approach should only be considered when other options are not feasible.

In terms of the surgical technique, laparoscopic principles for access and exposure to the kidney remain the same as with other intracorporeal kidney surgeries. A laparoscopic ultrasound can aid in identifying the diverticulum. The parenchyma overlying the diverticulum is incised with electrocautery scissors to reveal the diverticular cavity, followed by the removal of stones using graspers and placement in an endoscopy bag. The diverticular cavity is then obliterated with Argon beam coagulation, and the renal defect is sutured closed. Drain placement is at the surgeon's discretion based on the complexity of the case.

4.4 *Percutaneous Nephrolithotomy*

Perhaps the most versatile and effective method for addressing calyceal diverticula is PCNL. Percutaneous access in PCNL allows for treatment of large calyceal diverticula with high stone burden and can be performed for both posterior and anterior diverticula (Parkhomenko et al. 2017). Additionally, it allows for fulguration of the urothelium and ability to dilate the diverticular neck if desired. PCNL offers the advantage of being both minimally invasive while offering very high stone-free and symptom-free rates. Percutaneous management of calyceal diverticular calculi has shown remarkable outcomes, with stone-free rates ranging from 87.5 to 100% and diverticular cavity obliteration rates ranging from 76 to 100% (Patodia et al. 2017). Additionally, more than 90% of patients report relief from symptoms after percutaneous therapy. Long-term studies have shown that these results remain durable.

5 Steps to Percutaneous Treatment of Calyceal Diverticular Stones

5.1 *Step 1: Patient Positioning*

Traditionally, percutaneous access to calyceal diverticular stones have been executed in the prone position as it provides the shortest access tract, especially in posterior calyceal diverticulum. However, with growing comfort of supine PCNL amongst urologists, modified supine positions have been described and considered safe in select cases. We have found that the prone position is ideal for upper pole and more medially located diverticula, especially when the diverticular cavity lies above the

11th rib, but that the supine position is suitable for the majority of cases. We prefer the Bart's Flank-Free position in supine cases and a split leg table for prone cases.

The patient is brought into the operating room and general anesthesia is induced. The patient is placed into supine position on the OR table or flipped into prone position with all pressure points padded. The patient is prepped and draped in a sterile fashion ensuring easy access to the urethral catheter and the flank. A flexible cystoscope is then placed into the bladder and a ureteral catheter is advanced into the affected collecting system. A Foley catheter is then placed for continuous bladder drainage.

5.2 Step 2: Percutaneous Access

The prone percutaneous approach is typically achieved through the use of ultrasonography or biplanar fluoroscopy if the surgeon is not comfortable with US-guided access or if the diverticulum cannot be visualized adequately with ultrasound. The supine approach in our experience is most amenable to ultrasound access, which provides a precise real time roadmap to the stone. Ultrasound can be especially useful for supine access because the kidneys are more mobile in the supine position. Diverticular cavities can have an indurated lining and very little space internally due to impacted stones which allows the kidney to move away more readily compared to accessing a normal collecting system. The real time aspect of ultrasound allows adjustments in trajectory to gain puncture into the cavity.

5.3 Fluoroscopic Access

In order to facilitate this, a scout fluoroscopic image is first obtained. If the stones are clearly visible on x-ray within the diverticula, retrograde injection of contrast may be omitted (see Fig. 6).

Retrograde instillation of fluid has the potential to cause distension of the collecting system, increasing the likelihood of inadvertent entry into the system. Additionally, contrast medium has the potential to obscure visualization of small diverticula. However, in cases where the exact diverticulum location is not readily apparent, a retrograde pyelogram may be performed to opacify the calyceal diverticulum, which can then serve as the puncture target. On occasion we have found it useful to mix contrast solution with indigo carmine or methylene blue to opacify the collecting system, and then drain the collecting system so that only the diverticulum remains opacified. The dye makes it more obvious when the trocar of the needle is removed that the correct target has been entered. The triangulation technique described previously and elsewhere in this book is then used to establish direct access to the diverticulum using an 18G diamond-tipped percutaneous needle (Miller et al. 2012; Bernardo et al. 2019).

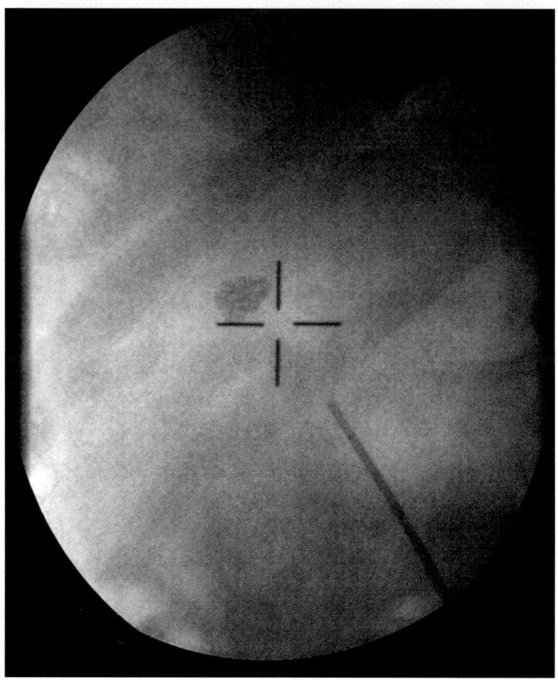

Fig. 6 Fluoroscopically apparent calyceal diverticulum cavity. Note The mulberry appearance of numerous stones within the cavity and the location between 11 and 12th ribs

5.4   Ultrasound Access

Percutaneous access can also be achieved with the aid of ultrasound guidance, particularly in cases where a fluoroscopic target is not visible, such as when the diverticular stones are radiolucent, and the diverticular cavity cannot be filled with contrast. An ultrasound-guided puncture requires a curved array ultrasound transducer in the 3.5–5.0 MHz range. Ultrasound scanning begins posteriorly and continues until the posterior axillary line is reached. To obtain a full longitudinal view of the kidney, the ultrasound probe should be parallel to the paraspinal muscles. Rib shadowing may often appear to crosscut the ultrasound image of the kidney, which can be overcome by rotating the probe until it is parallel to the ribs. The kidney is thoroughly scanned, and the calyceal diverticulum and associated shadowing stones are brought into view. A percutaneous access needle is then inserted directly onto the stone target through the ultrasound probe guide or free-hand approach.

Confirmation of proper needle placement can be achieved through biplanar fluoroscopy. Subsequently, the stylet is removed from the needle and a 0.035-inch J-wire or angled guidewire is meticulously inserted until resistance is encountered.

Once within the diverticular cavity, the floppy distal end of the guidewire is radiographically visualized, conforming to the dimensions and shape of the diverticulum (see Fig. 7). The stiffer segment of the guidewire is then utilized as the working wire.

Fig. 7 J-wire coiled in diverticular cavity through access needle. Note No need for retrograde contrast

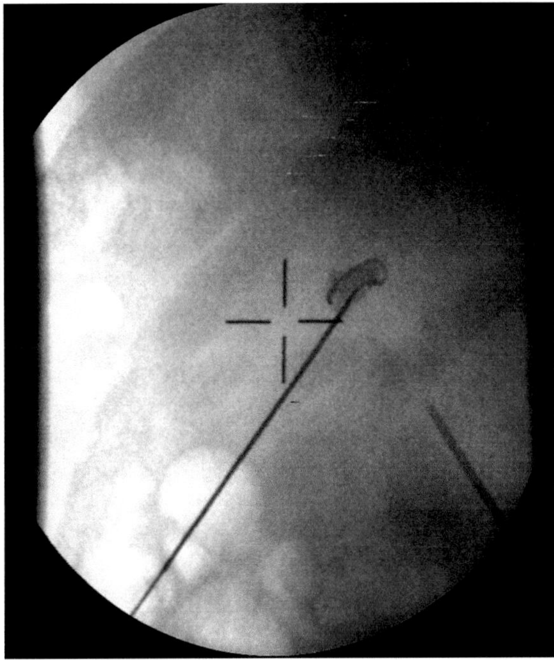

While the wire and needle are still in position, a #15 blade is utilized to incise the skin and underlying fascia, preparing the tract for subsequent dilation.

Compared to accessing a normal or dilated collecting system, there may be very little egress of fluid from the needle. This is because the cavity may be small or filled with stones, with very little fluid being present. Another caveat is that the needle shaft can sometimes become clogged with stone particles, making it difficult to place a guidewire. Should this happen, the stiff end of the guidewire sometimes is successful in clearing the channel. In other cases, a few drops of saline can be inserted to clear the channel.

5.5   Step 3: Dilation

Dilating a tract into a calyceal diverticulum cavity can be one of the most difficult and frustrating challenges percutaneous renal surgeons face. This is because these diverticula are often peripherally located, with very little supporting parenchyma. Thus, a guidewire can slip out very easily during the dilation process, even with a perfect puncture. In addition, diverticula are often located very high in the kidney, even above the most superior calyx, making transpleural access a real possibility. If the diaphragm has been traversed during puncture, the tract will not be straight due to respiratory motion, and during dilation the wire can easily slip out. In addition, there is a higher chance of pleural injury, hemothorax, and hydrothorax with these extreme upper pole punctures. The wall of the cavity may be indurated and difficult to puncture through with a dilator, with the kidney moving away or rotating away during attempted dilation. Finally, there may be very little space in the cavity to coil a wire, due to the stones within, and only the floppy tip of the wire may be in the diverticulum, again making for an unstable dilation. For these reasons, we have found the unconventional approach of using the stiff end of a guidewire to puncture through the back wall of the diverticulum to create a stable tract for dilation to be useful (see Fig. 8). A similar solution to obtain secure access to the diverticular cavity was described by Bennett et al. in 1992. Rather than puncturing through the back wall of the diverticulum, a transdiverticular puncture into the collecting system is made using a needle which is then exchanged for a guidewire to establish a stable tract for dilation (Bennett et al. 1992).

Of course, these techniques should only be done by very experienced surgeons, and in no case should dilation of the tract ever go beyond the diverticulum cavity. These cases are not the ones to minimize radiation. Every step of the dilation process should be monitored carefully with fluoroscopy. A 10Fr Teflon fascial dilator is passed over the guidewire under fluoroscopic guidance until it contacts and passes through the proximal diverticular wall, taking care to avoid distal wall perforation. The dilator is removed, leaving the guidewire in place. If a standard PCNL is being performed, a 24Fr balloon dilating device is inserted and inflated to a pressure of 16–18 atm over the working wire, with caution taken to avoid rear wall perforation (see Fig. 9).

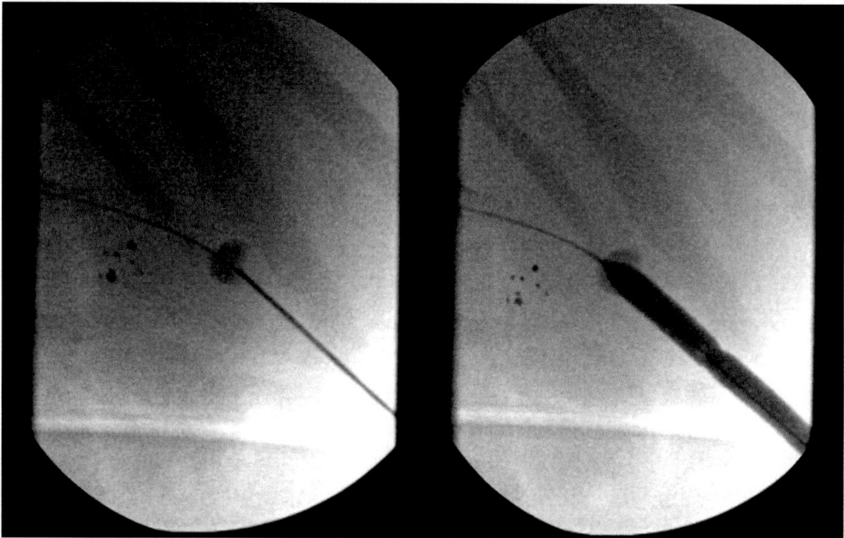

Fig. 8 Images showing diverticulum, placement of stiff wire through back wall of diverticulum, and precise balloon placement and inflation into diverticulum cavity

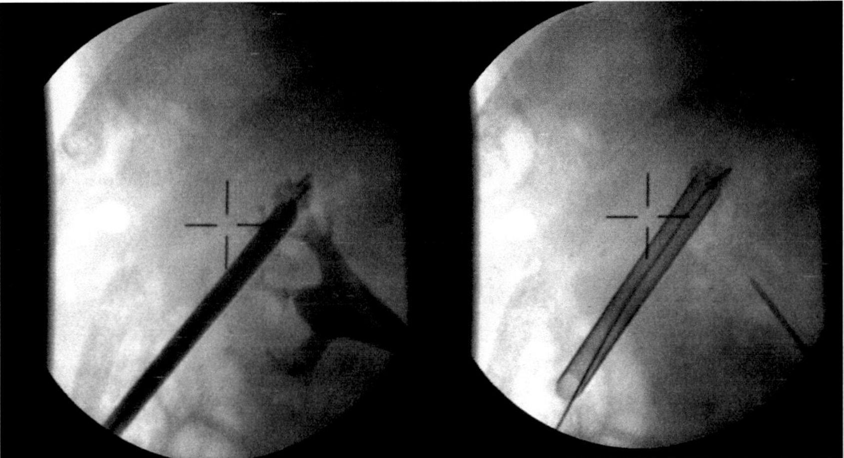

Fig. 9 Standard balloon dilation to 24Fr and sheath placement to stone-bearing calyceal diverticulum

A 24Fr Amplatz renal access sheath is then passed over the balloon dilator under fluoroscopic supervision. Note that introduction of the sheath straight into the diverticular space may be impeded by the tapered section on the distal end of the balloon dilator unless the diverticulum is large enough. The distance between the catheter tip and the balloon may prevent the balloon from entering the diverticulum cavity altogether, which can happen with small cavities and diverticula that are so impacted with stones that there is no space for dilation. In these cases, the balloon is forced retrograde, so it is not residing in the diverticular cavity. When a sheath is placed, it is outside the cavity, and often not even in the kidney, and finding a way back in can be difficult or impossible, especially if the wire slips out of the cavity. With the guidewire remaining in place, an offset 24Fr rigid nephroscope is inserted into the access sheath, and alligator forceps can be utilized through the working channel of the nephroscope to manually dilate the section of the tract immediately adjacent to the diverticulum, allowing for advancement of the scope and subsequent sheath into the diverticular lumen (Thummar et al. 2015). On occasion this entire situation can be prevented by using Amplatz sequential dilators or the Alken metallic dilator system because the distance between the tip and the dilator is much shorter than with balloon dilators.

Although access to miniaturized instruments is variable throughout the world, mini-PCNL (14-20Fr sheath), if available, can be particularly useful for treatment of calyceal diverticula and associated stones. The stone burden in calyceal diverticula tends to consist of numerous, tiny stones and thus can often be removed without the need for a standard sized sheath or large lithotrite device. In fact, a lithotrite device can occasionally be completely omitted as the small-sized stones may be amenable to evacuation using vortex effect only. The vortex effect may be more pronounced in mini-PCNL, as a smaller sheath with the same sized nephroscope will create a larger pressure gradient (Ito et al. 2023). One of the largest studies published regarding mini-PCNL was performed by Ding et al. in which 21 patients with calyceal diverticular calculi underwent mini-PCNL with a stone free rate of 90.5% (Ding et al. 2016). When a mini-PCNL is being done, we still prefer pre-dilating the tract with the 10Fr Teflon fascial dilator, as this facilitates placement of a one-step dilator in these challenging cases. Mini-PCNL can be selectively utilized for cavities that are smaller and for smaller stone burdens.

5.6   *Step 4: Stone Extraction*

Once the access sheath is seated appropriately within the diverticular cavity and the stone burden has been identified, stone extraction can ensue. The author prefers to extract smaller stones via a combination of employing the vortex effect technique and using graspers to extract fragments efficiently. The stones tend to be small, round and smooth and composed of calcium phosphate.

If a larger stone is present, a lithotrite device should be used. There are many lithotripsy devices on the market for percutaneous renal surgery including laser devices, pneumatic/ballistic, ultrasonic, and combination lithotrites as described elsewhere in this book. The author prefers a combined ballistic/ultrasonic lithotripter with suction capabilities as it very efficient at stone clearance with minimal to no collateral damage. When choosing a mini-PCNL, the stones should be small enough to vortex or suction out through the sheath, as trying to laser fragment a large number of stones can be inefficient. Fluoroscopy should be used to make sure all stones have been cleared and none have migrated behind the sheath (see Fig. 10).

5.7   *Step 5: Handling of the Diverticular Neck*

After removal of all stone material the entire cavity should be inspected for presence of a flattened renal papilla which would indicate an obstructed hydrocalyx rather than a calyceal diverticulum. If indeed a flattened renal papilla is identified, establishing continuity with the remaining collecting system is warranted as the calyx will inherently continue to excrete urine. This may be accomplished via dilation of the calyceal neck and placing a ureteral stent across the defect to re-establish continuity. In select cases, where the infundibulum cannot easily be traversed with a wire, or no infundibulum can be found but a hydrocalyx has been diagnosed, the diagnosis of a completely excluded calyx can be made and a neoinfundibulotomy can be performed (Mues et al. 2010) as described in our previous publication. If a true diverticulum has been diagnosed and the diverticular neck is readily apparent, a wire is placed across it and the neck is incised with a laser or balloon dilated (see Figs. 11 and 12).

If a neck is not readily apparent, and the diverticulum is a posterior diverticulum, indigo carmine or methylene blue solution can be placed via the ureteral catheter to

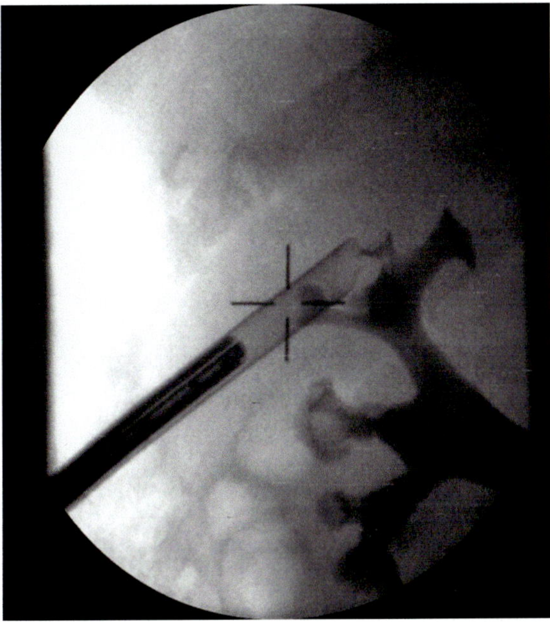

Fig. 10 Fluoroscopic confirmation of complete stone clearance in stone-bearing diverticulum

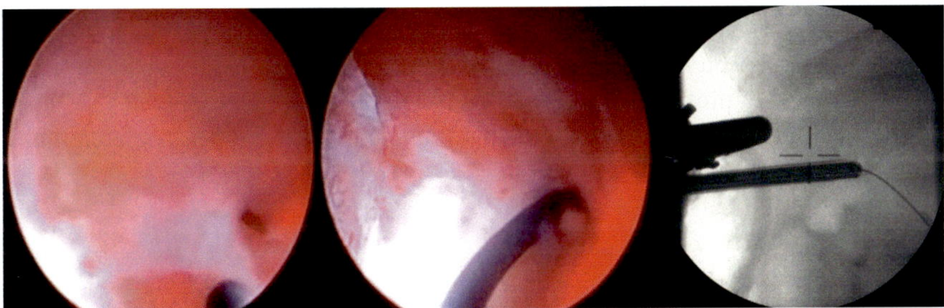

Fig. 11 Endoscopic and fluoroscopic images showing antegrade placement of guidewire under direct vision through diverticular neck

help identify the neck. If the neck is behind the sheath or the diverticulum is anterior, dilating the neck, even if it can be traversed, can cause bleeding due to the torque placed on the parenchyma and is not advisable. It is controversial whether dilating the neck is necessary for successful resolution of the diverticulum. In our previous publication, we did not see a difference in successful resolution when comparing treatment versus nontreatment (Parkhomenko et al. 2017). In our series, however, fulguration of the cavity was performed in all patients, and we feel that this is an essential part of the treatment to prevent recurrence.

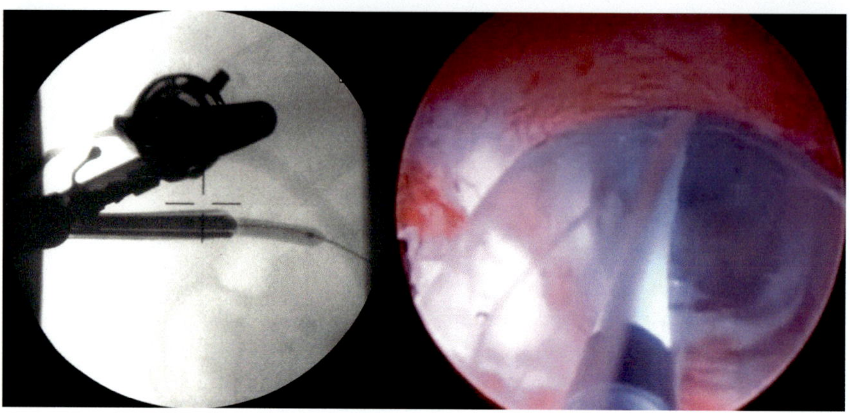

Fig. 12 Endoscopic and fluoroscopic images of nephroscope into diverticulum with balloon inflated across the diverticular neck

5.8 *Step 6: Treatment of the Diverticular Lining*

Fulguration of the diverticular mucosa is essential and can be performed many ways. Traditionally, when using a 30Fr sheath, this could be done with a resectoscope using bipolar energy and saline for irrigation with either a loop, roller ball, or plasma electrode of any kind including a button electrode. With 24Fr sheaths, resectoscopes will not fit, so a monopolar Bugbee electrode can be used with 1.5% glycine for irrigation. Sterile water should be avoided due to the risk of water absorption and hyponatremia. We prefer a very large and round Bugbee electrode because this is the least likely to cause perforation of the lining and the large surface area makes treatment more expeditious with less fluid absorption (see Fig. 13).

Fig. 13 Large round Bugbee electrode used to fulgurate diverticulum lining

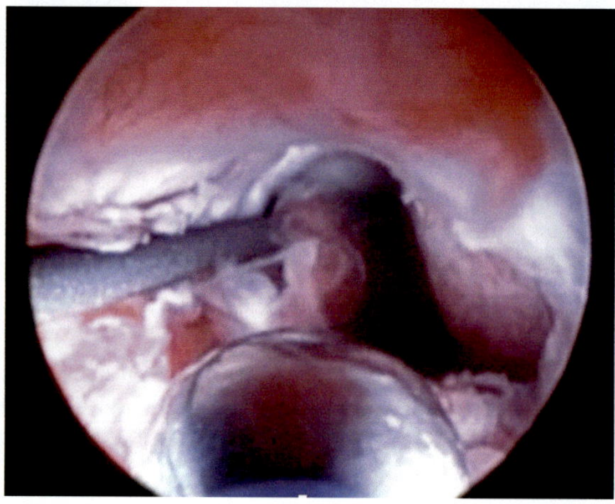

Fig. 14 Appearance post partial fulguration. Note Superficial charring and blanching of mucosa without perforation

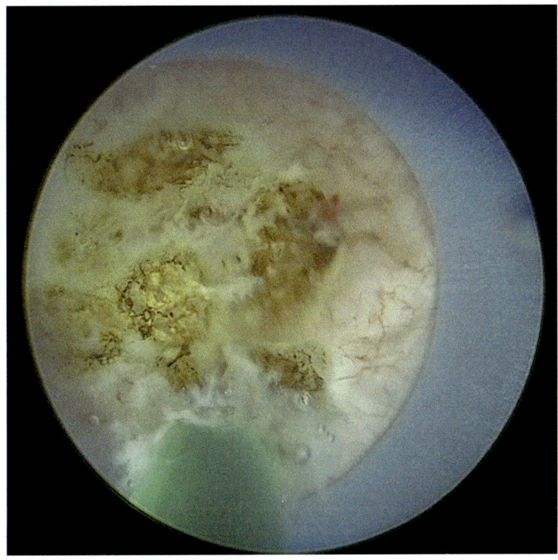

Figure 13 Gentle and superficial fulguration is used to prevent parenchymal bleeding (see Fig. 14). When a miniPCNL has been done, laser fulguration can be done of the diverticular cavity. We prefer the Thulium Fiber Laser for this, due to its superior hemostatic properties compared to the Holmium:YAG laser, but almost any laser, including a Neodynium:YAG laser or a Thulium:YAG can be utilized. In addition, a 2Fr or 3Fr Bugbee electrode can be used, but this has the disadvantage of requiring non-saline solution for irrigation (see Fig. 14).

5.9 Step 7: Drainage

Traditionally, once the cavity has been fulgurated, the surgeon would leave a nephrostomy tube or red rubber catheter within the cavity at the conclusion of the procedure (see Fig. 15).

We have found that drainage of the cavity is not necessary, whether the diverticular neck has been incised or dilated, nor have we found that a ureteral stent is necessary. We prefer to leave the ureteral catheter and foley catheter to gravity drainage for one hour post-operatively, remove them both simultaneously, and then discharge the patient home totally tubeless. Using this algorithm for the last 11 patients, we have not had issues with obstruction or flank drainage (Thomas et al. 2020). However, the choice of drainage should be left to surgeon discretion.

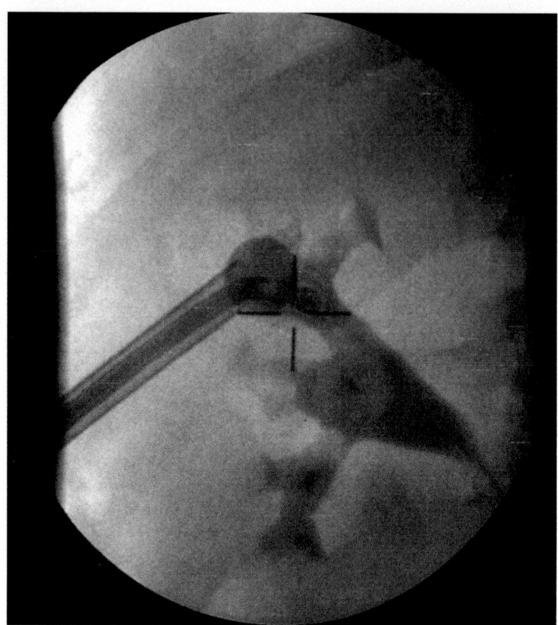

Fig. 15 Placement of a red rubber catheter into fulgurated diverticular cavity. Note: we have found this is no longer necessary

6 Complications

PCNL for calyceal diverticula treatment are similar as when utilized for nephrolithiasis. Potential complications include pleural effusion, hemothorax, pneumothorax, perirenal hematoma, hematuria, arrhythmia, acute renal failure, and ureteral edema (Krambeck and Lingeman 2009). Ito et al. reported an 11.9% complication rate in a cohort of 487 patients who underwent PCNL for calyceal diverticula treatment as compared to 8% in ESWL and 3.3% in ureteroscopic intervention (Ito et al. 2018). Krambeck et. al. had a 9.4% overall complication rate in their series but demonstrated a lower complication rate using diverticular fulguration (Krambeck and Lingeman 2009). Although PCNL can effectively treat both anterior and posterior calyceal diverticula, management of anterior diverticula may be challenging due to the longer distance traversed through the renal parenchyma. Tepeler et. al. found a greater severity of hemorrhaging in PCNL management of anterior calyceal stones as opposed to posterior calyceal stones (Tepeler et al. 2013). However, Parkhomenko et al. demonstrated a low complication rate of 4% (2 out of 51) and found no differences in blood loss or complication rates between anterior versus posterior calyceal diverticula PCNL management (Parkhomenko et al. 2017). With meticulous technique and extensive experience, PCNL can be both highly successful and have minimal complication rates for any type of calyceal diverticulum.

7 Conclusion

Calyceal diverticula are a rare pathology that are diagnosed most commonly with cross-sectional imaging. While the majority of patients do not require treatment, those with symptoms such as pain, hematuria, and infection may require intervention. There is a high concurrence of urolithiasis and calyceal diverticula, and in addition to calyceal location, stone size may dictate treatment choice and approach. Surgical techniques have made significant advances over the past few decades and patients and surgeons now have a variety of options when treating diverticula. PCNL is a versatile option for calyceal diverticula as it has been proven successful amongst many different diverticula locations and size. The stone-free and symptom-free rates are exceptional and overall morbidity rates have shown to be low. Significant advancements have been made in both technique and technology in the last several decades. The introduction of supine positioning and ultrasonography provides additional safety and efficacy benefits in PCNL treatment for calyceal diverticula. Much work is left to be done in the clinical treatment and research of calyceal diverticula, and future prospective trials are needed to solve currently unanswered questions. The future advancements of PCNL for calyceal diverticula will rely on continued cultivation of technique by surgeons, improvements in surgical technology, and an expansion of relevant research.

References

Batter SJ, Dretler SP. Ureterorenoscopic approach to the symptomatic caliceal diverticulum. J Urol. 1997;158(3 Pt 1):709–13. https://doi.org/10.1097/00005392-199709000-00006.

Bennett JD, Brown TC, Kozak RI, Sales J, Denstedt JD. Transdiverticular percutaneous nephrostomy for caliceal diverticular stones. J Endourol. 1992;6(1):55–7. https://doi.org/10.1089/end.1992.6.55.

Bernardo NO, Silva ML. Percutaneous nephrolithotomy access under fluoroscopic control. In: Smith AD, Preminger GM, Kavoussi LR, Badlani GH, Rastinehad AR, editors. Smith's textbook of endourology. Hoboken: Wiley Blackwell; 2019. p. 210–20.

Ding X, Xu S-T, Huang Y-H, Wei X-D, Zhang J-L, Wang L-L, et al. Management of symptomatic caliceal diverticular calculi: minimally invasive percutaneous nephrolithotomy versus flexible ureterorenoscopy. Chronic Dis Transl Med. 2016;02(04):250–6. https://doi.org/10.3760/cma.j.issn.2095-882X.2016.04.109.

Dretler SP. A new useful endourologic classification of calyceal diverticula. J Endourol. 1992;6(suppl):81.

Estrada CR, Datta S, Schneck FX, Bauer SB, Peters CA, Retik AB. Caliceal diverticula in children: natural history and management. J Urol. 2009;181(3):1306–11. https://doi.org/10.1016/j.juro.2008.10.043.

Gross AJ, Herrmann TR. Management of stones in calyceal diverticulum. Curr Opin Urol. 2007;17(2):136–40. https://doi.org/10.1097/MOU.0b013e328011bcd3.

Ito H, Aboumarzouk OM, Abushamma F, Keeley FX Jr. Systematic review of caliceal diverticulum. J Endourol. 2018;32(10):961–72. https://doi.org/10.1089/end.2018.0332.

Ito W, Prokop D, Valadon C, Whiles B, Neff D, Duchene D, et al. The vortex effect in mini-PCNL: improved understanding with a phantom model & computational fluid dynamics. J Urol. 2023;209(Supplement 4): e168. https://doi.org/10.1097/JU.0000000000003232.01.

Jones JA, Lingeman JE, Steidle CP. The roles of extracorporeal shock wave lithotripsy and percutaneous nephrostolithotomy in the management of pyelocaliceal diverticula. J Urol. 1991;146(3):724–7. https://doi.org/10.1016/s0022-5347(17)37906-5.

Krambeck AE, Lingeman JE. Percutaneous management of caliceal diverticuli. J Endourol. 2009;23(10):1723–9. https://doi.org/10.1089/end.2009.1541.

Middleton AW Jr, Pfister RC. Stone-containing pyelocaliceal diverticulum: embryogenic, anatomic, radiologic and clinical characteristics. J Urol. 1974;111(1):2–6. https://doi.org/10.1016/s0022-5347(17)59872-9.

Miller N, Lingeman JE. Percutaneous renal access. In: Smith JA, Howards SS, Preminger GM, Hinman F, editors. Hinman's atlas of urologic surgery. 3rd ed. Philadelphia: Elsevier Saunders; 2012. p. 845–53.

Monga M, Smith R, Ferral H, Thomas R. Percutaneous ablation of caliceal diverticulum: long-term followup. J Urol. 2000;163(1):28–32.

Mues AC, Landman J, Gupta M. Endoscopic management of completely excluded calices: a single institution experience. J Endourol. 2010;24(8):1241–5. https://doi.org/10.1089/end.2009.0663.

Parkhomenko E, Tran T, Thai J, Blum K, Gupta M. Percutaneous management of stone containing calyceal diverticula: associated factors and outcomes. J Urol. 2017;198(4):864–8. https://doi.org/10.1016/j.juro.2017.05.007.

Patodia M, Sinha RJ, Singh S, Singh V. Management of renal caliceal diverticular stones: a decade of experience. Urol Ann. 2017;9(2):145–9. https://doi.org/10.4103/ua.Ua_95_16.

Patriquin H, Lafortune M, Filiatrault D. Urinary milk of calcium in children and adults: use of gravity-dependent sonography. AJR Am J Roentgenol. 1985;144(2):407–13. https://doi.org/10.2214/ajr.144.2.407.

Rathaus V, Konen O, Werner M, Shapiro Feinberg M, Grunebaum M, Zissin R. Pyelocalyceal diverticulum: the imaging spectrum with emphasis on the ultrasound features. Br J Radiol. 2001;74(883):595–601. https://doi.org/10.1259/bjr.74.883.740595.

Tepeler A, Bozkurt OF, Resorlu B, Silay MS, Ozyuvali E, Ersoz C, et al. Is the percutaneous nephrolithotomy procedure complicated in patients with anterior caliceal stones? Urol Int. 2013;90(4):389–93. https://doi.org/10.1159/000345711.

Thomas DN, Atallah W, Chandhoke R, Bamberger JN, Gupta M. Ultrasound-guided totally tubeless mini-percutaneous nephrolithotomy for a completely excluded caliceal diverticulum associated with challenging anatomy. J Endourol Case Rep. 2020;6(3):121–3. https://doi.org/10.1089/cren.2019.0151.

Thummar HG, Khater U, Gupta K, Gupta M. Capsule to calculus optical dissection for tract creation during difficult percutaneous nephrolithotomy. J Endourol Part B, Videourol. 2015;29(5). https://doi.org/10.1089/vid.2015.0009

Waingankar N, Hayek S, Smith AD, Okeke Z. Calyceal diverticula: a comprehensive review. Rev Urol. 2014;16(1):29–43.

Wulfsohn MA. Pyelocaliceal diverticula. J Urol. 1980;123(1):1–8. https://doi.org/10.1016/s0022-5347(17)55748-1.

York NE, Lingeman JE. Percutaneous nephrolithotomy of calyceal diverticula, infundibular stenosis, and simple cysts. In: Smith AD, Preminger GM, Kavoussi LR, Badlani GH, Rastinehad AR, editors. Smith's textbook of endourology. Hoboken: Wiley Blackwell; 2019. p. 341–52.

Percutaneous Nephrolithotomy in the Horseshoe Kidney

Ryan L. Buettner and Bradley Schwartz

Abstract The horseshoe kidney (HSK) presents specific challenges when planning percutaneous intervention. The significant anatomic variation of the HSK requires the urologist to have a unique understanding of the altered anatomy in order to provide treatment that is both safe and effective. Variation in blood supply, malrotation of the HSK unit, relation to adjacent structures, and ectopic location must all be considered when undertaking percutaneous nephrolithotomy (PCNL) in the HSK. Because of the alteration in the percutaneous access tract required, flexible endoscopy should be performed at the conclusion of all PCNLs in the HSK. The expected complications and post-operative course for PCNL in the HSK is similar to that of the anatomically normal kidney. This chapter provides guidance to the urologist faced with the challenge of performing PCNL in the HSK. The primary purpose of this chapter is to describe the unique considerations required when performing PCNL in the HSK.

Keywords Percutaneous nephrolithotomy · Horseshoe kidney · Endoscopic technique · Nephrolithiasis · PCNL

1 Introduction

Horseshoe kidneys (HSK) are defined as bilateral functional renal moieties on both sides of the vertebral column which are fused together by an isthmus. The lower poles of the kidneys are connected by this isthmus, which may be positioned midline or slightly laterally. Lateral positioning will result in an asymmetric HSK. The isthmus is comprised of renal parenchyma in roughly 80% of cases, with the rest being comprised of fibrous connective tissue. The ureters remain uncrossed from the renal hilum to the urinary bladder and follow an anterior course up and over the isthmus, occasionally resulting in obstruction (Cook and Stephens 1977). Fusion occurs at the lower pole in 90% of cases (Khougali et al. 2021). The incidence of HSK is

R. L. Buettner · B. Schwartz (✉)
Division of Urology, Southern Illinois University School of Medicine, 747 N. Rutledge 5th Floor, Springfield, IL 62704-9665, USA
e-mail: bschwartz@siumed.edu

© The Author(s), under exclusive license to Springer Nature Switzerland AG 2023
J. D. Denstedt and E. N. Liatsikos (eds.), *Percutaneous Renal Surgery*,
https://doi.org/10.1007/978-3-031-40542-6_19

approximately 1:500 in the general population (0.25%) and is twice as common in males (Schiappacasse et al. 2015).

HSK can be associated with cardiovascular, gastrointestinal, skeletal, and genitourinary (GU) abnormalities. This chapter will briefly discuss GU abnormalities, as they are most common. These abnormalities include: vesicoureteral reflux (50%), ureteropelvic junction obstruction (35%), ureteral duplication (10%), cryptorchidism and hypospadias in 4% of male patients, and vaginal septum and bicornuate uterus in 7% of female patients (Schiappacasse et al. 2015). HSK has also been associated with Patau and Gardner syndromes (trisomy 13 and deletion q15q22), up to 20% of Down and Edwards (trisomies 21 and 18) syndromes, and 60% of Turner syndrome patients (Natsis et al. 2014).

The primary purpose of this chapter is to describe the unique considerations required when performing percutaneous nephrolithotomy in the horseshoe kidney.

2 Embryology

The normal embryological development of the kidney and ureter are well described. Three distinct structures are responsible for proper development: the pronephros, mesonephros, and metanephros. The pronephros and mesonephros degenerate in utero, and the metanephros ultimately develops into the mature kidney (Tanagho et al. 2013). During this process, the developing kidneys ascend from the pelvis to the upper lumbar region. As they ascend, the kidneys rotate medially approximately 90 degrees. This results in hila that are directed anteromedially (Muttarak and Sriburi 2012). Abnormal fusion of the developing kidneys causes an early arrest of the ascension process as cranial migration is prevented by the inferior mesenteric artery (IMA) (Baskin and Cunha 2021). This arrest is key to understanding the anatomic position and relationships of HSKs. Figure 1 illustrates these important anatomic differences.

Two theories have been described for HSK development. Classically, mechanical fusion of the metanephric blastema has been attributed to abnormal flexion or growth of the developing spine and pelvic organs. This is thought possible because the immature kidneys have no renal capsule, and this contact fusion results in a fibrous isthmus. Alternatively, it has been proposed that a teratogenic event occurs that results in abnormal migration of posterior nephrogenic cells that then fuse, creating an isthmus. It has been postulated that this process results in a parenchymatous isthmus (Schiappacasse et al. 2015; Natsis et al. 2014).

Fig. 1 Horseshoe Kidney. Note the relationship to the IMA (divided), the malrotation of the renal pelvises, and the ureters anterior course over the isthmus (Hansen 2022)

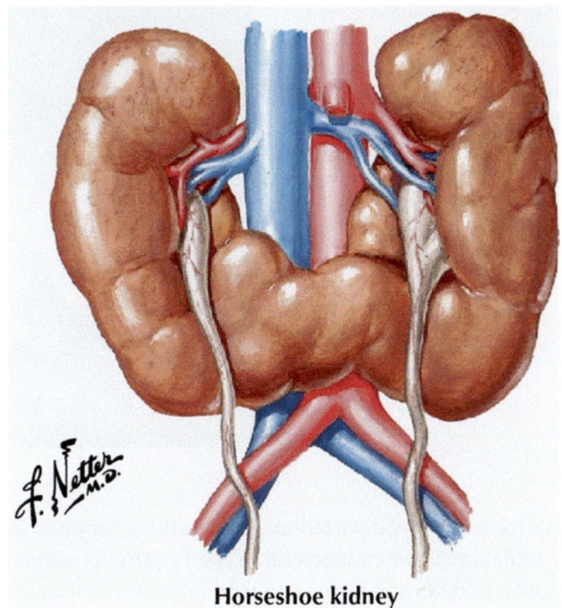

3   Anatomic Considerations

Abnormal fusion of bilateral kidneys across the midline creates significant anatomic variation from normal. Most commonly, the isthmus lies anterior to the great vessels at the level of the third to fifth lumbar vertebra, just inferior to the IMA (Muttarak and Sriburi 2012). The abnormal fusion also prevents normal renal rotation. This leaves the inferior poles oriented medially, with the renal pelvis located more anteriorly and/or laterally than normal (Schiappacasse et al. 2015; Muttarak and Sriburi 2012).

The calyces are located in the upper two-thirds of each kidney and often point medially towards the spinal column, downwards, or both. The isthmus may be drained by an extrarenal calyx or an independent ureter. The ureteropelvic junction (UPJ) is positioned more superior than normal at the inner rim of the superior part of the kidney (Natsis et al. 2014). The ureters cross anterior to the isthmus and then course inferiorly towards the bladder (Schiappacasse et al. 2015; Muttarak and Sriburi 2012). An example of these anatomic abnormalities is provided by the contrasted CT scan in Fig. 2.

The blood supply of HSK is widely variable (Schiappacasse et al. 2015; Natsis et al. 2014; Muttarak and Sriburi 2012). The isthmus is commonly supplied by a single vessel derived from the abdominal aorta (AA) (Natsis et al. 2014). The renal arteries can originate from the AA, common iliac arteries (CIA), and/or the IMA (Muttarak and Sriburi 2012).

Graves' classification was developed in attempt to characterize the most common variations in blood supply. This system classifies HSK arterial anatomy into one of

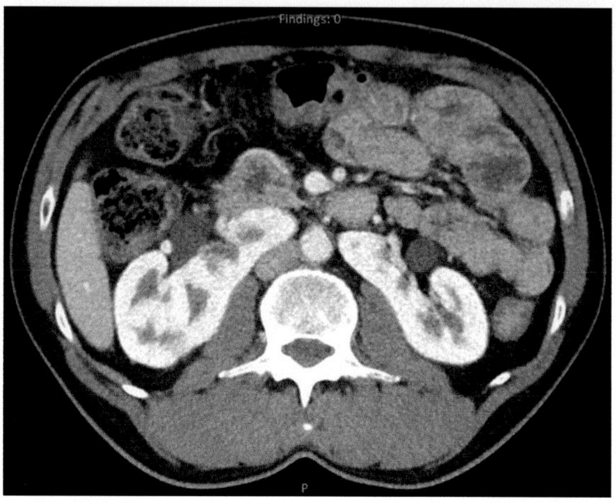

Fig. 2 CT abdomen/pelvis with contrast demonstrating common anatomic variation seen in HSKs. Note the position of the UPJs, malrotation of both renal units, and inferior displacement [original image]

six most observed variations. Each artery supplies its own area, with no collateral circulation between segments. Type 1a exhibits normal renal arterial pattern, with the upper, middle, and lower segments supplied by a single renal artery arising from AA. Type 1b occurs when the upper and middle segments are supplied by a single artery from the AA, while the lower segments are supplied by separate, single vessels from the AA. The lower segment arteries can arise from the AA by a common trunk, while the upper and middle segments are supplied by either a single (type 1c) or multiple (type 1d) RAs on either side. The isthmus may also be supplied by arteries that arise inferior to the fused segment, which can be unilateral or bilateral and may originate from the AA independently or via common trunk (type 1e). Lastly, the fused lower segments may derive supply on one or both sides from the CIA, hypogastric, or middle sacral arteries (type 1f) (Boatman et al. 1971). Figure 3 demonstrates these variations in arterial supply. Literature review demonstrates that most cases are types 1e (28%) and 1f (24%) (Natsis et al. 2014). It is worth mentioning that HSK is often associated with IVC abnormalities. These include double IVC, left IVC, and pre-isthmic IVC. Pre-isthmic IVCs cause retrocaval ureters, which are a direct cause of hydronephrosis and UPJ obstruction (Natsis et al. 2014).

Classically, urologists have been concerned by the potential of a retrorenal colon in HSK. However, studies have shown this occurs in < 1% of HSKs and has not been shown to affect PCNL outcomes in in these patients (Ding et al. 2015).

4 Stone Disease in the Horseshoe Kidney

Nephrolithiasis is the most common complication in HSK and essentially all stone types have been described. The incidence ranges from 21 to 60% (Yohannes and Smith 2002). Anatomic urinary stasis arising from the anterior orientation of the renal pelvis, abnormal ureteral course over the isthmus, and high ureteral insertion is

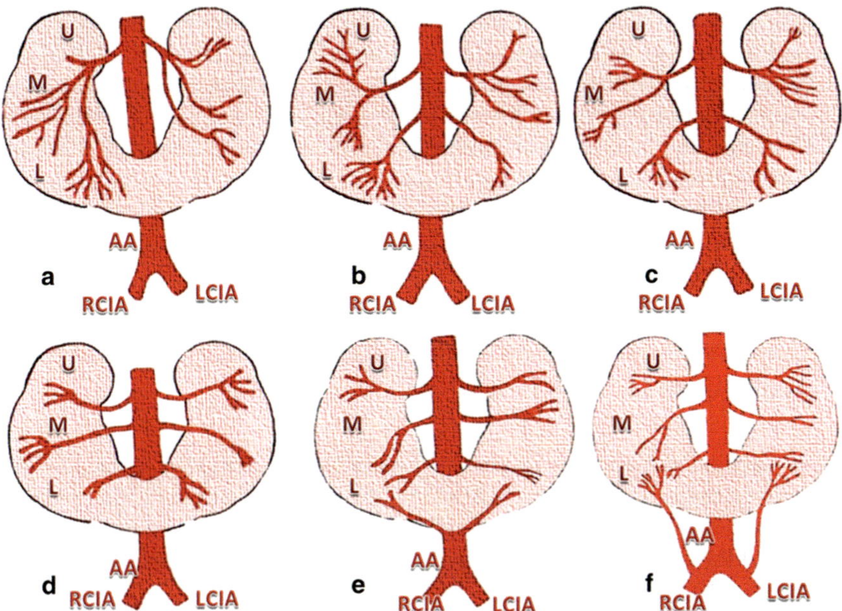

Fig. 3 Graves' classification of arterial variation in HSK. *U* upper, *M* middle, *L* lower, *AA* abdominal aorta, *RCIA* right common iliac artery, *LCIA* left common iliac artery (Natsis et al. 2014)

believed to contribute to urinary tract infection and stone formation (Yohannes and Smith 2002). It has also been proposed that the orientation of the calyces impairs drainage, resulting in stasis and stone formation. Stones are often multiple and there is significant increase in large staghorn stones (Natsis et al. 2014). While stones can form anywhere within the upper urinary tract, the most common locations for stone formation are the renal pelvis and lower pole. It is also quite common to have multiple stones in multiple locations (Pawar et al. 2018).

5 Other Surgical Management

The same treatment modalities used in the management of nephrolithiasis in normal kidneys can be considered in the HSK (Lavan et al. 2020). However, some unique considerations must be made given the anatomic challenges.

Shockwave lithotripsy presents a reasonable option for management of small renal stones in HSK. Stone free rates range from 28%-80%, however many patients require > 1 intervention after SWL (Ding et al. 2015; Stein and Desai 2007). This has been attributed to problems with energy localization for pelvic stones combined with poor fragment clearance secondary to impaired renal drainage. It is thus imperative to rule out coexisting UPJ obstruction when considering SWL. Stones greater than 15 mm appear less likely to achieve stone-free status after SWL (Stein and Desai 2007).

The use of ureteroscopy for the management of stones in HSK has been well described. Limited case series have reported stone free rates ranging from 70%-88.2%. Generally, these required multiple procedures, were for stones < 2.0 cm, and were not assessed with postoperative computed tomography. Technical challenges arise during retrograde access of the collecting system due to the angle of deflection required by the more superolateral positioning of the ureteral insertion into the renal pelvis (Geavlete et al. 2022).

6   Indications for PCNL in HSK

The main consideration when approaching stone disease in the HSK is the difficulty in gaining retrograde access that arises from the acute angle of deflection required by the more superolateral positioning of the ureteral insertion into the renal pelvis. Because of this, retrograde ureteroscopic single session stone-free rates in HSKs are typically < 60% (Ding et al. 2015).

If retrograde management is ineffective, unsuccessful, or deemed impossible, antegrade management is the preferred approach. Stone-free rates for PCNL in the HSK range from 65.5% to 87.5%, further supporting antegrade management as the preferred initial approach (Vicentini et al. 2021). Therefore, based on most data, antegrade management is preferred for most patients with nephrolithiasis in HSK to achieve stone-free status in a single operation. It should be noted that AUA guidelines currently recommend percutaneous nephrolithotomy as first-line therapy for staghorn stones and total renal stone burden > 20 mm (Assimos et al. 2016). However, given the unique challenges associated with retrograde access in HSK, indications for PCNL in HSK can be expanded to include smaller renal stone burden.

7   Preoperative Evaluation

A complete history and physical is essential prior to proceeding with percutaneous access. Identification of contraindications precluding percutaneous access is paramount. Active urinary tract infection (UTI) and bleeding disorders are especially important to identify. It is also important to obtain a thorough surgical history when planning percutaneous access.

Regarding preoperative urine testing, both AUA and EAU guidelines state that urinalysis is required prior to any stone intervention and a urine culture should be obtained with clinical or laboratory signs of infection. Positive urine cultures should be treated with antibiotics until a sterile culture is obtained (Assimos et al. 2016).

It is prudent to obtain a baseline complete blood count and serum electrolytes with renal function testing prior to proceeding with PCNL in HSK. This establishes a baseline that can be followed post-operatively and could potentially identify pre-operative conditions that may increase operative complications.

Preoperative imaging is required for proper surgical planning. AUA guidelines recommend clinicians obtain a non-contrast CT scan prior to performing PCNL (Assimos et al. 2016). We prefer a CT stone-protocol on every patient prior to attempting PCNL in HSK. If planning a prone approach, ideally this CT is obtained with the patient in a prone position. This allows for evaluation of total stone burden, prone relationship to adjacent structures, and anatomic assessment of the HSK. Per AUA guidelines, in patients with complex stones or anatomy, clinicians may obtain additional contrast imaging if further definition of the collecting system and the ureteral anatomy is needed (Assimos et al. 2016). Therefore, vascular contrast enhancement and/or CT urogram can also be considered in select patients.

8 Operating Room Setup

While recognizing that each surgeon will have preferences regarding the specific operating room set up for PCNL, we believe we can provide some general recommendations that we have found beneficial in our practice.

Surgeon safety and ergonomic considerations are fundamental for any endoscopic operating endeavor, and PCNL is no different. Radiation protection via lead impregnated aprons, thyroid shields, eyeglasses, etc. is imperative for any endourological surgery that uses fluoroscopic image guidance. All monitors used for the procedure (endoscope, X-ray) should be placed at eye level and in a location that requires minimal turning of the surgeon's head.

Our operating room set up is as follows. The surgeon, surgical assistant, and back table are positioned on the side to be treated. The endoscopic video monitor is positioned opposite the surgeon, near the patient's head. The X-ray monitor is positioned opposite the surgeon, near the patient's feet. The C-arm is positioned between these two monitors, above the patient's knees. Irrigation, lithotripter and/or LASER generators, suction, and other devices that may be required are placed at the foot of the bed.

9 Patient Positioning

The specific details regarding positioning for PCNL are covered in a separate chapter. For this reason, we provide limited commentary on positioning for PCNL in HSK. For both prone and supine positions, it is essential to ensure the patient is perfectly centered on the table. Deviations from center can cause difficulty with image interpretation as the C-arm orbits the patient, as well as possible instability and fall risk (Smith et al. 2019).

Prone position is most commonly used for HSK as it provides several advantages, which include larger surface area for puncture site, more room for instrument movement, and possibly a lower risk of visceral organ injury. It also allows upper pole puncture to be performed more easily in the HSK (Osther et al. 2011; Pérez Fentes 2021). Several disadvantages with prone positioning exist. Increased radiologic hazard to the urologist, patient discomfort, number of operating room staff needed for correct positioning, risk of pressure point injury, difficulty with retrograde access, circulatory and ventilator difficulties, as well as alteration in endocrine and pharmacokinetic effects have all been associated with prone positioning (Pérez Fentes 2021). These are uncommon and we have rarely encountered positioning complications, even in the morbidly obese.

While supine PCNL in HSK is gaining popularity, it is still relatively uncommon (Osther et al. 2011). Therefore, the data on supine PCNL in HSK is quite limited, and most commentary is extrapolated from PCNL in anatomically normal kidneys.

Generally, supine PCNL appears to be as safe and effective as prone PCNL regarding stone free rates, transfusion, and complications. For a variety of factors related to repositioning, supine PCNL has been associated with reduced operative times. Supine positioning also provides easier access to the urethral meatus for retrograde access (Kumar et al. 2012).

Five common supine positions have been described. Valdivia supine PCNL was the first described supine position for PCNL. Modifications to this position include: Galdakao-modified supine Valdivia (GMSVP), Barts Modified Valdivia, complete supine, and complete supine flank-free (Kumar et al. 2012).

The data on supine PCNL specifically in the HSK is quite limited. Pérez-Fentes described a case report of one 42F with a complete staghorn stone in the right moiety of a HSK. The patient was treated with endoscopic combined intrarenal surgery and positioned in GMSVP and required 3 separate procedures to achieve stone-free status (Pérez Fentes 2021).

Gupta et al. have described a case series of 5 supine tubeless PCNLs in HSKs. This series included 4 patients (one with BL nephrolithiasis) and all were operated on in GMSVP (Gupta et al. 2022).

Sohail et al. published a case report of one 45 M with two 1.5 cm renal stones. Stone-free status was achieved with one puncture and one procedure in "complete supine flank-free" position (Sohail et al. 2017).

Vincentini et al. reported a multicentric retrospective analysis of 106 PCNLs in HSKs. Approximately 37% were treated in supine position. There was no difference in transfusion, complication, and immediate success rates when compared to prone. Surgical time was significantly longer in the prone group (Geavlete et al. 2022). Based on this literature, supine PCNL is considered a safe and effective in HSK while carrying a low complication rate. It may be considered an option for treating stones in patients with HSK (Vicentini et al. 2021; Pérez Fentes 2021; Kumar et al. 2012; Gupta et al. 2022; Sohail et al. 2017).

10 Retrograde Injection

An open-ended ureteral catheter is placed via cystoscopy on the side to be treated. The timing of this placement depends on the planned operative position, as well as the type of operating table used. The ureteral catheter is then used to aid in retrograde imaging for identification of calyces when planning percutaneous puncture. It may also help reduce migration of stone fragments down the ureter during lithotripsy. We use a combination of contrast and air to completely characterize the calyceal anatomy. We have found air to be particularly useful in delineating the posterior calyces.

11 Percutaneous Puncture

The optimal calyx of entry is determined based on the preoperative CT scan, retrograde imaging, anatomic considerations, and stone location. The preoperative CT scan is useful for identifying a safe percutaneous window to avoid adjacent structures, while the intraoperative imaging guides percutaneous placement of the puncture needle.

The ultimate goal is to target a calyx that affords maximum stone clearance with a single puncture. Because of the downward displacement and malrotated axis of the HSK, calyxes tend to be oriented more inferiorly and posterolaterally, making subcostal puncture preferred in most cases (Stein and Desai 2007). The malrotated HSK and its relationship to adjacent structures also results in a more medial cutaneous puncture site than in anatomically normal kidneys. Cutaneous puncture is generally made near the posterior axillary line or slightly medial. Upper pole access is most often chosen in HSKs as this allows access to upper pole calyces, renal pelvis, ureteropelvic junction, and proximal ureter, with minimal torque on the renal parenchyma and lower risk of injury to adjacent structures. Figure 4 demonstrates fluoroscopic upper pole puncture yielding maximal collecting system access with minimal deflection angles. It should be noted that the puncture site is more medial than in a normal kidney, but access to the calyx is more lateral than in a normal kidney. This results in a longer than normal access tract, which is discussed in a later section.

As previously mentioned, the vascular anatomy of HSK is highly variable. However, blood vessels typically enter the kidney anteromedially and thus risk of vascular injury during percutaneous access is equivalent to that of a normal kidney. The exceptions to this are the arteries supplying the isthmus, which can arise laterally off the common iliac vessels (Boatman et al. 1971).

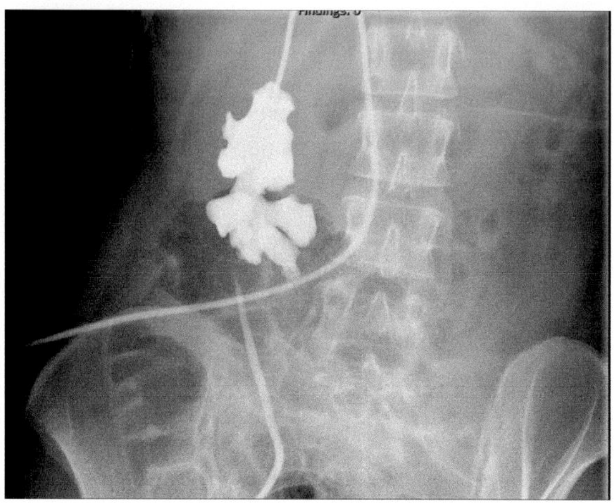

Fig. 4 Intraoperative fluoroscopic image demonstrating upper pole puncture in a HSK. Note the minimal deflection angles required to access the entire collecting system [original image]

12 Fluoroscopic Guidance

The use of C-arm is imperative to understanding the 3-dimensional anatomy of the collecting system. The C-arm is orbited around the patient, both towards and away from the surgeon. A combination of spot and live images are used to understand the 3-dimensional anatomy of the collecting system.

Generally, the collecting system is opacified and distended with a combination of contrast and air. A scout film is then obtained in the anterior–posterior plane. A target calyx is chosen based on this image and the preoperative CT scan. A percutaneous access needle is then advanced slightly into the subcutaneous tissue in a straight line towards the desired calyx. Live rotation between different views can aid in understanding of the 3-dimensional relationships between calyxes and the renal pelvis. The C-arm is then rotated to an appropriate axis as to provide a direct, end-on view of the needle hub, shaft, and target calyx in a "bull's-eye" fashion. Once the appropriate trajectory is established, the C-arm is rotated to an axis that allows the surgeon to monitor the depth of needle insertion into the target calyx. Ideally, access is obtained along the axis of the calyx and through the papilla, thus avoiding the vascular infundibulum (Smith et al. 2019). The inner stylet is removed, and access is confirmed by return of urine and/or contrast.

13 Tract Dilation

A hydrophilic, angled-tip guidewire is advanced through the lumen of the puncture needle. This wire should advance relatively easily. Aggressive probing should be avoided, as false tracts can be created. Because of the malrotated nature of the HSK and resultant acute angle of the UPJ, it can be exceedingly difficult to place the wire down the ureter. Thus, the luxury of having a wire down the ureter might have to be sacrificed due to the technical difficulty that arises from the altered anatomy. Instead, one may have to accept a wire coiled in the renal pelvis as adequate access for tract dilation. It is imperative that the wire is at least in the renal pelvis prior to tract dilation. This can be confirmed with repeat pyelogram as needed.

Dilation of the tract can then be performed via the operative surgeon's preferred method. In our practice, a balloon dilator is inflated to a pressure of 20–30 atm with contrasted material. Periodic spot fluoroscopic images are obtained to ensure all "waists" have been fully expanded.

The nephrostomy sheath is then advanced over the balloon under live fluoroscopy until the tip of the sheath rests at the distal end of the balloon. Given the more anterior position of the HSK, the renal pelvis may be deeper in relation to the skin than in the anatomically normal kidney. This can result in the inability to reach the middle and lower calyces with rigid instruments, especially in obese patients. Preoperative measurements can help determine if an extra-long nephroscope and/or nephrostomy sheath may be needed to overcome this problem. If there is concern that the sheath will become buried in the subcutaneous tissue, another option is to place a stay suture through the end of the nephrostomy sheath. The sheath can then be buried in the subcutaneous tissue to achieve extra reach. The previously placed stay suture is then used to retrieve the buried nephrostomy sheath at conclusion. Additionally, extra-long rigid scopes may be necessary.

14 Nephroscopy

Once the nephrostomy sheath is in place, the balloon is deflated, removed, and the nephroscope is inserted with the lithotripter and suction deployed. The rigid nephroscope is used to remove as much stone as possible. As previously mentioned, the lower pole calyces can be very difficult to visualize in the HSK. Therefore, the rigid nephroscope may not be effective in removing the entire stone burden. It should be emphasized that use of the flexible endoscopy is mandatory to assure all calyces are interrogated, which is discussed in more detail in a later section.

15 Stone Extraction

We use a wide variety of methods for stone extraction. These include manual basket extraction, ballistic lithotripters, ultrasonic lithotripters, and combination lithotripters. In special cases requiring treatment via flexible nephroscopy, Ho:YAG LASER is our preferred energy for laser lithotripsy.

The presence of a HSK neither necessitates nor limits the use any specific lithotripter. Lithotripsy technique is determined more by stone location than overall stone burden. Given that HSKs tend to have increased stone burden and stones in multiple calyces, there is increased requirement for flexible endoscopy to achieve stone-free status (Raj et al. 2003). Thus, LASER is used more commonly when treating stones in the HSK. It is our opinion that this could increase the use of dusting technique as manual stone extraction via flexible endoscopy is not ideal. Suction devices can then be used after completion of dusting to increase stone-free rates.

16 Flexible Endoscopy

AUA guidelines state that flexible nephroscopy should be a routine part of standard PCNL, and we strongly believe PCNL in HSKs to be no different (Assimos et al. 2016). Upper pole access in HSKs results in a tract that is longer than normal, which causes difficulty in reaching the middle and lower calyces (Stein and Desai 2007; Gupta et al. 2022). It has been demonstrated that > 80% of PCNL in HSKs require flexible nephroscopy to adequately access stones in all calyces (Raj et al. 2003). Ideally, flexible nephroscopy is used to reposition stones for removal via rigid nephroscopy. If repositioning is not feasible or unsuccessful, flexible nephroscopy can then be used to treat stones via laser lithotripsy. It is our recommendation and practice that flexible endoscopy should be performed at the conclusion of all PCNLs in HSKs.

17 Exit Strategy

In our opinion, drainage is required after any PCNL in HSKs. This is ultimately at the discretion of the operative surgeon and the type of drainage should be whatever is preferred. In our practice, a 16Fr tipless Foley catheter is left with the balloon inflated in the access tract. This provides a few advantages. Re-establishment of the access tract is easier if subsequent procedures are required. The larger diameter of the Foley provides maximal drainage, but generally causes the patient less pain than a larger or more rigid nephrostomy tube.

18 Complications

The expected complications that arise from PCNL in HSKs are similar to those with PCNL in anatomically normal kidneys. Complications include: bleeding, bleeding requiring transfusion, fever, and collecting system perforation. Less commonly, vascular injury, hydrothorax, sepsis, and visceral injury are seen. Current literature suggests that PCNL in HSK complication rates are comparable to PCNL in the anatomically normal kidney (Vicentini et al. 2021; Osther et al. 2011). It could be argued that, given the high rate of subcostal access, there is less risk of injury to the plural space when performing PCNL in the HSK as compared to PCNL in the anatomically normal kidney. Based on the current literature and our experience, we believe PCNL to be a safe and effective approach to the management of stone disease in HSKs.

19 Postoperative Considerations

Patients are observed in the hospital overnight after surgery. While it is our practice to obtain a non-contrasted CT of the abdomen/pelvis and an antegrade nephrostogram the morning of post-operative day one, these may not be required in all cases. The CT scan is useful in proving stone-free status and helps guide patient counseling if there are residual stone fragments. If stone fragments reside at the UPJ and/or renal pelvis, the kidney often will not drain postoperatively. In patients where there is concern for postoperative drainage, a nephrostogram may be of benefit prior to removing the nephrostomy tube. If the patient is deemed stone free, the drain is removed and the patient is discharged home on postoperative day one.

If residual stone is revealed on follow up imaging, these findings are discussed with the patient. Depending on the patient, stone burden, and other factors, we offer immediate or delayed antegrade versus retrograde ureteroscopy. In appropriate situations, observation may also be offered. Shared-decision making is imperative in this discussion and is often the most important factor when deciding how to proceed.

20 Follow up

Patients are seen in our clinic for a routine post-operative visit to perform a wound check and review stone analysis results. All patients are then seen at 6 month follow up intervals with renal ultrasound for stone surveillance.

21 Conclusion

The horseshoe kidney presents a unique operative challenge to the urologist when managing stone disease in this patient population. A thorough understanding of the embryology and anatomic variation that arises is crucial to the safe and effective treatment of these patients. With careful consideration of these differences, percutaneous intervention is safe and effective in the horseshoe kidney. Key points of percutaneous nephrolithotomy in the horseshoe kidney include: gaining upper pole access is preferred, ensuring the guidewire is within the renal pelvis or ureter prior to tract dilation is paramount, and performing flexible endoscopy at the conclusion of any percutaneous intervention in the horseshoe kidney is required. By understanding the anatomic variations and adhering to the principles described in this chapter, the urologist can safely and effectively approach stone disease percutaneously in most any patient with a horseshoe kidney.

References

Assimos D, Krambeck A, Miller NL, et al. Surgical management of stones: American Urological Association/Endourological Society Guideline, part II. J Urol. 2016;196:1161.

Baskin L, Cunha G. Campbell-Walsh-Wein urology: embryology of the genitourinary tract. 12th ed. Philadelphia: Elsevier; 2021. p. 305–40.

Boatman D, Cornell S, Kölln C. The arterial supply of horseshoe kidneys. Am J Roentgenol Radium Ther Nucl Med. 1971;113:447–51.

Cook W, Stephens F. Fused kidneys: morphologic study and theory of embryogenesis. Birth Defects. 1977;13(5):327–40.

Ding J, Huang Y, Gu S, Chen Y, Peng J, Bai Q, Ye M, Qi J. Flexible ureteroscopic management of horseshoe kidney renal calculi. Int Braz J Urol. 2015;41(4):683–9.

Geavlete B, Mareș C, Mulțescu R, Georgescu D, Geavlete P. Hybrid flexible ureteroscopy strategy in the management of renal stones—a narrative review. J Med Life. 2022;15(8):919–26.

Gupta S, Kasim A, Pal D. Supine tubeless PCNL in horseshoe kidney (a series of cases). Urologia. 2022;89(4):559–63.

Hansen M. Netter's clinical anatomy. 5th ed. Philadelphia: Elsevier; 2022.

Khougali S, Alawad O, Farkas N, Ahmed M, Abuagla A. Bilateral pelvic kidneys with upper pole fusion and malrotation: a case report and review of the literature. J Med Case Rep. 2021;15(1):181.

Kumar P, Bach C, Kachrilas S, Papatsoris A, Buchholz N, Masood J. Supine percutaneous nephrolithotomy (PCNL): 'in vogue' but in which position? BJU Int. 2012;110(11 Pt C):E1018–21.

Lavan L, Herrmann T, Netsch C, Becker B, Somani B. Outcomes of ureteroscopy for stone disease in anomalous kidneys: a systematic review. World J Urol. 2020;38(5):1135–46.

Muttarak M, Sriburi T. Congenital renal anomalies detected in adulthood. Biomed Imaging Interv J. 2012;8(1): e7.

Natsis K, Piagkou M, Skotsimara A, Protogerou V, Tsitouridis I, Skandalakis P. Horseshoe kidney: a review of anatomy and pathology. Surg Radiol Anat. 2014;36(6):517–26.

Osther P, Razvi H, Liatsikos E, et al. CROES PCNL Study Group. Percutaneous nephrolithotomy among patients with renal anomalies: patient characteristics and outcomes; a subgroup analysis of the clinical research office of the endourological society global percutaneous nephrolithotomy study. J Endourol. 2011;25(10):1627–32.

Pawar A, Thongprayoon C, Cheungpasitporn W, Sakhuja A, Mao M, Erickson S. Incidence and characteristics of kidney stones in patients with horseshoe kidney: a systematic review and meta-analysis. Urol Ann. 2018;10(1):87–93.

Pérez Fentes D. Case of the Month' from the University of Santiago de Compostela, Spain: challenging the status quo in percutaneous stone surgery for horseshoe kidneys, the Galdakao-modified supine Valdivia position is a safe alternative for complex cases. BJU Int. 2021;127(5):520–3.

Raj G, Auge B, Weizer A, Denstedt J, Watterson J, Beiko D, Assimos D, Preminger G. Percutaneous management of calculi within horseshoe kidneys. J Urol. 2003;170(1):48–51.

Schiappacasse G, Aguirre J, Soffia P, Silva C, Zilleruelo N. CT findings of the main pathological conditions associated with horseshoe kidneys. Br J Radiol. 2015;88(1045).

Smith J, Howards S, Preminger G, Dmochowski R, Hinman F. Hinman's atlas of urologic surgery. Philadelphia: Elsevier; 2019. p. 215–34.

Sohail N, Albodour A, Abdelrahman K, Bhatti K. Supine percutaneous nephrolithotomy in horseshoe kidney. J Taibah Univ Med Sci. 2017;12(3):261–4.

Stein R, Desai M. Management of urolithiasis in the congenitally abnormal kidney (horseshoe and ectopic). Curr Opin Urol. 2007;17(2):125–31.

Tanagho E, Nguyen H, McAninch J, Lue T. Smith and Tanagho's general urology: Chapter 2: embryology of the genitourinary system. 18th ed. New York: McGraw-Hill; 2013.

Vicentini F, Mazzucchi E, Gökçe M, Sofer M, Tanidir Y, Sener T, de Souza MP, Eisner B, Batter T, Chi T, Armas-Phan M, Scoffone C, Cracco C, Perez B, Angerri O, Emiliani E, Maugeri O, Stern K, Batagello C, Monga M. Percutaneous nephrolithotomy in horseshoe kidneys: results of a multicentric study. J Endourol. 2021;35(7):979–84.

Yohannes P, Smith A. The endourological management of complications associated with horseshoe kidney. J Urol. 2002;168(1):5–8.

PCNL for Lower Pole Calyceal Stones

Eduardo Mazzucchi, Alexandre Danilovic, and Fabio Carvalho Vicentini

Abstract Lower pole calyceal stones (LPCS) constitute approximately 35% of all renal stones, and 50% of these stones will require some kind of intervention within five years. Percutaneous nephrolithotripsy (PCNL) and its variants (miniperc, ultra miniperc, and microperc) are comparable to flexible ureteroscopy (FURS) in the treatment of LPCS between 10 and 20 mm, presenting a slightly better stone-free rate but is more invasive with higher blood loss and more pain. For stones > 20 mm, PCNL has a significantly higher stone-free rate than FURS. A one-week antibiotic regimen is recommended for high-risk patients. No significant differences have been found between the prone and supine decubitus positions. The lower pole is accessed directly by fluoroscopy or ultrasound-guided puncture, and after dilation of the tract, a nephroscope is introduced. Stones can be fragmented or removed using forceps. Nephrostomy can be left if necessary, or a ureteral stent is inserted at the end of the procedure and removed on the first or second postoperative day. Complications of PCNL occur in approximately 7% of patients and include bleeding, injury to the adjacent organs, and infection. Ambulatory PCNL is reported to be both safe and effective.

Keywords Percutaneous nephrolithotripsy · Renal stones · Lower calyceal stones

1 Introduction

Lower pole calyceal stones (LPCS) constitute approximately 35% of all renal stones (Gurocak et al. 2008) and can remain asymptomatic; however, 75% of the stones will progress (increase in size, cause pain, or require intervention) and 50% will require some kind of intervention within five years. The treatment of LCPS has been a subject

E. Mazzucchi (✉)
Urology and Head of Endourology Section, Clinicas Hospital, University of São Paulo Medical School, São Paulo, Brazil
e-mail: emazzucchi20@gmail.com

A. Danilovic · F. C. Vicentini
Urology, Clinicas Hospital, University of São Paulo Medical School, São Paulo, Brazil

© The Author(s), under exclusive license to Springer Nature Switzerland AG 2023
J. D. Denstedt and E. N. Liatsikos (eds.), *Percutaneous Renal Surgery*,
https://doi.org/10.1007/978-3-031-40542-6_20

of debate owing to the great variability in the anatomy of the lower pole, which makes it difficult to reach such stones using retrograde approaches and to eliminate the residual fragments, especially when associated with an acute infundibulopelvic angle and a narrow and long infundibulum (Donaldson et al. 2015).

Watchful waiting, extracorporeal lithotripsy (SWL), retrograde intrarenal surgery (RIRS or FURS), and percutaneous nephrolithotripsy (PCNL) and its variations are the primary treatment modalities for LPCS.

Herein, we focus on the indications, technical aspects, and results of PCNL for the treatment of LCPS.

2   Percutaneous Nephrolithotripsy

The development of PCNL began in the last century after the first publication of a successful renal stone removal through percutaneous nephrostomy under radiological control by Johansson and Fernstrom in 1976 (Fernstrom and Johansson 1976). Since then, PCNL has undergone many changes and has been the gold standard for the treatment of renal stones > 20 mm or > 15 mm if located in the lower renal calyx (AUA Guidelines—Surgical management of urinary stones; EAU—Guidelines on urolithiasis). Other indications for PCNL include stones located in the calyceal diverticula, stones in horseshoe kidneys, and as an alternative for upper ureter stones > 15 mm.

PCNL has undergone many changes in recent years, including a reduction in the calibers of rigid nephroscopes. Traditionally, PCNL was performed using a 26 Fr rigid nephroscope inserted into the collecting system through a 28 or 30 Fr Amplatz sheath. PCNL has always been considered a difficult procedure by surgeons, and the risk of intraoperative bleeding has been a constant source of concern among all patients who undergo PCNL. To reduce bleeding and injury to the renal parenchyma, smaller nephroscopes have been introduced in clinical practice, and more liberal use of the flexible nephroscope during the procedure has become routine. The term mini-percutaneous nephrolithotomy (miniperc) was introduced by Jackmann et al. for treating renal stones in children, but it has been used in adults also (Jackman et al. 1998). Miniperc refers to all percutaneous surgeries performed with a tract smaller than 20 Fr. Similarly, there are variations such as miniperc (16–20 Fr), ultra-miniperc (12–14 Fr), super-miniperc (12 Fr) and microperc (4.8 Fr- All-seeing-needle®). The miniaturization of instruments resulted in less aggression to the kidney and significantly less bleeding, transfusion, and pain, among other complications, in the postoperative period (Wan et al. 2022). In this setting, PCNL and miniperc gained an additional role in the treatment of lower calyceal stones, particularly those > 15 mm or when the lower calyx could not be reached by a flexible ureteroscope.

3 Anatomy of the Inferior Calyx of the Kidney

The anatomy of the collecting system may influence the treatment outcome for kidney stones, especially for SWL (Perlmutter et al. 2008). In 1992, Sampaio and Aragão described the lower pole spatial calyceal anatomy using endocasts and suggested that some anatomical features could impact fragment clearance (Sampaio and Aragao 1992). Among 146 endocasts obtained from 73 adult cadavers, 74% had an obtuse infundibulopelvic angle in the lower pole, 60.3% had lower pole infundibula with diameters $\geq$ 4 mm, and 56.8% of the lower poles drained multiple calyces (Sampaio and Aragao 1994). Sampaio et al. showed that the angle between the calyx where the stone is located and the renal pelvis (infundibulopelvic angle) influences stone elimination after lithotripsy In a study of 74 patients who underwent SWL for LPCS, 52 presented an infundibulopelvic angle $> 90°$, and 75% of them eliminated the fragments within 3 months, while in patients with an infundibulopelvic angle $< 90°$, the clearance rate was 23% (Sampaio et al. 1997). Although Elbahnasy et al. (Elmansy and Lingeman 2016) used a slightly different method to measure the infundibulopelvic angle, in their cohort of 34 patients, significantly larger infundibulopelvic angles were identified in stone-free patients following SWL ($75°$ vs. $51°$, $p = 0.009$), corroborating the studies of Sampaio. A retrospective study of 116 patients comparing five different anatomic characteristics demonstrated that infundibulopelvic angle was the only significant factor to predict stone-free rates after SWL (34% in patients with an acute angle vs. 66% for obtuse angle, $p = 0.012$) (Albala et al. 2001).

Although the results of PCNL are less affected by the anatomy of the lower pole, surgeons recognize that lower pole calyces with a very acute infundibulum-pelvic angle and a long and narrow infundibulum can be difficult to access percutaneously, even in experienced hands.

4 Overview of the Treatment of Lower Pole Calyceal Stones

All the currently known minimally invasive treatment modalities for renal stones can be used and are recommended for treating LPCS. These include watchful waiting, SWL, FURS or RIRS, and PCNL with its variations.

Watchful waiting is recommended for asymptomatic LPCS < 10 mm (or up to 15 mm in selected cases according to European guidelines) (Assimos et al. 2016; Türk et al. 2020). Patients with solitary kidneys, those with comorbidities, airplane pilots, frequent travelers, and other special situations are not suitable candidates for watchful waiting.

Extracorporeal lithotripsy is performed under sedation and in an outpatient setting with a low complication rate (Chaussy et al. 1982). The success of SWL is highly affected by stone burden (the likelihood of success decreases for stones > 20 mm), composition, location, and obesity. Hard stones (monohydrate oxalate and cystine) and very soft stones (struvite) present poor results. When the stone composition is unknown, stone density (as measured by Hounsfield units on CT) can predict stone fragility and response to SWL. According to Joseph et al., the stone-free rate (SFR) for stones with less than 500 HU, between 500–1000 HU, and more than 1000 HU is 100%, 87.5%, and 54.5%, respectively (Joseph et al. 2002). Another factor influencing the results of SWL is the anatomy of the inferior calyx. LPCS presents a challenge to SWL, particularly when the infundibulopelvic angle is acute; the results are poorer when compared to stones located in the upper pole or renal pelvis. In the multicentric trial study Lower Pole I, conducted by Albala et al., postoperative SFR at 3 months for LPCS treated with SWL in comparison to PCNL was 95% for PCNL versus 37% for SWL (Albala et al. 2001). Results of SWL for LPCS are highly variable, and stone-free rates of 37–90% (Torricelli et al. 2015; Pareek et al. 2005) for stones < 10 mm have been reported.

FURS is a minimally invasive method that has gained popularity among urologists owing to its high success rates and low incidence of complications. The method is not affected by obesity and can be performed in anticoagulated patients or during pregnancy, under general or spinal anesthesia, and in outpatient or short hospitalization settings. The anatomy of the lower calyx can influence the results of FURS. According to Danilovic et al., an infundibulopelvic angle of 41° results in a significantly higher occurrence of residual fragments (Danilovic et al. 2019). The major drawback of FURS is its cost; many disposables such as guide wires, baskets, access sheaths, and laser fibers are required in a regular procedure, although their use is not mandatory in all situations. SFR of FURS for LPCS ranges from 50 to 80% but can reach up to 95% in experienced hands (Knoll et al. 2012; Salvadó et al. 2019).

PCNL and its variations are the most efficient methods in terms of stone-free rates; however, it is the most invasive and has the highest morbidity among all the above-mentioned methods. The main complications include bleeding, injury to adjacent organs, pleural effusion, urinary extravasation, and sepsis.

5 Indications and Results of PCNL in the Treatment of Lower Pole Calyceal Stones

PCNL has been used in the treatment of LPCS between 10 and 20 mm, and mainly in those > 20 mm. PCNL for treating LPCS less than 10 mm is exceptional and is done only for very special cases.

Patients with medium-sized LPCS, between 10 and 20 mm, can be treated with SWL, FURS, and PCNL, including its variants (miniperc, ultra-miniperc, super-miniperc, and microperc).

Many studies have compared SWL, FURS, and PCNL, the results of some of these studies are summarized in Table 1.

Stone-free rates, which indicate the complete absence of residual fragments, were higher for patients who underwent PCNL and FURS when compared to SWL in most

Table 1 Stone-free rates for LPCS 10–20 mm at two or three months after treatment

	Type study	No of patients	SWL (%)	FURS (%)	Miniperc (%)	p-value
Bozkurt et al. (2011)	Retrospective	79	–	89.2	92.8	0.571
El-Nahas et al. (2012)	Retrospective	89	67.7	86.5	–	0.038
Kumar et al. (2015a)	Prospective	180	78.4	85.4	–	0.34
Vilches et al. (2015)	Prospective	55	41.2	75.0	–	< 0.05
Kumar et al. (2015b)	Prospective	126	73.8	86.1	95.1	0.01
Chan et al. (2017)	Retrospective	225	48.5	42.9	66.7	0.59
Zeng et al. (2018)	Prospective	160	–	82.5	93.8	0.028
Ozgor et al. (2018)	Retrospective	241	77.9	89.0	–	0.029
Jin et al. (2019)	Prospective	220		97.1	99.3	0.622
Shabana et al. (2021)	Retrospective	136		81.7	91.7	0.1

[*] Stone-free was defined as the occurrence of fragments < 3 mm

of the studies, but no significant difference was found when FURS was compared to miniperc.

Kumar et al. compared the operative times of SWL, FURS, and miniperc. Operative time was 43.6 ± 1.4 min, 47.5 ± 1.1 min, and 61.1 ± 1.3 for SWL, FURS, and mini PCNL, respectively with no significant differences among the three modalities (Vilches et al. 2015) which corroborates the data from Jin which also stated no significant difference in operative time (Table 2) (Jin et al. 2019). The re-treatment rate (63.4% vs. 2.1% and 2.2%, $p < 0.001$) and the need for auxiliary procedures (20.2% vs. 8.8% and 6.6%, $p < 0.02$) were significantly higher for patients submitted to SWL when compared to those treated with FURS or miniperc (Vilches et al. 2015). The mean hospital stay was 3.1 h, 1.3 days, and 3.1 days for SWL, FURS, and miniperc, respectively (Vilches et al. 2015). Jin et al. compared postoperative pain using the VAS score and found that FURS was significantly less painful (Jin et al. 2019).

Microperc (all-seeing needle, 4.8 Fr) is another variant of PCNL used for treating LPCS 10–20 mm in diameter. In a study published by Tok comparing microperc with miniperc, the SFR was 86.2% and 82.5% ($p = 0.66$), respectively. In this study, no significant differences were found regarding complications; however, microperc was associated with a significantly shorter operative time, fewer fluoroscopy times, less intraoperative bleeding (although transfusion was not necessary for any procedure), and a shorter hospital stay (Tok et al. 2016).

Table 2 Intra and postoperative data comparing flexible ureteroscopy and miniperc

	FURS (n = 110)	Miniperc (n = 110)	p
Operative time (min)	87.2 ± 13.34	79.6 ± 14.86	0.124
Complication Clavien- Dindo 2 (Dindo et al. 2004)	3 (2.7%)	3 (2.7%)	ns
Blood loss (ml)	14.35–7.96	31.67–23.72	0.002
Urosepsis	0 (0%)	1 (0.9%)	0.491
Pain at 6 h PO (VAS score 1–10)	3.86–1.10	6.53–1.35	< 0.001
Pain at 48 h PO (VAS score 1–10)	1.04–0.75	2.12–0.92	0.004

Adapted from Jin et al. (2019)

The conclusion is that Miniperc has a better SFR than FURS and SWL but is more invasive. FURS has a better SFR than SWL, fewer complications, and shorter hospitalization than miniperc. FURS is less affected by obesity and can be performed in patients with coagulopathies. Additionally, it has a short hospital stay and delivers less radiation to patients and the surgical team (Bozzini et al. 2017). Microperc is a good alternative, with results comparable to those of miniperc. Decisions must be made on a case-by-case basis according to the stone, patient, and surgeon aspects.

Traditionally, PCNL has been the most effective method for stones > 2 cm. Pardalidis et al. published results using the traditional 26 Fr rigid nephroscope for treating LPCS in the prone position using a flexible nephroscope as an adjunct to reach difficult calyces. A 98% SFR was observed after a single session of treatment in 48 patients with LPCS > 2 cm. The mean length of hospital stay was 2.3 days. Fever was the most common complication, occurring in 6.9% of patients, and no cases of hemorrhage or sepsis were reported (Qin et al. 2022).

Qin et al. recently published a meta-analysis comparing miniperc with standard PCNL. When compared to the traditional 30 Fr access, miniperc achieved a similar SFR with less blood loss, a lower transfusion rate, and a shorter hospital stay. Miniperc did not show significant advantages regarding SFR, blood loss, and transfusion and presented a longer operation time when compared to the 24 Fr (Pardalidis et al. 2010).

Flexible ureteroscopy has been used as an alternative method to treat LPS > 2 cm. In a meta-analysis where the results of the treatment of 445 patients were evaluated, the mean SFR was 93.7% (77–96.7%), with an average of 1.6 procedures per patient. The mean stone size was 2.5 cm. The complication rate was 10.1% (5.3% were major complications). A subgroup analysis showed that FURS had a 95.7% SFR with stones 2–3 cm and 84.6% with stones > 3 cm ($P = 0.01$). The authors stress that these results were obtained with experienced hands, and more than one procedure is generally necessary to render the patients stone-free (Aboumarzuk et al. 2012). SWL is not recommended for the treatment of lower pole stones > 2 cm, according to the AUA and EAU guidelines (Assimos et al. 2016; Türk et al. 2020).

6 Technical Aspects of PCNL in the Treatment of Lower Pole Calyceal Stones

Preoperative antibiotics are recommended before PCNL. In cases of positive urinary culture, infection stones, a previous history of urinary infection, patients with a nephrostomy or an internal stent, immunosuppressed patients, or other important comorbidities (called high-risk patients) should receive a seven-day course of antibiotics immediately before the surgery plus an intravenous dose of antibiotic at anesthesia induction. This regimen reduces the incidence of SIRS and sepsis (Jung et al. 2022). Patients not included in the above-mentioned categories received a prophylactic dose of cephalosporin, fluoroquinolone, or even a combination of gentamycin plus ampicillin at the induction of anesthesia that can be maintained for 24 h according to the hospital protocol (Jung et al. 2022). Danilovic et al. recently published a metanalysis suggesting one-week preoperative antibiotics for all patients independent of low or high risk for infection in the PO (Danilovic et al. 2022).

Anticoagulants and antiplatelet agents should be discontinued before surgery, according to Table 3 (Türk et al. 2020; Baron et al. 2013).

It must be emphasized that resuming or not using anticoagulants four days after surgery depends on the occurrence or absence of hematuria in the postoperative period.

Positioning the patient on the operating table in the prone or supine position has been a topic of discussion in recent years among endourologists. Both conventional PCNL and miniperc can be safely performed in the supine or prone position with good results. Recently, Perrela et al. published the results of a prospective study comparing conventional PCNL in the supine and prone positions for complex stones and not only for lower-pole stones. In their study, there was no significant difference in stone-free rates, but PCNL in the supine position had a shorter operative time and fewer high-grade complications (Perrella et al. 2022). To date, no studies have shown a clear advantage of any position over another, and it is quite consensual that every surgeon should operate according to the position he feels more comfortable.

The lower renal calyx is generally accessed by direct and accurate puncture of the desired calyx using an 18 Gauge × 12 cm or an 18 Gauge × 20 cm needle. Traditionally, a fluoroscopy-guided puncture is the most commonly used method to access the calyx. Fluoroscopy allows accurate identification of the desired calyx but does not allow the visualization of organs adjacent to the kidney, increasing the risk

Table 3 Management of anticoagulants and antiplatelet agents before and after PCNL

Aspirin	Discontinue 5–7 days before surgery	Resume 4 days after the procedure
Clopidogrel, Prasugrel, Ticagrelor, Warfarin	Discontinue 5 days before surgery	Resume 4 days after the procedure
Rivaroxaban, Dabigatran, Apixaban	Discontinue 1–3 days before surgery	Resume 4 days after the procedure

of lesions in these organs, particularly the colon. In contrast, the ultrasound-guided approach allows real-time tracking of the puncture, avoiding accidental injuries to adjacent organs. A flexible ureteroscope positioned in the lower pole can be used as an auxiliary procedure to guide the puncture. Ultrasound (US)-guided PCNL results are comparable to those of fluoroscopy-guided PCNL in terms of SFR, complications, intraoperative bleeding, transfusion rates, operative times, and hospital stay (Corrales et al. 2021). Currently, both US and fluoroscopy are used in a complementary fashion to facilitate access, particularly in difficult cases.

After puncturing the desired calyx, a guidewire must be inserted into the collecting system, and if possible, positioned in the bladder or even exteriorized through the urethra. A second guidewire can be inserted, working as a safety guidewire. Dilation of the tract can be accomplished by using a balloon dilator, fascial sequential dilators, or metallic coaxial dilators (Alken dilators). Generally, a 28 or 30-Fr tract is established for a traditional 26-Fr rigid nephroscope. In miniperc, dilation is achieved according to the modality of the miniaturized percutaneous choice. In many cases, a "single-shot" dilation is used. Dilation of the lower pole may be more challenging owing to higher kidney mobility, especially when the patient is supine. In some cases, the surgeon can attempt to hold the kidney by pushing it medially to prevent dislodgement. A through-and-through guidewire also reduces kidney movement during lower pole dilation.

After dilation and positioning of the Amplatz sheath in the calyx, to avoid forcing it into the infundibulum, particularly if using a larger nephroscope, a rigid nephroscope is introduced, and the stone can be removed with forceps or disintegrated using any energy source.

Different energy sources can be used for lithotripsy. Traditionally, ultrasonic lithotripters or combined ultrasonic and ballistic lithotripters, which have the advantage of suctioning fragments during the procedure, have been used in conventional or mini-PCNL. Holmium lasers and, more recently, Thulium fiber lasers have been used more frequently in miniperc and ultra-miniperc. In miniperc, fragments are eliminated by the vacuum cleaner effect; however, suctioning access sheaths are being introduced in clinical practice to reduce residual fragments.

At the end of the procedure, complete inspection of the excretory system is mandatory, preferentially using a flexible nephroscope or a flexible ureteroscope inserted through the urethra. This maneuver provenly increases the SFR and provides better results when the nephroscopy is performed retrograde using a flexible ureteroscope when compared to the nephroscopy performed antegrade with a flexible nephroscope (Gökce et al. 2019). This is particularly true when treating lower-pole stones when the flexible nephroscope movement can be limited.

A nephrostomy can be inserted to drain the urinary system and prevent bleeding. The use of nephrostomy at the end of PCNL has been reduced, and a nephrostomy tube is currently indicated in selected cases where perforation of the collecting system occurs, or when a second-look procedure is planned through the existing tract, or when massive bleeding or purulent secretion occurs. Currently, a ureteral stent can be used as a drainage method after PCNL or miniperc. Tubeless PCNL (ureteral stent, no nephrostomy) has a shorter operative time and hospital stay (Gauhar et al.

2022). In selected cases, where no residual fragments are left and manipulation of the excretory system is minimal, no drainage can be left (totally tubeless procedure). When used, the nephrostomy tube can be removed on the first or second postoperative day if no additional procedures are foreseen, and the patient is discharged home.

Complications of PCNL include bleeding, injury to adjacent organs (colon, liver, and spleen), lesions in the pleura, and infection. Bleeding is related to dilation size. Lesions to the pleura are less frequent in lower-pole stones, as access is generally performed through the inferior calyx.

Ambulatorial PCNL has been proven safe even in patients with an ASA grade 3 anesthetic risk. In a series of 500 patients operated in the prone position using Endoscopic Combined Intrarenal Surgery at an ambulatory surgery center, Chong et al. reported a 2.4% complication rate that required patients to transfer to the hospital and a 4.2% 30-day readmission rate (Chong et al. 2021). Thakker et al. compared 53 patients who underwent conventional or mini-PCNL in a same-day discharge setting retrospectively with 54 patients with similar clinical and stone characteristics who stayed at the hospital overnight. The complication rates for same-day discharge patients and one-day admission were 0 and 7% ($p = 0.045$), respectively. The 30-day ER visit rates were 4 and 6% ($p = 0.66$), and the 30-day re-admission rates were 2 and 4% ($p = 0.560$) for same-day discharge patients and one-day admission patients, respectively (Thakker et al. 2022). Other articles published in the literature also corroborate that ambulatory PCNL is safe and cost-effective.

References

Aboumarzuk O, Monga M, Kata SG, Traxer O, Somani BK. Flexible ureteroscopy and laser lithotripsy for stones > 2 cm: a systematic review and meta-analysis. J Endourol. 2012;26:1257–63.

Albala DM, Assimos DG, Clayman RV, et al. Lower pole I: a prospective randomized trial of extracorporeal shock wave lithotripsy and percutaneous nephrostolithotomy for lower pole nephrolithiasis-initial results. J Urol. 2001;166:2072–80.

Assimos D, Krambeck A, Miller NL, et al. Surgical management of stones: American Urological Association/Endourological Society Guideline, PART I. J Urol. 2016;196:1153–60.

AUA Guidelines—Surgical management of urinary stones. https://www.auanet.org/guidelines-and-quality/guidelines/kidney-stones-surgical-management-guideline.

Baron TH, Kamath PS, McBane RD. Management of antithrombotic therapy in patients undergoing invasive procedures. N Engl J Med. 2013;368:2113–24.

Bozkurt OF, Resorlu B, Yildiz Y, Can CE, Unsal A. Retrograde intrarenal surgery versus percutaneous nephrolithotomy in the management of lower-pole renal stones with a diameter of 15–20 mm. J Endourol. 2011;25:1131–5.

Bozzini G, Verze P, Arcaniolo D, et al. A prospective randomized comparison among SWL, PCNL and RIRS for lower calyceal stones less than 2 cm: a multicenter experience: A better understanding on the treatment options for lower pole stones. World J Urol. 2017;35:1967–75.

Chan LH, Good DW, Laing K, et al. Primary SWL is an efficient and cost-effective treatment for lower pole renal stones between 10 and 20 mm in size: a large single center study. J Endourol. 2017;31:510–6.

Chaussy C, Schmiedt E, Jocham D, Brendel W, Forssmann B, Walther V. First clinical experience with extracorporeally induced destruction of kidney stones by shock waves. J Urol. 1982;127:417–20.

Chong JT, Dunne M, Magnan B, Abbott J, Davalos JG. Ambulatory percutaneous nephrolithotomy in a free-standing surgery center: an analysis of 500 consecutive cases. J Endourol. 2021;35:1738–42.

Corrales M, Doizi S, Barghouthy Y, Kamkoum H, Somani B, Traxer O. Ultrasound or fluoroscopy for percutaneous nephrolithotomy access, is there really a difference? A review of literature. J Endourol. 2021;35:241–8.

Danilovic A, Rocha BA, Torricelli FCM, et al. Size is not everything that matters: preoperative CT predictors of stone free after RIRS. Urology. 2019;132:63–8.

Danilovic A, Talizin TB, Torricelli FCM, et al. One-week pre-operative oral antibiotics for percutaneous nephrolithotomy reduce risk of infection: a systematic review and meta-analysis. Int Braz J Urol. 2022;48 (ahead of print).

Dindo D, Demartines N, Clavien PA. Classification of surgical complications: a new proposal with evaluation in a cohort of 6336 patients and results of a survey. Ann Surg. 2004;240:205–13.

Donaldson JF, Lardas M, Scrimgeour D, et al. Systematic review and meta-analysis of the clinical effectiveness of shock wave lithotripsy, retrograde intrarenal surgery, and percutaneous nephrolithotomy for lower-pole renal stones. Eur Urol. 2015;67:612–6.

EAU—Guidelines on urolithiasis. https://uroweb.org/guidelines/urolithiasis/chapter/guidelines.

Elmansy HE, Lingeman JE. Recent advances in lithotripsy technology and treatment strategies: A systematic review update. Int J Surg. 2016;36:676–80.

El-Nahas AR, Ibrahim HM, Youssef RF, Sheir KZ. Flexible ureterorenoscopy versus extracorporeal shock wave lithotripsy for treatment of lower pole stones of 10–20 mm. BJU Int. 2012;110:898–902.

Fernstrom I, Johansson B. Percutaneous pyelolithotomy. A new extraction technique. Scand. J Urol Nephrol.1976; 10: 257–9.

Gauhar V, Traxer O, García Rojo E, et al. Complications and outcomes of tubeless versus nephrostomy tube in percutaneous nephrolithotomy: a systematic review and meta-analysis of randomized clinical trials. Urolithiasis. 2022;50:511–22.

Gökce Mİ, Gülpinar O, Ibiş A, Karaburun M, Kubilay E, Süer E. Retrograde versus antegrade flexible nephroscopy for detection of residual fragments following PNL: a prospective study with computerized tomography control. Int Braz J Urol. 2019; 45:581–7.

Gurocak S, Kupeli B, Acar C, Tan MO, Karaoglan U, Bozkirli I. The impact of pelvicaliceal features on problematic lower pole stone clearance in different age groups. Int Urol Nephrol. 2008;40:31–7.

Jackman SV, Hedican SP, Peters CA, Docimo SG. Percutaneous nephrolithotomy in infants and preschool age children: experience with a new technique. Urology. 1998;52:697–701.

Jin L, Yang B, Zhou Z, Li N. Comparative efficacy on flexible ureteroscopy lithotripsy and miniaturized percutaneous nephrolithotomy for the treatment of medium-sized lower-pole renal calculi. J Endourol. 2019;33:914–9.

Joseph P, Mandal AK, Singh SK, Mandal P, Sankhwar SN, Sharma SK. Computerized tomography attenuation value of renal calculus: can it predict successful fragmentation of the calculus by extracorporeal shock wave lithotripsy? A preliminary study. J Urol. 2002;167:1968–71.

Jung HD, Cho KS, Moon YJ, Chung DY, Kang DH, Lee JY. Antibiotic prophylaxis for percutaneous nephrolithotomy: an updated systematic review and meta-analysis. PLoS ONE. 2022;17: e0267233.

Knoll T, Buchholz N, Wendt-Nordahl G. Extracorporeal shockwave lithotripsy versus percutaneous nephrolithotomy vs. flexible ureterorenoscopy for lower-pole stones. Arab J Urol. 2012;10:336–41.

Kumar A, Vasudeva P, Nanda B, Kumar N, Das MK, Jha SK. A prospective randomized comparison between shock wave lithotripsy and flexible ureterorenoscopy for lower caliceal stones ≤ 2 cm: a single-center experience. J Endourol. 2015a;29:575–9.

Kumar A, Kumar N, Vasudeva P, Kumar Jha S, Kumar R, Singh H. A prospective, randomized comparison of shock wave lithotripsy, retrograde intrarenal surgery and miniperc for treatment of 1 to 2 cm radiolucent lower calyceal renal calculi: a single center experience. J Urol. 2015b;193:160–4.

Ozgor F, Sahan M, Yanaral F, Savun M, Sarilar O. Flexible ureterorenoscopy is associated with less stone recurrence rates over shockwave lithotripsy in the management of 10–20-millimeter lower pole renal stone: medium follow-up results. Int Braz J Urol. 2018;44:314–22.

Pardalidis NP, Andriopoulos NA, Sountoulidis P, Kosmaoglou EV. Should percutaneous nephrolithotripsy be considered the primary therapy for lower pole stones? J Endourol. 2010;24:219–22.

Pareek G, Armenakas NA, Panagopoulos G, Bruno JJ, Fracchia JA. Extracorporeal shock wave lithotripsy success based on body mass index and Hounsfield units. Urology. 2005;65:33–6.

Perlmutter AE, Talug C, Tarry WF, Zaslau S, Mohseni H, Kandzari SJ. Impact of stone location on success rates of endoscopic lithotripsy for nephrolithiasis. Urology. 2008;71:214–7.

Perrella R, Vicentini FC, Paro ED, et al. Supine versus prone percutaneous nephrolithotomy for complex stones: a multicenter randomized controlled trial. J Urol. 2022;207:647–56.

Qin P, Zhang D, Huang T, Fang L, Cheng Y. Comparison of mini percutaneous nephrolithotomy and standard percutaneous nephrolithotomy for renal stones > 2 cm: a systematic review and meta-analysis. Int Braz J Urol. 2022;48:637–48.

Salvadó JA, Cabello JM, Moreno S, Cabello R, Olivares R, Velasco A. Endoscopic treatment of lower pole stones: is a disposable ureteroscope preferable? Results of a prospective case-control study. Cent European J Urol. 2019;72:280–4.

Sampaio FJ, Aragao AH. Inferior pole collecting system anatomy: its probable role in extracorporeal shock wave lithotripsy. J Urol. 1992;147:322–4.

Sampaio FJ, Aragao AH. Limitations of extracorporeal shockwave lithotripsy for lower caliceal stones: anatomic insight. J Endourol. 1994;8:241–7.

Sampaio FJ, D'Anunciacao AL, Silva EC. Comparative follow-up of patients with acute and obtuse infundibulum-pelvic angle submitted to extracorporeal shockwave lithotripsy for lower caliceal stones: preliminary report and proposed study design. J Endourol. 1997;11:157–61.

Shabana W, Oquendo F, Hodhod A, et al. Miniaturized ambulatory percutaneous nephrolithotomy versus flexible ureteroscopy in the management of lower calyceal renal stones 10–20 mm: a propensity score matching analysis. Urology. 2021;156:65–70.

Thakker P, Mithal P, Duta R, Carreno G, Gutierrez-Aceves J. Comparative outcomes and cost of ambulatory PCNL in select kidney stone patients. Urolithiasis. 2022;51:22.

Tok A, Akbulut F, Buldu I, et al. Comparison of microperc and mini-percutaneous nephrolithotomy for medium-sized lower calyx stones. Urolithiasis. 2016;44:155–9.

Torricelli FC, Marchini GS, Yamauchi FI, et al. Impact of renal anatomy on shock wave lithotripsy outcomes for lower pole kidney stones: results of a prospective multifactorial analysis controlled by computerized tomography. J Urol. 2015;193:2002–7.

Türk C, Neisius A, Petrik A, et al. EAU guidelines on urolithiasis. Eur Urol. 2020. Retrieved from: http://uroweb.org/guidelines/compilations-of-all-guidelines/

Vilches RM, Aliaga A, Reyes D, et al. Comparison between retrograde intrarenal surgery and extracorporeal shock wave lithotripsy in the treatment of lower pole kidney stones up to 15 mm. Prospective, randomized study. Actas Urol Esp 2015;39:236–42.

Wan C, Wang D, Xiang J, et al. Comparison of postoperative outcomes of mini percutaneous nephrolithotomy and standard percutaneous nephrolithotomy: a meta-analysis. Urolithiasis. 2022;50:523–33.

Zeng G, Zhang T, Agrawal M, et al. Super-mini percutaneous nephrolithotomy (SMP) versus retrograde intrarenal surgery for the treatment of 1–2 cm lower-pole renal calculi: an international multicentre randomised controlled trial. BJU Int. 2018;122:1034–40.

Percutaneous Nephrolithotomy in Pediatric Patients

Jun Li, Bo-Yu Yang, and Hui-Min Zhao

Abstract Pediatric urolithiasis is a relatively rare disease in urology. According to the American Urological Association (AUA) 2016 Surgical Treatment Guidelines, surgery is recommended for patients who are unable to pass stones spontaneously after 4–6 weeks of observation and who are unresponsive to 4–6 weeks of medical therapy. Extracorporeal shock wave lithotripsy (ESWL) is the treatment of choice in most cases involving upper urinary tract stones, while percutaneous nephrolithotripsy (PCNL) is appropriate for more complex or unique types of kidney stones. Pediatric patients require a thorough assessment and preparation prior to undergoing PCNL. Age is not a limiting factor for surgery and infants as young as a few months can safely undergo PCNL as long as appropriate surgical equipment and adjunctive therapy are used. As 75%–84% of kidney stones in children are associated with genetic metabolic disorders, and 50% of children have symptomatic recurrences within three years of their first occurrence, the number of surgeries performed throughout a child's lifetime should be minimized. Since children are growing and developing, an ultrasound-guided technique is preferred because it avoids the harmful effects of radiation. The literature reports stone-free rates after PCNL ranging from 68 to 100%. Any remaining stones can be treated with a second phase of surgery or a combination of extracorporeal shock wave lithotripsy and flexible ureteroscopy lithotripsy.

Keywords Percutaneous nephrolithotom · Kidney stones · Nephrolithiasis · Urolithiasis · Minimally invasive surgery · Stone removal · Renal calculi · Percutaneous access · Nephroscope · Endourology · Lithotripsy · Stone fragmentation · Kidney anatomy · Renal pelvis · Calyces · Staghorn calculi · Fluoroscopy · Ultrasound-guided access · Tubeless percutaneous nephrolithotomy · Postoperative care

J. Li (✉) · B.-Y. Yang · H.-M. Zhao
Department of Urology, Capital Medical University Affiliated Beijing Friendship Hospital, Beijing 100050, China
e-mail: lljun@yeah.net

© The Author(s), under exclusive license to Springer Nature Switzerland AG 2023
J. D. Denstedt and E. N. Liatsikos (eds.), *Percutaneous Renal Surgery*,
https://doi.org/10.1007/978-3-031-40542-6_21

1 Indications and Contraindications

Indications and contraindications for PCNL in children are similar to those in adults (Grivas et al. 2020).

(1) Indications
(2) Staghorn calculi
(3) Renal pelvis stone > 2 cm
(4) Lower calyceal stones > 1 cm
(5) Cystine stones unsuitable for flexible ureteroscopy lithotripsy (FURS)

For special types of kidney stones, such as cystine or uric acid stones, the effectiveness of extracorporeal lithotripsy is often limited due to a high recurrence rate. In cases where being stone-free is critical, PCNL may be a preferred option. PCNL can also be used for upper ureteral stones with severe obstruction or a diameter greater than 1.5 cm in patients who have failed ureteroscopy or extracorporeal lithotripsy. It is important to select surgical instruments and PCNL methods appropriate for children, considering factors such as stone location, stone burden, age, and kidney size.

(B) Contraindications

In summary, contraindications for PCNL surgery in children are similar to those in adults:

1. Uncorrected systemic bleeding;
2. Patients with medical comorbidities precluding aanethesia;
3. Patients with untreated severe urinary tract infection;
4. Patients with renal tuberculosis;
5. Patients with untreated primary hyperoxaluria (PHO) type I/II.

2 Operative Position

PCNL can be performed in a variety of surgical positions, including prone, supine, and lateral. The prone position allows a wider range of equipment to be used and is the most common position for children with PCNL in China. However, it can be difficult for anesthesiologists to control tracheal intubation and is not convenient for resuscitation. The supine position was first used in adults by Valdivia et al. in 1987 and has many potential advantages in pediatric PCNL techniques. Data on the use of supine PCNL in children support its safety and high efficacy in stone clearance rates, even for infants under 1 year of age Vaddi et al. (2021). The modified Valdivia position, used in a small number of pediatric patients with the MicroPerc technique, has also shown satisfactory success and safety. In supine PCNL, the urinary tract is level or slightly upwardly inclined relative to the operating table, allowing rapid drainage of irrigating fluid and stone debris from the body, reducing the risk of hypothermia and severe postoperative infection. This position also addresses anesthesia limitations associated with the prone position. Lateral lithotomy at PCNL was first performed in morbidly obese patients in 1994 and has proven anesthetic advantages in patients with severe medical risk factors or comorbidities, as well as in patients with morbid obesity or kyphosis (Sultan et al. 2019).

3 Preoperative Preparation

In pediatric patients, it is critical to minimize bleeding during surgery due to smaller kidneys and correspondingly lower blood volume, making them less tolerant to bleeding. The use of adult surgical instruments can result in renal injury and massive bleeding, emphasizing the need for minimally invasive techniques in pediatric PCNL. Technological advances have led to the development of several minimally invasive PCNL techniques with reduced surgical channel size, including mini-PCNL (14–20 Fr), ultra-mini PCNL (11–13 Fr), ultra-mini PCNL (14 Fr) and micro-PCNL (4.8Fr), have all been successfully used in the treatment of children with kidney stones. Smaller tracts result in less renal injury and less bleeding. Standard PCNL (sPCNL) using 24–30 Fr channels is associated with high stone clearance rates (>90%) but also carries the risk of kidney injury and excessive bleeding requiring blood transfusion, particularly in children (Sultan et al. 2019). While sPCNL is recommended for staghorn stones in adults, it is not suitable for the growing and developing kidneys of children, especially those of infants with a renal size of only 5 to 6 cm. Compared to mini PCNL associated complications with standard PCNL are more common and more severe according to some studies (Tefekli et al. 2008). Therefore, minimally invasive techniques such as mini-PCNL and micro-PCNL are preferred in pediatric patients to minimize bleeding and reduce the risk of complications.

Mini-PCNL is a modified version of sPCNL, which utilizes a smaller access channel of 14 to 20 Fr, compared to the larger 24–30 Fr channel used in sPCNL. Surgical endoscopes typically consist of 8.0–9.8 Fr rigid ureteroscopes or 8.5–12.5 Fr nephroscopes with high-pressure endoscope perfusion pumps. Fascial dilators are used to dilate the percutaneous renal channel, starting at 8 Fr and gradually expanding to 14 to 20 Fr. Compared with sPCNL, mini-PCNL has several advantages, including reduced incidence of complications such as bleeding, less perioperative pain, shorter hospital stay, and lower treatment costs (Bodakci et al. 2014). Mini-PCNL is recommended for the management of kidney stones smaller than 2.5 cm, although multiple tracts can be established to treat larger stones (Ganpule et al. 2016a). Studies (Utangac et al. 2016) have shown that mini-PCNL has a much lower complication rate than sPCNL, with an overall complication rate of 12% compared to 24% in sPCNL (P = 0.048). The incidence of bleeding requiring blood transfusion is also significantly lower in mini-PCNL patients (2.4% vs. 12.9%, P = 0.013). Even with the smaller channel size, mini-PCNL has a high stone clearance rate, making it a safe and effective treatment option for pediatric patients with kidney stones.

To improve the safety and efficacy of mini-PCNL while minimizing complications, Desai et al. (2013) introduced Ultra-Mini-PCNL (UMP). UMP adopts 3 Fr optical system, 7.5 Fr nephroscope and 11–13 Fr metal channel, with high stone-free rate and low complication rate. Desai et al. (2013) compared UMP with RIRS for the treatment of kidney stones ranging from 1.0 to 3.5 cm, and both techniques were found to have a high stone-free rate and a low rate of complications. Additionally, Dede et al. (2015) reported that UMP achieved a final SFR of 87.1% in the treatment of 39 children with renal calculi, with no children requiring blood transfusions during the perioperative period. In 2015, Zeng et al. (2016) suggested the use of a super mini PCNL {SMP} involving an 8 Fr micronephroscope, and 12 Fr and 14 Fr irrigation and suction sheaths. The unique design of the flushing suction sheath tube allows for separate irrigation and aspiration, thereby improving the efficiency of stone clearance despite the use of a smaller instrument. With an incision size of only 3 mm, the stone can be directly aspirated through the suction device after being fragmented to 2 mm using a laser. The SMP's suction sheath is double-layered, with the sandwich filling the patient's pelvis while also absorbing water and debris without the need for additional tubing. Bleeding in the kidney is stopped through autologous tissue compression and an autologous coagulation mechanism after the operation, and pain is minimized for the patient, making SMP a minimally invasive surgery. The procedure is performed under fluoroscopic guidance in the prone position using a 7 Fr nephroscope with an outer channel sheath ranging from 10 to 14 Fr. SMP has been successfully performed on 141 adult patients with a mean stone size of 2.2 cm, resulting in a reported SFR of 90.1% (Zeng et al. 2016). No major complications were reported, and 72.3% of the patients were catheter-free.

MicroPerc is a novel hybrid surgical instrument, which consists of a 4.8 Fr puncture needle and a surgical channel. The first part is the working outer sheath with a circumference of 4.8 Fr. The second part is the connection device, equipped with three channels that can simultaneously accommodate the imaging fiber, the perfusion device, and the 200–270 μm laser fiber. The preoperative preparation for MicroPerc surgery is similar to conventional nephroscopic surgery, and the patient is placed in a prone position after ureteral catheter or ureteral stent placement. The needle-shaped nephroscope (all-seeing needle) allows for direct visualization of the puncture route after insertion of the optical fiber. Under B-ultrasound guidance, the target renal calices are punctured and the position of the needle is monitored in real time. Once the needle enters the collection system, the working path is established and the working outer sheath is maintained. The inner needle portion is then retracted and a cross connector installed to allow placement of the 200–270 μm holmium laser fiber and lithotripsy perfusion device. The use of MicroPerc's small working channel reduces intraoperative bleeding and injury, thereby eliminating the need for external drainage tubes after surgery. Internal stents can be placed retrogradely according to the intraoperative situation. In comparison to traditional PCNL, MicroPerc minimizes the risk of kidney injury, bleeding, infection, and other surgical complications Ganpule et al. (2016b).

When MicroPerc is combined with holmium laser lithotripsy, a channel can be established through one-step puncture, so that the stones can be crushed and then fragmented and discharged. If the pulverization is complete and the ureter is in good condition, only a 5 Fr ureter catheter is necessary 24–48 hours after the operation.

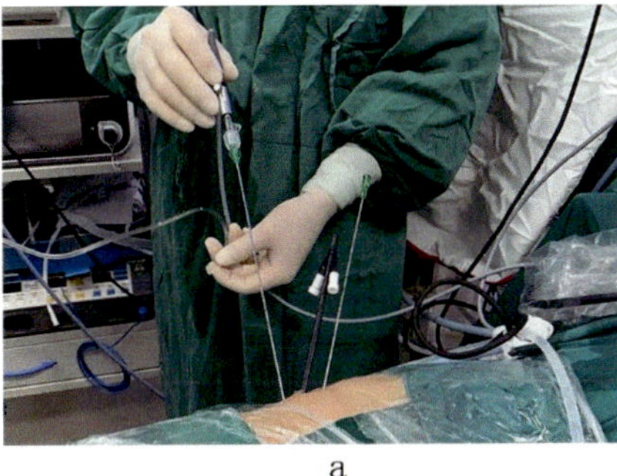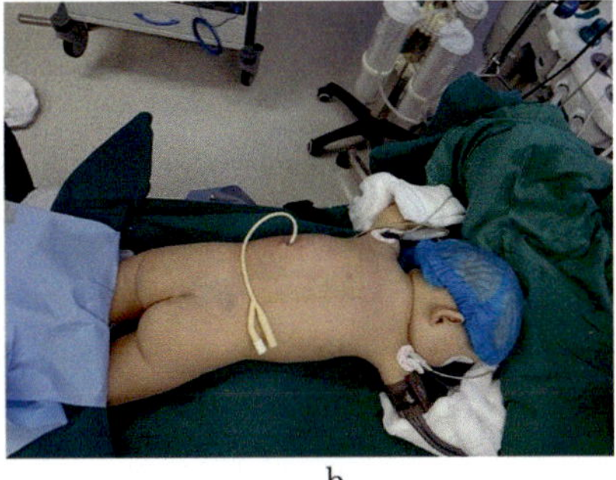

a   b

Fig. 1 a, b: Multi-channel pediatric PCNL, a 14Fr peel-away sheath and two MicroPerc channels, during operation (1a), only a 12Fr nephrostomy tube was needed after operation (1b)

This eliminates the need for stents and external drains after surgery, greatly reducing potential damage to the kidneys and risk of bleeding (Fig. 1). Additionally, secondary anesthesia to remove the stent is not required. Previous clinical research has demonstrated the potential of this approach to improve the quality of life for children, save money on treatment and be effective. For stones smaller than 2 cm in diameter, mPCNL, UMP, and SMP are more appropriate treatment options. These stones can be crushed by pneumatic ballistics or holmium lasers, and then quickly removed from the body using water pressure or a negative pressure device. For older children, children with large volume of hydronephrosis collection system, or children with large stone load and long operation time, the standard channel combined with negative pressure stone removal system can also be used to quickly remove stones, which improves the operation efficiency, shorten the operation time and reduce the incidence of postoperative complications. For relatively simple calculi with a small stone burden, it is possible to avoid the use of an indwelling nephrostomy tube or even a ureteral stent to improve postoperative comfort (Choi et al. 2014).

For conventional percutaneous nephrolithotomy, the following surgical instruments are needed:

1. The renal puncture and dilation set contain a puncture needle with an outer sheath, metal guide wire, fascia dilator, peel-away sheath, nephrostomy tube and cap.
2. Nephroscope and ureteroscope.
3. Lithotripsy equipment and instruments: holmium laser, pneumatic ballistic, stone-removal basket, and stone-removal forceps.
4. Liquid infusion pump.
5. Video observation system, camera system, video conversion system, and monitor.

4 Surgical Procedures

(1) Preoperative preparation

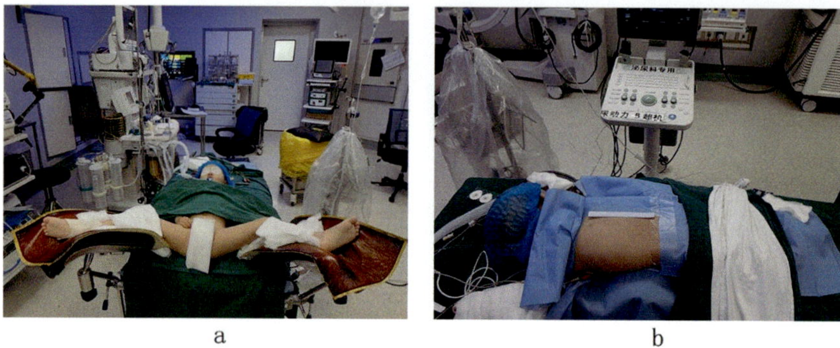

Fig. 2 a, b: Position during pediatric PCNL, lithiotomy position (2a), prone position (2b)

The patient is placed in the lithotomy position, and a 5 Fr ureteral catheter is inserted into the ipsilateral ureter leading to the kidney under the guidance of a cystoscope. The catheter is secured, and the end is connected to an infusion device for continuous perfusion and filling the collection system. Additionally, a 5 Fr double pigtail stent may be inserted according to the patient's body length and estimated ureter length (age number + 10 cm). The bladder (volume estimated as (number of age + 2) * 30 ml) is then filled with saline to provide reflux hydronephrosis. Finally, the chest and abdomen are elevated and the surgical field is exposed (Fig. 2).

(B)   Puncture under ultrasound guidance

To prepare for the procedure, the B ultrasound probe is directed parallel to the long axis of the kidney in order to observe the overall outline of the kidney, the location of the stone, and its relationship with the collecting system. Usually, the area between the posterior axillary line and the scapular line is the best area for puncture, and the posterior calyx puncture in the middle group is usually selected first. The needle can be inserted within the plane of B-ultrasound (both end parts of the probe), and for patients with a high stone position, the needle can be inserted from outside the plane of B-ultrasound (lateral part of the probe). The direction of puncture was chosen to be the dorsal calices closest to the dorsal skin, providing the shortest access. Pediatric patients typically have less subcutaneous and perinephric fat, making it easier to lose access when the needle is outside the kidney. During the puncture process, B-ultrasound is used to clarify the path of the puncture needle and prevent deviation. When the puncture needle is successfully inserted into the renal calyceal, urine overflow can be seen after retracting the core of the needle. For some patients with low renal pelvis pressure or mild hydronephrosis, the correct position of the needle tip can be determined by negative pressure suction with a syringe.

(C)   Establishment of tracts

Once the needle position is confirmed by B-ultrasound, an ultrastiff guide wire with a "J" tip is inserted along the outer sheath of the puncture needle. The skin and subcutaneous tissue are then incised with a sharp knife, approximately 0.5–1 cm in length. After removing the outer sheath of the indwelling guidewire, the channel is gradually expanded along the guidewire using a fascial dilator. There are two methods to expand the channel: the "step-by-step method" and the "one-step" dilation with a high-pressure balloon. The former involves gradual enlargement of the channel to the desired size using a fascial dilator or a telescoping antenna-style metal dilator. The latter involves expanding the channel to the desired size in one step using a high-pressure balloon. Kidney stones in children form quickly, have a brittle texture, and have a good crushing effect. As a result, after channel establishment, the procedure is usually straightforward. The specific channel specifications should be determined based on the patient's individual circumstances.

(D)   Stone removal

After the peel-away sheath is established, a nephroscope or ureteroscope is placed in an antegrade manner, and continuous saline perfusion is used to flush the visual field maintain a clear field of view. The location and general texture of the stones are observed, and the stones are fragmented and removed using lithotripsy devices. Any remaining stones should be extracted. If a ureteral catheter is used for artificial hydronephrosis before the operation, a ureteral stent will be placed at the conclusion of the procedure. Additionally, a nephrostomy tube will be placed.

5   Operation Tips and Tricks

Children have a lower body weight and lower blood volume, and their tolerance to blood loss is poor. During the access procedure, it is critical to emphasize the accuracy of the target and the direction of the needle. The accuracy of the puncture needle point is the key factor in preventing severe bleeding during the perioperative period of percutaneous nephrolithotomy.

When performing infant nephropuncture under ultrasound guidance, the quality of the imaging device is crucial. High-frequency linear array probes are superior to low-frequency convex array probes for infant puncture guidance. Due to the short distance between the kidney and the skin, a high-frequency linear array probe can offer a clear visualization of the kidney structure, particularly the vessels, with the assistance of Doppler technology (Tzeng et al. 2011) (Fig. 3). However, in older and obese children, high-frequency probes may not provide any significant visualization advantage.

When performing infant nephropuncture, it is important to consider the unique anatomical features of children, especially infants, such as their thin skin, subcutaneous tissue, and perirenal tissue. The short distance between the target calyx and the skin provides limited space for adjusting the needle direction and securing the ultra-stiff guidewire. Thus, it is crucial to accurately determine the direction of the needle from the target calyx to the uretero-pelvic junction and ensure that the puncture pathway is long enough to securely hold the guidewire and prevent the loss of the channel during the operation. When expanding the channel, the principle of

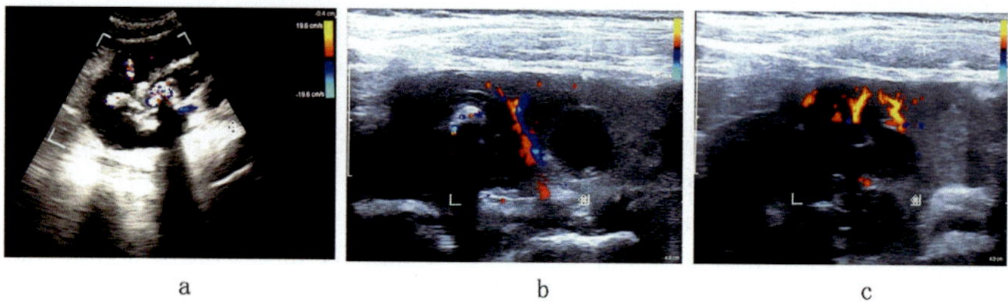

a   b   c

Fig. 3 a, b, c: Infant kidney structure and vessels under ultrasound san. Image from low-frequency convex array probe (3a), image from high-frequency linear array probe (3b, c)

"prefer shallow rather than deep" should be followed. Children have smaller kidney volumes than adults, and basing dilation depth on experience in adults may result in a deep channel that could damage the contralateral collecting system or even the renal pedicle. Therefore, when using facial dilators for channel expansion, it is important to avoid creating channels that penetrate too deeply.

Children's kidneys are more brittle in texture but more compliant, and often multiple adjacent calices can be explored through the target calices. During lithotripsy, attention should be given to solving the main problem through a single channel. If the calyx where the stone is located cannot be explored due to a challenging angle, another channel should be established if necessary to prevent laceration of the renal parenchyma or a calyceal neck caused by excessive exploration.

To ensure the health of children during PCNL, special care must be taken to maintain their body temperature. It is important to note that children are more susceptible to rapid temperature drops due to the use of hypothermic saline during the procedure, which can lead to decreased blood pressure, heart rate, and even endanger their lives. To prevent this, all fluids used during the procedure, including perfusion saline, must be heated to 37 °C. Additionally, a warm blanket should be used to maintain a steady temperature. If possible, the monitor should be equipped with a body temperature monitoring module to allow for continuous tracking of any changes in the child's body temperature (Fig. 4).

6 Postoperative Management

Perioperative management in children is a team effort with physicians and allied health members familiar with the special needs of pediatric patients. Infant patients are unable to express their feelings, and they need to rely on their parents to relay their wishes. Postoperative complications need to be addressed by professional pediatricians and nursing teams.

In pediatric patients, fever, bleeding, and pain are common complications following PCNL. The external drainage tube is typically thin in children, and regular monitoring is necessary to detect any potential obstructions caused by blood clots or

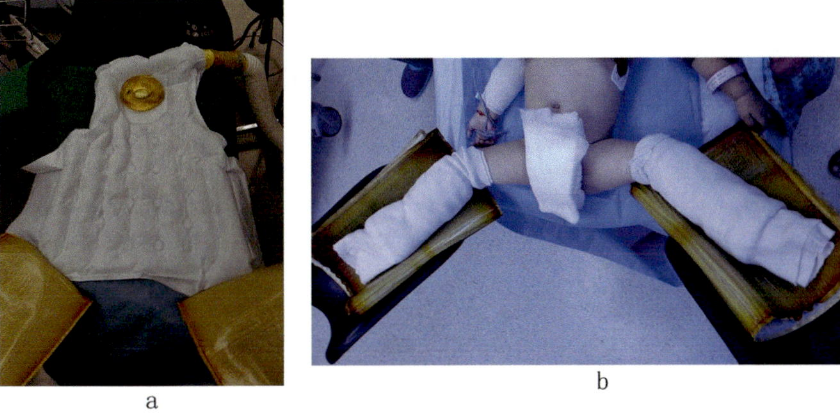

Fig. 4 a, b: Insulation measure, warm blanket for children (4a), arms and legs proof (4b)

stone fragments. Infants and young children have low immune resistance, which can easily cause postoperative fever. Inadequate drainage should be excluded first, and symptomatic drug treatment should be provided according to the cause. Children have low pain tolerance and may require analgesic medication to prevent postoperative pain-induced uncooperative behavior.

When the general condition of the child is stable, the imaging data can be reviewed to observe the position of the internal stent and the residual stone. If reoperation is not needed, the nephrostomy tube and urinary catheter can be removed. The ureteral stent can be removed 2 to 4 weeks after surgery. After the drainage tube is removed, patients and their families should be advised to rest and not engage in strenuous activities to reduce the occurrence of delayed bleeding.

7   Complications and Their Prevention

In children, bleeding, postoperative fever or infection, and persistent urinary fistula are the most frequently reported complications following percutaneous nephrolithotomy. Bleeding is generally associated with stone burden, location, operation time, size of the working sheath, and number of working channels. The need for blood transfusions is reported to be less than 10% in the literature (Ozden et al. 2011; Onal et al. 2014). The proportion of severe bleeding requiring blood transfusion is gradually decreasing with the miniaturization of current access. Accurate puncture and appropriate channel size remain the most important strategies to prevent intraoperative and postoperative bleeding. The use of B-ultrasound-guided puncture not only avoids radiation exposure but also identifies possible blood vessels along the puncture path, which helps the surgeon avoid and prevent injury. In infants with small kidney volumes, a larger channel increases the risk of bleeding and exacerbates kidney injury. Conversely, smaller access reduces the probability and risk of major bleeding. Recent studies have shown that postoperative fever generally occurs in less than 15% of patients, and most early-onset fever is often unrelated to urinary tract infection. Compared to adults, children have poorer self-immunity and resistance, lower tolerance to trauma, and are more likely to develop a fever after surgery. For children, maintaining urine drainage unobstructed after surgery and administering timely and sufficient antibiotics to prevent infection are critical. Adequate drainage during surgery and open drainage after surgery can help prevent a persistent urinary fistula.

8 Recent Advances in PCNL

Nephrostomy is the most commonly employed drainage method following PCNL. Some surgeons also insert a double-J tube in the ureter to enhance drainage into the bladder. The presence of a nephrostomy tube may result in increased postoperative pain and prolonged hospital stay for patients. To address this issue, some surgeons have introduced the concept of tubeless mini-PCNL. Completely tubeless PCNL in children was evaluated and found to be a safe procedure (Softness and Kurtz 2022). A controlled trial comparing tubeless mini-PCNL with mini-PCNL in 70 children under 3 years of age concluded that tubeless mini-PCNL had similar outcomes and safety (such as stone clearance rate, postoperative fever, and hemoglobin decrease) but significantly reduced recovery time (Song et al. 2015).

Endoscopic combined intrarenal surgery (ECIRS) is a novel and promising surgical approach for the treatment of urolithiasis. ECIRS combines RIRS with PCNL and requires two surgeons to operate simultaneously. Specifically, RIRS is utilized to identify stones that may have been missed by PCNL, and these stones are subsequently flushed or grasped and delivered to the renal pelvis for removal via the PCNL channel. This technique leverages the strengths of both PCNL and RIRS, which results in a reduction of the bleeding risk associated with multiple channels and an improvement in stone clearance rates. ECIRS is a viable option for the treatment of complex kidney stones. In a systematic review published in 2020, Cracco and Scoffone (2020) reported that ECIRS boasts a high stone-free rate and a low incidence of Clavien-Dindo grade I and II complications. Moreover, the incidence of grade III, IV, and V complications is minimal. In this study, postoperative bleeding risk was also low, with hemoglobin decreases ranging from 0.8 to 2.1 g/dL.

9 Summary and Future Prospects

The development of pediatric PCNL technology has mainly focused on miniaturization. This is of significant importance in the surgical treatment of pediatric calculi as it can avoid large renal parenchyma injuries in children. Its safety and effectiveness have been established in the pediatric population. PCNL has proven beneficial in the treatment of staghorn and large kidney stones, and pediatric PCNL technology offers a variety of surgical access, locations, and combinations of endoscopic and intrarenal procedures that can eliminate the need for tubes. However, the success rates of stone-free rate (SFR) and stone clearance rate (CR) remain critical factors that surgeons must consider when applying PCNL technology to children with urinary calculi. Currently, there is a lack of expert consensus or an appropriate risk prediction model to help surgeons choose the most suitable surgical approach for individual children. The choice of surgical position will also affect the postoperative SFR and CR of children. Future technical improvements should not only increase the efficiency of existing procedures but also reduce the incidence of complications. Additionally, research on the applicability of various surgical methods for PCNL and the exploration of prediction models for children with stones can assist clinicians in making informed decisions and achieving accurate, personalized treatment. Furthermore, future studies should investigate whether the choice of surgical method needs to be tailored to the stone composition and improved surgical methods for patients with recurrent stones.

References

Bodakci MN, Daggulli M, Sancaktutar AA, Soylemez H, Hatipoglu NK, Utangac MM, Penbegul N, Ziypak T, Bozkurt Y. Minipercutaneous nephrolithotomy in infants: a single-center experience in an endemic region in Turkey. Urolithiasis. 2014;42(5):427–33.

Choi SW, Kim KS, Kim JH, Park YH, Bae WJ, Hong SH, Lee JY, Kim SW, Hwang TK, Cho HJ. Totally tubeless versus standard percutaneous nephrolithotomy for renal stones: analysis of clinical outcomes and cost. J Endourol. 2014;28(12):1487–94.

Cracco CM, Scoffone CM. Endoscopic combined intrarenal surgery (ECIRS)—Tips and tricks to improve outcomes: a systematic review. Turk J Urol. 2020;46(Supp. 1):S46–57.

Dede O, Sancaktutar AA, Dagguli M, Utangac M, Bas O, Penbegul N. Ultra-mini-percutaneous nephrolithotomy in pediatric nephrolithiasis: both low pressure and high efficiency. J Pediatr Urol. 2015;11(5):253 e251–256.

Desai J, Zeng G, Zhao Z, Zhong W, Chen W, Wu W. A novel technique of ultra-mini-percutaneous nephrolithotomy: introduction and an initial experience for treatment of upper urinary calculi less than 2 cm. Biomed Res Int. 2013;2013:490793.

Ganpule A, Chhabra JS, Kore V, Mishra S, Sabnis R, Desai M. Factors predicting outcomes of micropercutaneous nephrolithotomy: results from a large single-centre experience. BJU Int. 2016b;117(3):478–83.

Ganpule AP, Vijayakumar M, Malpani A, Desai MR. Percutaneous nephrolithotomy (PCNL) a critical review. Int J Surg. 2016a;36(Pt D):660–4.

Grivas N, Thomas K, Drake T, Donaldson J, Neisius A, Petrik A, Ruhayel Y, Seitz C, Turk C, Skolarikos A. Imaging modalities and treatment of paediatric upper tract urolithiasis: a systematic review and update on behalf of the EAU urolithiasis guidelines panel. J Pediatr Urol. 2020;16(5):612–24.

Onal B, Dogan HS, Satar N, Bilen CY, Gunes A, Ozden E, Ozturk A, Demirci D, Istanbulluoglu O, Gurocak S, Nazli O, Tanriverdi O, Kefi A, Korgali E, Silay MS, Inci K, Izol V, Altintas R, Kilicarslan H, Sarikaya S, Yalcin V, Aygun C, Gevher F, Aridogan IA, Tekgul S. Factors affecting complication rates of percutaneous nephrolithotomy in children: results of a multi-institutional retrospective analysis by the Turkish pediatric urology society. J Urol. 2014;191(3):777–82.

Ozden E, Mercimek MN, Yakupoglu YK, Ozkaya O, Sarikaya S. Modified Clavien classification in percutaneous nephrolithotomy: assessment of complications in children. J Urol. 2011;185(1):264–8.

Softness KA, Kurtz MP. Pediatric stone surgery: what is hot and what is not. Curr Urol Rep. 2022;23(4):57–65.

Song G, Guo X, Niu G, Wang Y. Advantages of tubeless mini-percutaneous nephrolithotomy in the treatment of preschool children under 3 years old. J Pediatr Surg. 2015;50(4):655–8.

Sultan S, Aba Umer S, Ahmed B, Naqvi SAA, Rizvi SAH. Update on surgical management of pediatric urolithiasis. Front Pediatr. 2019;7:252.

Tefekli A, Ali Karadag M, Tepeler K, Sari E, Berberoglu Y, Baykal M, Sarilar O, Muslumanoglu AY. Classification of percutaneous nephrolithotomy complications using the modified clavien grading system: looking for a standard. Eur Urol. 2008;53(1):184–90.

Tzeng BC, Wang CJ, Huang SW, Chang CH. Doppler ultrasound-guided percutaneous nephrolithotomy: a prospective randomized study. Urology. 2011;78(3):535–9.

Utangac MM, Tepeler A, Daggulli M, Tosun M, Dede O, Armagan A. Comparison of scoring systems in pediatric mini-percutaneous nephrolithotomy. Urology. 2016;93:40–4.

Vaddi CM, Ramakrishna P, Pm SS, Anandan H, Ganesan S, Babu M. Supine percutaneous nephrolithotomy in a 9-month infant. Urol Case Rep. 2021;34:101424.

Zeng G, Wan S, Zhao Z, Zhu J, Tuerxun A, Song C, Zhong L, Liu M, Xu K, Li H, Jiang Z, Khadgi S, Pal SK, Liu J, Zhang G, Liu Y, Wu W, Chen W, Sarica K. Super-mini percutaneous nephrolithotomy (SMP): a new concept in technique and instrumentation. BJU Int. 2016;117(4):655–61.

Endoscopic Technology for PCNL

Zachary E. Tano, Andrei D. Cumpanas, Ahmad Abdel-Aziz, and Ralph V. Clayman

Abstract The endoscope used daily by urologists has a 200-year history of technologic innovation progressing from a simple tube and candle to today's digital semi-conductors. Herein, we review the history of technologic evolution that led to the modern endoscope and proceed to review the latest technologic advances in endoscopy for percutaneous nephrolithotomy (PCNL).

Keywords Percutaneous nephrolithotomy · Nephroscopy · Robotic surgery · Rigid endoscopy · Flexible endoscopy

The Lichleiter Era

The earliest records of purposeful, successful endoscopy dates to 1806, when Philip Bozzini presented his *"Lichtleiter"* (German word meaning *light guide* or *conductor*) to the Academy of Medicine in Vienna. The light guide consisted of a candle holder for a light source and a rigid tube that would allow the physician to inspect the female bladder through the urethra (Ramai et al. 2018; Berci and Forde 2000; Shah 2002; Gow 1998; Nicholson 1982). The combination of a skeptical audience and an imperfect prototype resulted in severe criticism of Bozzini's *lichtleiter* as a "mere toy" (Ramai et al. 2018; Berci and Forde 2000; Shah 2002). The Academy's pejorative reception largely halted further development of the *lichtleiter* (Ramai et al. 2018; Berci and Forde 2000; Shah 2002) (Fig. 1).

Z. E. Tano · A. D. Cumpanas · A. Abdel-Aziz · R. V. Clayman (✉)
Department of Urology, University of California, Irvine, CA, USA
e-mail: rclayman@uci.edu

Z. E. Tano
e-mail: ztano@hs.uci.edu

A. D. Cumpanas
e-mail: acumpana@hs.uci.edu

A. Abdel-Aziz
e-mail: aabdela1@hs.uci.edu

© The Author(s), under exclusive license to Springer Nature Switzerland AG 2023
J. D. Denstedt and E. N. Liatsikos (eds.), *Percutaneous Renal Surgery*,
https://doi.org/10.1007/978-3-031-40542-6_22

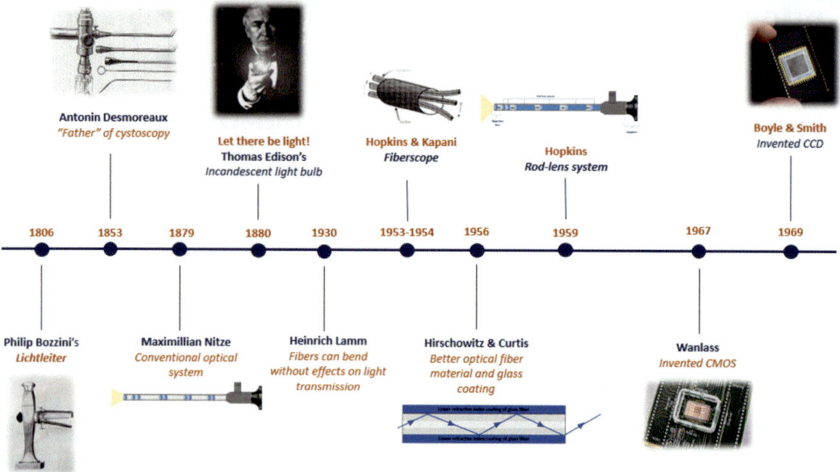

Fig. 1 Timeline of major technological advancements in the field of endourology

Bozzini died three years later but his visionary concept continued (Ramai et al. 2018; Berci and Forde 2000; Shah 2002). In 1853, Antonin Jean Desormeaux presented his novel cystoscope concept in Paris that consisted of a kerosene lamp at the base of the telescope that illuminated the female bladder by way of a 45-degree mirror (Shah 2002; Gow 1998). Desormeaux would later be referred to as the "father of cystoscopy" not only for devising the term "endoscopy" but also for being the first to use the concept of the *"lichtleiter"* for the clinical purpose of excising a papilloma from the urethra (Shah 2002).

The Conventional Optic System for the *Rigid* Endoscope

A major shortcoming of the first endoscopes was the poor illumination due to their reliance on an **external** light source (Shah 2002). In 1879, based on the concept, "to light up a room one must carry the lamp inside", Maximillian Nitze designed the first conventional optical system endoscope using a water-cooled, platinum filament lamp at the tip of the telescope (Shah 2002; Das 1987; Zada et al. 2013; Ieva et al. 2014). His design incorporated an objective lens at the distal end, which transmitted and magnified an inverted image along a series of relay lenses with large air gaps in-between them, ending in a focusing eyepiece that would display the final, upright image to the surgeon (Fig. 2A) (Ieva et al. 2014; Liang 2010).

Light source innovation continued with the Mignon lamp that was developed in the wake of Edison's invention of the incandescent lightbulb in 1886. It was a less expensive, small, non-heat generating vacuum lamp, that was inserted in the tip of the cystoscope to visualize the bladder (Shah 2002; Moran 2010). At that time, this was the most reliable source of lighting for medical imaging while mitigating any thermal damage to the urothelium (Shah 2002; Moran 2010). Apart from minor

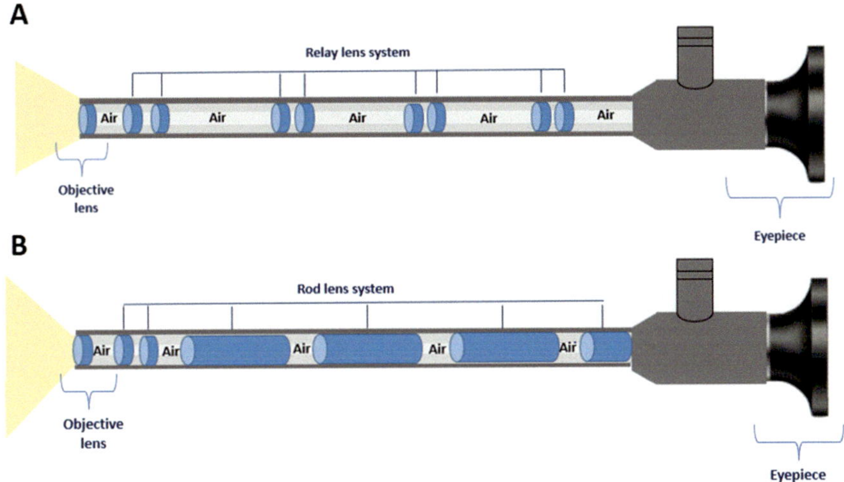

Fig. 2 **A.** Layout of the conventional optical system in a rigid endoscope designed by Maximillian Nitze in 1879; **B-**Layout of the rod-lens optical system developed by Howard Hopkins in 1967. (Adapted from Karl Storz, Inc.)

modifications to the instruments, the design of the rigid endoscope remained largely unchanged between the 1880s and the 1960s (Gow 1998).

Hopkins' Rod Lens Era

In 1959, James G. Gow, a urologist, approached Harold Hopkins, a physicist specializing in optics at the University College of London, and asked him if it was possible to improve the current design of the rigid cystoscope to better visualize bladder tumors and, if possible, to photographically document cystoscopic findings. After Gow secured a 3,000 £ grant from the British Medical Research Council, Hopkins agreed to proceed (Gow 1998; Ieva et al. 2014).

In the 1960s, the conventional optical lens system consisted of a tube of air with internalized thin glass lenses (Fig. 2A). Hopkins realized that he could vastly improve the quality of the endoscopic image by doing just the opposite; specifically, he constructed long tubes of glass with internalized thin air spaces (Fig. 2B) (Shah 2002; Gow 1998; Zada et al. 2013; Ieva et al. 2014; Liang 2010; Cockett and Cockett 1998). This new design revolutionized light transmission by increasing it 80-fold (Gow 1998).

Hopkins, like Bozzini, was ahead of the times, and thus American and British companies had no interest in Hopkins' innovation (Gow 1998; Ieva et al. 2014). It was, Karl Storz, a Tuttlingen-based precision medical instrument maker, recognized the promise of the rod-lens endoscope and decided to finance Hopkins' rod-lens endoscope (Gow 1998; Zada et al. 2013; Ieva et al. 2014; Cockett and Cockett 1998; Zajaczkowski and Zamann 2004; Maciolek et al. 2018). In short order, it became obvious that the Hopkins-Storz endoscope's rod-lens system was far superior to

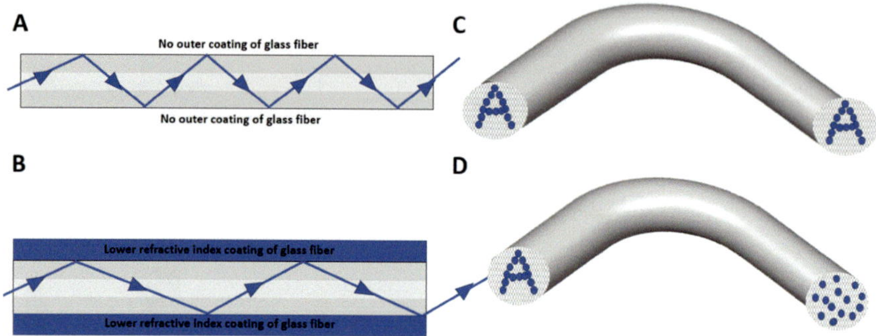

Fig. 3 Evolution of the fiberoptic scope. **A**- Lamm (1930), Hopkins and Kapany (1948) demonstrated that bundles of glass optical fibers could transmit an image while bent. **B**- Refinement of the fiberscope by Hirschowitz and Curtis increased the reflection critical angle resulting in increased light transmission efficiency by adding a low-refractive index glass cladding. **C**-Hirschowitz and Curtis's "**coherent**" glass fiber bundles aligning each fiber at the proximal end of the bundle with the fiber's position at the distal end of the bundle for image transmission. **D**- Storz's "**incoherent**" glass fiber bundles contain random glass fibers positions for light transmission

the traditional cystoscope due to improved light transmission, brighter and sharper images, and a wider viewing angle (Shah 2002; Gow 1998; Cockett and Cockett 1998).

The Birth of Flexible Endoscopy

In 1930, Heinrich Lamm, a medical school student, showed that bundled glass fibers could be bent while preserving light and image transmission (Berci and Forde 2000; Shah 2002; Zajaczkowski and Zamann 2004; Maciolek et al. 2018; Lau et al. 1997; Marshall 1964). Figure. 3A He investigated whether the image of a lightbulb at one end of glass bundle optical fibers could be seen at the opposite end (Berci and Forde 2000; Shah 2002; Zajaczkowski and Zamann 2004; Maciolek et al. 2018; Lau et al. 1997; Marshall 1964). Similar to Bozzini's rejection by the "leading, senior" minds of the day, so too Lamm's report was shunned by his medical school professors who refused to be listed as co-authors on his first manuscript describing his work (Maciolek et al. 2018).

Eighteen years later, Dr. Hugh Gainsborough, a gastroenterologist dissatisfied with the current rigid gastroscope, approached Hopkins to discuss the poor visualization of the gastric mucosa and extreme patient discomfort with rigid endoscopy (Gow 1998). Hopkins, along with one of his graduate students, Narinder Kapany, proceeded to improve on Lamm's idea by incorporating multiple 0.1 mm diameter glass fibers, with a high central refraction index, into a fiber bundle and demonstrated that the fiber bundle could indeed transport light and an image (Gow 1998; Ieva et al. 2014). Subsequently, they decreased the size of the glass fibers to 0.025 mm which resulted in an even sharper image (Gow 1998; Ieva et al. 2014). They named this instrument the *flexible fiberscope* and published their results in 1954 in the form of two letters sent to *Nature* (Hopkins and Kapany 1954) (Fig. 3A). Although Hopkins was one of the pioneers in glass fibers, lack of interest and lack of financial support from the British industry prevented further development (Gow 1998; Ieva et al. 2014).

Basil Hirschowitz, a South African gastroenterologist, working as a fellow at the University of Michigan, read about Hopkin's work in *Nature* and realized its potential (Gow 1998; Hirschowitz 1979, 1961; Hirschowitz et al. 1962; Morgenthal et al. 2007). In 1956, with the help of an Ann Arbor physicist, Larry Curtis, Hirschowitz refined Hopkins' design by coating the core glass fibers with an extra layer of glass of lower refractive index. This cladding process increased the critical angle between the coating and the core glass fiber, which resulted in overall fewer reflections along the length of the bundle, less energy loss and faster light transmission (Fig. 3B) (Zada et al. 2013; Ieva et al. 2014) (Maciolek et al. 2018). They also determined that a high-fidelity image transmission required the glass fiber bundle to be organized in a **"coherent bundle"**, meaning that the glass fibers are alligned from distal to proximal in the endoscope (Fig. 3C) (Shah 2002; Ieva et al. 2014; Zajaczkowski and Zamann 2004).

Storz attended a presentation of Hirschowitz's flexible fiberscope at a medical conference in Holland (Zajaczkowski and Zamann 2004). He realized that while for accurate imaging, the glass fibers had to be organized in "coherent" bundles, but for light transmission alone, the glass fibers could be packed together randomly into **"incoherent"** bundles (Fig. 3D) (Shah 2002; Ieva et al. 2014; Zajaczkowski and Zamann 2004). After attending this conference, Storz proceed to patent the idea of incoherent fiberoptic bundle light transmission (Zajaczkowski and Zamann 2004).

The Rise of Flexible Endoscopy in Urology (1980s)

While throughout the 1960s and 1970s, other medical specialties were incorporating flexible endoscopes more and more into their daily practice, urologists seemed reluctant to move from rigid to flexible endoscopy because the fiberoptic image was considered too granular (Maciolek et al. 2018; Fowler et al. 1984). It wasn't until 1984 that two groups of urologists, Clayman and colleagues in the United States, and Fowler and colleagues in Great Britain, published their studies in the Journal of Urology and the British Journal of Urology, respectively, showing that although not nearly as clear as the image displayed by the Hopkins-Storz rod-lens system, the flexible fiberoptic image was sufficient to identify normal anatomy as well as pathological lesions in the bladder (Fowler 1984; Clayman et al. 1984a). This deficiency was counterbalanced by the atraumatic nature of the flexible endoscopic procedure allowing cystoscopy to be performed in the outpatient setting under urethral anesthesia (Maciolek et al. 2018; Fowler et al. 1984; Fowler 1984; Clayman et al. 1984a).

The Digital Endoscope Revolution: "Chip on the Tip" Camera Techology

As postulated by Bozzini in his *Lichtleiter* thesis, there were two obstacles to creating the ideal endoscope: (**1**) sufficient illumination in the body, and (**2**) a clear, true image for the user (Bush et al. 1806). While Hopkins and Storz solved the problem of light transmission by developing fiberoptic light transmission, the flexible fiberoptic endoscope image remained pixelated and of low resolution (Natalin and Landman 2009).

In 1969, Williard Boyle and George Smith, from AT&T Bell Labs developed the diminutive charge-coupled device (CCD), a silicon chip for which they were awarded the 2009 Nobel Prize in Physics (Natalin and Landman 2009; Tejas et al. 2020). CCD chips contain an array of millions of "passive" photodiodes, or pixels (Natalin and Landman 2009; Tejas et al. 2020). At each pixel level, incident light is converted into an electric charge (electron) proportional to the intensity of the light source to which the chip is exposed (Fig. 4A). The generated charge is transferred down to the next row in the chip sequentially, until reaching the very edge of it, where the horizontal read-out register is located. This sequential electrical charge transfer occurs through an electron bucket brigade system, consisting of couples of negatively charged and positively charged capacitators. After passing through the read-out register, the transported electrical charge is converted into actual voltage.

The large photoactive surface per pixel of the CCD chip results in high sensitivity, low noise, and enhanced visualization, but it comes at a cost. The CCD system complexity is expensive, has a high energy consumption, and due to the centralized analog-to-digital conversion that occurs at the edge of the chip and it has a relatively slow read-out speed (Natalin and Landman 2009; Tejas et al. 2020; Jorden et al. 2014; Bohndiek et al. 2008).

Predating the CCD chip by two years was the development of complementary metal oxide semiconductor (CMOS) chips by Frank Wanlass (Natalin and Landman 2009; Tejas et al. 2020). While CMOS chips also rely on the photoelectric effect, each photodiode, or pixel in the CMOS chip, is its own "active" integrated circuit that can convert photons to electrons and electrons to voltage (Fig. 4B) (Natalin and Landman 2009; Tejas et al. 2020). This integrated architecture results in a smaller, more compact chip with lower power consumption (almost one fourth of that needed by a CCD), a higher image processing speed, and low risk of pixel saturation resulting in less image smearing or blooming (Natalin and Landman 2009; Tejas et al. 2020; Kempainen 1997; Hillebrand et al. 2000). Importantly, the CMOS chip is far less costly to produce (Natalin and Landman 2009; Tejas et al. 2020; Bohndiek et al. 2008).

The digital revolution was not isolated to imaging; it also took hold of illumination with the advent of Light Emitting Diodes (LEDs). The physical basis of the LED is the reversal of the previously discussed semiconductor principle of transforming light into electrical current, to transforming electrical current into light. Historically, Henry J. Round discovered the principle of electroluminescence, but it was Oleg Vladimirovich Losev who is credited with the invention of the LED in 1927 (Zheludev 2007). LED production of white light that is used for endoscope illumination requires mixing of various colors which was not possible until Shuki Nakamura developed the functional blue LED light, for which he was awarded the 2014 Nobel Prize in physics. The value of LEDs compared to other endoscopic light sources are their relatively low heat production, efficiency, low cost, and long life. Moreover, the LED provides improved shadow sharpness, better brightness, flicker reduction, and augmented perception of peripheral detail (Lee et al. 2009). The combination of

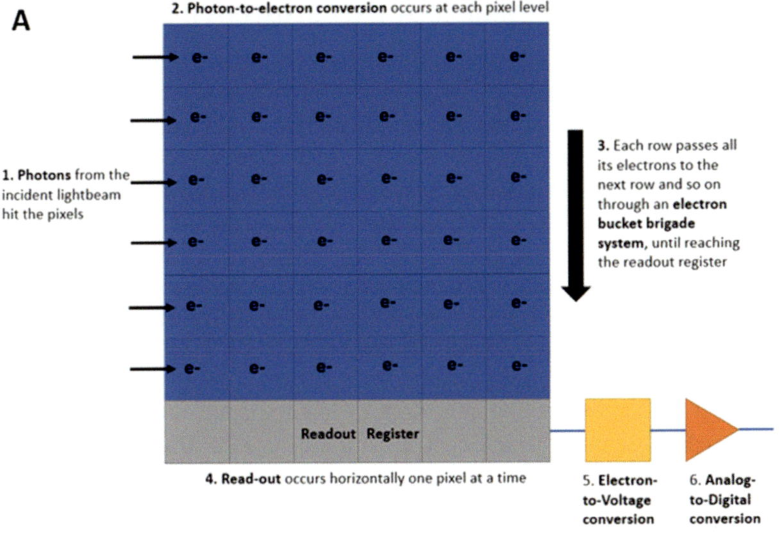

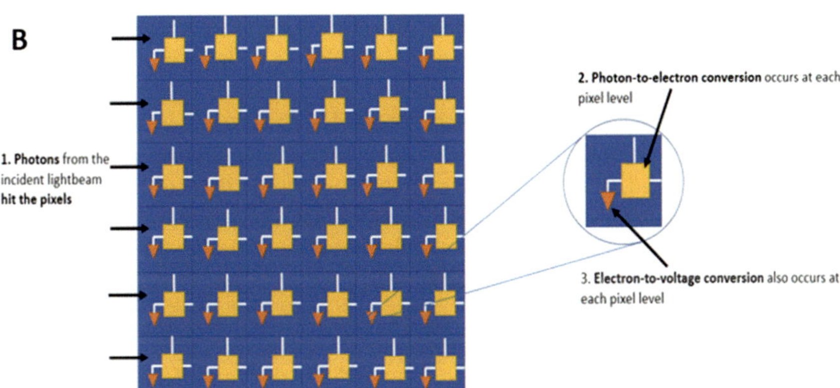

Fig. 4 The digital endoscope revolution. A-Mechanism of action of the charge-coupled device (CCD)-chip for which Williard Boyle and George Smith won the Nobel Prize in Physics in 2009; **B**-Mechanism of action of the low-cost complementary metal oxide semiconductor (CMOS) chip

the inexpensive LED and CMOS chip has led to the current interest in single use endoscopes.

1 Percutaneous Renal Endoscopy (Nephroscopy): Past to Present

Unlike cystoscopy and ureteroscopy, for which a natural orifice exists, nephroscopy mandates the creation of a percutaneous tract (i.e., nephrostomy). While the surgical creation of a nephrostomy had been in place since 1863 when a "renal cyst" was drained using a "trochar" (Hillier 1865; Bloom et al. 1989), the use of the tract other than to drain urine did not occur until 1941, when Rupel and Brown first reported the passage of a rigid cystoscope into the kidney to recover a stone through an open nephrostomy tube tract created to stabilize a patient with an infected stone (Rupel and Brown 1941). In the same decade, Trattner developed a rigid endoscope to be placed via an open pyelotomy for viewing the calyces during surgery (Trattner 1948). In 1950, Leadbetter, taking advantage of fiberoptic technology, created an angled rigid endoscope thereby making it easier to traverse the infundibulae via the open pyelotomy incision (Leadbetter 1950).

The percutaneous revolution began in 1955 when Willard Goodwin performed the first antegrade nephrostogram and reported on the first percutaneous placement of a nephrostomy tube (Goodwin et al. 1955). Twenty-one years later, in 1976, Fernström and Johansson proceeded to perform the first percutaneous stone removal (Fernström I, Johansson 1976). Subsequently in the late 1970's, the technique of percutaneous stone removal was further refined by a host of pioneers in the United States (i.e. Arthur Smith, Kurt Amplatz, Joseph Segura) and Europe (i.e. Peter Alken, Michael Marberger, John Wickham) (Patel and Nakada 2015). The endoscopes employed were initially all rigid, until the introduction of a purpose built flexible nephroscope in 1979 by American Cystoscope Makers Inc. (ACMI). The advent of flexible cysto-scopes with LED and CMOS/CCD technology replaced the flexible nephroscope and thus has come to serve both purposes.

Rigid Nephroscopes

Rigid nephroscopes (Table 1) are commonly used due to their excellent optical quality (attributed to the use of the rod lens system), irrigation, and working channels. More-over, the ease of sterilization and their durability further enhance their practicality. In particular, the McCarthy panendoscope was initially employed given its straight, angled beak which made it easier to traverse the nephrostomy tract alongside a guidewire (Clayman et al. 1984b). To maintain a straight working channel necessary for the passage of rigid lithotrites (e.g. ultrasonic or pneumatic), the nephroscope had to be fitted with a parallel or angled offset arm to which an eyepiece could be affixed. Two distinct designs of nephroscopes have evolved: the Wickham model, characterized by a 130° angle between the eyepiece and the endoscope's sheath and the Amplatz model, featuring a 90° angle between the eyepiece and the endoscope's sheath (Fig. 5) (Mulţescu et al. 2016). The typical rigid nephroscopes for use in adults were matched to the size of the nephrostomy tract which was typically 24–30 Fr; as such 20 Fr and 24 Fr endoscopes, respectively, have predominated to the present day.

Table 1 Rigid Nephroscopes (conventional, mini, ultra-mini and micro PCNL) comparison

Manufacturer	Model	PCNL approach	Instrument sheath size (Fr)	Working channel diameter (Fr)	Working channel length (cm)	Direction of view (°)	Eyepiece	Imaging
Karl Storz	Conventional	Conventional	24 / 26	N/A	22	6	Parallel	Hopkins® rod-lens system
	Conventional	Conventional	24 / 26	N/A	22	6	Angled	Hopkins® rod-lens system
	MIP L	Mini	19.5	12.4	22	12	Angled	Hopkins® rod-lens system
	Slender	Mini	18	13.7	20	6	Parallel	Hopkins® rod-lens system
	Slender	Mini	18	13.7	20	6	Angled	Hopkins® rod-lens system
	MIP XS/S	Ultra-mini	7.5	2	24	6	Angled	Fiberoptic
	MIP M	Ultra-mini	12	6.7	22	12	Angled	Fiberoptic
Richard Wolf	Low-pressure universal nephroscope	Conventional	27	10.5	17.5	20	Parallel	PANOVIEW rod-lens system
	Low-pressure universal nephroscope	Conventional	27	10.5	17.5	20	Angled	PANOVIEW rod-lens system
	Long Compact nephroscope	Conventional	24	10.5	20.5	20	Parallel	PANOVIEW rod-lens system
	Long Ultrathin Nephroscope	Mini	20.8	10.5	20.5	N/A	Parallel	PANOVIEW rod-lens system

(continued)

Table 1 (continued)

Manufacturer	Model	PCNL approach	Instrument sheath size (Fr)	Working channel diameter (Fr)	Working channel length (cm)	Direction of view (°)	Eyepiece	Imaging
	Mini Percutaneous Nephroscope	Mini	18	6	22.5	12	Angled	PANOVIEW rod-lens system
	Mini Percutaneous Nephroscope	Mini	15	6	22.5	12	Angled	PANOVIEW rod-lens system
	UMP Nephroscope	Ultra-mini	11	3	26	0	Parallel	N/A
Olympus	OES Pro High Flow Nephroscope	Conventional	25	14.5	23	30	Angled	Rod-lens system
	Mini Nephroscope	Mini	18/20	7.5	22	7	Angled	Rod-lens system

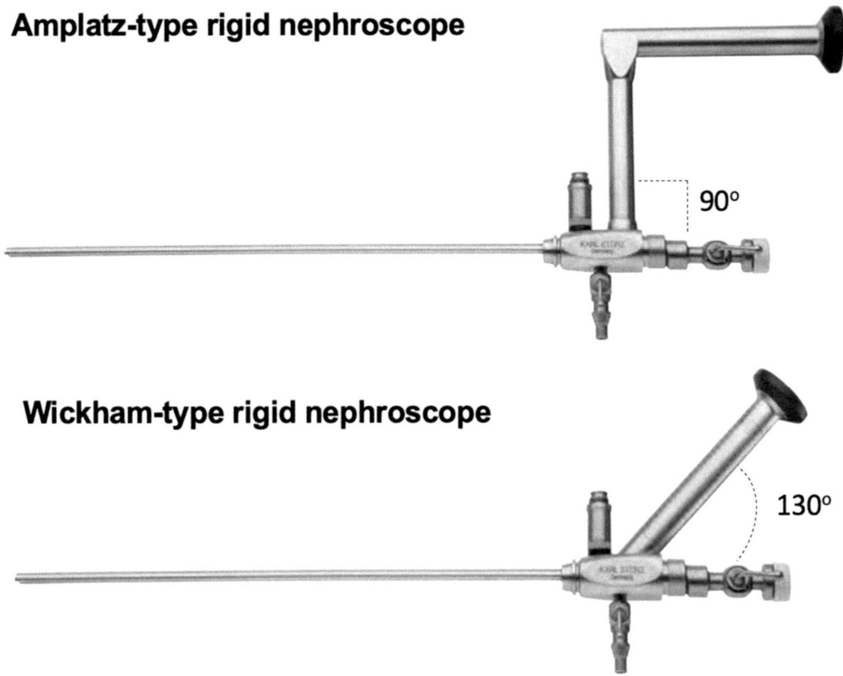

Fig. 5 Rigid nephroscope configuration (Adapted from Karl Storz, Inc.)

Flexible Nephroscopes

Flexible nephroscopy arose as a logical extension of flexible cystoscopy; however, it was of greater need in the kidney than in the bladder given the more complex, convoluted anatomy of the upper urinary tract (Table 2). The original ACMI flexible nephroscope never became widely accepted and thus disappeared from the scene replaced by first the flexible choledochoscope and later by flexible cystoscopes (Wilbur 1981). While the 16Fr size of the flexible cystoscope is perhaps not ideal, it appears to suffice in most circumstances for traversing the infundibulae and as such, to this day, a renal specific nephroscope based on the anatomy of the collecting system has yet to be developed. An endoscope of this nature would ideally have a length of only 25–35 cm, and be equipped with a 12 Fr tip/shaft in order to enter nearly all infundibulae (Clayman et al. 1982).

Miniaturized PCNL: Reducing the Diameter of the Nephrostomy Tract

Performing a percutaneous stone removal in the pediatric population using adult instruments was problematic since the 24 Fr access sheath used in adults was the equivalent of a 72 Fr access sheath when used in the smaller kidney of a child (Jackman et al. 1998). To decrease the morbidity associated with PCNL in the pediatric population, Jackman sought to miniaturize the conventional equipment for percutaneous renal access (Jackman et al. 1998). With stone free rates of 85%

Table 2 Flexible nephroscopes (i.e., cystoscopes)

Manufacturer	Model	Sheath size	Working channel diameter (Fr)	Working channel length (cm)	Deflection (°) (down/up)	Angle of view (°)	Imaging
Karl Storz	Flexible video cystoscope HD-VIEW	16	7	37	140/210	100	Digital-CMOS
	Video cysto-urethroscope C-VIEW®	15.6	7	37	140/210	100	Digital-CMOS
	Cysto-urethro fiberscope	15.5	7	37	140/210	110	Fiberoptic
Richard Wolf	Flexible fiber-urethro-cystoscope	15	7.5	40	150/210	120	Fiberoptic
	MAMBA vision flexible sensor cystoscope	16.2	7.5	40	210/210	110	Digital-N/A
Olympus	HD flexible cysto-nephro videoscope	16.5	6.6	38	130/220	120	Digital-proprietary system
	CYF-V2: VISERA flexible cysto-nephro videoscope	16.2	6.6	38	120/210	120	Digital-CCD
	CYF-5: flexible cysto-nephro fiberscope	16.5	7.2	38	120/210	120	Fiberoptic
ACMI-Gyrus	ACN 2-flexible cystoscope	14.6 (at the tip)	6.4	37	170/180	110	Fiberoptic

achieved in children, it was only natural to extrapolate the use of smaller devices to the adult population. In 2001, findings associated with the use of a miniaturized 12 Fr nephroscope with a 15 Fr Amplatz sheath in a cohort of adult patients were first reported by Lahme et al. (Lahme et al. 2001).

The idea that a smaller tract size would minimize the morbidity and complications associated with PCNL, most specifically bleeding and renal parenchymal injury, has led to further miniaturization of surgical instruments with the evolution of "mini", "ultra-mini" and even "micro" PCNL. Indeed, a multivariate regression analysis by Kukreja et al. revealed that the size of the dilation tract is a significant predictor for blood loss (Kukreja et al. 2004). Whether a smaller nephrostomy tract results in less parenchymal damage is debatable based on studies that compared standard PCNL to mini-PCNL in terms of acute-phase reaction markers as well as histologically-assessed renal scarring showing no difference between the groups (Li et al. 2010; Traxer et al. 2001; Clayman et al. 1987).

Despite the expansion of miniaturized PCNL over the globe, the terms of "mini", "ultra-mini" and "micro"-PCNL have yet to be standardized, as such the terminology overlaps in terms of the size of the access sheath used. (Fig. 6) (Table 1) (Wright et al. 2016). Regardless of the terminology, the miniaturization of the nephroscopes reduces the features available, and the urologist must weigh the real or perceived reduction in morbidity to the ability to render the patient truly stone free (i.e. no fragments). Flexible nephroscopy ability diminishes with reduction in tract size. For sheaths used for a mini-PCNL (13–22 Fr size), the tract size, if 16Fr or larger allows for flexible nephroscopy with the flexible cystoscope. In contrast, the ultra mini-PCNL sheath (11–14 Fr) precludes the use of the flexible cystoscope; however, a flexible ureteroscope can still be employed to examine the renal calyces via the nephrostomy tract. More problematic is the micro-PCNL sheath (4.75 Fr) which precludes antegrade, flexible nephroscopy. The method of stone removal also varies based on nephroscope size as for the micro-PCNL only laser lithotripsy can be performed.

Finally, nephroscope size has been related to the concern of pyelovenous backflow. An intra-pelvic pressure of 30 mmHg is safe in terms of the risk of pyelovenous

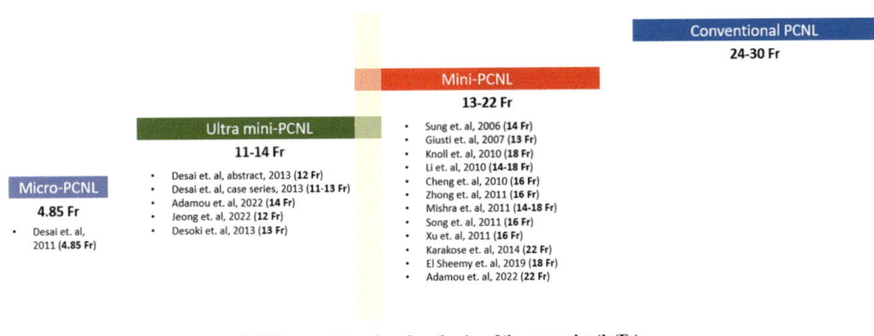

Fig. 6 Percutaneous nephrolithotomy nomenclature based on the size of the access sheath used

backflow and potential for subsequent urosepsis. Given the larger nephroscopes and sheaths, this concern is mitigated. In contrast, with micro-PCNL higher intrapelvic pressures have been noted during all phases of the procedure. This is even more of a concern during the irrigation phase of the procedure (Tepeler et al. 2014; Hinman and Redewill 1926; Mulvaney 1963; Stenberg et al. 1988).

Endoscopic Innovation in PCNL: Vacuum and Needle Endoscopy

In 2008, Udo Nagele introduced a novel approach for mini-PCNL. This technique involved using an 18 Fr metal sheath with a tight-fitting rigid endoscope allowing for removal of stone fragments with a "vacuum cleaner" effect, which occurred as the endoscope was removed from the sheath (Lahme 2020; Nicklas et al. xxxx; Tokas and Nagele 2022). This concept is applied in the Minimally Invasive PCNL (MIP) system from Karl Storz, with the system available in three different sizes: XS/S (7.5 Fr nephroscope outer sheath size), M (12 Fr nephroscope outer sheath size) and L (19.5 Fr nephroscope outer sheath size). Each nephroscope has separate irrigation and working channel ports that combine into a common channel through the body of the nephroscope. A custom, reusable, metallic dilator allows for the metal access sheath to be placed in one (Fig. 7). Stones can be lasered at the tip of or inside of the access sheath as they are sucked out of the body. At the end of the case, a custom applicator can be used to facilitate the placement of hemostatic agents.

Another innovation is the "all-seeing" 4.85 Fr micro-PCNL needle endoscope. In this case the goal is to reduce the stone to dust using the holmium laser. Stone clearance is dependent upon subsequent passive passage of the fragments.

Retrograde Renal Endoscopy During PCNL: Use of the Flexible Ureteroscope

Flexible ureteroscopy is being used more and more often in conjunction with PCNL. On the one hand, it may be used at the outset of the procedure to identify the optimal calyx for entry and then to guide the passage of the nephrostomy needle

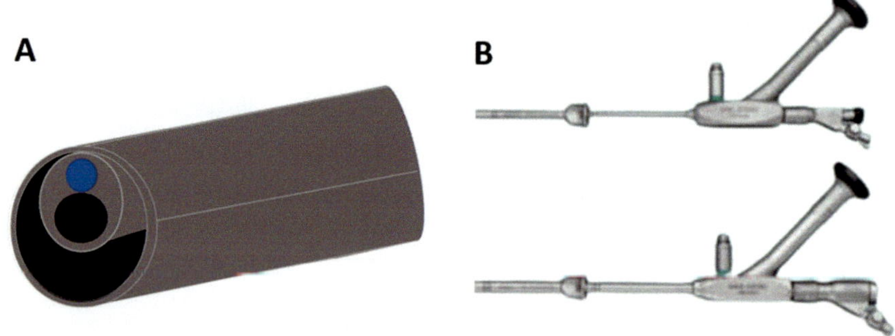

Fig. 7 Minimally Invasive Percutaneous Nephrolithotomy (MIP) system. A-Close-up view of the distal tip of the operating sheath with the nephroscope within it. B-Side views of the MIP-M (upper) and MIP-L (lower) system. (Adapted from Udo Nagele-Minimally Invasive Percutaneous Nephrolitholapaxy (Nagele 2017))

and monitor dilation of the nephrostomy tract. Furthermore, the early passage of the flexible ureteroscope allows the surgeon to more easily secure a through-and-through guidewire (Isac et al. 2013). At the end of the procedure, retrograde ureteroscopy allows for the examination of the calyx juxtaposed to the nephrostomy sheath as well as viewing the area around the sheath itself possibly providing for a higher stone free rate (Widyokirono et al. 2022).

Flexible ureteroscopy has evolved significantly its inception in 1964 by Marshall (Marshall 1964). Subsequent developments brought the benefits of active tip deflection and fiberoptics into play as championed in the late 1980s and 1990s independently in the works of Drs. Bagley, in the United States (Bagley 1987; Grasso M, Bagley 1994), and Aso, in Japan (Aso et al. 1990). In the past 20 years, major advances have occurred in flexible ureteroscopy with the incorporation of CMOS and CCD digital imaging technology and LED light transmission. To date, there has been only one innovation in the realm of multiuse flexible ureteroscopes. Richard Wolf Inc. introduced the first dual channel flexible ureteroscope which allowed for more rapid intraoperative stone clearance and improved stone free rates (Brevik et al. 2022).

The multiuse flexible ureteroscope has been plagued by its excessive fragility, providing the user with an estimate of as few as 15 uses prior to requiring repair (Table 3) (Rindorf et al. 2022). Furthermore, repair of the endoscope has failed to return it to its original state; indeed, after repair, only an average of 11 uses occur before the endoscope again fails (Carey et al. 2006).

The expensive scenario of the multiuse flexible ureteroscope in combination with the inexpensive nature of CMOS and LED technology has led to the rise of a robust market in single use ureteroscopes (Taguchi et al. 2018). Today, in many operating rooms ureteroscopes are treated similar to guidewires and ureteral access sheaths, with the entire lot being disposed at the end of the case (Table 4). Given the transition to a disposable endoscope, there is the opportunity for rapid iteration and the evolution of endoscopes with enhancements to facilitate the performance and the safety of the ureteroscopic procedure. Endoscopes have now been developed that allow for one-handed opening and closure of the stone basket as well as for measuring the pressure in the renal pelvis.

2 Future Directions and Perspectives

The Multifunctional Rigid Endoscope

The Virtuoso System (Virtuoso Surgical, Nashville, TN) incorporates concentric tube technology in its instruments—rigidity is achieved through a series of concentric tubes that are the basis for lateral movement of the arms and force delivered. The result increases tip stiffness enough to handle tissue while leaving space in the lumen for mechanical structures that control articulated instruments (Bergeles et al. 2015). The Virtuoso endoscope has a light source, camera, irrigation system, and a pair of tools

Table 3 Multi-use flexible fiberoptic and digital ureteroscopes

	Tip/Sheath size (Fr)	Working channel diameter (Fr)	Working channel length (cm)	Deflection (down/up) (°)	Angle of view (°)	Imaging
Karl Storz Flex-X^2	6.6/7.5	3.6	67	270/270	88	Fiberoptic
Karl Storz Flex-X^c	8.5 (tip size not specified)	3.6	70	270/270	105	Digital-N/A
Richard Wolf's Boa Vision	6.6/8.7	3.6	68	270/270	90	Digital-N/A
Richard Wolf's Cobra Vision	5.2/9.9	3.6 working channel and 2.4 Fr laser channel	68	270/270	90	Fiberoptic
Richard Wolf's The Cobra	6/9.9	3.3 × 2 (1st flexible 2-channel laser uretero-renoscope)	68	270/270	85	Fiberoptic
Richard Wolf's The Viper	6/9.6	3.6	68	270/270	85	Fiberoptic
Olympus URF-P7 (P7R)	4.9/7.95	3.6	67	275/275	90	Fiberoptic
Olympus URF-P6 (PS6)	4.9/7.95	3.6	67	275/275	90	Fiberoptic
Olympus URF-P5	5.3/8.4	3.6	70	275/180	90	Fiberoptic
Olympus URF-V	8.5/9.9	3.6	67	275/180	90	Digital-CCD
Olympus URF P3	8.1/8.4	3.6	70	180/180	100	Fiberoptic
Olympus URF-V3/V3R	8.5/8.4	3.6	67	275/275	80	Digital-CCD
Stryker Flexvision U500	6.9/7.1	3.6	N/A	275/275	90	Fiberoptic
ACMI-Gyrus AUR-7	7.2/11	3.6	67	120/160	80	Fiberoptic
ACMI-Gyrus DUR 8—Elite	8.7/9.4	3.6	64	270/270	80	Fiberoptic

(continued)

Table 3 (continued)

	Tip/Sheath size (Fr)	Working channel diameter (Fr)	Working channel length (cm)	Deflection (down/up) (°)	Angle of view (°)	Imaging
ACMI-Gyrus DUR 8—Ultra	8.6/9.36	3.6	N/A	270/270	80	Fiberoptic
ACMI-Gyrus DUR D	8.7/9.3	3.6	65	250/250	80	Digital-CMOS

Table 4 Disposable flexible ureteroscopes

	Lithovue (Boston Scientific)	Uscope (Pusen)	Axis (Dornier)	NeoFlex (Neoscope)
Tip (Fr)/Sheath size (Fr)	7.7/9.5	9.0/9.5	8.5/8.5	9.0/9.0
Working channel diameter (Fr)	3.6	3.6	3.6	3.6
Working length (cm)	95.5	65	65	65
Deflection (°)	270/270	270/270	275/275	280/280
Image type (Fiberoptic, CCD, CMOS chip)	CMOS	CMOS	CMOS	CMOS
Light source (Fiberoptic or LED)	LED	Fiberoptic	LED	LED

that allow the surgeon to simultaneously gasp, manipulate, and cut tissue through a port less than 1 cm in diameter (Virtuoso Surgical 2022). To date this technology has been limited to the bladder, but one could easily envision its application during PCNL to provide for simultaneous basketing and laser lithotripsy of a stone.

Robotic Flexible URS (rfURS): An Evolution Toward Robotic PCNL

The age of robotic assisted PCNL is in the process of realization following on the heels of forays into the realm of robotic ureteroscopy (Table 5). In 2011, the Sensei-Magellan robot (Hansen Medical, Mountainview, CA), was first used to perform clinical ureteroscopy (Desai et al. 2011). The Sensei set the standard for rfURS with the robot's ability to improve ergonomics and reduce radiation exposure while offering safe treatment of stones and incorporating an increased range of instrument motion and stability. The Sensei robot and all subsequent rfURS robots function as a master–slave system, similar to the DaVinci (Intuitive Surgical, Sunnyvale, CA, USA) robot. Key features of the Sensei consist of three components: a custom ureteroscope, a single 3D joystick, and multiple video displays for live image, fluoroscopy, and instrument position. The ureteroscope is a 7.5 Fr passive fiberoptic ureteronephroscope that is part of a 10 Fr/12 Fr catheter guide with a 12 Fr/14 Fr outer sheath. Contrary to typical ureteroscope designs, pressurized fluid flows into the body between the ureteroscope and catheter guide and the working channel serves as the outflow conduit. Some disadvantages include the fixed size of the custom ureteroscope, assistants required for instrument management, limited ability to examine the ureter, lack of haptic feedback, and paucity of memory for rapid repositioning (Desai et al. 2008). A clinical study was conducted in 2011 on 18 patients who had a mean renal stone size of 12 mm, half of which were in the lower pole. The stones were basketed and moved to a more favorable position, if necessary, and then laser-fragmented to 1 mm to 2 mm fragments. Mean procedure time was 91 min and the stone free rate was 56% at two months (based on CT). Users had favorable subjective ratings for control, stability, and ease of fragmentation (Desai et al. 2011). Despite these sanguine results, the Sensei robot was not brought to the general Urology market.

The next iteration in rfURS was reported in 2016 with the advent of the Roboflex Avicenna (ELMED, Ankara, Turkey). Key differences from the Sensei included reduction in the footprint of the robot from three units to two, use of universally compatible, off-the-shelf ureteroscopes, two joysticks, a wheel for fine control of flexion, a touch screen monitor, adjustable movement speeds, user-controlled laser fiber and irrigation flow, a memory feature for rapid re-positioning, and force limitation, capping pressure at 1 N/mm^2. The main drawbacks of the Roboflex Avicenna are lack of haptic feedback and the time required to basket stones due to thee need to undock the robot. In clinical studies, 81 patients with a mean stone size of 1296 mm^3 had a total procedure time of 74 min. Overall, 80% of patients were stone-free on plain film radiographs and ultrasound evaluation at three months (Saglam et al. 2014). This robotic system is not currently available for purchase in the United States.

A third robotic system, described by Shu et al. in December of 2021, adds many of the "wish-list" features described in the critiques of prior robotic systems, in particular, haptic feedback. Other features include the ability to control the laser fiber, control the built-in irrigation system, and monitor the intra-renal pressure (Shu et al. 2022). As this robot was unnamed, these authors could not verify that the robot was available for purchase.

In October 2022, Park et al. described a fourth robotic system for ureteroscopy, easyUretero (ROEN Surgical Inc., Daejeon, Korea) that incorporated automated basketing. Other design modifications include a TV remote-like gimbal handle with a preserved wheel to control fine motion (Park et al. 2022). To our knowledge, the easyUretero is not available for clinical implementation in the United States.

PCNL Combined with rfURS

These endoscopic advancements in rfURS are relevant to the future performance of PCNL since endoscopic combined intrarenal surgery (ECIRS) may lead to higher stone-free rates (Gökce et al. 2019). In this regard, Tokatli et al. published a retrospective study utilizing the combination of rfURS and PCNL access with the Roboflex

Table 5 Advances in rfURS systems

Robotic system	Publication year (earliest)	Floor components	Ureteroscope	Human interface	Automated laser and basket control	Irrigation control	Position memory	Unique features	Reference
Sensei	2011	Three	Custom	Single 3D joystick	No	No	No	n/a (initial design)	Desai et al. (2011)
Roboflex	2016	Two	Universal	Two joysticks/ wheel	Yes (laser)/no (basket)	Yes	Yes	Force limit	Saglam et al. (2014); Geavlete et al. (2016); Klein et al. (2021)
Shu robot	2021	Two	Universal	Two haptic devices	Yes (laser)/yes (basket, translational motion)	No	No	AI enhanced haptic feedback, irrigation pressure sensor	Shu et al. (2022); Shu et al. (2021)
easyUretero	2022	Two	Universal	Gimbal handle (TV remote)/ wheel	Yes (laser)/yes (basket, translational motion and open/close)	Yes	Yes	Large stone and UAS contact alarm	Park et al. (2022); Han et al. (2022)

on 42 patients (44 renal units) in what they termed, robot-assisted mini-ECIRS from 2019–2020 for stones that were a mean size of 28 mm. The mini-PCNL was done with a 16.5 Fr access sheath and a 12 Fr mini-nephroscope. Surgeons worked simultaneously both antegrade and retrograde; at the end of the procedure, the calyces were examined with the Roboflex to identify any residual stones. Results were excellent—96% of patients were considered stone-free on CT scan. The authors also noted less of a drop in hemoglobin, and a shorter hospital stay compared to a standard PCNL procedure (Tokatli et al. 2022).

Totally Robotic PCNL: Robotic PCNL Combined with rfURS

The Monarch robot (Ethicon, Johnson and Johnson, Raritan, NJ, USA), originally developed for bronchoscopy procedures, has been modified to combine rfURS with electromagnetic guided renal access and totally robotic control of a percutaneously placed flexible aspiration instrument. The first totally robotic PCNL combined with rfURS was completed on February 7, 2023, at the University of Califiornia, Irvine by Drs. Landman and Desai. The surgeon had the ability to perform simultaneous percutaneous and ureteroscopic tasks (Robotic-Assisted Removal 2023).

Conclusions

Over the past two centuries, the technology applied for endoscopy in PCNL has advanced to encompass flexible endoscopes, digital imaging, LED illumination, and most recently, robotics. Whether PCNL stone surgery will follow the path of prostate surgery into the realm of robotics remains an open question, but clearly the first steps along that path have already been taken.

References

Aso Y, Ohta N, Nakano M, Ohtawara Y, Tajima A, Kawabe K. Treatment of staghorn calculi by fiberoptic transurethral nephrolithotripsy. J Urol. 1990;144(1):17–9.

Bagley DH. Active versus passive deflection in flexible ureteroscopy. J Endourol. 1987;1(1):15–8.

Berci G, Forde KA. History of endoscopy: what lessons have we learned from the past? Surg Endosc. 2000;14(1):5–15.

Bergeles C, Gosline AH, Vasilyev NV, Codd PJ, Del Nido PJ, Dupont PE. Concentric tube robot design and optimization based on task and anatomical constraints. IEEE Trans Robot. 2015;31(1):67–84.

Bloom DA, Morgan RJ, Scardino PL. Thomas Hillier and percutaneous nephrostomy. Urology. 1989;33(4):346–50.

Bohndiek SE, Cook EJ, Arvanitis CD, Olivo A, Royle GJ, Clark AT, et al. A CMOS active pixel sensor system for laboratory-based x-ray diffraction studies of biological tissue. Phys Med Biol. 2008;53(3):655.

Brevik A, Peta A, Okhunov Z, Afyouni AS, Bhatt R, Karani R, et al. Prospective, randomized comparison of dual-lumen versus single-lumen flexible ureteroscopes in proximal ureteral and renal stone management. J Endourol. 2022;36(7):921–6.

Bush RB, Leonhardt H, Bush IV, Landes RR. Dr. Bozzini's Lichtleiter. A translation of his original article (1806). Urology. 1974;3(1):119–23.

Carey RI, Gomez CS, Maurici G, Lynne CM, Leveillee RJ, Bird VG. Frequency of ureteroscope damage seen at a tertiary care center. J Urol. 2006;176(2):607–10; discussion 10.

Clayman RV, Miller RP, Reinke DB, Lange PH. Nephroscopy: advances and adjuncts. Urol Clin North Am. 1982;9(1):51–60.

Clayman RV, Reddy P, Lange PH. Flexible fiberoptic and rigid-rod lens endoscopy of the lower urinary tract: a prospective controlled comparison. J Urol. 1984a;131(4):715–6.

Clayman RV, Hunter D, Surya V, Castaneda-Zuniga WR, Amplatz K, Lange PH. Percutaneous intrarenal electrosurgery. J Urol. 1984b;131(5):864–7.

Clayman RV, Elbers J, Miller RP, Williamson J, McKeel D, Wassynger W. Percutaneous nephrostomy: assessment of renal damage associated with semi-rigid (24F) and balloon (36F) dilation. J Urol. 1987;138(1):203–6.

Cockett WS, Cockett AT. The Hopkins rod-lens system and the Storz cold light illumination system. Urology. 1998;51(5A Suppl):1–2.

Das HH. urologische Erbe: Maximilian Nitze (1848–1906). Seine Bedeutung für die Entwicklung der Urologie [Our urologic heritage: Maximilian Nitze (1848–1906). His importance in the development of urology]. Z Urol Nephrol. 1987;80(9).

Desai MM, Aron M, Gill IS, Pascal-Haber G, Ukimura O, Kaouk JH, et al. Flexible robotic retrograde renoscopy: description of novel robotic device and preliminary laboratory experience. Urology. 2008;72(1):42–6.

Desai MM, Grover R, Aron M, Ganpule A, Joshi SS, Desai MR, et al. Robotic flexible ureteroscopy for renal calculi: initial clinical experience. J Urol. 2011;186(2):563–8.

Di Ieva A, Tam M, Tschabitscher M, Cusimano MD. A journey into the technical evolution of neuroendoscopy. World Neurosurg. 2014;82(6):e777–89.

Fernström I, Johansson B. Percutaneous pyelolithotomy. A new extraction technique. Scand J Urol Nephrol. 1976;10(3):257–9.

Fowler CG. Fibrescope urethrocystoscopy. Br J Urol. 1984;56(3):304–7.

Fowler CG, Badenoch DF, Thakar DR. Practical experience with flexible fibrescope cystoscopy in out-patients. Br J Urol. 1984;56(6):618–21.

Geavlete P, Saglam R, Georgescu D, Mulţescu R, Iordache V, Kabakci AS, et al. Robotic flexible ureteroscopy versus classic flexible ureteroscopy in renal stones: the initial Romanian experience. Chirurgia (bucur). 2016;111(4):326–9.

Gökce M, Gülpinar O, Ibiş A, Karaburun M, Kubilay E, Süer E. Retrograde vs. antegrade fl exible nephroscopy for detection of residual fragments following PNL: a prospective study with computerized tomography control. Int Braz J Urol. 2019;45(3):581–7.

Goodwin WE, Casey WC, Woolf W. Percutaneous trocar (needle) nephrostomy in hydronephrosis. J Am Med Assoc. 1955;157(11):891–4.

Gow JG. Harold Hopkins and optical systems for urology–an appreciation. Urology. 1998;52(1):152–7.

Grasso M, Bagley D. A 7.5/8.2 F actively deflectable, flexible ureteroscope: a new device for both diagnostic and therapeutic upper urinary tract endoscopy. Urology. 1994;43(4):435–41.

Han H, Kim J, Moon YJ, Jung HD, Cheon B, Han J, et al. Feasibility of laser lithotripsy for midsize stones using robotic retrograde intrarenal surgery system easyUretero in a porcine model. J Endourol. 2022;36(12):1586–92.

Hillebrand M, Stevanovic N, Hosticka B, Conde JS, Teuner A, Schwarz M, editors. High speed camera system using a CMOS image sensor. Proceedings of the IEEE intelligent vehicles symposium 2000 (Cat No 00TH8511). IEEE; 2000.

Hillier T. Congenital hydronephrosis in a boy four years old, repeatedly tapped. Recovery Med Chir Trans. 1865;48:73–87.

Hinman F, Redewill FH. Pyelovenous back flow. J Am Med Assoc. 1926;87(16):1287–93.

Hirschowitz BI. Endoscopic examination of the stomach and duodenal cap with the fiberscope. Lancet. 1961;1(7186):1074–8.

Hirschowitz BI. A personal history of the fiberscope. Gastroenterology. 1979;76(4):864–9.

Hirschowitz BI, Balint JA, Fulton WF. Gastroduodenal endoscopy with the fiberscope–an analysis of 500 examinations. Surg Clin North Am. 1962;42:1081–90.

Hopkins HH, Kapany NS. A flexible fibrescope, using static scanning. Nature. 1954;173(4392):39–41.

Isac W, Rizkala E, Liu X, Noble M, Monga M. Endoscopic-guided versus fluoroscopic-guided renal access for percutaneous nephrolithotomy: a comparative analysis. Urology. 2013;81(2):251–6.

Jackman SV, Hedican SP, Peters CA, Docimo SG. Percutaneous nephrolithotomy in infants and preschool age children: experience with a new technique. Urology. 1998;52(4):697–701.

Jorden PR, Jordan D, Jerram PA, Pratlong J, Swindells I, editors. e2v new CCD and CMOS technology developments for astronomical sensors. High energy, optical, and infrared detectors for astronomy VI; 2014: SPIE.

Kempainen S. CMOS image sensors: eclipsing CCDs in visual information? EDN. 1997;42(21):101–10.

Klein J, Charalampogiannis N, Fiedler M, Wakileh G, Gözen A, Rassweiler J. Analysis of performance factors in 240 consecutive cases of robot-assisted flexible ureteroscopic stone treatment. J Robot Surg. 2021;15(2):265–74.

Kukreja R, Desai M, Patel S, Bapat S, Desai M. First prize: factors affecting blood loss during percutaneous nephrolithotomy: prospective study. J Endourol. 2004;18(8):715–22.

Lahme S, Bichler K-H, Strohmaier WL, Götz T. Minimally invasive PCNL in patients with renal pelvic and calyceal stones. Eur Urol. 2001;40(6):619–24.

Lahme S. Minimal-invasive PCNL (mini-PCNL). Percutaneous nephrolithotomy; 2020. p. 137–49.

Lau WY, Leow CK, Li AK. History of endoscopic and laparoscopic surgery. World J Surg. 1997;21(4):444–53.

Leadbetter WF. Instrumental visualization of the renal pelvis at operation as an aid to diagnosis. Presentation of a new instrument*. J Urol. 1950;63(6):1006–12.

Lee ACH, Elson DS, Neil MA, Kumar S, Ling BW, Bello F, et al. Solid-state semiconductors are better alternatives to arc-lamps for efficient and uniform illumination in minimal access surgery. Surg Endosc. 2009;23(3):518–26.

Li LY, Gao X, Yang M, Li JF, Zhang HB, Xu WF, et al. Does a smaller tract in percutaneous nephrolithotomy contribute to less invasiveness? A prospective comparative study. Urology. 2010;75(1):56–61.

Liang RB. Wash. Society of photo-optical instrumentation engineers. Optical design for biomedical imaging. SPIE Press; 2010.

Maciolek KA, Best SL. History of Optics in endourology. In: Patel SR, Moran ME, Nakada SY, editors. The History of technologic advancements in urology. Cham: Springer; 2018. p. 21–35.

Marshall VF. Fiber optics in urology. J Urol. 1964;91:110–4.

Moran ME. The light bulb, cystoscopy, and Thomas Alva Edison. J Endourol. 2010;24(9):1395–7.

Morgenthal CB, Richards WO, Dunkin BJ, Forde KA, Vitale G, Lin E. The role of the surgeon in the evolution of flexible endoscopy. Surg Endosc. 2007;21(6):838–53.

Mulțescu R, Georgescu D, Geavlete PA, Geavlete B. Chapter 2—equipment and instruments in percutaneous nephrolithotomy. In: Geavlete PA, editor. Percutaneous surgery of the upper urinary tract. San Diego: Academic Press; 2016. p. 3–24.

Mulvaney WP. The hydrodynamics of renal irrigations: with reference to calculus solvents. J Urol. 1963;89(6):765–8.

Nagele U. Minimally invasive percutaneous nephrolitholapaxy (MIP). Endo Press; 2017.

Natalin RA, Landman J. Where next for the endoscope? Nat Rev Urol. 2009;6(11):622–8.

Nicholson P. Problems encountered by early endoscopists. Urology. 1982;19(1):114–9.

Nicklas AP, Schilling D, Bader MJ, Herrmann TR, Nagele U, Training, et al. The vacuum cleaner effect in minimally invasive percutaneous nephrolitholapaxy. World J Urol. 2015;33:1847–53.

Park J, Gwak CH, Kim D, Shin JH, Lim B, Kim J, et al. The usefulness and ergonomics of a new robotic system for flexible ureteroscopy and laser lithotripsy for treating renal stones. Investig Clin Urol. 2022;63(6):647–55.

Patel SR, Nakada SY. The modern history and evolution of percutaneous nephrolithotomy. J Endourol. 2015;29(2):153–7.

Ramai D, Zakhia K, Etienne D, Reddy M. Philipp Bozzini (1773–1809): the earliest description of endoscopy. J Med Biogr. 2018;26(2):137–41.

Rindorf DK, Tailly T, Kamphuis GM, Larsen S, Somani BK, Traxer O, et al. Repair rate and associated costs of reusable flexible ureteroscopes: a systematic review and meta-analysis. Eur Urol Open Sci. 2022;37:64–72.

Robotic-assisted removal of kidney stones for first patient using MONARCH platform for urology [press release]. Ethicon, Johnson and Johnson surgical technologies 2023 Feb 07.

Rupel E, Brown RS. Nephroscopy with removal of stone following nephrostomy for obstructive calculous anuria. J Urol. 1941;46:177–82.

Saglam R, Muslumanoglu AY, Tokatlı Z, Caşkurlu T, Sarica K, Taşçi A, et al. A new robot for flexible ureteroscopy: development and early clinical results (IDEAL stage 1–2b). Eur Urol. 2014;66(6):1092–100.

Shah J. Endoscopy through the ages. BJU Int. 2002;89(7):645–52.

Shu X, Chen Q, Xie L. A novel robotic system for flexible ureteroscopy. Int J Med Robot. 2021;17(1):1–11.

Shu X, Hua P, Wang S, Zhang L, Xie L. Safety enhanced surgical robot for flexible ureteroscopy based on force feedback. Int J Med Robot. 2022;18(5): e2410.

Stenberg A, Bohman SO, Morsing P, Müller-Suur C, Olsen L, Persson A. Back-leak of pelvic urine to the bloodstream. Acta Physiol Scand. 1988;134(2):223–34.

Taguchi K, Usawachintachit M, Tzou DT, Sherer BA, Metzler I, Isaacson D, et al. Micro-costing analysis demonstrates comparable costs for LithoVue compared to reusable flexible fiberoptic ureteroscopes. J Endourol. 2018;32(4):267–73.

Tejas R, Macherla P, Shylashree N. Image sensor—CCD and CMOS. Microelectronics, communication systems, machine learning and internet of things: select proceedings of MCMI 2020. Springer; 2022. p. 455–84.

Tepeler A, Akman T, Silay MS, Akcay M, Ersoz C, Kalkan S, et al. Comparison of intrarenal pelvic pressure during micro-percutaneous nephrolithotomy and conventional percutaneous nephrolithotomy. Urolithiasis. 2014;42:275–9.

Tokas T, Nagele U. Intrarenal pressure, fluid management, and hydrodynamic stone retrieval in mini-PCNL. Minimally invasive percutaneous nephrolithotomy: Springer; 2022. p. 181–90.

Tokatli Z, Ibis MA, Sarica K. Robot-assisted mini-endoscopic combined intrarenal surgery for complex and multiple calculi: What are the real advantages? J Laparoendosc Adv Surg Tech A. 2022;32(8):890–5.

Trattner HR. Instrumental visualization of the renal pelvis and its communications: proposal of a new method; preliminary report[1]. J Urol. 1948;60(6):817–34.

Traxer O, Smith TG 3rd, Pearle MS, Corwin TS, Saboorian H, Cadeddu JA. Renal parenchymal injury after standard and mini percutaneous nephrostolithotomy. J Urol. 2001;165(5):1693–5.

Virtuoso Surgical I. Device promotion material; 2022. Available from: https://virtuososurgical.net/technology/.

Widyokirono DR, Kloping YP, Hidayatullah F, Rahman ZA, Ng AC-F, Hakim L. Endoscopic combined intrarenal surgery vs percutaneous nephrolithotomy for large and complex renal stone: a systematic review and meta-analysis. J Endourol. 2022;36(7):865–76.

Wilbur HJ. The flexible choledochoscope: a welcome addition to the urologic armamentarium. J Urol. 1981;126(3):380–1.

Wright A, Rukin N, Smith D, De la Rosette J, Somani BK. 'Mini, ultra, micro'—nomenclature and cost of these new minimally invasive percutaneous nephrolithotomy (PCNL) techniques. Ther Adv Urol. 2016;8(2):142–6.

Zada G, Liu C, Apuzzo ML. "Through the looking glass": optical physics, issues, and the evolution of neuroendoscopy. World Neurosurg. 2013;79(2 Suppl):S3-13.

Zajaczkowski T, Zamann AP. Julius Bruck (1840–1902) and his influence on the endoscopy of today. World J Urol. 2004;22(4):293–303.
Zheludev N. The life and times of the LED—a 100-year history. Nat Photonics. 2007;1(4):189–92.

Ancillary Devices for Percutaneous Nephrolithotomy

M. Binbay, F. Sendogan, and F. Yanaral

Abstract Urolithiasis is one of the most common urologic diseases with an increasing incidence and prevalence. There are various minimally invasive surgical techniques used in the treatment of urolithiasis. Percutaneous nephrolithotomy (PNL) is a well-defined procedure in the treatment of large and complex kidney stones with a high stone-free rate. The main purpose of percutaneous nephrolithotomy, as in all stone surgeries, is to provide complete stone clearance with minimal morbidity. For this, a variety of ancillary devices are employed. In the world of medicine, there are always new innovations and tools making their way to the forefront every year. Technique and instrumentation advances have been made over time to reduce morbidity and increase efficacy in PNL. In this section, we reviewed the ancillary devices used in PNL.

Keywords Urolithiasis · Percutaneous nephrolithotomy · Kidney stone · Ancillary devices

1 Introduction

In 1976, Fernström et al. succeeded in removing stones from the renal pelvis by creating a percutaneous canal, using a nephroscope and a stone basket, and described the PNL technique Fernström and Johansson (1976). This landmark publication paved the way for the development of endourology. From the past to the present, the PNL technique has developed rapidly. Currently, PNL is a well-known, widely accepted and innovative minimally invasive surgical procedure stone removal within urological procedures. The current European Association of Urology guidelines

M. Binbay (✉) · F. Sendogan
School of Medicine, Department of Urology, Bahcesehir University, Istanbul, Turkey
e-mail: muratbinbay@yahoo.com

F. Yanaral
School of Medicine, Department of Urology, Arel University, Istanbul, Turkey

© The Author(s), under exclusive license to Springer Nature Switzerland AG 2023   335
J. D. Denstedt and E. N. Liatsikos (eds.), *Percutaneous Renal Surgery*,
https://doi.org/10.1007/978-3-031-40542-6_23

recommend PNL as first-line therapy for complex and larger than 2 cm kidney stones Skolarikos et al. (2022).

The main goal of PNL is to achieve maximal stone clearance with minimal morbidity. The key to stone clearance is to use a correct surgical technique and appropriate expertise and instrumentation provided by up-to-date technology. In this section, ancillary devices for PNL surgical steps such as access, tract dilatation, stone fragmentation, stone removal will be discussed.

2 Instruments for Access/Puncture

The optimal access should be planned preoperatively according to the characteristics of the stone, the anatomy of the collecting system, and the location of adjacent organs Yu et al. (2018). Whether in the prone, supine, or modified positions, obtaining adequate access to the renal collecting system is the general principle to performing successful PNL. Imaging modalities are the most important key providing access. However, the ancillary access devices are just as important as the imaging modalities. Ancillary devices providing access in PNL are discussed in this section.

2.1 Needle Holder

During PNL operations, the surgeon's hands are the most exposed to radiation. Needle holder is designed to prevent the hands from being directly exposed to radiation during the puncture procedure. In addition, while accessing under C arm fluoroscopy particularly using bull-eye technique, a much better view is obtained if a needle holder is used as the hands will stay away from the operation area. The silicone insert holds the needle in place while preventing the stylet from backing out of the cannula during introduction. The silicone inserts are designed to accommodate an 18 gauge trocar needle and a 22 gauge Chiba needle.

2.2 Needles

Standard options for an access needle are a 21 gauge and 18 gauge needle. A guide wire of 0.018 inch and 0.035 inch is passed through these needles, respectively. The needles used for accessing the pyelocaliceal system consist of two or three pieces. The central mandrel has oblique edges and exceeds the external sheath in length. After removing the central part, the tip is often cut straight to avoid damaging the wall of the upper urinary tract Mulţescu et al. (2016).

The advantage of the 21 gauge needle is that it causes relatively minor injuries as it passes through tissue. Multiple accesses can be made due to the low risk of needle-related hemorrhage. However, in patients with scarred kidneys or obese patients, the 21 gauge needle does not adequately protect trajectory. A thicker 18 gauge needle should be preferred in these patients. In addition, a 0.018 inch guidewire passing through a 21 gauge needle may not provide sufficient stability for subsequent tract dilatation or catheter placement. In this case it should be replaced with a standard 0.035 inch guidewire. This requires an extra step, which adds to the complexity of the procedure and increases the risk for access failure.

The impact of puncture needles on bleeding complications of PNL is often ignored. Actually, the conventional needle tip used in standard PNL is sharp and can easily injure the renal vessels. In a study by Sampaio et al. reported that the interlobar or segmental artery was injured in 13.6–26.5% of patients in punctures performed with an 18 gauge needle Sampaio et al. (1992). Bleeding risk is less in blunt surgeries due to the elastic structure of major arteries. The majority of devices used in PNL are blunt-tipped due to possible major injuries. Based on these ideas, Hou et al. provided the first proposal of the concept of blunt puncture in PNL. The blunt needle consists of two parts, a blunt needle core and a needle sheath Hou et al. (2022). The tip of the needle core looked like an elongated semi-ellipsoid. The distal end of the needle sheath was designed with dense echo holes, and the needle sheath was marked with a scale line to enable real-time monitoring and allow the depth of needle penetration to be determined by ultrasound (Fig. 1).

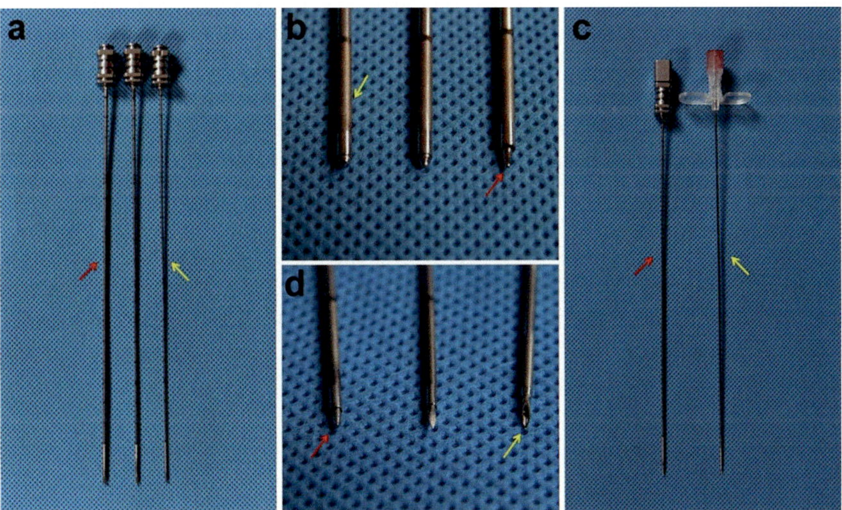

Fig. 1 Characteristics of the needles. **a** 16-gauge (red arrow), 17-gauge and 18-gauge (yellow arrow) needle sheaths. **b** Needle core tips with three different degrees of bluntness (red arrow); echo holes (yellow arrow). **c** The selected blunt needle (red arrow) and conventional needle (yellow arrow). **d** The tips of the selected blunt needle (red arrow), auxiliary sharp needle and conventional needle (yellow arrow)

Visibility of needles differs between fluoroscopy-guided access and ultrasound-guided access. In fluoroscopic access, the needle is only visible during fluoroscopy. Echotip needle provides enhanced visualization of needle tip when used with ultrasonic access Alken (2022). The Echotip needle typically consists of a blunt 1.3 mm diameter cannula with a special grid for enhanced ultrasound reflection and a 1.0 mm diameter stylet with a diamond-shaped cutting tip van Gerwen (2014).

2.3 Guidewires

The usage of guidewires is a cornerstone in the field of endourology. In urology, guidewires are generally used for two main purposes: to access the upper urinary tract and to serve as navigation tools for catheters, stents, ureteral access sheaths, and endoscopes Clayman et al. (2004). Each guidewire is designed with different structural features to perform certain surgical procedures. Guidewires used for percutaneous access traditionally have soft J-shaped ends to reduce the risk of peripheral injury and perforation. The diameters of the guide wires range from 0.018 inches to 0.039 inches. However, thin guide wires can be deformed more easily and cannot navigate to ureter. Therefore, radiopaque hybrid guidewires, combination of hydrophilic flexible tip with stiff nitinol core, are more preferred for initial access to pelvicalyceal system. Hybrid guidewires facilitates passage beyond obstructions and negotiates tortuous anatomy with the hydrophilic flexible tip as well as provides enhanced instrumentation and device placement (Fig. 2). Whole hydrophilic coated guidewires are less frequently used during percutaneous procedures due to the increased risk of extraction or easy displacement. Mulțescu et al. (2016) Loach smooth polytetrafluoroethylene (PTFE) guidewires can be used by surgeons who have cost concerns. However, faulty placement of loach wire is common during percutaneous nephrolithotomy, resulting in incorrect dilation and complications Ding et al. (2023).

Dilation of the puncture tract is usually performed on 0.038–0.039 inch guidewires with increased axial rigidity LeRoy et al. (2006). The Amplatz super-stiff wire® (Boston Scientific Microvasive, USA) is one such example. Amplatz Super Stiff guidewire is made up of PTFE coated superstiff shaft. The rigidity of the flat wire design allows advancement of drive instruments such as dilation catheters and ureteral access sheaths Kolvatzis et al. (2022). In this way, dilatation of the percutaneous nephrolithotomy tract is facilitated.

2.4 Angled Catheters

An angled catheter is often preferred after obtaining access to pelvicaliceal system whenever the guidewire is unable to reach a desired calyx or ureter. It is useful for negotiating the guidewire around an obstructing stone of the calyx or for directing the guidewire towards ureter. Angled catheters are usually designed in single lumen,

Fig. 2 Sensor® Guidewire (Boston-Scientific Microvasive, USA) is one of the examples of hybrid guidewires

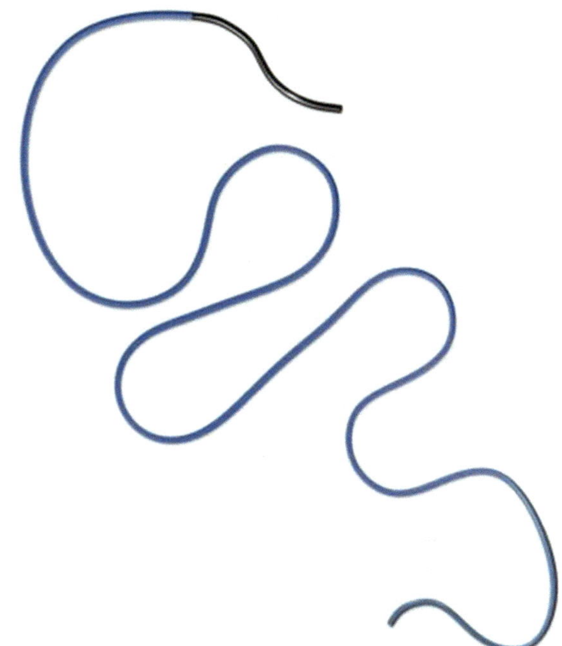

composed of radioopac materials and a 45° angled tip. Kumpe catheter® (Cook Medical, USA) and Imager™ II (Boston Scientific Microvasive, USA) are brand examples of angled catheters.

2.5 *Dual Lumen Catheters*

A dual lumen catheter is an indispensable instrument in the urologist's toolkit, provides two important functions during percutaneous nephrolithotomy. Firstly, dual lumen catheter is placed in kidney on the guidewire located in the kidney and through the second lumen a contrast media injection system allows the surgeon to accurately visualize the pelvicalyceal system and location of the stone under a fluoroscopic image. Secondly, a safety guidewire can be placed in the pelvicalyceal system where the initial guidewire is located.

3 Dilation Instruments

Tract dilation is one of the crucial steps in PNL, and it is mandatory to create a safe and effective percutaneous tract. Various techniques (Balloon dilation, Amplatz dilation) for establishing a percutaneous tract have been defined. Studies have shown that as tract diameter increases, the probability of bleeding in PNL increases Akman et al. (2011). For this reason, over the years, the technique has evolved to include instruments with smaller tracts. PNL operations are classified as standard, mini, ultra-mini and micro PNL according to the tract diameter created. The surgeon should decide which size tract to use in a balance by considering the patient's stone load, estimated operation time, and the patient's anatomical structure.

3.1 Nephrostomy Balloon Catheter

Nephrostomy balloon dilation catheter is designed for radial dilatation of nephrostomy tract in a single step over a guidewire. Radiopaque marker band on the tip of balloon catheter guides navigation and assure the correct placement. After inflation of balloon to manufacturer's proposed pressure, working sheath is placed under fluoroscopic view. If a balloon dilator is preferred, surgeon should be sure that a high-pressure inflation device is present in the operating room. Kit forms of balloon dilators includes the inflator device.

The use of a balloon catheter shortens the duration of fluoroscopy and dilatation Tepeler et al. (2009). It provides convenience to the surgeon by providing a single-step tract dilation in hypermobile kidneys. On the other hand, in patients who had previous kidney surgeries, balloon dilators could fail to create a tract because of low burst pressure at 17 ATM. In recent years, this problem has been solved with the introduction of new nephrostomy balloon catheters that apply higher inflation force up to 20–30 atm pressure (Fig. 3).

Different sizes of balloon catheters (18Fr, 24 Fr, 30Fr) and catheters with longer balloon and working sheath length for obese patients are available in the market. Renal sheath is available in PTFE and Clear materials. Clear Renal Sheath facilitates visualization of calculi surrounding the sheath.

3.2 Amplatz Type Renal Dilator

The Amplatz Renal Dilator is a set of firm dilators, used for sequential dilatation of the nephrostomy tract. The Amplatz Renal Dilator works by progressively expanding the desired calyces. Initially 8 Fr stylet is placed in the pelvicalyceal system over the guidewire; following progressive dilation is performed over 8 Fr stylet. Graduated dilator set includes 12 dilators (8F to 30F) and 8 Fr stylet. The Amplatz Renal Dilator

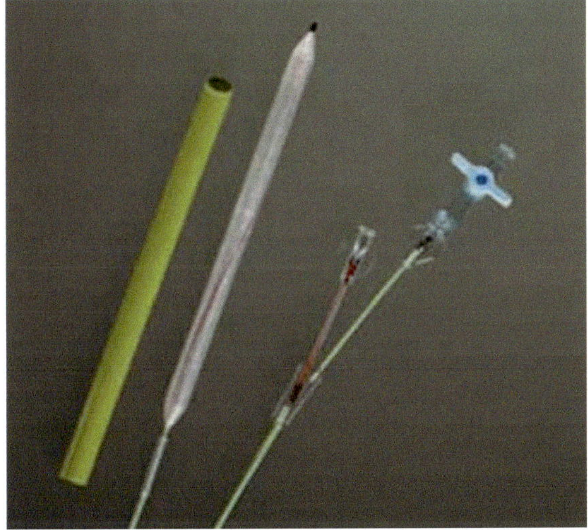

Fig. 3 X-Force® N30 high pressure nephrostomy balloon catheter

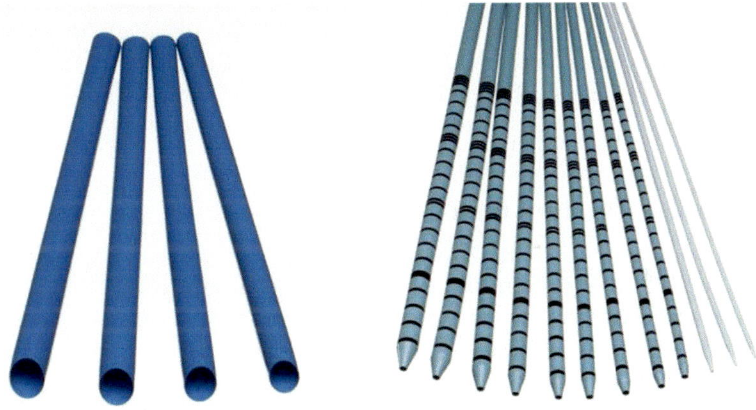

Fig. 4 Different sizes of Amplat sheath dilators and percutaneous access sheaths

set also includes various sizes of Amplatz sheaths from 24 to 30 Fr (Fig. 4). Moreover, smaller sizes Amplatz sheaths from 14 to 24 Fr is available in the market. The diversity in dilator sizes allows for individualized dilatation, considering anatomical characteristics of the patients and stone size.

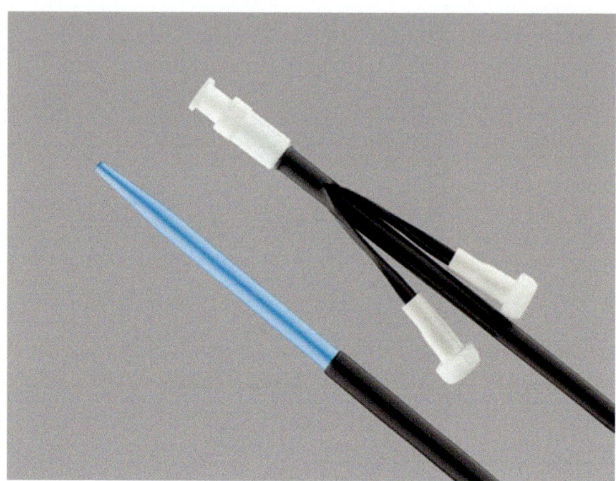

Fig. 5 Peel-Away®
Introducer Set

3.3 Peel Away Introducer

Another option in tract dilation has been the introduction of the pathway access sheath (PAS), a device that allows for tract dilation and sheath placement at the same time for mini PNL. Peel Away introducer has a 32 cm, relatively longer working sheath. Various diameters of Peel-Away® Introducer (Cook) in 9 Fr, 10 Fr and 12 Fr are available in the market (Fig. 5).

4 Stone Extraction Instruments

Many ureteroscopic instruments are especially applicable to PNL when a flexible scope is inserted; however, percutaneous access also enables various unique stone-removal techniques. During the procedure, a variety of stone instruments are used to effectively remove the stones. Stone extraction baskets and stone-grasping forceps are the tools used in PNL for stone extraction. They can be rigid (thicker and more robust) or flexible (typically of a lower caliber and imply more fragile). The flexible ones can be used on flexible as well as rigid nephroscopes. In comparison to the retrograde approach, the flexible nephroscope with wider working channel allows for the insertion of instruments of a higher caliber, which are both more durable and more effective at extracting stones.

4.1 Forceps

Alligator forceps, tripod (or tetrapod) graspers, and smooth graspers are the three main types of rigid extractors. The profile of the alligator forceps' jaws allows for

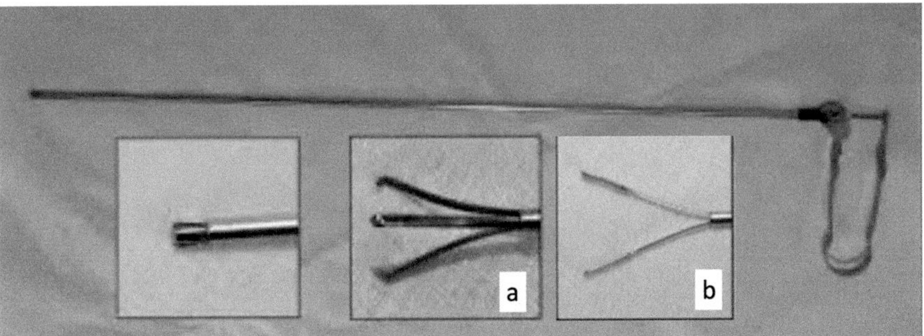

Fig. 6 Tripod grasper (a) and grasper with smooth jaws (b)

a firm hold on the stone fragments. However, because of the scissors-like way they open, they need space around the stones, and if more pressure is put on the actioning mechanism, it becomes relatively brittle. The jaws' significant force makes it possible for stones with a reduced consistency to fragment uncontrollably. Alligator graspers with curved jaws that define a small space between them can be used for these kinds of stones.

Tripod graspers have three sturdy arms with curved, claw-like ends (Fig. 6). They are among the most effective extracting tools, having a firm hold on the fragments while only requiring a small opening space. The walls of the pyelocaliceal system can be easily penetrated by the arms' thin and rough ends, though. Additionally, there are four-arm graspers, which are thought to be less effective.

Smooth graspers rarely manage to get a strong grip. Additionally, their full opening implies that they protrude from the extractor's working channel and exterior sheath, which is another reason it must be done carefully to avoid damaging the tissues. A movement of anteriorly pushing the instrument must be combined with that of closing the jaws, as in the case of the tripod, to ensure that the stone is caught.

The distal portion of a basket probe and a grasper's actioning mechanism are combined in the Cook Medical Perc N Circle®. Squeezing a handle causes a lightweight 10 F probe to release a 2 cm, tipless basket. The tipless design of the Perc NCircle is positioned directly against the mucosal lining with minimal trauma. In bleeding cases Perc NCircle is a unique instrument for safely removal of blood clots. Perc NCircle® has a special design, opening the basket with an angle of 45° allows to safely collect small stones in the calyx that cannot be reached with a rigid nephroscope. A tripod grasping forceps and the Perc NCircle were compared, and it was discovered that the Perc NCircle had a quicker stone extraction time. Additionally, it was linked to a lower chance of dislodging the percutaneous access sheath Hoffman et al. (2004). Subsequently, the Perc N Compass and Perc N Gage, which have different basket models, have been added to the Perc extractor line (Fig. 7).

The PerkX Stone Extractor (Rocamed) is a 10 Fr basket catheter with nitinol 4 wires and a tipless design. Its ergonomic handle and Tuohy Borst connected design allow for efficient insertion of a 272 μm fiber. The tipless basket of PerkX enables direct positioning against the mucosal lining during procedures. It offers both stone

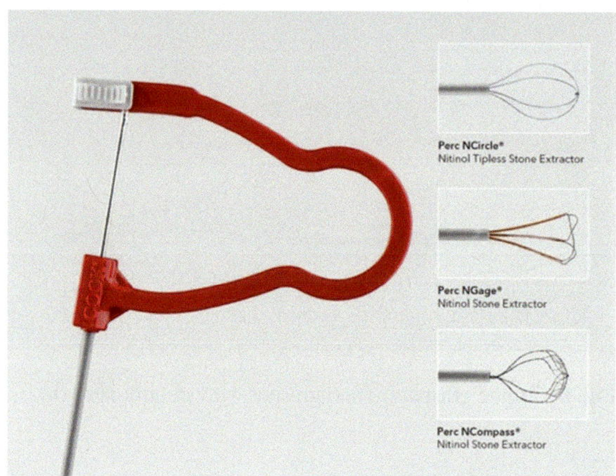

Fig. 7 Perc nitinol stone extractors

fixation and laser lithotripsy, with the possibility for stone displacement particularly in hydronephrotic systems.

Graspers are good for obtaining a strong grip on stones and for removing large fragments. However, they can be difficult to use in smaller spaces and may cause tissue damage. Baskets, on the other hand, are useful for capturing small stones and fragments. They are gentle on tissue and cause less trauma. However, they are not as effective at gripping larger stones and may cause fragmentation.

4.2 Basket Catheters

Basket catheter, also known as a stone retrieval basket, is a small wire mesh device designed to capture and remove stone fragments. There are different types of basket catheters used in PNL. Old baskets were made of stainless steel and could be reused. Nitinol, a metal alloy made of titanium and nickel, is used in modern baskets so that the surgeon can remove stones more successfully and with less trauma. They are all single-use, and due to their various sizes, shapes, and designs, the surgeon can use them in different situations. 4.5 French baskets are utilized in larger scopes with wider working channels, such as flexible cystoscopes and mini-nephroscopes. Tipped baskets are not preferred for PNL as tip of the basket may damage the urothelial lining and cause bleeding.

There are two different categories of baskets for PNL: tipless baskets and special design baskets.

Tipless Baskets

They are typically made of four nitinol wires with twisted or flower design to increase the radial dilating force while minimizing trauma to the urothelium. In addition, they frequently have the ability to alter the calyx's shape and access stones that may be just beyond the endoscope's tip's reach. They are the most widely used across the globe because of the design, which enables the surgeon to use it in a variety of settings without risking a traumatic tip effect. French sizes range from 1.3 to 4.5.

Bard (1.9/2.4/3.0 Fr), Boston Scientific (1.9/2.4/3.0 Fr), Cogentix Medical/ Laborie (1.3/1.9/2.2 Fr), Coloplast (1.5/2.2/3 Fr, twisted wire with flower design), Cook (1.5/2.2/3.0/4.5 Fr), Olympus (1.8/2.2/3.0 Fr, twisted wires to maintain shape, rotation control handle), Sacred Heart (1.5/2.4 Fr, with rotation control handle) are the manufacturers of 4-wire round tipless baskets. There are also manufacturers of unique tipless baskets, such as Olympus (1.8/2.2/3.0 Fr, cross-paired wires for increased radial dilating force, rotatable handle) and Sacred Heart (1.5 Fr, 6-wire round).

There are some front-opening, tipless special baskets. These baskets are useful in some situations where the surgeon wants to catch the stone from the front with wires closing from the laterals. When you are in front of the stone and want to simply catch and release it (for instance, to move it from the inferior to the superior calyx), this is incredibly helpful. French sizes are range from 1.7 to 2.2. Manufacturers of tipless end engaging baskets include Cook (1.7/2.2 Fr) and Boston Scientific (1.9 Fr, OpenSure handle capable of secondary opening to ensure release).

Special Design Baskets

There are also some special design baskets. Bard has 2.4/3.0 Fr baskets with articulated basket position at handle. The 2.6/3.3 Fr basket from Boston Scientific has serrated nitinol wire edges and is shaped like a grasping forceps. Cook's 1.5/2.4 Fr basket has a 16-wire mesh construction that is intended for retrieving small stone fragments. It is recommended that urologists who frequently perform endoscopic stone surgery to have a variety of stone extraction instruments in their armamentarium.

5 Instruments for Preventing Complication

5.1 Ureteral Occlusion Device

Ureteral occlusion devices are used during percutaneous nephrolithotomy (PNL) to prevent the migration of stone fragments into the ureter and to facilitate stone clearance. These devices can be used when there is a risk of larger stone fragments being created during the PNL or when there is concern that smaller fragments may migrate into the ureter and cause obstruction. By blocking the ureter, the catheter allows for the safe use of nephroscopy and laser lithotripsy. The catheter is typically removed at the end of the PNL procedure.

Ureteral occlusion balloons are inflatable devices typically made of silicone or latex, which are temporarily placed within the ureter to block its lumen. Once inflated, the balloon prevents stone fragments from passing into the ureter. It is important to note that the choice of an occlusion device depends on several factors, including the size and location of the stone, the patient's anatomy, and the surgeon's experience and preferences. Additionally, not all PNL procedures require the use of ureteral occlusion devices, and their use may be determined on a case-by-case basis.

There are several types of ureteral occlusion balloons available in the market: Cook Ureteral Balloon Catheter, Bard Ureteral Balloon Catheter, Boston Scientific Occluder™ Occlusion Balloon Catheter, Coloplast Ureteral Balloon Catheter, Teleflex Ureteral Catheter, Olympus Balloon Catheter (Fig. 8).

There are advantages and disadvantages to the use of ureteral balloon occlusion devices. The device can be placed quickly and is easy to use. It reduces the risk of stone migration by providing good occlusion. Whereas the balloon may cause irritation or injury to the ureter or renal pelvis. There is a risk of balloon rupture, which can lead to complications. In some cases, it may be difficult to achieve adequate occlusion with the balloon device.

While the types of ureteral occlusion balloons used in PNL are not directly compared, the studies show that the success of the ureteral occlusion balloons used in PNL is related to the size of the stones. A review article published in 2021 provides guidance on the optimal use of ureteral occlusion catheters based on patient and stone characteristics, as well as the surgeon's preference and experience Sadiq et al. (2021).

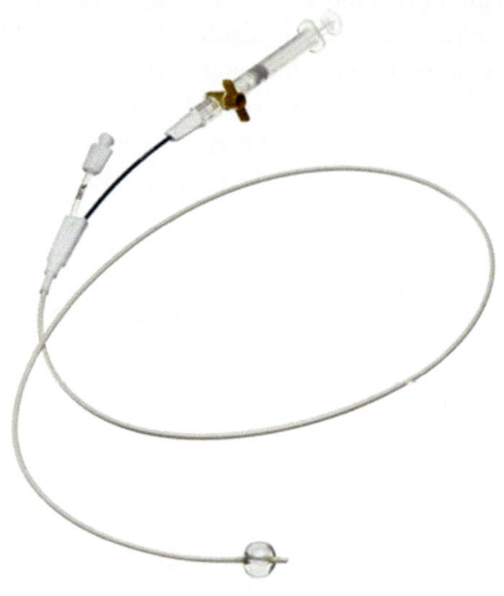

Fig. 8 Boston scientific occluder™ occlusion balloon catheter

The importance of careful patient selection, appropriate catheter placement, and close intraoperative monitoring to minimize the risk of complications was emphasized by the authors. The decision should be made after careful consideration of the risks and benefits.

Another occlusion device is the Accordion Stone Management Device, a microcatheter-based tool with a hydrophilic coating that creates an occlusion to stop stone fragments from being retropelled. During ureteroscopic lithotripsy, its effectiveness at preventing retrograde fragment migration has been well described Ahmed et al. (2009). Retrospective evaluating of the Accordion®'s capacity to stop antegrade stone migration during PNL was conducted by Wosnitzer et al. (2009). Comparatively, 17 patients (57%) in the control group and 13 patients (43%) in the Accordion® group needed ureteral stenting (there is a statistically significant difference). This device is comparable to the majority of conventional ureteral balloon occlusion devices and appears to be effective in preventing stone migration. However, it is unknown if this device increases stone free rates.

5.2 *Tamponade Balloon Device*

Serious bleeding requiring blood transfusion is seen 3–20% of PNL cases. Since most of the bleedings are due to venous injuries, applying pressure on the percutaneous tract would undoubtedly control the bleeding.

Kaye tamponade balloon device is an instrument produced by Cook company. It is a 14 Fr radiopaque balloon catheter; 15 cm length balloon reaches 12 mm (36 Fr) diameter when inflated. The balloon is able to withstand an inflation pressure of 2.5 atm.

In case of serious hemorrhage from the percutaneous tracts 18Fr or larger, placing a Kaye tamponade balloon catheter not only immediately tamponades the nephrostomy tract but effectively drains the renal pelvis, while maintaining ureteral access.

6 Conclusion

PNL is one of the most important options in the treatment of kidney stones. Nowadays, PNL is performed with high success and lower complication rates due to newly developed techniques, combining different types of surgery, and increasing experience among urologists. The use of high quality and advanced products in PNL surgeries, as well as the fact that urologists know which product to use at what stage is one of the subjective criteria affecting the safety of surgery.

References

Ahmed M, Pedro RN, Kieley S, Akornor JW, Durfee WK, Monga M. Systematic evaluation of ureteral occlusion devices: insertion, deployment, stone migration, and extraction. Urology. 2009;73(5):976–80.

Akman T, Binbay M, Sari E, Yuruk E, Tepeler A, Akcay M, Muslumanoglu AY, Tefekli A. Factors affecting bleeding during percutaneous nephrolithotomy: single surgeon experience. J Endourol. 2011;25(2):327–33.

Alken P. Percutaneous nephrolithotomy—the puncture. BJU Int. 2022;129(1):17–24.

Clayman M, Uribe CA, Eichel L, Gordon Z, McDougall EM, Clayman RV. Comparison of guide wires in urology. Which, when and why? J Urol. 2004;171(6 Pt 1):2146–50.

Ding X, Hou Y, Wang C, Wang Y. Super-stiff guidewire or loach guidewire during percutaneous nephrolithotomy? BJU Int Compass. 2023. https://doi.org/10.1002/bco2.219.

Fernström I, Johansson B. Percutaneous pyelolithotomy: a new extraction technique. Scand J Urol Nephrol. 1976;10(3):257–59.

Hoffman N, Lukasewycz SJ, Canales B, Botnaru A, Slaton JW, Monga M. Percutaneous renal stone extraction: in vitro study of retrieval devices. J Urol. 2004;172(2):559–61. https://doi.org/10.1097/01.ju.0000129195.71871.17.

Hou B, Wang M, Song Z, He Q, Hao Z. Renal puncture access using a blunt needle: proposal of the blunt puncture concept. World J Urol. 2022 Apr;40(4):1035-1041

Kolvatzis M, Sierra A, Corrales M, Traxer O. Stiff guidewires in endourology: What is stiffness? J Endourol. 2022;36(11):1475–82.

LeRoy AJ, second edition. Percutaneous access, tract dilation, and maintenance of the nephrostomy tract, 2nd ed. Hamilton, London: BC Decker Inc.; 2006, p. 107–15.

Mulţescu R, et al. Equipment and instruments in percutaneous nephrolithotomy, in percutaneous surgery of the upper urinary tract. Elsevier; 2016. p. 3–24.

Sadiq AS, Atallah W, Khusid J, Gupta M. The surgical technique of mini percutaneous nephrolithotomy. J Endourol. 2021;35(S2):S68–74.

Sampaio FJ, et al. Intrarenal access: 3-dimensional anatomical study. J Urol. 1992;148(6):1769–73.

Skolarikos AAN, Petřík A, Somani B, Thomas K, Gambaro G, Davis NF, Geraghty R, Lombardo R, Tzelves L. EAU guidelines on urolithiasis; 2022. ISBN 978-94-92671-16-5.

Tepeler A, Binbay M, Yuruk E, Sari E, Kaba M, Muslumanoglu AY, Tefekli A. Factors affecting the fluoroscopic screening time during percutaneous nephrolithotomy. J Endourol. 2009;23(11):1825–9.

van Gerwen DJ, Dankelman J, van den Dobbelsteen JJ. Measurement and stochastic modeling of kidney puncture forces. Ann Biomed Eng. 2014;42(3):685–95.

Wosnitzer M, Xavier K, Gupta M. Novel use of a ureteroscopic stone entrapment device to prevent antegrade stone migration during percutaneous nephrolithotomy. J Endourol. 2009;23(2):203–7.

Yu X, Xia D, Peng EJ, Yang H, Li C, Yuan HX, Cui L, Wu BL, Zhang JQ, Wang S, Wei C, Ye ZQ, Wang SG. Clinical investigation of ultrasound-guided percutaneous nephrolithotomy accessed by SVOF-principle and two-step puncture techniques. Zhonghua Wai Ke Za Zhi. 2018;56(10):764–67.

Intracorporeal Lithotripsy Devices for PCNL

Cesare Marco Scoffone and Cecilia Maria Cracco

Abstract "Intracorporeal lithotripsy" literally means "fragmentation of stones occurring within the body". Intracorporeal lithotripsy devices for percutaneous nephrolithotomy (PCNL) vary in terms of energy source, mechanism of action, probe features, comminution potential, stone retropulsion, side effects on surrounding tissues, versatility of use, and costs. The choice of the best intracorporeal lithotripter in terms of efficacy, safety and cost-effectiveness can be tailored case by case on the features of the urolithiasis and of the collecting system containing the calculi. Referring to their mechanism of action and at the same time to their order of appearance in the clinical practice, intracorporeal lithotripters for PCNL can be classified into electrohydraulic, ultrasonic, ballistic, combination, and laser devices. More than ten years ago standard PCNL resorted to ballistic, ultrasonic, and combined ballistic/ultrasonic lithotripsy most of the times. Nowadays, considering the current trend towards miniaturization and flexible endoscopy, intracorporeal lithotripters with suction and thinner probes as well as different lasers are used more and more, while electrohydraulic technology has largely been discontinued. History, mechanism of action, technique of lithotripsy, pros and cons, and future developments of each intracorporeal lithotripter for PCNL are described.

Keyword Ballistic · Electrohydraulic · Electrokinetic · Intracorporeal lithotripsy · Laser · Lithotripter · PCNL · Percutaneous nephrolithotomy · Pneumatic · Ultrasonic

1 Introduction

"Intracorporeal lithotripsy" means fragmentation (from the Ancient Greek $\tau\rho\acute{\iota}\psi\iota\varsigma$, *trípsis*) of stones (from the Ancient Greek $\lambda\acute{\iota}\vartheta o\varsigma$, *líthos*) occurring within (from the Latin *intra*) the body (from the Latin *corpus-corporis*)". Going beyond the literal etymology, "intracorporeal lithotripsy" is a minimally invasive approach to stone

C. M. Scoffone (✉) · C. M. Cracco
Department of Urology, Cottolengo Hospital, Turin, Italy
e-mail: scoof@libero.it

J. D. Denstedt and E. N. Liatsikos (eds.), *Percutaneous Renal Surgery*,
https://doi.org/10.1007/978-3-031-40542-6_24

management, consisting in the endoscopically controlled generation of a volume of stone fragments which is equivalent to the initial stone volume, in our case contextualized to percutaneous nephrolithotomy (PCNL).

Intracorporeal lithotripsy devices for PCNL vary in terms of energy source, mechanism of action, probe features, comminution potential, stone retropulsion, side effects on surrounding tissues, versatility of use, and costs. The choice of the best intracorporeal lithotripter in terms of efficacy, safety and cost-effectiveness can be tailored case by case on the features of the urolithiasis (number, size, location, shape, composition, hardness) and of the collecting system containing the calculi (morphology, elasticity, presence of hydronephrosis, concomitant infection, previous surgeries, presence of foreign bodies).

Referring to their mechanism of action and at the same time to their order of appearance in the clinical practice, intracorporeal lithotripters for PCNL can be classified into electrohydraulic, ultrasonic, ballistic, combination, and laser devices. Ballistic and electrohydraulic lithotripters crack stones turning them into fragments, ultrasonic and laser lithotripters offer both fragmentation and dusting (Scotland et al. 2017; Alken 2018).

More than ten years ago standard PCNL resorted to ballistic, ultrasonic, and combined ballistic/ultrasonic lithotripsy in almost 85% of the cases, whereas laser and electrohydraulic lithotripsy covered only 7% and 1% of the cases respectively (Tailly and Denstedt 2016). Nowadays, considering the current trend towards miniaturized PCNL on one hand and the widespread use of antegrade and retrograde flexible endoscopes (also simultaneously like in Endoscopic Combined IntraRenal Surgery, ECIRS) on the other hand, intracorporeal mechanical lithotripters with suction and thinner probes are required more and more, as well as different lasers with their ultra-thin and flexible fibers, while electrohydraulic technology has largely been discontinued (Tailly and Denstedt 2016; Axelsson et al. 2021; Castellani et al. 2022).

2 Electrohydraulic Lithotripsy

2.1 History

Electrohydraulic lithotripsy (EHL) was the very first method designed for intracorporeal lithotripsy, applied to bile duct stones and urolithiasis since the early Seventies using the Soviet device Urat-1. The electrohydraulic impact was discovered in 1955 by the Soviet physicist Lev Aleksandrovich Yutkin, who was out of favor with the Stalinist government and thus banished, therefore the use of his invention was delayed for at least ten years (Grocela and Dretler 1997).

Electrohydraulic technology has been applied not only in medicine, but also in mechanical engineering, agriculture, construction, hydrometallurgical production, and oil industry (for instance, to destroy large boulders in alternative to explosives, reduce residual stresses in the weld, create organic fertilizers, disinfect water, clean field pipelines) (Drozdov et al. 2019).

In the Eighties EHL, first applied to PCNL with the durable 9 Fr probes, became available for semirigid ureteroscopy passing to the thinner 5 Fr and 3 Fr probes, and finally for flexible ureteroscopy with the 1.9 Fr flexible probes (Scotland et al. 2017; Alken 2018; Grocela and Dretler 1997; Zheng and Denstedt 2000).

2.2 *Mechanism of Action*

The principle behind EHL-induced stone fragmentation is based on the effect of an electric discharge produced in a liquid medium, vaporizing the surrounding fluid, and creating a cavitation bubble that rapidly expands, symmetrically collapses, and finally rebounds. Consequently, a hydraulic shock wave impacts on the stone and causes its fragmentation (Fig. 1).

The working component of EHL consists in a pair of concentric metallic electrodes maintained at different voltages and separated by an insulating layer. When the current applied is stronger than the insulating gap between the electrodes, an electric spark jumps between the two, producing a shock wave from the spark itself, and a cavitation bubble from the superheated steam around the electrode (Scotland et al. 2017; Alken 2018; Grocela and Dretler 1997; Zheng and Denstedt 2000).

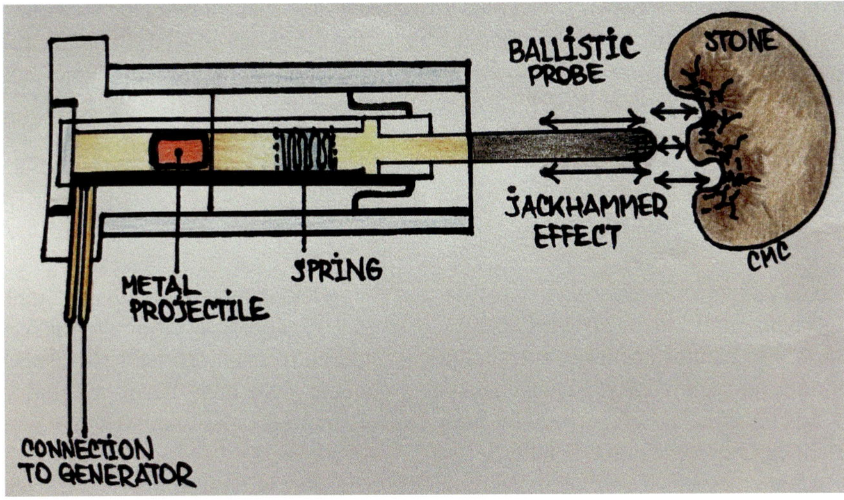

Fig. 1 Mechanism of action of electrohydraulic lithotripsy

2.3 Technique of Lithotripsy

The probe should not be held directly on the stone, because in this case the shock wave from the spark is too small, minimal water is vaporized, the stone only slightly heated, and the cavitation bubble not produced. The tip of the probe should rather be placed about 1 mm from the stone to allow water to cavitate, remembering that the generated shock wave is not focused. For this reason, the probes should be extended at a distance of 2–5 mm from the distal tip of the scope, to protect the lens and avoid expensive instrument repairs.

Before starting lithotripsy, the probe must be inspected to ensure the tip is smooth and that insulation layers are intact. In fact, overuse of the probe can result in shedding of the insulation or the entire probe tip.

Power output and spark frequency can be regulated. Energy settings should begin with low voltages (50–60 V) and be titrated up as needed to fragment the stone. A short burst of electrical discharge is applied to the stone only when the tip of the probe is clearly visible and away from the urothelium (Grocela and Dretler 1997; Zheng and Denstedt 2000).

2.4 Advantages

EHL is the cheapest lithotripter available, although disposable probes increase the costs because one or two might be used in each case, and even more for harder stones. The rougher the surface of the stone the better the efficiency of EHL (Grocela and Dretler 1997; Zheng and Denstedt 2000). EHL also produces the highest percentage of inactivated bacteria in models of infected stones (Gutiérrez et al. 2008).

2.5 Disadvantages

EHL is known to be less effective in uric acid stones and in those larger than 15 mm.

Having EHL the narrowest margin of safety of all forms of intracorporeal lithotripsy, careful attention to technique is required to maximize stone fragmentation and minimize tissue injury. The major concern is the high risk of perforation of the collecting system, especially when treating harder stones with high energies, producing large cavitation bubbles.

Another issue is the retropulsion of the stone fragments, requiring further manipulations or second look procedures (Scotland et al. 2017; Alken 2018; Grocela and Dretler 1997; Zheng and Denstedt 2000).

2.6 *Latest Evolutions*

The Nanosecond ElectroPulse Lithotripsy (NEPL) uses a nanosecond duration electrical discharge through a reusable flexible coaxial probe to endoscopically fragment urinary stones. With direct contact to the stone, higher voltage, and faster discharge than with conventional EHL the energy passes directly into the stone and not in the surrounding liquid, causing the stone to fragment. We have no recent news of this device (Alken 2018). In any case, nowadays EHL technology has largely been discontinued, owing to its poor fragmentation efficacy, the increased risk of injury to adjacent tissues, and the high costs of probe replacement (Tailly and Denstedt 2016).

3 Ultrasonic Lithotripsy

3.1 *History*

In 1794 the Italian biologist Lazzaro Spallanzani demonstrated that bats used inaudible sound instead of vision to hunt and navigate.

During the First World War a Russian engineer named Constantin Chilowski proposed to excite a cylindrical mica condenser by a high-frequency Poulsen arc at approximately 100 kHz, and thus to generate an ultrasound beam for detecting submerged objects. Something similar was proposed by L. F. Richardson after the Titanic disaster, but his high-frequency hydraulic whistle was not suitable for the purpose.

In 1917 the Director of the School of Physics and Chemistry in Paris Paul Langevin, having become acquainted with the piezoelectric effect as a student in the laboratories of Jaques and Pierre Curie, built an ultrasound transducer comprising a thin sheet of quartz sandwiched between two steel plates, activated it by the Poulsen arc, and produced high frequency sound waves useful for the underwater detection of submarines.

Nowadays, ultrasonic devices are used as motion sensors (like for parking sensors), and to measure distances in the context of web guiding systems (drones included). Industrially, ultrasound is used for cleaning, mixing, and accelerating chemical processes, as well as in metallurgy and engineering like for nondestructive testing of wood and cement (Klein 1948).

Although the use of ultrasound vibrational energy (acoustic waves with a frequency of about 20,000 vibrations per second, higher than that of the human audio spectrum) to break renal stones was described in 1953 by William P. Mulvaney and studied in vitro in 1955 by T. L. Coates, its clinical use in the percutaneous treatment of a renal staghorn stone was described more than twenty years later by K. H. Kurth and coworkers. The first such lithotripter was the Aachen model developed by Karl Storz in Germany, the father of all pure ultrasonic lithotripters. The Storz Calcuson®, in the market since 1976, had two different probes, one with a movable tip and one without it. Jackhammer movement of the movable tip were initiated by the ultrasound probe, thus combining both ultrasound and ballistic effects in one probe (Scotland et al. 2017; Alken 2018; Axelsson et al. 2021; Grocela and Dretler 1997; Zheng and Denstedt 2000).

3.2 Mechanism of Action

An alternating electric current field excites a piezoceramic crystal within the ultrasound transducer. The crystal vibrates at a specific frequency and generates an acoustic wave with a frequency of 23–25 kHz, inaudible to the human ear.

The vibrational energy of the transducer is transmitted to a hollow steel probe, which in turn vibrates longitudinally and transversally. The probe in direct contact with the non-compliant stone stimulates it to resonate at a high frequency, acting on it (Fig. 2).

Soft stones are preferably dusted, hard ones fragmented (Scotland et al. 2017; Alken 2018; Axelsson et al. 2021; Grocela and Dretler 1997; Zheng and Denstedt 2000).

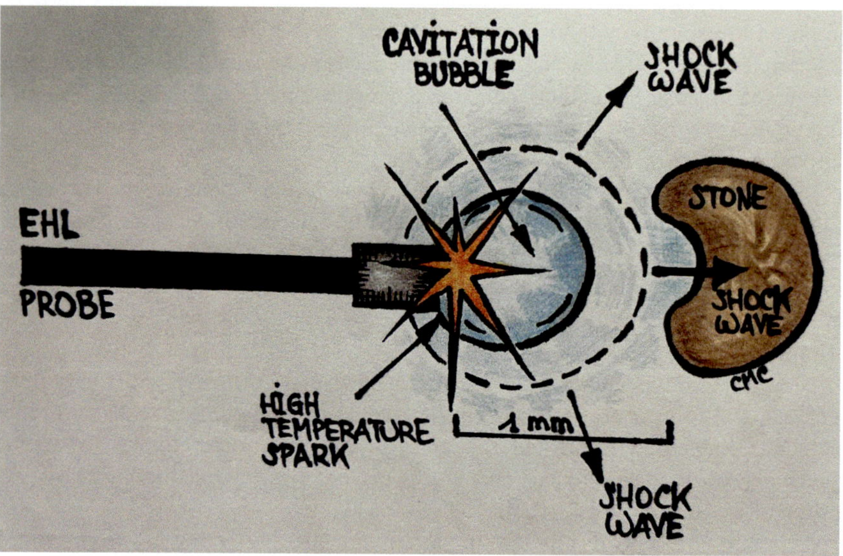

Fig. 2 Mechanism of action of ultrasonic lithotripsy

3.3 Technique

Ultrasonic lithotripters work best when used through a rigid endoscope, therefore the rigid probes (from 2.5 Fr to 12 Fr) should not be bent for optimal efficacy and safety. In PCNL the stone should be gently pinned by the tip of the probe against the urothelium under direct visualization, refraining from excessive force to avoid perforation of the collecting system, although the risk is lower than with EHL.

If the probe drills a hole within the stone and gets stuck, reduced oscillations may reduce efficiency, so the probe must be retracted and repositioned on the stone.

The heat generated by ultrasonic lithotripsy needs cooling of both handpiece and probe, provided by continuous irrigation and a suction device activated when the lithotripter is working, also maintaining the pressure steady to optimize endoscopic vision and removal of blood, dust, and debris.

All probes are hollow except the 2.5 Fr, which is solid with no suction capability and increased risk of overheating (thus intermittent firing might be useful in this case). Larger probes have better suction, enabling more efficient heat dispersion.

At the same time, more suction may also cause more collapse of the collecting system containing the urolithiasis and worse endoscopic vision, therefore adequate irrigation inflow must be provided (for instance, elevating the height of irrigation bags) (Scotland et al. 2017; Alken 2018; Axelsson et al. 2021; Grocela and Dretler 1997; Zheng and Denstedt 2000; Liatsikos et al. 2001; Feng et al. 2020).

3.4 Advantages

Ultrasonic lithotripsy is particularly successful with less dense stones with a rough surface, but overall success rates are as high as 97% (Liatsikos et al. 2001).

The hollow probes can evacuate stone material during fragmentation (also usable for stone analysis), and stone propulsion is negligible. Operating costs are relatively low. Finally, when the probe encounters the compliant urothelium of the collecting system, the damage is minimal because soft tissues do not resonate, and a negligible edema is the worst consequence (Scotland et al. 2017; Alken 2018; Liatsikos et al. 2001).

A good balance between irrigation inflow and suction allows a good endoscopic view, and at the same time avoids distension of the collecting system, with the risk of increased intrarenal pelvic pressure, resorption of bacteria and endotoxins, and developing infectious complications including urosepsis (Feng et al. 2020).

3.5 Disadvantages

Harder stones like calcium oxalate monohydrate, cysteine, and brushite are more difficult to be fragmented by this lithotripter, as well as those with a smooth surface.

With this vibrational energy transmission, loss of energy is dissipated as heat. Therefore, a good deal of irrigation and a well-functioning suction device are needed, otherwise thermal damage might occur to patient, surgeon, and device itself.

The rigid probe design is a disadvantage. A bend in the probe may dissipate enough heat to damage surrounding tissues at the site of the bend, rendering the tip ineffective.

Malfunctions of ultrasonic lithotripters are not infrequent, especially dealing with cooling and suction. Probes are vulnerable to clogging and heating, and if bended may also break (Scotland et al. 2017; Alken 2018; Grocela and Dretler 1997; Zheng and Denstedt 2000; Patel et al. 2017).

3.6 Latest Evolutions

UreTron® is a single-handle, single-probe ultrasonic lithotripter approved in 2012, available with rigid, semi-flexible, and flexible probes to suit different surgical requirements and equally effective treating hard stones. The lithotripsy system has three functions: ultrasonic lithotripsy, "similar" ballistic lithotripsy (via adjustment of the mechanical force or amplitude through unique electric-kinetic energy conversion using a different ultrasound frequency), and negative pressure suction on a single lithotripter rod. The vibration along the probe is transmitted to the tip to produce an axial 20–100 μm motion to optimally distribute the energy when acting on the stones. There is no recent news on this device, especially for PCNL (Scotland et al. 2017; Alken 2018; Tailly and Denstedt 2016; Grocela and Dretler 1997).

4 Ballistic Lithotripsy

4.1 History

The term "ballistic" stems from the Greek word βάλλειν (ballein), meaning thrust, hurl, or throw. In fact, the mechanical force producing stone disintegration is intermittently supplied through vibrating metallic probes, thanks to compressed air for pneumatic lithotripsy or electromagnetic impulses for electrokinetic lithotripsy, propelling a projectile inside the handpiece at the stone of interest. In both cases the resulting action is like that of a jackhammer.

The first available percutaneous ballistic lithotrite introduced in 1991 was the Swiss LithoClast by EMS, a pneumatic machine as most ballistic lithotripters.

Another low-cost device was the Browne pneumatic impactor, using a nitinol (nickel-titanium ally) probe to mechanically impact the stones, accelerated by compressed air (Scotland et al. 2017; Alken 2018; Axelsson et al. 2021; Grocela and Dretler 1997; Zheng and Denstedt 2000; Keeley et al. 1999; Denstedt 1993).

4.2 Mechanism of Action

Compressed air (pneumatic lithotripsy) or electromagnetic/-mechanic impulses (electrokinetic lithotripsy, EKL) are used to accelerate an inner mobile metal body attached to the external probe, passing through the endoscope, and touching the stone. Return movement of the metal body is provided by simultaneously compressed springs of elastic material within the handpiece (Fig. 3).

For pneumatic lithotripsy the generator is connected to a clean air supply or compressed air tank. A foot pedal triggers activation by providing compressed air to propel the metal probe at a pressure of 3 atmospheres. EKL uses electromagnetic energy to accelerate the projectile.

The Swiss LithoClast by EMS uses precisely controlled bursts of compressed air to accelerate to a high speed a metallic bullet that is central to its fragmentation mechanism. Ballistic lithotripsy uses the harnessed energy from the motion of a projectile,

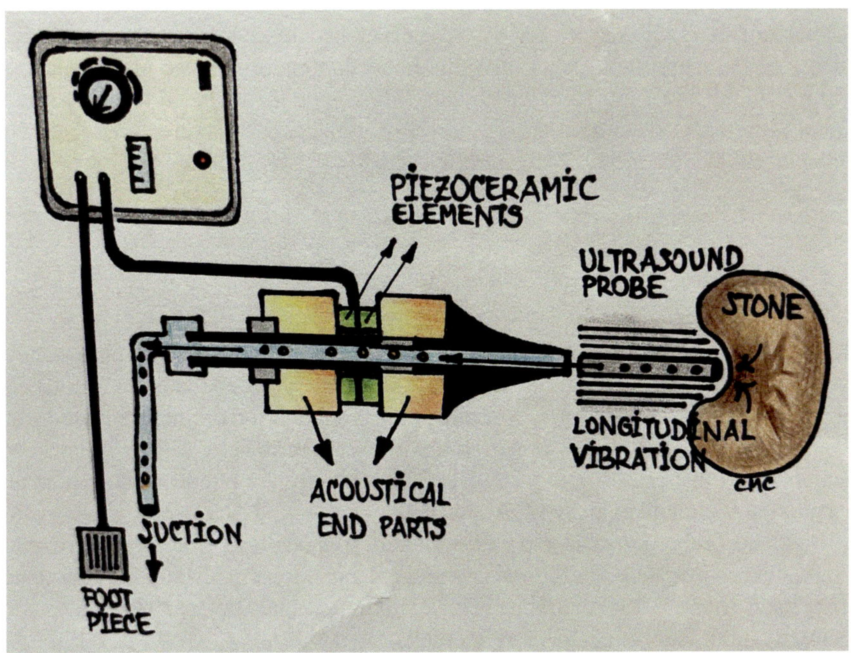

Fig. 3 Mechanism of action of ballistic lithotripsy

guided within precision of one micrometer, that transfers its ballistic energy through the probe to the stone, thus resulting in fragmentation.

Two cordless, portable ballistic devices have also been developed: the Cook LMA™ StoneBreaker, a pneumatic lithotripter with self-contained CO_2 pressure cartridges, each delivering 80–100 shots, and the EMS Swiss LithoBreaker, an electromechanic device with the power pack situated in the handle of the device and consisting of 4 rechargeable NiL AAA batteries, able to deliver up to 3,000 shots (Scotland et al. 2017; Alken 2018; Tailly and Denstedt 2016; Axelsson et al. 2021; Grocela and Dretler 1997; Zheng and Denstedt 2000).

4.3 Technique

Probes of different diameters and lengths are available (6–2.5 Fr and 40–57 cm). The probe should be in direct contact with the stone before activating the pedal, possibly in a place where it is unable to move. Pneumatic-ballistic lithotripters have multiple firing modes, ranging from single pulses to continuous firing. Frequency (0.5–3.4 Hz), extent (0.8–25 mm) and velocity (10–30 m/s), and thereby intensity of the probe tip displacement, can be regulated to optimize ballistic stone disintegration, obtaining fast stone fragmentation and short lithotripsy time.

Usually, smaller fragments undergo spontaneous evacuation through the Amplatz sheath, while larger ones are manually extracted with graspers or baskets. In 1995 special probes (LithoVac by EMS) were developed to counteract the propulsive energy of ballistic lithotripsy with variable suction energy. These probes vary in width (1.6, 3.5 and 4 mm) and length, depending upon the intended location of use (kidney, ureter, bladder) (Scotland et al. 2017; Alken 2018; Axelsson et al. 2021; Grocela and Dretler 1997; Zheng and Denstedt 2000; Denstedt 1993).

4.4 Advantages

Ballistic lithotripters are simple and reliable, safe, and efficient also on hard stones. There is a low risk of perforation of the collecting system because rigid objects like a stone are fragmented, while flexible targets such as the urothelium absorb the momentum. Minimal heat is produced, and in an experimental setting it has been demonstrated that after 6 min of direct application to the ureteral wall there is no perforation (Scotland et al. 2017; Alken 2018).

Being the probes reusable and with a long lifespan, ballistic lithotripters are relatively inexpensive, and thus a good economical and cost-effective option (Scotland et al. 2017; Alken 2018; Axelsson et al. 2021; Grocela and Dretler 1997; Zheng and Denstedt 2000; Patel et al. 2017; Denstedt 1993).

4.5   Disadvantages

Ballistic lithotripsy is less efficient in ureteroscopes because of the smaller diameter, and when the rigid probe is flexed or torqued because a good deal of power is lost for every small degree of bowing. Flexible ballistic probes do exist but are not the first choice in the current clinical practice.

Stone retropulsion in absence of suction, and large fragmenting instead of dusting with need for baskets or forceps for litholapaxy are further disadvantages (Scotland et al. 2017; Alken 2018; Axelsson et al. 2021).

4.6   Latest Evolutions

The PercSac is an interesting novel ancillary device that consists of an internally deployed polyethylene bag used to entrap the stones. In vitro tests have shown promising results towards a better stone-free rates (Tailly and Denstedt 2016).

The ClearPetra is a 16 Fr nephrostomic sheath for vacuum-assisted mini-PCNL. Variable suction allows to use this aid when required for efficient and progressive clearance of the stone fragments, also reducing intrarenal pelvic pressure and possibly the risk of infectious complications (Tominaga et al. 2023).

5   Combined Ultrasonic and Ballistic Lithotripsy

5.1   History

Combination models were born from the idea to join lithotripsy modalities to improve the overall efficiency of stone treatment, being the ballistic energy more efficient for harder stones and the ultrasonic approach for softer stones.

The very first combined lithotripter was the Waltz Lithotron EL27, previously marketed in 1996 as Combilith, with electrohydraulic and electrokinetic energies combined in one device. It was very economical, with probes working for 1–3 operations (Scotland et al. 2017; Alken 2018; Axelsson et al. 2021).

5.2   Two-Probe Dual-Modality Lithotripsy

The Swiss LithoClast® Master by EMS, introduced in 2001, combines ultrasonic and pneumatic-ballistic probes. The ballistic probe is a metallic rod inside the hollow ultrasonic probe, projecting its tip 1 mm past the end of the ultrasonic probe when activated. The two modes can be used individually or in combination. The need for constant probe changing is user-unfriendly, lowering surgeon satisfaction (Hofmann et al. 2002). The LithoClast Ultra introduced by Boston Scientific shortly afterwards was similarly efficient and safe.

The CyberWand™ by ACMI/Olympus has two ultrasound probes. The inner hollow probe vibrates at 21 kHz, the larger ballistic outer probe moves at a lower frequency of 10 Hz. Vibration of the inner fixed probe results in the sliding movement of a piston whose motion pushes the movable outer probe forward, improving the perforation rate (Scotland et al. 2017; Alken 2018; Tailly and Denstedt 2016; Axelsson et al. 2021).

5.3 Single-Probe Dual-Modality Lithotripsy

Single-probe dual-energy (SPDE) lithotripters have emerged as a promising treatment modality with greater ergonomics, combining simultaneous application of different forms of energy through a single probe during PCNL for a cumulative efficacy in terms of stone clearance and safety. Despite the initial encouraging findings of preclinical and isolated clinical studies, it seems that SPDE lithotripters provide similar efficiency compared to older generation devices, but for sure are more user-friendly, with no need for constant probe changing.

The Shock-Pulse-SE lithotripter by Olympus was launched in 2017 and was the first available SPDE lithotripter that used constant ultrasonic energy with intermittent ballistic force (300 Hz). The device is controlled by buttons on the handpiece or by foot pedals, but the hand-activated suction has been very appreciated, as well as low level of noise during activation. The lumen is larger than that of the two-probe combined devices, which are partially occupied by the ballistic probe. The 3.76 mm probe is the largest lumen of any existing device, in absence of a luminal pneumatic probe.

The EMS LithoClast® Trilogy was introduced in 2018 and went a step further by combining ultrasonic and ballistic energy, as well as concomitant vacuum suction, all in one probe. A foot pedal controls suction and lithotripsy. The handpiece is heavier than that of other lithotripters, however it has no impact on the surgical outcomes (Scotland et al. 2017; Alken 2018; Tailly and Denstedt 2016; Axelsson et al. 2021; Mykoniatis et al. 2023).

6 Laser Lithotripsy

6.1 History

For sure, the application of lasers in the treatment of urolithiasis is among the most important developments in urology in the last fifty years. Laser is the acronym of Light Amplification of Stimulated Emission of Radiation: an energy source stimulates defined atoms, elevating their electrons to an excited metastable state; when the electrons relax and return to their natural state they emit energy in the form of photons, i.e., a discrete amount of light energy. The emitted radiation is monochromatic, coherent, and collimated.

The first laser ever operated was a ruby laser built by Theodore Maiman in 1960, with xenon flashtubes discharging several thousand volts, a silver-plated cylindrical reflector, a crystal of aluminum oxide (i.e., sapphire), also containing chromium atoms in a small percentage and with gold-reflecting coatings on its ends. The ruby laser emitted a visible red radiation at a wavelength of 695 nm, significantly absorbed by melanin and hemoglobin, and delivered as a series of irregular spikes within the pulse duration. For this reason, in 1961 Robert W. Hellwarth invented the method of Q-switching, to concentrate the output into a single pulse. In 1962 Willard Boyle (the Canadian physicist who shared the 2009 Nobel prize in Physics for the invention of the CCD sensor, the charge-coupled device) produced the first continuous output from a ruby laser. In 1966 Ralph L. Parsons was the first to experiment the ruby laser in urology, in canine bladders; in 1968 William P. Mulvaney and Carl W. Beck reported that the ruby laser was able to fragment urinary stones, although clinically unsafe because of excessive heat generation and unacceptable tissue damage.

Since then, both continuous-wave (like the 1064 nm neodymium:Yttrium–Aluminium-Garnet (Nd:YAG), poorly absorbed by water and stones, and the 960–1060 nm carbon dioxide, one of the earliest gas lasers to be developed and applied in urology by Mulvaney and Beck) and pulsed lasers (like the 750 nm Alexandrite laser with strong plasma and cavitation effects, the 2940 nm erbium:YAG (Er:YAG) laser with efficient photothermal effects, and the ultrashort-pulse femtosecond laser with a high peak power causing catastrophic damage of the optical fiber and too low plasma-mediated ablation rates) were tested for lithotripsy but had little success, mainly due to excessive collateral thermal damage to soft tissues or limitations in fiber-optic delivery systems.

In 1987 the first successful pulsed laser lithotripsy system, the short-pulse dye laser, was commercialized. The wavelength was 504 nm, well absorbed by hemoglobin, and the pulse length short, allowing shock wave production and stone fragmentation without excessive heat. To improve absorption of this laser by harder stones, otherwise unresponsive to fragmentation, in 1988 Andrea Tasca developed a method of coating stones with rifamycin, making them absorb more energy at their surface. In 1989 G. M. Watson used the FLPDL (Flashlamp-Pumped Pulsed Dye Laser) for laser fragmentation, monitoring their plasma and acoustic signals in absence of direct endoscopic vision. Unfortunately, the green coumarin dye used as liquid laser medium was highly toxic, the costs high, and the effects on the stones too violent, with stone extrusion and retromigration.

In 2001 the frequency-doubled double-pulse YAG (FREDDY) laser, incorporating a KTP crystal into the resonator of a Nd:YAG laser, produced two simultaneous pulses, one at 532 nm in the green spectrum, initiating plasma formation at the stone surface, and another at 1064 nm, heating the preformed plasma, causing expansion and contraction, and thus stone fragmentation. It was not very efficient on hard stones, but costs were low and intrinsic safety on soft tissues reasonable because of its photomechanical effect.

Currently, Holmium:YAG (Ho:YAG) is the most used laser in urology. Because of the relative ease of delivering pulses of laser energy through rigid and flexible endoscopes, and its cost-effectiveness in comparison with other lasers and non-laser technologies, this method by the late Nineties had emerged as the dominant tool for laser lithotripsy, being currently the gold standard laser. Initial ex-vivo experiments were described by J. Sayer in 1993 and the first clinical outcomes were published by J. D. Denstedt in 1995 (Scotland et al. 2017; Alken 2018; Castellani et al. 2022; Grocela and Dretler 1997; Zheng and Denstedt 2000).

6.2   Ho:YAG Laser, General Features

Ho:YAG is a compromise between the ultraprecise Er:YAG laser (using a wavelength of 2940 nm for tissue ablation and incision), and the Nd:YAG laser (using a wavelength of 1064 nm for thermal coagulation and hemostasis). Ho:YAG is an infrared laser that uses a solid YAG crystal doped with holmium ions, emits a 2120 nm wavelength radiation, close to the 1940 nm absorption peak of water and thus strongly absorbed by water, has an optical penetration depth of 0.4 mm. It is pulsed with the possibility to reach long pulse durations and is available in the 20W to 150W range. Pulse energy varies from 0.2 to 6 J, pulse frequencies from 5 to 80 Hz; the pulse peak power (i.e., the amount of energy a laser pulse contains in comparison to its pulse width) may reach thousands of Watts.

The flashlamp pumping scheme for the Ho:YAG laser is relatively inexpensive in comparison with other diode-pumped laser systems; on the other hand, more powerful Ho:YAG lasers are bulky and more expensive with a higher initial capital cost, because more complex, requiring more water cooling units, dedicated electrical plugs and high-voltage power supply. The wall-plug efficiency is limited, being about 1–2% (Scotland et al. 2017; Alken 2018; Castellani et al. 2022; Fried and Irby 2018; Kronenberg and Traxer 2019; Andreeva et al. 2020).

New technological advances allowed for changing the way of delivering the energy pulse, creating the concept of pulse modulation. Initially, pulse modulation consisted in regulating the pulse length once it became tunable from the standard 350 µs duration, with the possibility to stretch the laser pulse up to 1500 µs or compress it to 50 µs. The Moses Technology, known since the Eighties but commercialized by Lumenis since 2017, is a pulse modulation which modified the pulse shape into two subpulses. The first is a short, low-energy pulse, creating a vapor bubble and "parting the water", the second is a longer, higher energy pulse, more efficiently delivered to the stone for enhanced ablation with reduced retropulsion. Previous Moses Contact (to be used at a 1 mm distance) and Moses Distance (to be used at 2 mm distance) modes were overtaken in 2020 by the Moses 2.0 system which introduced the new predefined pulse modulation called Optimized Moses when using high frequencies in high-power lasers. Other manufacturers developed pulse modulation techniques, like the Vapor Tunnel™, Virtual Basket™ and Bubble Blast™ by Quanta System, Advanced Mode™ by Dornier, and Stabilization Mode™ by Olympus (Sánchez-Puy et al. 2022).

Ho:YAG wavelength can be delivered through traditional, low-hydroxyl (OH-) silica optical fibers. The silica core is biocompatible, robust, flexible, resistant to corrosion in the urine environment and to sterilization for medical use, affordable both as multiuse and disposable, single-use fiber-optic delivery system, being mass produced for use in telecommunications and industrial applications. The laser fiber consists of this silica core whose diameter characterizes the fiber technically, a first coating named cladding that keeps the light into the core, and a colored plastic cover named jacket for better visualization. Each fiber has a specific connector to the generator and the sizes vary from 200 to 550 and 1000 μm (Fried and Irby 2018). Smaller fibers are better for flexible scopes, allowing a simultaneous adequate irrigation and nor interfering with the scope deflection. They can be cut with metal scissors and cleaved every 15 minutes of lithotripsy/10 kJ. Fibers should not be stripped for better vision and less tip degradation, while the better fragmenting efficiency is under discussion. The fiber should not be kept too near to the optics of the scope (about 1/4 of the screen diameter), to avoid its inadvertent damage (Alken 2018; Fried and Irby 2018; Kronenberg and Traxer 2019).

6.3 Ho:YAG Laser, Mechanism of Action

Two are the primary and well recognized mechanisms of stone ablation, possibly occurring in parallel: (1) photothermal ablation: the direct infrared laser absorption by the stone produces a rise in stone temperature, with subsequent chemical decomposition of stone components heated with laser irradiation or by boiling/vaporizing water; (2) thermomechanical ablation: the interstitial water inside stone pores, fissures and lamellations of the stone surface absorbs infrared laser energy, causing microexplosions during thermal expansion and vaporization, leading to stone bursting from inside causing mechanical stress on the surrounding structure as part of the ablation mechanism (Fig. 4).

A plasma-induced shockwave destruction has also been described (Fig. 4). Absorption of a laser pulse with short pulse duration and high pulse energy by molecules of stone composites results in free electrons in front of the stone. This aqueous cloud, also containing a mixture of urine and irrigation fluid, absorbs the remaining laser pulse energy (plasma shielding) and induces a cavitation bubble in

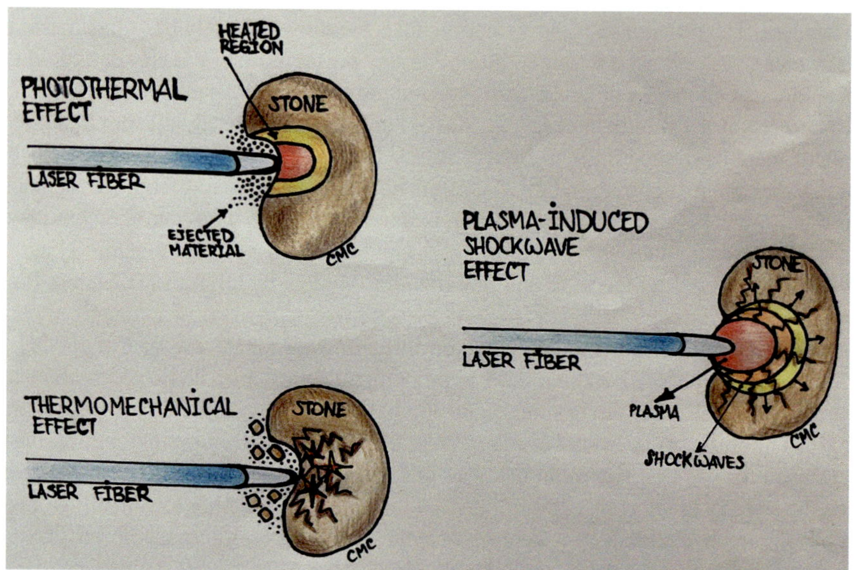

Fig. 4 Mechanisms of action of laser lithotripsy

front of the calculus. A shockwave with high-pressure emits immediately after its collapse. Usually, the induced pressure wave is weak and contributes little to the mechanical destruction of the stone, but significantly to stone retropulsion (Fried and Irby 2018; Kronenberg and Traxer 2019; Andreeva et al. 2020; Taratkin et al. 2021).

6.4 Ho:YAG Laser, Technique of Lithotripsy

Contact lithotripsy constitutes the first (and sometimes the only) stage of a lithotripsy procedure. The dusting approach (low energy, high frequency, long pulse) or the fragmenting strategy (high energy, low frequency, short pulse) can be chosen, exploiting the different sizes and shapes of the vapor bubbles produced with the combination of the settings of the three tunable parameters. However, fragment size may not only be related to laser lithotripter settings, but also on the surgical technique employed (chipping versus dancing or painting the stone, working uniformly or tangentially on the surface). Even the best dusting setting, when used improperly, can produce large stone fragments.

However, when numerous smaller fragments result, which are still big enough to need treatment but too time-consuming to chase individually, a second stage non-contact lithotripsy can be performed. The aim is to pulverize these fragments and allow their spontaneous passage, preferably in a smaller and enclosed space such as a calix to increase the efficiency. The laser fiber is activated in bursts, away from the stone fragments resulting in a whirlpool-like effect that causes stones to collide and fragment further. Additionally, laser vaporization of stone fragments occurs as they swirl around. Two different techniques can be employed. One is the pop-corn technique, with moderate to high pulse energy and frequency ($\approx$ 1.5 J, 20–40 Hz) and long pulse mode. The other one is the pop-dusting technique, quite like the pop-corn technique but using a lower pulse energy (0.5 J), resulting in finer fragments without compromising fiber tip burn-back (Scotland et al. 2017; Alken 2018; Castellani et al. 2022; Fried and Irby 2018; Kronenberg and Traxer 2019; Andreeva et al. 2020; Taratkin et al. 2021; Hardy et al. 2017).

6.5 Ho:YAG Laser, Advantages

The Ho:YAG laser is effective on all stone types and compositions, with stone-free rates approaching 95% in experienced hands, depending on stone size, location, patient anatomy, and surgical technique, although the good stone-free rates do not depend only on the laser features but rather on the surgeon's technique, lithotripsy strategy and skills. It can be used in both rigid and flexible endoscopes, especially the miniaturized ones, with both antegrade and retrograde accesses. Long pulse duration reduces retropulsion, while moderate to high energies can transect guidewires and the wires of a basket if needed (Scotland et al. 2017; Alken 2018; Castellani et al. 2022; Fried and Irby 2018; Kronenberg and Traxer 2019; Andreeva et al. 2020; Taratkin et al. 2021; Hardy et al. 2017).

Additionally, Ho:YAG is very versatile, and apart from being used for the treatment of urolithiasis, is very efficient in a variety of applications like prostate endoscopic enucleation, incision of urethral and ureteral strictures, en-bloc resection of bladder tumors, and ablation of upper tract urothelial tumors (Scotland et al. 2017; Alken 2018; Castellani et al. 2022; Grocela and Dretler 1997; Zheng and Denstedt 2000).

6.6 Ho:YAG Laser, Disadvantages

High-power devices are expensive, delicate, and potentially dangerous. Dedicated electrical plugs are required, and installation is complex. The multimode beam profile of Ho:YAG laser prohibits coupling of high laser power into small core fibers less than 200 μm in diameter. High energy and short pulse length produce more fiber burnback. The ability to ablate, however, is poor.

High intrarenal temperatures (up to 70 °C or more), potentially causing tissue injury, are developed with high-energy settings and laser emission in long bursts, even at lower power settings, particularly when irrigation is closed. The heat energy flows beyond the region of direct laser absorption during the laser pulse because the pulse duration is longer than the thermal diffusion period. This action leads to coagulation, carbonization, and denaturation of surrounding tissues (Scotland et al. 2017; Alken 2018; Castellani et al. 2022; Grocela and Dretler 1997; Zheng and Denstedt 2000).

6.7 Present Developments: The Superpulse Thulium Fiber Laser

The TFL technology was born more than twenty years ago and studied as lithotripsy energy since 2005, although with a modulated 100W continuous wave device. The superpulse thulium fiber laser (TFL) lithotripter has been cleared for clinical use in the Russian Federation and launched in that market in 2018. TFL can operate either in a continuous mode or adopt a pulsed mode within a large range of energy, frequency, and pulse shape settings, with a higher peak power (500W) (Fried and Irby 2018; Kronenberg and Traxer 2019; Andreeva et al. 2020).

As its name suggests, the gain medium of the TFL consists of trivalent Thulium ions that are doped within a very thin (10–20 μm core diameter) and 10–30 m long silica fiber. The Thulium ions are pumped by multiple diode lasers. The resulting laser beam emits at 1940 nm, closely matching a major water absorption peak. For this reason, TFL has over Tm:YAG a twofold and over Ho:YAG a fourfold higher absorption coefficient in water, facilitating conversion of laser energy into mechanical and thermal energy during laser lithotripsy with very little energy release as heat.

Absorption of infrared energy by water is believed to have a major role in stone ablation, in addition to direct absorption of laser energy by the stone material. Lower peak powers lead to effective heating of the stone compounds, but water in pores is not vaporized at a rate necessary for stone destruction. On the other hand, the higher water absorption and the prolonged TFL peak allow for uniform heating of the stone, leading to rapid water vaporization and photomechanical damage (Taratkin et al. 2021). This also explains the fourfold lower TFL ablation thresholds for the most common stone compositions (Fried and Irby 2018). TFL vapor bubbles are smaller and stream-like, translating into an improved safety profile with a 1 mm working distance, reduced stone retropulsion and less fiber burnback (Hardy et al. 2017).

Further advantages of TFL include smaller operating laser fibers (50–150 μm core diameter) because of the uniform and focused output beam, lower energy per pulse (as low as 0.025 J), higher maximal pulse repetition rate (up to 2000 Hz), no need for dedicated electrical plugs in the operating room, smaller size and lower weight of the laser device, more unlikely misalignment of the very small mirrors at the end of the fiber, a 12% wall-plug efficiency enabling simple air cooling for heat dissipation.

6.8 Latest Evolutions: The Pulsed Thulium:YAG Laser

The novel diode-pumped solid-state Thulium:YAG (Tm:YAG) laser should not be confused with the TFL laser, nor with the continuous wave Tm:YAG laser, known for its usefulness in prostate ablation but also for its unsuitability for lithotripsy. Now such devices (by Dornier and by LISA Laser), with a 2013 nm wavelength, offer 120–150 W of power with frequencies of 1 Hz to 300 Hz and possible pulse energies as low as 0.1 J up to 3 J. Being capable of pulsed laser emission, Tm:YAG produces stone lithotripsy by a photothermal mechanism with a higher water absorption coefficient, as demonstrated back in 2005, additionally producing vapor bubbles at the tip of the laser fiber. To eliminate stone retropulsion the pulse peak power may be adjustable from 500 Watts to more than 1000 Watts. Pulsed Tm:YAG lithotripsy has shown to be fast, without any significant heat increase, additionally producing minimal stone retropulsion (and sometimes none at all). The new hybrid Thulium-YAG laser combines the desirable features of existing Tm:YAG (in continuous wave mode offering excellent tissue incision, vaporization, and haemostasis) and Ho:YAG lasers (in pulsed mode, with high frequencies for stone dusting). The bubble's shape is not spherical, and the hypothesis is that reduced lateral expansion of Tm: YAG could possibly translate to less collateral damage to the ureteral wall and renal cavities. Pulsed Tm:YAG lithotripsy looks promising; however, true clinical studies are still lacking (Kraft et al. 2022).

7 Conclusions

As kidney stone prevalence continues to rise, the importance of the development and evolution of lithotripsy technologies cannot be understated. Currently available intracorporeal lithotripters have advantages and disadvantages, often depending on the clinical situation, and the surgeon can customize stone treatment to maximize efficacy and safety, tailoring the procedure on the individual patient's needs. Continuous improvements in the incredible array of options for intracorporeal lithotripsy are guided by intense research in the field.

References

Alken P. Intracorporeal lithotripsy. Urolithiasis. 2018;46:19–29.

Andreeva V, Vinarov A, Yaroslavsky I, Kovalenko A, Vybornov A, Rapoport L, et al. Preclinical comparison of superpulse thulium fiber laser and a holmium:YAG laser for lithotripsy. World J Urol. 2020;38(2):497–503.

Axelsson TA, Cracco C, Desai M, Hasan MN, Knoll T, Montanari E, et al. Consultation on kidney stones, Copenhagen 2019: lithotripsy in percutaneous nephrolithotomy. World J Urol. 2021;39(6):1663–70.

Castellani D, Corrales M, Lim EJ, Cracco C, Scoffone CM, Teoh JY, et al. The impact of lasers in percutaneous nephrolithotomy outcomes: results from a systematic review and meta-analysis of randomized comparative trials. J Endourol. 2022;36(2):151–7.

Denstedt JD. Use of Swiss Lithoclast for percutaneous nephrolithotripsy. J Endourol. 1993;7(6):477–80.

Drozdov AN, Narozhnyy IM, Pak DX, Ludupov VB, Zamlianslii GS. Electrohydraulic effect as an example of electrophysical technologies application in the oil industry. IOP Conf Ser Mater Sci Eng. 2019;675: 012024.

Feng D, Zeng X, Han P, Wei X. Comparison of intrarenal pelvic pressure and postoperative fever between standard- and mini-tract percutaneous nephrolithotomy: a systematic review and meta-analysis of randomized controlled trials. Transl Androl Urol. 2020;9(3):1159–66.

Fried NM, Irby PB. Advances in laser technology and fibre-optic delivery systems in lithotripsy. Nat Rev. 2018;15:563–73.

Grocela JA, Dretler SP (1997) Intracorporeal lithotripsy. Instrumentation and development. Urol Clin North Am. 1997;24(1):13–23.

Gutiérrez J, Alvarez UM, Mues E, Fernandez F, Gomez G, Loske AM. Inactivation of bacteria inoculated inside urinary stone-phantoms using intracorporeal lithotripters. Urol Res. 2008;36:67–72.

Hardy LA, Kennedy JD, Wilson CR, Irby PB, Fried NM. Analysis of thulium fiber laser induced bubble dynamics for ablation of kidney stones. J Biophotonics. 2017;10(10):1240–9.

Hofmann R, Olbert P, Weber J, Wille S, Varga Z. Clinical experience with a new ultrasonic and LithoClast combination for percutaneous litholapaxy. BJU Int. 2002;90(1):16–9.

Keeley FX Jr, Pillai M, Smith G, Chrisofos M, Tolley DA. Electrokinetic lithotripsy: safety, efficacy, and limitations of a new form of ballistic lithotripsy. BJU Int. 1999;84(3):261–3.

Klein E. Some background history of ultrasonics. J Acoust Soc Am. 1948;20(5):601–4.

Kraft L, Petzold R, Suarez-Ibarrola R, Miernik A. In vitro fragmentation performance of a novel, pulsed Thulium solid-state laser compared to a Thulium fibre laser and standard Ho:YAG laser. Lasers Med Sci. 2022;37(3):2071–8.

Kronenberg P, Traxer O. The laser of the future: reality and expectations about the new thulium fiber laser - a systematic review. Transl Androl Urol. 2019;8(Suppl 4):S398–417.

Liatsikos EN, Dinlenc CZ, Fogarty JD, Kapoor R, Bernardo NO, Smith AD. Efficiency and efficacy of different intracorporeal ultrasonic lithotripsy units on a synthetic stone model. J Endourol. 2001;15:925–8.

Mykoniatis I, Pyrgidis N, Tzelves L, Pietropaolo A, Juliebø-Jones P, De Coninck V, et al. Assessment of single-probe dual-energy lithotripters in percutaneous nephrolithotomy: a systematic review and meta-analysis of preclinical and clinical studies. World J Urol. 2023;41(2):551–65.

Patel NH, Schulman AA, Bloom JB, Uppaluri N, Phillips JL, Konno S, et al. Device-related adverse events during percutaneous nephrolithotomy: review of the manufacturer and user facility device experience database. J Endourol. 2017;31(10):1007–11.

Sánchez-Puy A, Bravo-Balado A, Diana P, Baboudjian M, Piana A, Girón I, et al. Generation pulse modulation in holmium:YAG lasers: a systematic review of the literature and meta-analysis. J Clin Med. 2022;11(11):3208.

Scotland KB, Kroczak T, Pace KT, Chew BH. Stone technology: intracorporeal lithotripters. World J Urol. 2017;35:1347–51.

Tailly T, Denstedt J. Innovations in percutaneous nephrolithotomy. Int J Surg. 2016;36:665–72.

Taratkin M, Laukhtina E, Singla N, Tarasov A, Alekseeva T, Enikeev M, Enikeev D. How lasers ablate stones: in vitro study of laser lithotripsy (Ho:YAG and Tm-fiber lasers) in different environments. J Endourol. 2021;35(6):931–6.

Tominaga K, Inoue T, Yamamichi F, Fujita M, Fujisawa M. Impact of vacuum-assisted mini-endoscopic combined intrarenal surgery for staghorn stones: analysis of perioperative factors of postoperative fever and stone-free status. J Endourol. 2023;37(4):400–6.

Zheng W, Denstedt JD (2000) Intracorporeal lithotripsy. Update on technology. Urol Clin North Am. 2000;27(2):301–13.

Exit Strategies in PCNL

Kazumi Taguchi, Rei Unno, Tomonori Habuchi, and Takahiro Yasui

Abstract Percutaneous nephrolithotomy (PCNL) is a highly effective treatment option for large renal stones, staghorn stones, and complex renal calculi. The procedure has become safer and more effective over time, and techniques, such as miniaturization of the percutaneous tract and improvements in surgical techniques, have made the insertion of a nephrostomy tube (NT) for drainage less necessary. The possible exit strategies in PCNL include large-bore NT, small-bore NT, externalized ureteral catheter, double-J stents, and tubeless with or without the use of hemostasis agents. The literature shows the advantages of small-bore over large-bore NT, ureteral stent over NT insertion, and tubeless over the use of NT and stents in terms of postoperative pain, duration of hospital stay, and complications, such as urinary leakage and bleeding. However, from the physician's perspective, the patient's quality of life and the cost of consumables also need to be considered, especially in the use of ureteral stents and hemostasis agents. Tubeless PCNL is now widely accepted for uncomplicated cases and may be beneficial to both physicians and patients. Although there are preoperative factors that can predict the optimal exit strategy during PCNL, including device selection by surgeons, precise intraoperative decisions are key to reducing complications and for effective practice. Here we review the literature, summarize the different types of drainage methods, and present a flow chart for intraoperative decision-making with regards to PCNL exit strategy.

Keywords Percutaneous nephrolithotomy · Nephrostomy tube · Ureteral stent · Tubeless · Hemostasis agents · Drainage · Exit

K. Taguchi · R. Unno · T. Yasui (✉)
Department of Nephro-urology, Nagoya City University Graduate School of Medical Sciences, Nagoya, Japan
e-mail: yasui@med.nagoya-cu.ac.jp

T. Habuchi
Department of Urology, Akita University Graduate School of Medicine, Akita, Japan

     369
J. D. Denstedt and E. N. Liatsikos (eds.), *Percutaneous Renal Surgery*,
https://doi.org/10.1007/978-3-031-40542-6_25

1 Introduction

Percutaneous nephrolithotomy (PCNL) is the most effective treatment for staghorn stones, large renal stones, and complex renal calculi. Improvements in technology and techniques have made the procedure safer and more effective and lowered complication rates. However, reducing postoperative pain, preventing urine leakage, and shortening hospital stay remain important areas of focus. At the completion of the procedure, nephrostomy tube (NT) insertion is widely performed for drainage to aid in the healing of the percutaneous tract; it also provides access for future procedures in the case of staged surgery. However, recent studies have shown that miniaturizing the percutaneous tract size and improving surgical techniques allows us to perform NT-free PCNL, which is safe and associated with minimal complications. Ureteric catheters and double-J (DJ) stents are currently available as alternatives to NT drainage. Hemostatic agents may also help to reduce bleeding after PCNL.

In this chapter, we summarize the use of NT as an exit strategy in PCNL and discuss the current understanding of the different types of drainage after PCNL, including large-bore and small-bore NT, ureteral stents, and tubeless methods.

2 NTs: Large-Bore, Small-Bore, and Nephroureterostomy Catheter

Large-bore NTs have a diameter ≥ 18 Fr, and some common examples are council-tip, circle, and re-entry Malecot catheters. Small-bore NTs have a diameter ≤ 18 Fr, and include the Cope loop NT, pigtail NT, and nephroureterostomy catheter (NUC). All NTs share certain essential features, including openings for drainage, self-retaining loops, an effluent channel for urinary drainage, and a tap connected to a drainage bag. Three randomized trials compared small- with large-bore NT and found that smaller tubes caused less pain, reduced analgesic requirements, and resulted in less urine leakage without increasing bleeding rates. Patients with small-bore NT also had shorter hospitalization periods (Sundaram et al. 2022). In contrast, a study of the Clinical Research Office of the Endourological Society (CROES) PCNL database showed contradictory results, with small-bore NT having greater bleeding and higher rates of fever and complications than large-bore NT. However, this study included a heterogeneous population and an unmatched group. It was concluded that larger tubes are preferable in complex cases (Cormio et al. 2013).

Moreover, NUCs are feasible alternatives to both large- and small-bore NTs. Some studies have suggested that using NUCs minimizes postoperative pain, reduces the length of hospital stay, and maintains ureteral patency (Bolton and Hennessey 2019).

3   NT Versus Ureteral Stent in PCNL

The CROES PCNL Global Study surveyed NT insertion as an exit strategy in PCNL, between November 2007 and December 2009 (Cormio et al. 2013). Patients who received NT only were more likely to have had prior open renal surgery than those who received stent only, which was the only significant difference between the groups. The most commonly used NT size was 20 Fr, followed by 14 Fr. In terms of the operative procedure the only significant difference reported between the NT- and stent-only groups was in relation to the percutaneous access point. The stone-free rates and incidence of bleeding did not differ significantly between the groups. The mean duration of PCNL varied from 67 to 82 min across treatment groups, and was longer for patients who had NT only than for those who had stent only. Postoperative hospital stay was also longer for NT-only patients than for stent-only patients; however, no other significant differences were noted between the two matched groups. Therefore, the authors concluded that stent-only might be a less invasive exit strategy, but that the choice should be made based on the intraoperative course of PCNL. There are several studies that have compared the efficacy and safety of NT and ureteral stent in PCNL; these are summarized in Table 1.

Earlier in the CROES survey, Yates et al. (Yates et al. 2009) reported that compared to standard PCNL with 26 Fr, NT-free PCNL with a DJ stent significantly reduced the length of hospital stay, analgesia requirements, transfusion rate, and mean hemoglobin decrease. Shah et al. (2009) analyzed more than 800 PCNL cases and concluded that DJ stent usage was associated with less postoperative pain, a reduced requirement for analgesia, and earlier discharge compared with standard PCNL with a 24 or 28 Fr NT, but there were no significant differences in complication and stone-free rates. The same group conducted a randomized controlled trial (RCT) (Shah et al. 2008) that aimed to compare the effectiveness of DJ and small-bore nephrostomy drainage after PCNL. Patients in the DJ group experienced less postoperative pain, needed less analgesia, and were discharged 9 h earlier than those in the 8 Fr NT group. The two groups had comparable surgical outcomes; however, patients in the DJ group had more severe stent-related symptoms.

Another RCT by Agrawal et al. (2008) demonstrated that patients in the DJ group had less pain, required less analgesia, and had a shorter hospital stay and a faster recovery time than those in the 16 Fr NT group. The incidence of urinary leakage from the nephrostomy site was lower in the DJ group. However, there were no significant differences between the two groups in terms of blood loss or urinary tract infection. They also compared the outcomes of smaller-sized NT with those of DJ drainage in 166 patients who underwent PCNL (Agrawal et al. 2014). The results of the study showed that patients in the DJ group required significantly less postoperative analgesia, had no urinary leakage, and spent significantly less time in hospital than those in the 12 Fr NT group. In addition, an RCT assessed patients' quality of life using the Wisconsin Stone Quality of Life questionnaire (WISQOL). The study found that patients in the DJ group had significantly worse quality of life changes and negative responses on the WISQOL assessment 7–10 days after surgery compared with patients who received nephrostomy drainage. Both groups had similar WISQOL scores 30 days after surgery (Zhao et al. 2016).

Table 1 Studies have compared the postoperative outcomes between nephrostomy tubes and ureteral stent placement in percutaneous nephrolithotomy

Authors	Year	Journal	Study type	Number of NT cases	Number of stent cases	Size of NT	Type of stent	Favors in DJ and/or EUC groups over NT group
Agrawal et al.	2008	J Endourol	RCT	101	101	16Fr	DJ	Less pain/required analgesia, shorter hospital stay, faster recovery time, lower urinary leakage incidence
Shah et al.	2008	J Endourol	RCT	33	32	8Fr	DJ	Less postoperative pain/analgesia, earlier discharge
Shah et al.	2009	BJU Int	Retrospective cohort	386	454	24 or 28Fr	DJ	Less postoperative pain, a reduced requirement for analgesia, earlier discharge
Yates et al.	2009	Ann R Coll Surg Engl	Case control study	55	46	26Fr	DJ	Shorter hospital stay, less analgesia, lower transfusion rate/Hb decrease
Gonulalan et al.	2013	Urolithiasis	Retrospective cohort	180	148, 120	14Fr	DJ, EUC	Shorter hospitalization time, lower VAS scores, lower need for postoperative transfusion/narcotic analgesic
Agrawal et al.	2014	J Endourol	RCT	83	83	12Fr	DJ	Less postoperative analgesia and shorter hospital stay

(continued)

Table 1 (continued)

Authors	Year	Journal	Study type	Number of NT cases	Number of stent cases	Size of NT	Type of stent	Favors in DJ and/or EUC groups over NT group
Zhao et al.	2016	J Endourol	RCT	15	15	8 or 10Fr	DJ	Worse WISQOL at 7 to 10 days after surgery
Pimentel Torres et al.	2020	Minerva Urol Nephrol	Retrospective cohort	198	123	–	DJ, SJ	Lower complication rate and shorter hospitalization
Raharja et al.	2020	Urol J	Retrospective cohort	350	189, 227	8–10.5Fr	DJ, EUC	Shorter hospital stay and lower pain score in EUC group

DJ double-J stent; *SJ* single-J stent; *EUC* externalized ureteral catheter; *RCT* randomized controlled trial; *WISQOL* Wisconsin stone quality of life questionnaire

A retrospective study evaluated 707 patients who underwent PCNL with either 14 Fr NT, DJ, or externalized ureteral catheter (EUC) between 2004 and 2011. The results showed that patients in the NT group had longer hospitalization times, higher visual analog scale scores, and a greater need of postoperative transfusion and narcotic analgesics compared with the other two groups (Gonulalan et al. 2013). They found that NT was associated with a higher rate of complications (30.3 versus 13%) and longer hospitalization (4 versus 2 days) than ureteral stents. Both types of ureteral stent were associated with similar morbidities and lengths of hospital stay. Patients with a higher stone burden were more likely to undergo NT and DJ. In addition, Raharja et al. (2020) found that tubeless PCNL with EUC had a shorter postoperative hospitalization period and lower postoperative pain scores than PCNL with NT or DJ stent. The EUC group also had a lower urine leakage complication rate than that of the NT group.

4 NT Versus Tubeless in PCNL

The use of tubeless PCNL as an alternative to standard PCNL with NT has been evaluated in multiple studies, through systematic reviews and meta-analyses. These studies aimed to compare the outcomes of the two procedures and identify which method is safer and more effective for patients with urolithiasis. These studies are summarized in Table 2.

Table 2 Meta-analyses have compared postoperative outcomes between tubeless and nephrostomy tube placement in percutaneous nephrolithotomy

Authors	Year	Journal	Number of studies	Number of tubeless cases	Number of NT cases	Advantages of tubeless methods
Gauhar et al.	2022	Urolithiasis	26	907	932	Shorter operative time and hospital stay, lower postoperative urinary fistula rate
Li et al.	2020	Minim Invasive Ther Allied Technol	14	529	602	Shorter operative time and hospital stay, less postoperative pain medication use
Chen et al.	2020	Asian J Surg	15	470	477	Reduced postoperative pain, analgesia use, hospital stay, and urine leakage
Nouralizadeh et al.	2018	Urologia J	3	74	73	No difference among pediatric cases
Xun et al.	2017	BMC Urol	14	576	572	Shorter operative time/ hospital stay, faster recovery, lower postoperative pain scores, reduced analgesia requirement/ urine leakage
Lee et al.	2017	BMC Urol	16	476	485	Smaller hemoglobin changes/ pain scores, shorter operation time
Zhong et al.	2013	J Endourol	9	304	348	Shorter hospital stay, less pain medication requirement

(continued)

Table 2 (continued)

Authors	Year	Journal	Number of studies	Number of tubeless cases	Number of NT cases	Advantages of tubeless methods
Wang et al.	2012	BJU Int	7	705	660	Less analgesic requirement, shorter hospital stay
Shen et al.	2012	Urol Int	9	258	289	Less postoperative pain, shorter hospital stay
Yuan et al.	2011	Urol Res	14	776		Shorter hospital stay, less requirement of postoperative analgesic, lower rate of urine leakage
Ni et al.	2011	Urology	13	375	377	Shorter hospital stay, less pain medication, faster return to normal activity

NT nephrostomy tube

A review by Gauhar et al. analyzed 26 studies and found that total tubeless PCNL resulted in a shorter operative time and hospital stay, as well as a lower rate of postoperative urinary fistula, than standard PCNL. However, other factors, such as blood transfusions, pain scores, and infection rates, did not differ significantly between the two approaches (Gauhar et al. 2022).

Another analysis included 1365 cases from seven studies and found no differences in efficacy in terms of operation duration and hematocrit change. Tubeless PCNL had lower analgesic requirements and shorter hospital stays than standard PCNL with NT (Wang et al. 2012). An update on this analysis found no significant differences in postoperative hemoglobin reduction, stone-free rate, postoperative fever rate, or blood transfusion rate (Xun et al. 2017). A separate meta-analysis involving 947 patients from 15 randomized clinical trials found that tubeless PCNL was associated with reduced postoperative pain, analgesic use, hospital stay, and urine leakage compared to standard PCNL, but no significant differences were observed with regard to other outcomes such as drop in hemoglobin, stone-free status, blood transfusion, and pyrexia (Chen et al. 2020). No significant differences were observed in postoperative hemoglobin reduction, stone-free rate, postoperative fever rate, or blood transfusion rate.

A meta-analysis by Nouralizadeh et al. (2018) investigated the outcomes of tubeless PCNL and standard PCNL in the pediatric population and found that patients who underwent tubeless PCNL had a slightly shorter length of hospitalization than those who underwent standard PCNL; however, the difference was not statistically significant.

Network meta-analyses suggested that total tubeless PCNL may be better than PCNL with small-bore NT and PCNL with stents for hemoglobin changes, and PCNL with small-bore NT superior to PCNL with stents. Regarding the length of hospital stay, total tubeless and PCNLs with stents were better than PCNL with NT. PCNL with small-bore NT and total tubeless PCNLs were ranked higher than the other techniques in terms of operation time and pain scores (Lee et al. 2017). Another meta-analysis comparing an NT-free group, a small tube group (8–9 Fr), a middle tube group (16–18 Fr), and a large tube group (20–24 Fr) found that there were no significant differences in hospital stay and postoperative pain on day 1 between the NT-free group and the small tube group, but there were differences between the NT-free group and the middle and large tube groups (Shen et al. 2012).

Overall, most studies suggest that tubeless PCNL is safe and effective for carefully evaluated and selected patients. Tubeless PCNL requires significantly less pain medication and results in a shorter hospital stay and faster return to normal activity. However, there were no significant differences in the rates of complications and blood transfusions between the two procedures. While some studies have found similar outcomes between the two approaches, others have found significant differences in operative time, analgesia requirement, and urine leakage (Li et al. 2020; Zhong et al. 2013; Yuan et al. 2011; Ni et al. 2011). It is important for urologists to consider these findings when making exit decisions after PCNL.

5   Hemostasis Techniques and Agents in Tubeless PCNL

Achieving hemostasis may be more important in tubeless PCNL compared with PCNL with NT. Mechanical compression after the procedure, stitches in the deep fascia, direct diathermy of the visible bleeding vessels, and cryotherapy are techniques used to achieve hemostasis (Jou et al. 2004; Aron et al. 2004; Mouracade et al. 2008). Hemostatic agents such as oxidized cellulose, gelatin, and fibrin sealants have also been used to speed up this process (Aghamir et al. 2006; Shah et al. 2006; Gudeman et al. 2012; Noller et al. 2004; Mikhail et al. 2003; Ziaee et al. 2013; Nagele et al. 2006).

Gelatin matrix products expand and produce a compressive effect, whereas fibrin sealants contain both thrombin and fibrinogen, which form a clot regardless of patient factors. However, experimental studies have shown some adverse effects; gelatin matrix products can form a fine suspension of particles when in contact with urine, which may contribute to stone formation (Uribe et al. 2005). Although some studies found these techniques to be safe and associated with shorter hospital stays, they did not show any decrease in bleeding complication rates compared with control groups

(Aghamir et al. 2006; Shah et al. 2006; Gudeman et al. 2012; Noller et al. 2004). Gelatin matrix hemostatic sealants and thrombin-soaked absorptive gelatin sealants have also been successfully used in tubeless PCNL procedures (Mikhail et al. 2003; Ziaee et al. 2013).

These studies did not provide high-level evidence indicating the best treatment of the access tract in PCNL, but most agreed that sealing the tract could be omitted in uncomplicated procedures without increasing the risk of complications. In addition, using hemostatic sealants led to a significant increase in procedural costs (Hüsch et al. 2015). A summary of these studies is presented in Table 3.

Table 3 Studies have evaluated the use of hemostatic agents in tubeless PCNL

Authors	Year	Journals	Number of cases	Study type	Hemostasis	Results
Gudeman et al.	2012	BJU Int	107	Retrospective	Fibrin sealant	Shorter hospital stays, lower complication rates
Noller et al.	2004	J Urol	8	Consecutive	Fibrin sealant	Safe and feasible
Shah et al.	2006	J Endourol	70	Consecutive	Fibrin sealant	Safe, less analgesic requirement, shorter hospital stays
Mikhail et al.	2003	Urology	43	Retrospective	Fibrin sealant	Safe
Jou et al.	2004	J Endourol	51	Consecutive	Diathermy	Safe
Aron et al.	2004	Urol Int	40	Consecutive	Diathermy	Simple and easy procedure
Singh et al.	2008	J Endourol	50	Consecutive	Gelatin sealant	Shorter hospital stays, lower urinary extravasation, lower analgesia use
Nagele et al.	2006	Urology	11	Prospective	Gelatin sealant	Safe
Ziaee et al.	2013	Urol J	43	Randomized	Autologous fibrin glue	No significant difference
Aghamir et al.	2006	J Endourol	22	Randomized	Oxidized cellulose	Did not affect bleeding or urine leak rate

(continued)

Table 3 (continued)

Authors	Year	Journals	Number of cases	Study type	Hemostasis	Results
Hüsch T et al.	2015	World J Urol	–	Systematic review	Various	Not provide high-level evidence for the use of agents, increase in the immediate costs

6 Intraoperative Decision-Making for Appropriate Exit

Ultimately, the exit strategy during PCNL depends on intraoperative factors that surgeons face, some of which are predictable prior to surgery, and some of which are not. The most important factor is the need for a second procedure. If there are sufficient untreated residual fragments, a second-look procedure will be required, and in such cases, either an NT or EUC needs to be inserted. Additionally, the possibility of developing postoperative fever, urinary tract infection, bleeding, or intraoperative complications such as urinary injury or other organ injuries requires drainage with an NT, DJ stent, or EUC, depending on the patient's characteristics and medical history.

There may be a few unfortunate situations in which surgeons must decide to discontinue the procedure, owing to the following:

1. Inadequate visualization. To treat stones, surgeons must gain a clear endoscopic view. If the stone is not well visualized owing to anatomical, bleeding, or device malfunction issues, it may be difficult to safely continue.
2. Complications. PCNL is generally a safe procedure; however, similar to any surgical procedure, it can be associated with complications. If a patient experiences significant bleeding, infection, or other complications during the operation, the surgeon may decide to stop the procedure and manage the complications before continuing.
3. Patient discomfort. PCNL is generally performed under general anesthesia; however, patients may experience discomfort, pain, or sudden vital changes during the procedure. If the patient is unable to tolerate the procedure or experiences significant discomfort, the procedure may need to be discontinued and planned as staged surgery.

The decision to discontinue the procedure during PCNL depends on a variety of factors, including the patient's health status, size and location of the stone, and any complications that arise during the procedure. The surgeon works closely with the patient to ensure that the safest and most effective treatment plan is selected.

Figure 1 shows the flow chart for intraoperative decision making for PCNL exit. As described in the literature, (Veser et al. 2020) confirmation of residual fragments,

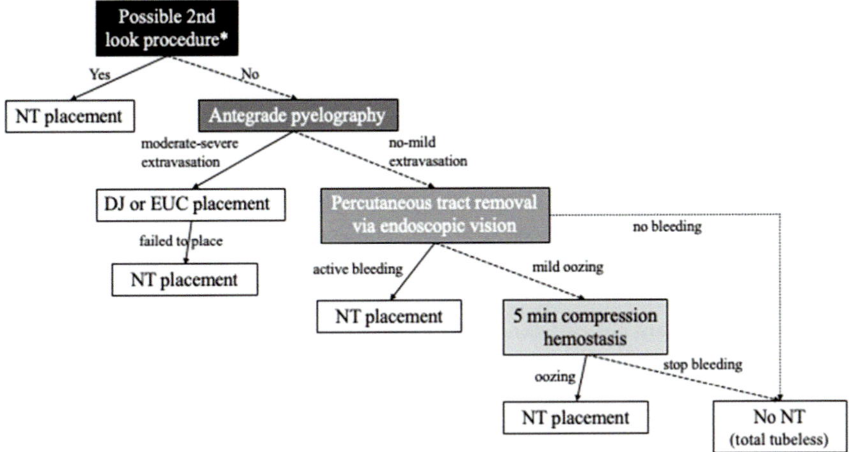

Fig. 1 Flow chart for intraoperative decision-making regarding drainage methods. * Residual fragments or intraoperative complications. NT, nephrostomy tube; DJ, double-J stent; EUC, externalized ureteral catheter

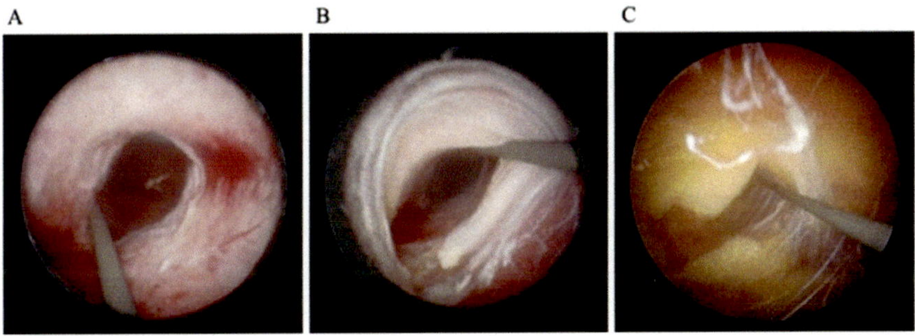

Fig. 2 Endoscopic images during percutaneous tract removal with a safety guidewire. A) Renal parenchyma just outside the renal collecting system, B) inside Gerota's fascia, and C) the subcutaneous tissue

extravasation, and parenchymal as well as interfascial bleeding (Fig. 2) are the most important factors in selecting NT or stent insertion for drainage.

7 Summary

An exit strategy for PCNL involves considering the placement of an NT, which is optional in uncomplicated, presumed stone-free cases. Opting for tubeless PCNL can result in less postoperative pain, reduced hospital stay, and similar complication rates. Tract sealing techniques such as electrocauterization, fibrin glue, and hemostatic matrix placement have been found to be safe and effective in controlling tract bleeding. However, further randomized controlled trials are necessary to determine the clinical significance of these results. Typically, an NT is required in PCNL to aid hemostasis, prevent urine leakage, and allow re-entry into the collecting system. Tubeless PCNL involves performing the procedure without using a postoperative NT. In early tubeless PCNL, an internal DJ stent or EUC was necessary; however, newer versions do not require either. Tubeless PCNL is recommended only for specific cases, including single-tract procedures with no collecting system perforation, complete stone removal, and no active bleeding from the tract. Although tubeless PCNL has been found to have similar stone-free and complication rates to standard PCNL, there are still concerns regarding tract bleeding, which may require additional hemostasis technique.

References

Aghamir SMK, Khazaeli MH, Meisami A. Use of surgical for sealing nephrostomy tract after totally tubeless percutaneous nephrolithotomy. J Endourol. 2006;20:293–5.

Agrawal MS, Agrawal M, Gupta A, Bansal S, Yadav A, Goyal J. A randomized comparison of tubeless and standard percutaneous nephrolithotomy. J Endourol. 2008;22:439–42.

Agrawal MS, Sharma M, Agarwal K. Tubeless percutaneous nephrolithotomy using antegrade tether: a randomized study. J Endourol. 2014;28:644–8.

Aron M, Goel R, Kesarwani PK, Gupta NP. Hemostasis in tubeless PNL: point of technique. Urol Int. 2004;73:244–7.

Bolton DM, Hennessey DB (2019) Exit strategies after percutaneous nephrolithotomy. In: Smith's textbook of endourology. p. 427–40.

Chen ZJ, Yan YJ, Zhou JJ. Comparison of tubeless percutaneous nephrolithotomy and standard percutaneous nephrolithotomy for kidney stones: a meta-analysis of randomized trials. Asian J Surg. 2020;43:60–8.

Cormio L, Preminger G, Saussine C, Buchholz NP, Zhang X, Walfridsson H, Gross AJ, de la Rosette J. Nephrostomy in percutaneous nephrolithotomy (PCNL): does nephrostomy tube size matter? Results from the Global PCNL study from the clinical research office endourology society. World J Urol. 2013;31:1563–8.

Cormio L, Gonzalez GI, Tolley D, Sofer M, Muslumanoglu A, Klingler HC, Stolzenburg JU, de la Rosette J. Exit strategies following percutaneous nephrolithotomy (PCNL): a comparison of surgical outcomes in the Clinical Research Office of the Endourological Society (CROES) PCNL Global Study. World J Urol. 2013;31:1239–44.

Gauhar V, Traxer O, García Rojo E, et al. Complications and outcomes of tubeless versus nephrostomy tube in percutaneous nephrolithotomy: a systematic review and meta-analysis of randomized clinical trials. Urolithiasis. 2022;50:511–22.

Gonulalan U, Cicek T, Istanbulluoglu O, Kosan M, Ozturk B, Ozkardes H. Tubeless percutaneous nephrolithotomy is effective and safe in short- and long-term urinary drainage. Urolithiasis. 2013;41:341–6.

Gudeman SR, Stroup SP, Durbin JM, Patino G, L'Esperance JO, Auge BK. Percutaneous stone surgery using a tubeless technique with fibrin sealant: report of our first 107 cases. BJU Int. 2012;110:E1048–52.

Hüsch T, Reiter M, Mager R, Steiner E, Herrmann TRW, Haferkamp A, Schilling D. The management of the access tract after percutaneous nephrolithotomy. World J Urol. 2015;33:1921–8.

Jou YC, Cheng MC, Sheen JH, te Lin C, Chen PC. Cauterization of access tract for nephrostomy tube-free percutaneous nephrolithotomy. J Endourol. 2004;18:547–9.

Lee JY, Jeh SU, Kim MD, Kang DH, Kwon JK, Ham WS, Choi YD, Cho KS. Intraoperative and postoperative feasibility and safety of total tubeless, tubeless, small-bore tube, and standard percutaneous nephrolithotomy: a systematic review and network meta-analysis of 16 randomized controlled trials. BMC Urol. 2017;17:1–16.

Li Q, Gao L, Li J, Zhang Y, Jiang Q. Total tubeless versus standard percutaneous nephrolithotomy: a meta-analysis. Minim Invasive Ther Allied Technol. 2020;29:61–9.

Mikhail AA, Kaptein JS, Bellman GC. Use of fibrin glue in percutaneous nephrolithotomy. Urology. 2003;61:910–4.

Mouracade P, Spie R, Lang H, Jacqmin D, Saussine C. Tubeless percutaneous nephrolithotomy: What about replacing the double-j stent with a ureteral catheter? J Endourol. 2008;22:273–5.

Nagele U, Schilling D, Anastasiadis AG, Corvin S, Seibold J, Kuczyk M, Stenzl A, Sievert KD. Closing the tract of mini-percutaneous nephrolithotomy with gelatine matrix hemostatic sealant can replace nephrostomy tube placement. Urology. 2006;68:489–93.

Ni S, Qiyin C, Tao W, Liu L, Jiang H, Hu H, Han R, Wang C. Tubeless percutaneous nephrolithotomy is associated with less pain and shorter hospitalization compared with standard or small bore drainage: a meta-analysis of randomized, controlled trials. Urology. 2011;77:1293–8.

Noller MW, Baughman SM, Morey AF, Auge BK. Fibrin sealant enables tubeless percutaneous stone surgery. J Urol. 2004;172:166–9.

Nouralizadeh A, Simforoosh N, Shemshaki H, Soltani MH, Sotoudeh M, Ramezani MH, Nikravesh M, Golshan A, Ansari A. Tubeless versus standard percutaneous nephrolithotomy in pediatric patients: a systematic review and meta-analysis. Urologia J. 2018;85:3–9.

Raharja PAR, Atmoko W, Rasyid N, Birowo P. Safety and effectiveness of externalized ureteral catheter in tubeless percutaneous nephrolithotomy. Urol J. 2020;17:456–61.

Shah HN, Kausik V, Hedge S, Shah JN, Bansal MB. Initial experience with hemostatic fibrin glue as adjuvant during tubeless percutaneous nephrolithotomy. J Endourol. 2006;20:194–8.

Shah HN, Sodha HS, Khandkar AA, Kharodawala S, Hegde SS, Bansal MB. A randomized trial evaluating type of nephrostomy drainage after percutaneous nephrolithotomy: small bore v tubeless. J Endourol. 2008;22:1433–9.

Shah H, Khandkar A, Sodha H, Kharodawala S, Hegde S, Bansal M. Tubeless percutaneous nephrolithotomy: 3 years of experience with 454 patients. BJU Int. 2009;104:840–6.

Shen P, Liu Y, Wang J. Nephrostomy tube-free versus nephrostomy tube for renal drainage after percutaneous nephrolithotomy: a systematic review and meta-analysis. Urol Int. 2012;88:298–306.

Sundaram P, Ramesh M, Mishra DK, Agrawal MS (2022) Exit strategy after PCNL. In: Minimally invasive percutaneous nephrolithotomy. p. 197–204.

Uribe CA, Eichel L, Khonsari S, et al. What happens to hemostatic agents in contact with urine? An in vitro study. J Endourol. 2005;19:312–7.

Veser J, Fajkovic H, Seitz C. Tubeless percutaneous nephrolithotomy: evaluation of minimal invasive exit strategies after percutaneous stone treatment. Curr Opin Urol. 2020;30:679–83.

Wang J, Zhao C, Zhang C, Fan X, Lin Y, Jiang Q. Tubeless versus standard percutaneous nephrolithotomy: a meta-analysis. BJU Int. 2012;109:918–24.

Xun Y, Wang Q, Hu H, Lu Y, Zhang J, Qin B, Geng Y, Wang S. Tubeless versus standard percutaneous nephrolithotomy: an update meta-analysis. BMC Urol. 2017;17:1–17.

Yates DR, Safdar RK, Spencer PA, Parys BT. "Nephrostomy-free" percutaneous nephrolithotomy: experience in a UK district general hospital. Ann R Coll Surg Engl. 2009;91:570–7.

Yuan H, Zheng S, Liu L, Han P, Wang J, Wei Q. The efficacy and safety of tubeless percutaneous nephrolithotomy: a systematic review and meta-analysis. Urol Res. 2011;39:401–10.

Zhao PT, Hoenig DM, Smith AD, Okeke Z. A randomized controlled comparison of nephrostomy drainage versus ureteral stent following percutaneous nephrolithotomy using the Wisconsin stone QOL. J Endourol. 2016;30:1275–84.

Zhong Q, Zheng C, Mo J, Piao Y, Zhou Y, Jiang Q. Total tubeless versus standard percutaneous nephrolithotomy: a meta-analysis. J Endourol. 2013;27:420–6.

Ziaee SAM, Sarhangnejad R, Abolghasemi H, Eshghi P, Radfar MH, Ahanian A, Parizi mehdi kardoust, Amirizadeh N, Nouralizadeh A (2013) Autologous fibrin sealant in tubeless percutaneous nephrolithotomy: a prospective study. Urol J. 2013 10:999–1003.

Outpatient Percutaneous Nephrolithotomy

Darren Beiko

Abstract Percutaneous nephrolithotomy (PCNL) is the gold standard for management of large renal calculi. Traditionally, PCNL has involved placement of a nephrostomy tube and admission to hospital. The rationale for this approach was to ensure optimal renal drainage and observe for the development of the two major potential acute life-threatening post-PCNL complications—sepsis and hemorrhage. At the present time, this standard approach remains the most prevalent among urologists performing PCNL. However, a shift toward ambulatory surgery across surgical specialties, the emergence of tubeless PCNL, widespread adoption of mini-PCNL (mPCNL) and the pressures to preserve valuable hospital resources have resulted in the rise of outpatient PCNL (oPCNL). Over the past several years, oPCNL has gained momentum across the globe as a safe and effective option in highly selected patients. In this chapter, a comprehensive review of the oPCNL literature—comparing it to standard PCNL (sPCNL) involving hospital admission where appropriate—is provided to understand the current state of oPCNL in 2023. The chapter will include sections on the history of oPCNL, practical advantages and disadvantages of oPCNL, patient selection for oPCNL, intraoperative considerations for oPCNL, outcomes of oPCNL, steps to build an oPCNL program and potential future advances in oPCNL.

Keywords Urolithiasis · Renal Calculi · Percutaneous nephrolithotomy · Tubeless · Outpatient surgery · Ambulatory surgery

Abbreviations

aPCNL	Ambulatory percutaneous nephrolithotomy
ASA	American Society of Anesthesiologists'
BMI	Body mass index
CROES	Clinical Research Office of the Endourological Society

D. Beiko (✉)
Department of Urology and Smith School of Business, Queen's University, Kingston, ON K7L 2V7, Canada
e-mail: beiko@queensu.ca

J. D. Denstedt and E. N. Liatsikos (eds.), *Percutaneous Renal Surgery*,
https://doi.org/10.1007/978-3-031-40542-6_26

ER   Emergency room
LOS   Length of stay
mPCNL   Mini-percutaneous nephrolithotomy
oPCNL   Outpatient percutaneous nephrolithotomy
OR   Operating room
PCNL   Percutaneous nephrolithotomy
PROM   Patient-reported outcome measure
QoL   Quality of life
SFR   Stone-free rate
sPCNL   Standard percutaneous nephrolithotomy (with hospital admission)
UCSD   University of California San Diego

1   History of Outpatient PCNL

Unbeknownst to many, the history of outpatient PCNL dates back almost 40 years
to the mid-1980s (Preminger et al. 1986). It may not surprise most readers to learn
that the true pioneers of oPCNL included two rising urologists who became giants
in the world of endourology—Drs. Glenn Preminger and Ralph Clayman. In their
1985 case series published in the Journal of Urology, they reported a series of 5
patients who underwent successful 1-stage percutaneous stone removal on an outpatient basis. Their patients were treated in the radiology procedure suite under assisted
local anesthesia, removing all stones intact. A 22F Councill catheter was used as a
nephrostomy tube and they placed an antegrade 5F ureteral catheter in each patient.
Patients remained in the day surgery unit for an average of 4.5 hours before being
discharged. Antegrade nephrostograms were performed on postoperative days 1–
4 and there were no complications. After Preminger et al.'s publication in 1985,
advances in oPCNL fell into a period of dormancy for almost a quarter century.

Twenty-four years after Preminger et al.'s initial report, oPCNL was resurrected
by a 2009 case report of totally tubeless oPCNL in which a patient was discharged
home 72 minutes after transferring out of the recovery room, without a nephrostomy
tube or stent or Foley catheter (Beiko et al. 2009). The next year, two small case series
of outpatient emerged from Canada (Beiko and Lee 2010; Shahrour and Andonian
2010). In 2018, Abbott and Davalos advanced the field of oPCNL by being the first
to report safe and effective ambulatory PCNL (aPCNL) in a freestanding ambulatory
surgery center, eliminating the hospital altogether (Abbott and Davalos 2018). The
first systematic review and meta-analysis on day case PCNL were published in 2019
Jones et al. (2019) and 2020 Gao et al. (2020), respectively. Since 2010, oPCNL
has slowly gained momentum across several continents, as evidenced by the surging
number of published abstracts and articles annually.

In the literature, the terms aPCNL and oPCNL are often used interchangeably, and
day care PCNL has been used to refer to both (Jones et al. 2019; Gao et al. 2020). For
the purposes of this chapter, aPCNL refers to discharge home within 24 hours home,

often from a short-stay surgical unit and sometimes on postoperative day 1. On the other hand, oPCNL refers specifically to same-day discharge, often a few short hours after surgery. In other words, all oPCNL cases are by definition aPCNL cases but not all aPCNL cases qualify as oPCNL. Although this chapter focuses on oPCNL, because some studies include a hybrid population of both same-day and < 24 hours discharges, it is impractical to ignore aPCNL studies when reviewing oPCNL.

2   Practical Advantages and Disadvantages of oPCNL

Advantages. There are several advantages to performing PCNL on a completely outpatient basis. These advantages are listed in Table 1. First, oPCNL is completely compatible with the high level shift toward ambulatory care across all surgical specialties. The Davalos group has taken it one step further, shifting PCNL from a hospital-based operation to a freestanding surgery center-based operation (Abbott and Davalos 2018; Chong et al. 2021). Second, shorter hospital stays are incentivized by reimbursement schedules in many jurisdictions. Third, even if done in a hospital setting, oPCNL minimizes the patient's time spent in a healthcare institution, thereby reducing their risk of nosocomial infections. Fourth, hospital resources can be conserved. With the advent of oPCNL, fewer hospital beds are required, nursing care requirements are lower and costly intravenous medication needs are decreased as well. Fifth, oPCNL usually avoids the need for a nephrostomy tube, which in turn eliminates the need for additional x-rays and/or trips to the interventional radiology suite for antegrade nephrostography. Sixth, oPCNL results in lower costs to the healthcare systems involved, mainly by eliminating the costs associated with hospitalization. This has been shown in several studies in different jurisdictions and will be presented below in the section on outcomes. Seventh, shifting from inpatient to oPCNL eliminates overnight hospital admission which directly results in an increased hospital operating margin, as shown by Thakker et al. (2022). Eighth, by avoiding an overnight stay in hospital and allowing the patient to sleep in the comfort of their own home, the patient experience is improved. This improvement in patient experience has been shown through the work of Abbott et al. in their freestanding ambulatory surgery center (Abbott and Davalos 2018). Finally, oPCNL facilitates earlier ambulation and a more rapid return to normal activities of daily living for the patient.

Disadvantages. There are several disadvantages to sending patients home a few short hours after PCNL. These disadvantages are summarized in Table 1. The first, and perhaps most significant, drawback is losing the ability to closely monitor the patient's clinical status and vital signs in the early postoperative period for potential septic shock or hemorrhagic shock. This may in fact be the biggest barrier for many urologists to starting oPCNL. After all, patient safety is of paramount importance and most urologists and endourologists currently performing PCNL trained during a time when post-PCNL hospital admission was a routine part of the patient care pathway. Second, oPCNL may result in inefficient care if the patient needs to return

Table 1 Practical advantages and disadvantages of outpatient PCNL

Advantages
Aligned with shift to ambulatory surgery
Aligned with reimbursement schedules
Lowers the risks associated with hospitalization
Conserves valuable hospital resources
Typically avoids nephrostomy tube
Lowers overall cost to healthcare system
Increases hospital operating margin
Improved patient experience
Earlier ambulation and return to activities of daily living
Disadvantages
Patient safety concerns (e.g., hemorrhage)
Inefficient care (e.g., return for imaging on postoperative day #1 or 2)
May limit postoperative options (e.g., 2nd look nephroscopy)
Patient stress/anxiety
Urologist stress/insomnia
Requires embracing change

on postoperative day 1 or 2 for bloodwork or imaging. Third, some potential postoperative interventions, such as 2nd look nephroscopy, may not be possible without nephrostomy tube access. Fourth, the thought of being discharged home a few hours after renal trauma may cause significant stress and anxiety for some patients. This may lead some patients to be very hesitant to follow a same-day discharge plan. Fifth, the wellbeing of the treating urologist may be at risk due to insomnia arising from wandering thoughts of the patient potentially suffering from acute hemorrhagic or septic shock at home. Finally, a major barrier to oPCNL for many treating urologists is the challenge of managing and embracing the change needed to succeed. Changing one's practice can be very difficult for experienced urologists with established practices that are safe and effective and, in many cases, associated with world class results. When an experienced urologist—one who routinely admits their patients postoperatively—is achieving excellent outcomes in their PCNL patients, how can anyone blame her/him for resisting oPCNL?

Despite the above drawbacks, the advantages of oPCNL outweigh the disadvantages, and this forms the rationale for oPCNL.

3   Patient Selection for Outpatient PCNL

When starting an oPCNL program, adherence to strict patient selection criteria is strongly recommended initially to minimize morbidity and ensure a successful oPCNL program is built. The two groups from Canada who resurrected oPCNL both clearly described their initial strict selection criteria in their case series (Beiko and Lee 2010; Shahrour and Andonian 2010). As can be seen from Schoenfeld et al.'s published inclusion and exclusion criteria (Schoenfeld et al. 2019), there are, understandably, significant similarities and overlap in the selection criteria for oPCNL across different institutions.

Preoperative Selection Criteria. The first step is to ensure the PCNL patient is medically fit for same-day discharge. Although most endourology practices focus primarily on adults, oPCNL should be safe and feasible in children if one or more reliable parent stays with the child. We would expect oPCNL to be performed in children in centers of excellence and/or high volume centers. According to literature review, Jackman et al. were the first to report safe and successful oPCNL in a child in 1998 (Jackman et al. 1998), and Chong et al. have reported effective aPCNL in their state-of-the-art freestanding surgery center in patients as young as 16 years old (Chong et al. 2021). When starting out, it is recommended that generally healthy adults with normal renal function, an American Society of Anesthesiologist's (ASA) score of 1 or 2 and a body-mass index (BMI) less than 35 kg/m^2 (class 1 obesity) be considered for oPCNL. As experience is gained and the treating urologist sees firsthand how safe and effective oPCNL is in this patient population, she or he can consider select ASA class 3 and more obese patients.

After the patient is determined to be medically fit for same-day discharge, the next step is to ensure the stone burden and renal anatomy are appropriate for same-day discharge. For example, when starting oPCNL, the urologist ideally chooses patients with small to medium stone burdens and uncomplicated intrarenal collecting system anatomy. For example, although large staghorn calculi and complex calyceal diverticular stones may eventually be appropriate for same-day discharge, the urologist may want to exclude these types of complicated situations in the early phases of adopting oPCNL.

Finally, the patient must be socially fit for oPCNL. Treating urologists will want to ensure the patient has adequate support of family or friends, including someone to stay overnight with them. The patient and/or family/friend should be reliable and able to understand and ensure compliance with postoperative instructions. Specifically, the urologist needs to be assured the patient and caregiver know the signs and symptoms of an urgent complication such as septic shock or hemorrhagic shock and know when to return urgently to the emergency room (ER) to mitigate risk to the patient. Ideally, the patient lives or stays close enough to the hospital to allow for rapid access to the ER.

Intraoperative Selection Criteria. Uncomplicated, relatively brief cases that appear to have achieved a stone-free state and lack evidence of purulent urine, hemorrhage, perforation can be considered for oPCNL. It is ill-advised to consider same-day discharge on a patient with any type of significant intraoperative complication. The intraoperative criteria for selecting candidates for oPCNL are perhaps the most important, especially considering the urologist has control over the criteria related to technique. The urologist controls the point at which the collecting system is accessed, the number of attempts to gain access, the number of tracts created, whether a long narrow infundibulum is dilated, and she/he impacts whether (and to what degree) collecting system perforation occurs.

Postoperative Selection Criteria. A patient may be considered for same-day discharge following PCNL when their pain, nausea and vomiting is adequately controlled with oral medication. Patients in the recovery room must be hemodynamically stable, and it is recommended that they have recovery room bloodwork showing an acceptable hemoglobin and hematocrit. If an upper pole and/or supracostal puncture was performed, then the patient should have a normal post operative chest x-ray in the recovery room showing no evidence of pneumothorax or any other thoracic complication. Once the patient has satisfied all the preoperative, intraoperative and postoperative discharge criteria, they can be considered for oPCNL.

Extended Selection Criteria. As experience is gained and acceptable safety and efficacy outcomes are realized, the urologist will naturally start extending their selection criteria. At the University of California at San Diego (UCSD), Bechis et al. were the first to assess outcomes of PCNL on a completely outpatient basis in a high volume stone center of excellence without strict patient selection criteria (Bechis et al. 2018). In their study, 72% (43 of 60) patients involving 61 renal units (1 bilateral case) were successfully discharged home the same day as planned. Importantly, only 1 of the 17 unplanned postoperative admissions—a small incisional urine leak requiring nephrostomy tube change—was due to a technical/surgical factor. The remaining unplanned admissions were due to symptom control (7 patients), social factors (6 patients), delayed respiratory function (2 patients) and urinary retention in one patient. Just as importantly, they showed that oPCNL could be safely performed, with excellent results, in patients with significant comorbidities (44% of their patients were ASA class 3 or 4), large/complex renal stones (24% had staghorn calculi and/or encrusted stents) and anomalous/complex renal anatomy (23% had anomalies, horseshoe or transplant kidney). More recently, Hosier et al. provided further support to the findings of Bechis et al. by similarly showing oPCNL is feasible in ASA class 3 and 4 patients, bilateral stones, solitary kidneys, transplant kidneys, large stone burdens including complete staghorn calculi, multiple tracts and preexisting nephrostomy tubes/stents (Hosier et al. 2022). Additionally, Hosier et al. extended the selection criteria further by reporting outcomes in morbidly obese patients and octogenarians.

Contraindications. Given the expanded selection criteria described above, there are relatively few absolute contraindications to oPCNL. American Society of Anesthesiologists' (ASA) class 5 is an absolute contraindication, as a moribund patient should not ever undergo PCNL or anything more than a nephrostomy tube or stent. For similar reasons, ASA class 4 is a strong contraindication to PCNL, although both studies cited above using extended selection criteria each reported successful oPCNL in a single ASA class 4 patient (Bechis et al. 2018; Hosier et al. 2022). Similarly, although morbid obesity is not an absolute contraindication, same-day discharge would be generally unwise in patients with class 4 obesity. Having said that, in Hosier et al.'s study, same-day discharge was performed in morbidly obese patients with BMIs as high as 82 kg/m^2 (Hosier et al. 2022). Any patient living alone, who lacks the support of a family member or friend to stay overnight with them, is not suitable for same-day discharge. Any intraoperative findings or complications related to major concern for infection, perforation or bleeding will require hospital admission. Any patient with evidence a significant pneumothorax, hydrothorax, hemothorax or urinothorax (particularly if it requires a chest tube) should not be discharged home. Finally, any ongoing symptoms (most commonly pain, nausea or vomiting) requiring intravenous therapy are considered contraindications to same-day discharge following PCNL. The absolute and strong relative contraindications to oPCNL are enumerated in Box 1.

Box 1 Contraindications to Outpatient PCNL

Absolute Contraindications

- ASA class 5
- Infected urine/sepsis/septic shock
- Hemorrhagic shock or hemorrhage requiring blood transfusion/Kaye catheter
- Renal pelvic perforation
- Unstable vital signs in recovery room
- Ongoing hypoxemia in recovery room (compared to baseline)
- Nobody available to stay with patient overnight
- Significant pneumothorax or other thoracic complication

Strong Relative Contraindications

- ASA class 4
- Class 4 obesity
- Pain requiring intravenous analgesics
- Nausea or vomiting requiring intravenous antiemetics

4   Intraoperative Considerations for Outpatient PCNL

Patient positioning, tract size and renal drainage are the three main reported factors related to surgical technique in oPCNL. Table 2 summarizes these factors for the ten studies involving PCNL done on a completely outpatient basis, with same-day discharge. As can be calculated from the table, oPCNL has been reported in more than 1000 patients globally to date.

Patient Positioning. As shown in Table 2, the majority of oPCNL procedures reported to date have involved the prone position. The systematic review by Jones et al. found that 6 of the 9 articles on day case PCNL reported prone positioning, 2 used the supine approach and 1 did not report positioning (Jones et al. 2019).

Tract Size. Although 7 of the 10 outpatient studies shown in Table 2 involved standard large 30F tract size in most or all study patients, there has been a recent

Table 2 The 10 pure outpatient (same-day discharge) PCNL studies to date, listed in descending order of number of cases performed

Authors	Year	N (F/M)	Mean stone size	Patient position	Tract size	Renal drainage
Chong et al. (2021)	2021	**500** (267/233)	30.3 mm	Prone	24-30F (77%) 17.5F (23%)	99.2% TL 0.4% NT 0.4% TTL
Fahmy et al. (2017)	2017	**146** (54/92)	504.5 mm^2	Prone	30F	20.5% TL 79.5% NT
Roberts et al. (2022)	2022	**134** (73/61)	18.5 mm	Prone (71%) Supine (29%)	24-30F (65%) 17.5F (35%)	94.8% TL 3.7% NT 1.5% TTL
Hosier et al. (2022)	2022	**118** (61/57)	24 mm	Prone	30F	98.3% TL 1.7% TTL
Shabana et al. (2021)	2021	**60** (20/40)	14.3 mm	Prone	17.5F	10.0% TL 90.0% TTL
Thakker et al. (2022)	2022	**53** (n/a)	1.4 cm^3	n/a	30F (19%) mini (81%)	n/a
Beiko et al. (2015)	2015	**50** (24/26)	19.6 mm	Prone	30F	94.0% TL 2.0% NT 4.0% TTL
Schoenfeld et al. (2019)	2019	**47** (23/24)	23 mm	Prone	30F	66.0% TL 34.0% TTL
Bechis et al. (2018)	2018	**43** (22/21)	26.3 mm	Prone	30F	88.4% TL 11.6% NT
Baboudjian et al. (2022)	2022	**32** (n/a)	15 mm	n/a	16F	n/a

N = number; F = female; M = male; F = French size; TL = tubeless; NT = nephrostomy tube; TTL = totally tubeless; n/a = not available surge in mini-PCNL (mPCNL). In assessing the data presented in Table 2, 4 of the 5 studies using only 30F tracts were published in earlier years (2015–2019), whereas the 5 studies involving miniaturized tracts were all published in 2021 or 2022. This is consistent with the rise in mPCNL we have seen across the globe and in the literature over the past few years and supports the belief that mPCNL will continue to facilitate the adoption of oPCNL globally.

Renal Drainage. In Jones et al.'s systematic review, 48%, 45% and 7% of patients underwent tubeless (stent only), nephrostomy tube and totally tubeless exit strategies, respectively (Jones et al. 2019). All studies in Table 2 that reported exit strategy utilized the tubeless approach, often in the majority of patients. There are certainly extremes seen across the studies. In Chong et al.'s impressive study involving PCNL done in a surgery center setting outside the hospital, 496 of 500 patients underwent tubeless oPCNL (Chong et al. 2021), whereas in Shabana et al.'s study using entirely 17.5F mPCNL, 90% of patients were managed in a totally tubeless fashion (Shabana et al. 2021). And although Fahmy et al. used nephrostomy drainage in most of their patients, it should be noted that nephrostomy tubes were removed 4–6 h postoperatively (Fahmy et al. 2017). These findings of increasing use of tubeless and totally tubeless approaches in oPCNL, when compared with the results from the Clinical Research Office of the Endourological Society (CROES) PCNL Global Study (where 91.2% of the 5803 patients received nephrostomy tube drainage) (de la Rosette 2011), illustrates how tubeless drainage drives oPCNL.

5 Outcomes of Outpatient PCNL

Since oPCNL is a relatively new field of study, most urologists have either not (yet) adopted oPCNL or are early in the adoption phase and using strict criteria for patient selection. The adherence to strict patient selection will naturally tend to expose studies to selection bias, as smaller, simpler stones and healthier patients are selected for oPCNL, leaving larger, complex stones and medically complicated patients for sPCNL. It is refreshing to see that some groups have started employing propensity score-matching analysis to compare oPCNL to sPCNL (Shabana et al. 2021; Lee et al. 2022). To date, the most reported outcomes of oPCNL include operating room (OR) times, length of stay (LOS) in hospital (particularly for ambulatory/day case surgery PCNL), complications, unplanned medical visits (ER visits, readmissions) and stone-free rates (SFR). For PCNL studies done on a completely outpatient basis, these outcomes are shown in Table 3. Other outcomes that have been less commonly reported include drop in hemoglobin, postoperative pain/analgesic requirements, costs and patient-reported outcome measures (PROMs) such as time to resumption of normal activity. Overall, the consensus in the literature to date is that oPCNL is associated with excellent outcomes.

OR times. Most comparisons of OR times between oPCNL and sPCNL are limited by selection bias, as many early studies on oPCNL select for smaller and less complex stone burdens. Notwithstanding this limitation, several studies have shown

Table 3 Outcomes for the 10 outpatient PCNL studies

Authors	OR time (minutes)	LOS (hours)	Complication rates	Readmission rates (%)	SFR (%)
Chong et al. (2021)	104	1.6	1.4% minor 1.0% major	4.2	84.0
Fahmy et al. (2017)	84	9.0	12.3% minor 1.4% major	1.3	88.9
Roberts et al. (2022)	154	6–10	21.6% total	13.4	56.3
Hosier et al. (2022)	104	n/a	15.3% minor 1.7% major	5.1	83.3
Shabana et al. (2021)	68	6.0	25.0% minor 0% major	n/a	91.7
Thakker et al. (2022)	n/a	n/a	0%	1.9	n/a
Beiko et al. (2015)	91	3.5	18.0% minor 0% major	4	92
Schoenfeld et al. (2019)	100	n/a	8.5% minor 0% major	2	85
Bechis et al. (2018)	141	n/a	16.3% minor 7.0% major	12	96
Baboudjian et al. (2022)	n/a	n/a	18.1% minor 4.1% major	12.5	75

OR = operating room; LOS = length of stay; SFR = stone-free rate; n/a = not available

that oPCNL is associated with shorter OR times compared to sPCNL (Gao et al. 2020; Fahmy et al. 2017). On the other hand, some studies did not find a significant difference in the mean OR time between day case PCNL and sPCNL (Tian et al. 2020; Kumar et al. 2016). Shabana et al. used propensity score-matching analysis to compare mini aPCNL to flexible ureteroscopy for 10–20 mm lower calyceal stones, finding that the OR times were significantly longer for the aPCNL group (Shabana et al. 2021), a finding that is understandable given PCNL is being compared to ureteroscopy. In the systematic review by Jones et al. the overall mean OR time was 65.6 minutes with a range of 38–106 minutes (Jones et al. 2019). The OR times published in oPCNL studies to date are generally the same or shorter than sPCNL, ranging between 1–2.5 hours as shown in Table 3.

Length of stay in hospital. Since aPCNL includes hospital stays of up to 24 h and oPCNL more strictly includes only same-day discharges, the length of stay (LOS) for oPCNL is by definition shorter than aPCNL. However, the literature clearly indicates that both oPCNL and aPCNL are associated with shorter LOS than sPCNL (Gao et al. 2020; Fahmy et al. 2017; Kumar et al. 2016). The systematic review by Jones et al. included both oPCNL and aPCNL, reporting an overall mean hospital stay of 17.5 hours with a range of 0.5–96 hours (Jones et al. 2019). Kumar et al. reported a significantly lower hospital LOS (0.48 vs 4.74 days) in the day care surgery group compared to the inpatient group (Kumar et al. 2016). Tian et al. reported a median LOS of 18.3 hours (Tian et al. 2020), clearly illustrating their focus was on aPCNL. The LOS of 9 h reported by Fahmy et al. on the other hand, shows the shorter LOS attainable through completely oPCNL (Fahmy et al. 2017). In a multicenter study from McGill University and Queen's University involving 50 oPCNL patients, a 3.5-hour LOS was safely achieved (Beiko et al. 2015). Shabana et al. reported a longer LOS (6 hours vs 4 hours) in their outpatient mPCNL group compared to their flexible ureteroscopy group (Shabana et al. 2021). By far the shortest LOS was found at a freestanding surgery center, where patients experienced a mean 1.6-hours postoperative recovery room stay (Chong et al. 2021).

Complications. Gao et al.'s meta-analysis found that day care PCNL was associated with a significantly lower complication rate (odds ratio = 0.47; P < 0.001) compared to standard inpatient PCNL in the 6 selected studies (3 pure oPCNL + 2 aPCNL + 1 hybrid) included in their meta-analysis (Gao et al. 2020). As shown in Table 3, however, when looking at the 10 pure oPCNL studies published to date, the overall complication rate of oPCNL is not significantly different than the expected complication rate following sPCNL (Baboudjian et al. 2022). As expected, the overall oPCNL complication rate ranges between 10–25%, with most complications being minor complications. Major complications certainly occur, ranging between 0–7%. The CROES PCNL Global Study reported an overall complication rate of 20.5%, including 16.4% minor and 4.1% major complication rates (de la Rosette 2011). Most importantly, as confirmed by literature review and a systematic review, there have been no reported deaths following oPCNL to date (Jones et al. 2019).

Unplanned medical visits. Unplanned postoperative ER visits and hospital admissions occur following any surgery and this is no different for oPCNL. When comparing ER visits and readmissions between the oPCNL and sPCNL groups, Schoenfeld et al. (2019) and Roberts et al. (2022) found no statistically significant difference between groups. Across the 10 oPCNL studies in Table 3, readmission rates ranged between 1.3–13.4%, no different than sPCNL, as shown in Gao et al.'s meta-analysis (Gao et al. 2020).

Stone-free rates. The mean overall SFR for the 10 oPCNL studies was 83.6%. Selection bias notwithstanding, this SFR represents a good outcome considering the overall SFR reported in the CROES PCNL Global Study was 75.7% (de la Rosette 2011). As we know from the PCNL literature in general, reported SFRs have historically been based on inconsistent timing and radiologic modalities, with clinical trials and systematic reviews/meta-analyses reporting varying use of plain radiography, ultrasonography and computed tomography.

Drop in hemoglobin/hematocrit. Most studies did not report changes in hemoglobin or hematocrit. Hosier et al. reported a hemoglobin drop of more than 20 g/L in 4.7% of their oPCNL patients (Hosier et al. 2022). Kumar et al. found their mean drop in hemoglobin was statistically significantly lower in their day care surgery group than the control group (10.5 vs. 13.0 g/L) (Kumar et al. 2016), but the clinical importance of this finding is debatable. Regardless, the reason most studies did not report this outcome is because an oPCNL patient would not qualify for same-day discharge if they experienced a significant drop in hematocrit or hemoglobin in the recovery room.

Postoperative Pain/Analgesia Requirements. Most studies comparing outpatient to standard inpatient PCNL show either no difference or a decrease in pain scores (less analgesia) for the outpatient cohorts. For example, in Kumar et al.'s study, they found significantly lower mean postoperative pain scores and analgesia requirements in their day care surgery group compared to the sPCNL group admitted with nephrostomy tube drainage (Kumar et al. 2016). In the McGill-Queen's study, the mean postoperative narcotic requirement was 41 mg of oral morphine equivalents (Beiko et al. 2015). Roberts et al. found that 14.6% of their "unsuccessful" oPCNL cases (required unplanned admission postoperatively) were admitted because of uncontrolled pain (Roberts et al. 2022).

Costs. On the surface, it is easy to understand why there is consensus that oPCNL decreases healthcare costs. After all, eliminating the need for a hospital stay and the attendant resources can only result in lower expenses. Although cost has not been addressed in most studies, there are a few studies that have looked at the financial implications of oPCNL. In a U.S. study by Thakker et al. aPCNL was found to be associated with a 30% decrease in total cost compared to sPCNL, resulting in a $2,817 USD savings per case (Thakker et al. 2022). In another U.S. study, Lee et al. found that, through no increase in 30-day ER visits or hospital readmissions between the aPCNL and sPCNL arms of their study, a total cost savings of $5,327 per case was realized (Lee et al. 2022). In Canada, Kroczak et al. published a research letter that reported a potential 35% cost savings of aPCNL over sPCNL, which translated to a cost savings of $3,348 CAD per case (Kroczak et al. 2018).

Patient-Reported Outcome Measures. Unfortunately, there remains a paucity of literature on PROMs regarding oPCNL. In a study comparing day case PCNL to sPCNL, Kumar et al. found it took a statistically significantly shorter time to resume normal activity in the day case PCNL group compared to the standard group. The difference, 8.1 days versus 18.4 days, is also clinically significant (Kumar et al. 2016). There is an opportunity to study quality of life (QoL) outcomes and additional PROMs in patients undergoing oPCNL. Patient preferences and satisfaction regarding oPCNL would be an obvious place to start.

Identifying Causes for Admission. A recent UCSD study by Roberts et al. has helped us gain a better understanding of causes for admission for planned oPCNL patients (Roberts et al. 2022). Although most of their patients were successfully discharged as planned, 23% (41 of 175) of patients required admission. There were several reasons for admission, including unexpected additional intraoperative procedures (34%), intraoperative complications (20%), social/administrative issues (19%), postoperative pain (15%) and postoperative complications (12%). On univariate analysis, ASA class 2, upper pole access, multiple tracts and nephrostomy tube drainage had a greater probability of requiring postoperative hospitalization. Nephrostomy tube was the only variable associated with hospital admission on multivariate analysis, however. The UCSD team is to be applauded for their work. More studies like this are needed to help us better determine the probability of admission for patients enrolled in oPCNL pathways.

6 Getting Started with Outpatient PCNL

Figure 1 shows 10 key steps that will help urologists navigate the start-up of their oPCNL programs. This is largely based on previously published lessons learned from two institutions where oPCNL was pioneered in Canada (Beiko and Andonian 2015). Many urologists will already have some of the steps covered in their practice, so it is for each individual urosurgeon to determine which steps require specific action plans or changes to practice. By following and achieving each step, the likelihood of successful adoption of oPCNL is maximized. In other words, each step could be thought of as a potential barrier to achieving a safe and successful oPCNL program. The 10 steps are described below.

Step 1: Remember trauma cases. PCNL is essentially an iatrogenic form of a grade IV renal trauma. However, a PCNL patient differs from an ER patient because the former is more accurately exposed to a "controlled" form of trauma because the highly precise location of the renal puncture at the calyceal tip helps minimize renal hemorrhage and urine leak. We know from experience that the majority of grade 4 renal trauma cases require either no intervention or ureteral stent (or rarely, a nephrostomy tube) at most. So, if we recall the outcomes of the traditional renal trauma cases we've seen over the years, it helps shift our mindset toward oPCNL

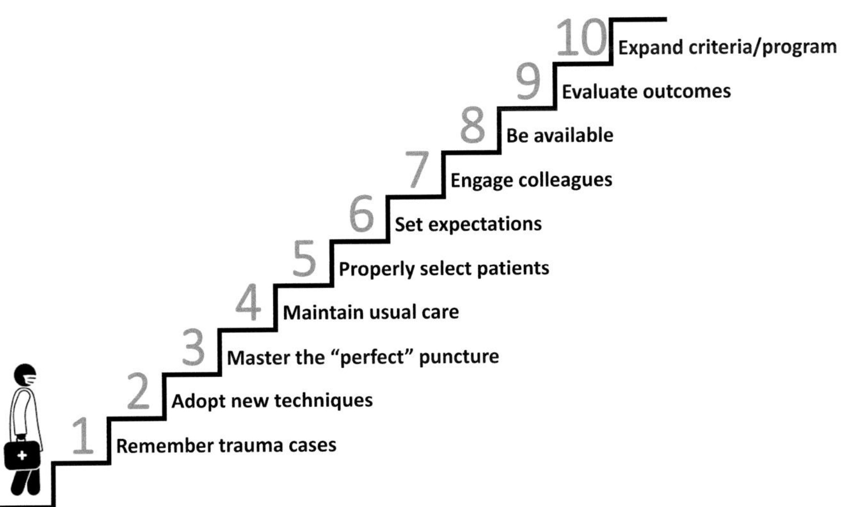

Fig. 1 Steps to building a successful outpatient PCNL program

and accepting that it is safe to send our patients home a few short hours after their PCNL.

Step 2: Adopt new techniques. The two most important techniques that will facilitate adoption of oPCNL are tubeless PCNL and mPCNL. Bellman et al. pioneered tubeless PCNL (Bellman et al. 1997) and this innovation is perhaps the single most important advance that has led to the uptake of oPCNL. Although there is no doubt that oPCNL can be performed in nephrostomized patients, we strongly recommend adoption of tubeless PCNL before starting an oPCNL program. Tubelessness helps the individual urologist see firsthand that their patients don't need a nephrostomy tube to tamponade the tract. In fact, one could argue that a nephrostomy tube (a type of foreign body that spans the entire wound from collecting system to skin) serves only to delay wound healing and sealing of the nephrotomy site. A natural step to facilitate same-day discharge is to convert to mini-PCNL. Since smaller tracts help facilitate oPCNL, micro-PCNL and ultra mPCNL would be particularly facilitative. Regardless of what size of tract is used, any mPCNL technique results in a smaller tract and nephrotomy, which can only serve to reduce the risk of hemorrhage. This lower risk translates to easier adoption by urologists who are, rightly so, concerned about sending patients home with the risk of potentially life-threatening hemorrhage.

Step 3: Master the "perfect" puncture. Like mPCNL, mastering the "perfect" puncture at the tip of the calyx serves to reduce intraoperative and postoperative bleeding. Any urologist should be able to readily determine their personal blood transfusion rate for PCNL. If she/he is not satisfied with their transfusion rate, then she/he can improve their technique by pursuing the "perfect" puncture. For those who are satisfied their blood transfusion rate is low enough (0.5–2%, for example), and for those who are able improve their technique and lower their transfusion rates, the transition to oPCNL can be safely pursued.

Step 4: Maintain usual care. For any urologist who has routinely admitted patients following PCNL, same-day discharge can be a disconcerting change. Furthermore, to get to the point of considering oPCNL, many urologists will have already adopted the new techniques of tubeless PCNL or mPCNL. In other words, the urologist has already engaged in a significant amount of change, altering their approach to PCNL patient care. At that point, it is imperative that the urologist otherwise maintain their usual clinical care/pathway for their PCNL patients and assess their outcomes of oPCNL before making other changes. Specifically, it is recommended that urologists use familiar endoscopic equipment, devices and techniques while making the transition to oPCNL and intentionally delay the trialing of new equipment until after they have gained adequate experience with same-day discharge. Where possible, it is recommended to avoid the hiring of new OR team members during the transition to oPCNL. Starting a program with engaged (see below) team members who have bought into the philosophy of same-day discharge is critical.

Step 5: Properly select patients. Any urologist considering an oPCNL program will absolutely need to adhere to strict selection criteria, especially for the first cohort of patients. This single recommendation is perhaps the most important to safely establish an oPCNL program. All it takes is one bad outcome early and the momentum for the program will be lost. To reduce the risk of a bad outcome, when choosing their early patients for same-day discharge—at least the first dozen patients or more—the urologist will need to be extremely strict and highly selective with respect to patient factors, stone factors and renal anatomy factors.

Step 6: Set expectations. Setting expectations with the patient and family starts in the clinic/office at the initial consultation. Unless they completely understand the postoperative plan for discharge home a few short hours after PCNL, the plan for an ambulatory procedure may fail. Having said that, it is important to be honest and realistic by preparing the patient and family—both physically and psychologically— that hospital admission may be required, especially early on as experience is gained. Physically, patients should be advised to bring an overnight bag in preparation for the possibility of hospital admission, while at the same time explaining that the probabilities favour same-day discharge.

Step 7: Engage colleagues. Engaging and empowering our nursing and anesthesiology colleagues is a crucial step. Often healthcare providers go into an "autopilot" mode in providing their care and this can lead to resisting any proposed change in the perioperative clinical care pathway. For better or worse, the COVID-19 pandemic has resulted in a significant shortage of hospital beds, so at the present time, many institutions may provide tailwinds to any proposed shift to outpatient care from a previously hospital-based care operation such as PCNL. Regardless, the earlier nurses and anesthesiologists are engaged, the better. Engaging anesthesiologists preoperatively by asking—and not telling—them what anesthetic agents are most likely to facilitate discharge home a few short hours after surgery. Postoperatively, after the patient has been reassessed in the recovery room, actively seeking the nurse's and anesthesiologist's professional assessment and impression of the patient's suitability for same-day discharge engages them in the decision-making process, promotes teamwork and ensures patient safety. Although nerve blocks are not routinely used in many institutions, asking our anesthesiology colleagues about their experience and opinions on nerve blocks is another way to potentially establish confidence in same-day discharge.

Step 8: Be available. Being available, particularly after-hours, is crucial. If a urologist is to take the plunge and start discharging PCNL patients home a few hours postoperatively, she/he must be prepared to be available for any potential acute complications presenting to the ER. One after-hours tactic that may prove to be of benefit to both the PCNL patient and the urologist is a quick phone call from the urologist on the evening of surgery to check in with patient. At the present time, the author does not routinely call ambulatory surgery patients at home the evening of surgery but when starting out, the author called the first several patients at home to check in with them. Truth be told, the author was calling to make sure the patients were still alive and had not bled to death. But the few minutes it took to make the phone call was well worth it and reassuring to the patients and author. The patients expressed appreciation for the call as it made them feel valued and cared for. Knowing each patient was fine and not bleeding to death allowed the author to sleep better at night.

Step 9: Evaluate outcomes. Community, private and academic urologists can and should periodically evaluate their outcomes. This is particularly important when adopting a new approach such as oPCNL. Unless one is planning on submitting their outcomes for publications in a journal (in which case a more comprehensive database of preoperative, intraoperative and postoperative variables should be pursued), a crude assessment of 5 basic data points such as postoperative ER visits, postoperative hospital admissions, postoperative complications, SFRs and stakeholder satisfaction (patients, family/friends, colleagues and urologists) would suffice in most cases.

Step 10: Expand criteria/program. As time passes and the number of cases increases, the urologist gains valuable experience and knowledge through evaluation of their outcomes. After the urologist reviews her/his outcomes and determines that oPCNL is safe and effective in her/his hands according to clinically relevant endpoints (such as the 5 basic data points listed above, for example) expansion of the oPCNL program by extending selection criteria to more complex patients and stones becomes an achievable goal.

7 Future Directions in Outpatient PCNL

Clinical. There is much more to learn and expand upon to improve the care of patients undergoing oPCNL. After all, oPCNL is a field in its infancy with an exciting future and several tailwinds. Access to hospital beds is becoming increasingly challenging in many centers, so a further shift to oPCNL is expected for hospital based PCNL. Furthermore, the shift toward ambulatory care outside hospitals is likely to continue. As a result, oPCNL is expected to be increasingly performed in ambulatory surgery centers across the globe in the future. This trend of expanding PCNL into surgery centers should help make PCNL care more efficient and further reduce costs. Urologists are likely to continue to embrace tubeless and mPCNL techniques. All these factors provide an opportunity for increasing adoption of oPCNL in the future.

Academic. There are several potential interesting avenues of research in oPCNL. Surveying patients to capture more PROMs related to QoL is critical but let us not forget the urologist. Surveying urologists for their concerns, ideas, preferences and satisfaction regarding oPCNL may provide insights on how to grow this nascent field of study and help guide potential new approaches in the future. The literature to date suffers from a lack of properly designed prospective randomized controlled trials (RCT) on oPCNL. We are aware of one such multicenter study that is underway involving U.S. and Canadian institutions. There may be RCTs being performed in other countries on oPCNL or aPCNL. Prospective RCTs will only improve the robustness of future systematic reviews and meta-analyses, thereby further advancing the field of oPCNL.

8 Conclusions

Same-day discharge following PCNL is a relatively new advance that has been shown to be safe and effective, especially in highly selected patients. The literature suggests that, with experience, patient selection criteria can be extended to more medically complex patients and more surgically complex stones. For most outcomes, oPCNL compares favorably to sPCNL. There are many tailwinds for oPCNL, and as urologists across the globe continue to shift to tubeless and mPCNL techniques, further adoption of this approach is expected. Higher quality studies, including prospective RCTs, are expected as oPCNL becomes more widely adopted.

References

Abbott JE, Davalos JG. Outpatient tubeless percutaneous nephrolithotomy performed in a free-standing ambulatory surgery center. J Endourol Case Rep. 2018;4(1):28–31. https://doi.org/10.1089/cren.2017.0136.PMID:29503872;PMCID:PMC5831992.

Baboudjian M, Negre T, Van Hove A, McManus R, Lechevallier E, Gondran-Tellier B, Boissier R. A multi-institutional experience of micro-percutaneous Nephrolithotomy (MicroPERC) for renal stones: results and feasibility of day case surgery. Prog Urol. 2022;32(6):435–41. https://doi.org/10.1016/j.purol.2022.02.002. Epub 2022 Apr 14 PMID: 35431123.

Bechis SK, Han DS, Abbott JE, Holst DD, Alagh A, DiPina T, Sur RL. Outpatient percutaneous nephrolithotomy: the UC San Diego health experience. J Endourol. 2018;32(5):394–401. https://doi.org/10.1089/end.2018.0056. Epub 2018 Apr 10 PMID: 29634376.

Beiko D, Lee L. Outpatient tubeless percutaneous nephrolithotomy: the initial case series. Can Urol Assoc J. 2010;4(4):E86-90. https://doi.org/10.5489/cuaj.886.PMID:20694090;PMCID:PMC2911986.

Beiko D, Elkoushy MA, Kokorovic A, Roberts G, Robb S, Andonian S. Ambulatory percutaneous nephrolithotomy: what is the rate of readmission? J Endourol. 2015;29(4):410–4. https://doi.org/10.1089/end.2014.0584. Epub 2014 Oct 23 PMID: 25221917.

Beiko D, Andonian S. Getting started with ambulatory PCNL: a CanMEDS perspective. Can Urol Assoc J. 2015;9(7–8):223–5. https://doi.org/10.5489/cuaj.3198. PMID: 26316901; PMCID: PMC4537328.

Beiko D, Samant M, McGregor TB. Totally tubeless outpatient percutaneous nephrolithotomy: initial case report. Adv Urol. 2009; 295825. https://doi.org/10.1155/2009/295825. Epub 2009 May 24. PMID: 19478955; PMCID: PMC2685914.

Bellman GC, Davidoff R, Candela J, Gerspach J, Kurtz S, Stout L. Tubeless percutaneous renal surgery. J Urol. 1997;157(5):1578–82 PMID: 9112480.

Chong JT, Dunne M, Magnan B, Abbott J, Davalos JG. Ambulatory percutaneous nephrolithotomy in a free-standing surgery center: an analysis of 500 consecutive cases. J Endourol. 2021;35(12):1738–42. https://doi.org/10.1089/end.2021.0159. PMID: 34036805.

de la Rosette J, Assimos D, Desai M, Gutierrez J, Lingeman J, Scarpa R, Tefekli A. CROES PCNL study group. The clinical research office of the endourological society percutaneous nephrolithotomy global study: indications, complications, and outcomes in 5803 patients. J Endourol. 2011;25(1):11–7. https://doi.org/10.1089/end.2010.0424. PMID: 21247286.

Fahmy A, Rhashad H, Algebaly O, Sameh W. Can percutaneous nephrolithotomy be performed as an outpatient procedure? Arab J Urol. 2017;15(1):1–6. https://doi.org/10.1016/j.aju.2016.11.006.PMID:28275511;PMCID:PMC5329725.

Gao M, Zeng F, Zhu Z, Zeng H, Chen Z, Li Y, Yang Z, Cui Y, He C, Chen J, Chen H. Day care surgery versus inpatient percutaneous nephrolithotomy: a systematic review and meta-analysis. Int J Surg. 2020;81:132–9. https://doi.org/10.1016/j.ijsu.2020.07.056. Epub 2020 Aug 12 PMID: 32795609.

Hosier GW, Visram K, McGregor T, Steele S, Touma NJ, Beiko D. Ambulatory percutaneous nephrolithotomy is safe and effective in patients with extended selection criteria. Can Urol Assoc J. 2022;16(4):89–95. https://doi.org/10.5489/cuaj.7527.PMID:34812729;PMCID:PMC9054338.

Jackman SV, Hedican SP, Peters CA, Docimo SG. Percutaneous nephrolithotomy in infants and preschool age children: experience with a new technique. Urology. 1998;52(4):697–701. https://doi.org/10.1016/s0090-4295(98)00315-x. PMID: 9763096.

Jones P, Bennett G, Dosis A, Pietropaolo A, Geraghty R, Aboumarzouk O, Skolarikos A, Somani BK. Safety and efficacy of day-case percutaneous nephrolithotomy: a systematic review from european society of uro-technology. Eur Urol Focus. 2019;5(6):1127–34. https://doi.org/10.1016/j.euf.2018.04.002. Epub 2018 Apr 12 PMID: 29657068.

Kroczak T, Pace KT, Andonian S, Beiko D. Ambulatory percutaneous nephrolithotomy in Canada: A COST-reducing innovation. Can Urol Assoc J. 2018;12(12):427–9. https://doi.org/10.5489/cuaj.5416.PMID:30273115;PMCID:PMC6261719.

Kumar S, Singh S, Singh P, Singh SK. Day care PNL using 'Santosh-PGI hemostatic seal' versus standard PNL: a randomized controlled study. Cent European J Urol. 2016;69(2):190–7. https://doi.org/10.5173/ceju.2016.792. Epub 2016 Jun 20. PMID: 27551557; PMCID: PMC4986304.

Lee MS, Assmus MA, Agarwal DK, Rivera ME, Large T, Krambeck AE. Ambulatory percutaneous nephrolithotomy may be cost-effective compared to standard percutaneous nephrolithotomy. J Endourol. 2022;36(2):176–82. https://doi.org/10.1089/end.2021.0482. PMID: 34663076.

Preminger GM, Clayman RV, Curry T, Redman HC, Peters PC. Outpatient percutaneous nephrostolithotomy. J Urol. 1986;136(2):355–7. https://doi.org/10.1016/s0022-5347(17)44867-1. PMID: 3735494.

Roberts JL, Sur RL, Flores AR, Girgiss CBL, Kelly EM, Kong EK, Abedi G, Berger JH, Chen TT, Monga M, Bechis SK. Understanding causes for admission in planned ambulatory percutaneous nephrolithotomy. J Endourol. 2022;36(11):1418–24. https://doi.org/10.1089/end.2021.0811. PMID: 35699065.

Schoenfeld D, Zhou T, Stern JM. Outcomes for patients undergoing ambulatory percutaneous nephrolithotomy. J Endourol. 2019;33(3):189–93. https://doi.org/10.1089/end.2018.0579. Epub 2019 Jan 2 PMID: 30489147.

Shabana W, Oquendo F, Hodhod A, Ahmad A, Alaref A, Trigo S, Hadi RA, Nour HH, Kotb A, Shahrour W, Elmansy H. Miniaturized ambulatory percutaneous nephrolithotomy versus flexible ureteroscopy in the management of lower calyceal renal stones 10–20 mm: a propensity score matching analysis. Urology. 2021;156:65–70. https://doi.org/10.1016/j.urology.2021.05.041. Epub 2021 Jun 17 PMID: 34097943.

Shahrour W, Andonian S. Ambulatory percutaneous nephrolithotomy: initial series. Urology. 2010;76(6):1288–92. https://doi.org/10.1016/j.urology.2010.08.001. PMID: 21130245.

Thakker PU, Mithal P, Dutta R, Carreno G, Gutierrez-Aceves J. Comparative outcomes and cost of ambulatory PCNL in select kidney stone patients. Urolithiasis. 2022;51(1):22. https://doi.org/10.1007/s00240-022-01392-5. .PMID:36571653;PMCID:PMC9791625

Tian Y, Yang X, Luo G, Wang Y, Sun Z. Initial prospective study of ambulatory mPCNL on upper urinary tract calculi. Urol J. 2020;17(1):14–8. https://doi.org/10.22037/uj.v0i0.4828. PMID: 30882168.

PCNL in Developing Countries

Mohammed Lezrek and Otas Durutovic

Abstract Percutaneous nephrolithotomy (PCNL) is an established and effective surgical procedure for the management of kidney stones. While PCNL has gained widespread popularity in developed countries, its application and challenges in developing countries require specific considerations. Limited resources, inadequate infrastructure, and economic constraints pose significant challenges in the implementation of PCNL in developing nations. However, despite these obstacles, PCNL continues to play a crucial role in the treatment of complex and large renal calculi. Factors such as patient selection, cost-effective instrumentation, and optimization of surgical techniques are discussed in the context of resource-limited settings. Training programs, skill development, and collaborative efforts to enhance surgical outcomes and expand the reach of PCNL in these regions are important areas covered along with the need for continuous improvement, knowledge sharing, and innovation to overcome the barriers and maximize the benefits of PCNL in resource-constrained environments. By understanding the unique challenges and experiences of PCNL in developing countries, healthcare providers and policymakers can work towards enhancing access to this effective treatment modality.

Keywords Percutaneous nephrolithotomy (PCNL) · Kidney stone surgery · Urolithiasis · Renal calculi · Developing countries · Resource-limited settings · Healthcare infrastructure · Cost-effective instrumentation · Surgical techniques · Patient selection · Skill development · Training programs · Collaborative efforts · Access to care · Surgical outcomes · Adaptations in PCNL · Economic constraints · Healthcare disparities · Knowledge sharing · Innovation in PCNL

M. Lezrek · O. Durutovic (✉)
Urology, Department for Urolithiasis, University Clinical Centre of Serbia, Belgrade, Serbia
e-mail: otas.durutovic@med.bg.ac.rs

© The Author(s), under exclusive license to Springer Nature Switzerland AG 2023   401
J. D. Denstedt and E. N. Liatsikos (eds.), *Percutaneous Renal Surgery*,
https://doi.org/10.1007/978-3-031-40542-6_27

1 Introduction

Since its introduction, percutaneous nephrolithotomy (PCNL) was associated with the innovative spirit of the founders and the need to adapt to specific circumstances. The first documented case of PCNL was published in 1976 by Fernstorm and Johansson, and was performed as a simple forceps stone extraction (Akenroye et al. 2013). Is it possible that so many decades after stones are still extracted due to a lack of fine dusting and fragmenting devices…we will see…

Technological improvements brought significant benefits in procedure efficacy and safety during its evolution, especially in the last decade. All these innovations are associated with increased costs and widely adopted only in developed countries.

The current population of Europe is 748,897,226 (9.78%), Northern America is 375,158,288 (4.73%), Australia is 26,319,190 (0.33%), as of Wednesday, April 12, 2023, based on the latest United Nations estimates. With Japan and other developed countries this constitutes around 17% of the global population, leaving 83% in developing or undeveloped countries.

Urolithiasis is a worldwide disease, with a rising incidence and significant impact on health care resources. In developed countries these costs are recognized as a potential barrier yet an opportunity for improvement and cost reduction.

Although data are limited, urinary stone disease incidence is high and rising in developing countries, especially in Sub-Saharan Africa (SSA) (Assimos et al. 2016; Bickler et al. 2010). In this region skills for open stone removal are still widely available and utilized. The outcome of open surgery may not necessarily be inadequate. In experienced hands, the entire stone burden can be removed, but at the cost of impaired renal function and a risk of strictures at the level of ureteropelvic junction (UPJ). UPJ stenosis when it occurs facilitates the risk of recurrence.

Aware of all these scenarios, but also possibilities and advancements in surgical modalities along with easier and free approach to information and education, urologists in developing countries are progressing towards a solution—how to use minimally invasive techniques in what are often challenging circumstances in their countries.

Being informed about possibilities is just a first step on the road of adopting new technique. With the guidance of tutors, attendance at workshops and accessing educational materials and models are necessary. The apprenticeship model known as—"see one, do one, teach one" has many disadvantages, even in countries without resources for proper training.

Precise diagnosis is a prerequisite for a safe and efficient treatment. Treating kidney stones implies the use of appropriate imaging tools preoperatively and the essential equipment for a treatment. Limitations and difficulties urologists face in developing countries can be divided as follows

1. Imaging
2. Teaching and training
3. Instruments, devices and procedure settings

In this chapter we will try to represent what is recognized or could be identified as a minimal imaging and instruments for performing PCNL safely. We shall present teaching activities, organized with a minimal resource, but a tremendous spirit and enthusiasm of both tutors and participants.

2 Imaging

Regardless of our setting, we can agree that advancements in imaging are often the cornerstone of improvements in medical care and facilitated the development of many minimally invasive techniques. PCNL is an excellent example of how being familiar with kidney anatomy and stone characteristics and distribution can improve procedural outcomes. According to all current recommendations, including guidelines on urolithiasis of the American Urological Association (AUA) and European Association of Urology (EAU), computed tomography (CT) is the gold standard imaging tool prior to PCNL surgery (Campain et al. 2022; Cassell et al. 2020).

Pursuing these recommendations may become a challenge in developing countries due to lack of access to modern technology including CT imaging. In other words, limitations are present even before introducing the patient into operating theatre, during diagnostic procedures and case preparation.

There is a significant difference in low- and middle-income countries (LMICs) health systems, from free public health service, but with limited resources, to a number of countries where no healthcare system exists or is rudimentary (Cracco and Scoffone 2011; Fernström and Johansson 1976), or is inaccessible for various cultural, religious, or logistic reasons (Geraghty et al. 2023). Computed tomography (CT) is sometimes available just in a few hospitals, perhaps only in capital cities. As distances are far and traveling is difficult due to numerous reasons, diagnosis must be made based on basic and low cost X-ray machines, performing only kidney, ureter and bladder (KUB) films and intravenous urography (IVU). The presence of ultrasound (US) imaging in these settings is of enormous value, as US helps and delivers safety in both, case preparation and surgery (Lezrek et al. 2016a).

Even when CT is available, lack of radiologists dedicated to uropathology including urolithiasis, is a reason why urologists have to be familiar with CT software and extract details for procedure planning. Sometimes collaboration with colleagues from different institutions, such as Electrical Engineering may be productive, using free software for creating semi 3D models (Lezrek et al. 2016b) These models can be useful for the evaluation of the best access route, but also as a tool in teaching (Fig. 1).

This is a scenario frequently seen in many African countries, where diagnostic procedures for urolithiasis are performed by simple use of X-rays, kidney, ureter and bladder (KUB) and intravenous urography (IVU).

According to the experience of urologists practicing in countries facing these limitations, PCNL cases can be safely prepared with use of these images. With addition of ultrasound (US), as an easily accessible and widely available tool, urologists can

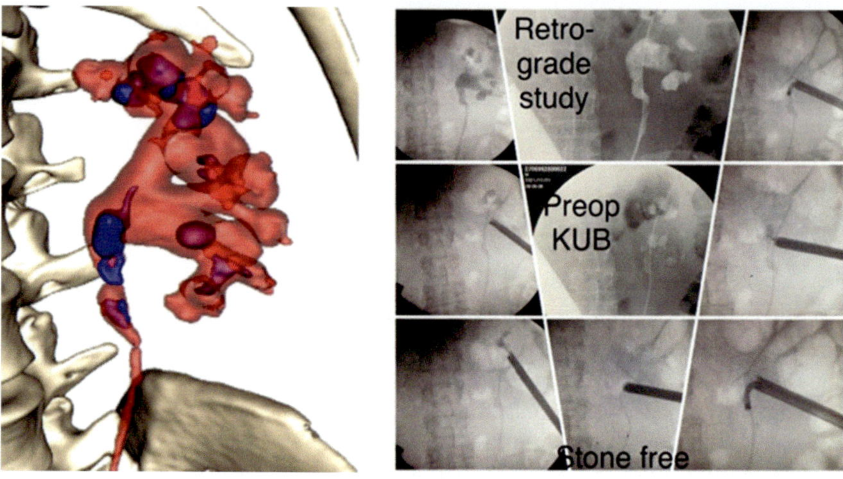

Fig. 1. 3D Gastro CT Ex tool as an open-source tool developed on Python 3. The software supports segmentation and 3D rendering of abdominal CT scans for individual phases and offers the option for 3D hybrid visualization of native and delayed phase. An example of its use in real case

create a clear and good plan and entry strategy for PCNL. Experience in use of US by urologists is crucial for simplifying puncture technique, as the depth of the puncture can be determined in this way, especially if just fixed, monoplane fluoroscopy is used. US is of an enormous significance in absence of CT, as it facilitates evaluation of the interposition of adjacent organs in a puncture route. US can be performed in all positions for PCNL surgery including prone or (modified) supine.

In experienced hands ultrasound guidance can replicate imaging for PCNL access exactly the same to those we collect in retrograde studies at the beginning of the procedure, when contrast is injected through a ureteral catheter. The combination of KUB and IVU can also typically provide the necessary information to perform PCNL.

Well into 21st Century, in developing countries PCNL is still planed and performed successfully after KUB and IVU imaging (Fig. 2). Being familiar with kidney and pelvicalyceal system anatomy contributes to better interpretation of IVU images. Rotation of the kidney in the retroperitoneal space and orientation of calices are useful details in determination of the best possible puncture, allowing access to most calices (Lezrek et al. 2018; Meara et al. 2015). So called "LAMP rule", lateral anterior, medial posterior, can be used in understanding how to plan anatomy based on IVU and compared to KUB, if patient is positioned in prone and not lateral/ oblique position.

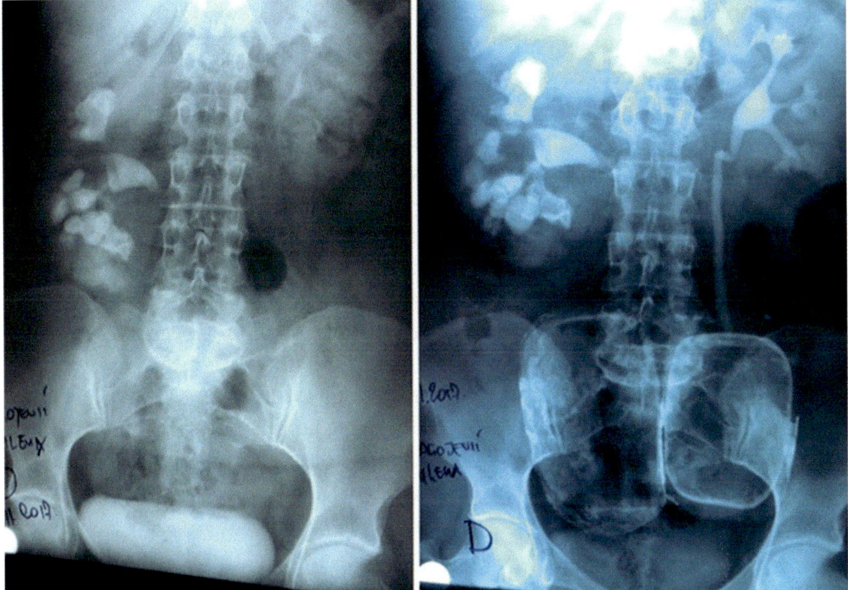

Fig. 2 IVU prior to PCNL for a staghorn stone

3   Teaching and Training

Precise and planned puncture is the key of for success of PCNL. This step is recognized also as critical from the point of view of complications which can be severe, including damage to surrounding organs or the kidney. This does not necessarily mean that other steps cannot be "critical". Tract formation and force used during dilation is also a point where experience is paramount. Every part of PCNL has its secrets and nuances, as a potential risk that have to be kept in mind when involving younger colleagues into the procedure during training.

PCNL is a procedure with several steps and techniques, so often comes with a long learning curve with at least 45–60 cases to be able to perform PCNL, and more than 100 cases to have excellent results (Osman et al. 2005; Payne and Chalwe 2022).

Teaching and learning on simulators became a standard approach in many countries with accessibility to it. Developing countries often cannot provide this tool and training must take into consideration available equipment in hospitals. As it is not a rare scenario, in some regions PCNL is not established procedure yet, so urologists from other countries are invited, with idea to present it in a simple and efficient way, appropriate to local circumstances.

One of the first initiatives to recognize local circumstances and availabilities in LMICs was the Commission on Global Surgery 2030 published in Lancet in 2015 (Sorokin et al. 2017). After estimating the burden of surgical conditions and the unmet need for surgical care in LMICs, initial strategies and frameworks for improvement were developed (Tanriverdi et al. 2007; Tatanis et al. 2023).

In the absence of expensive virtual simulators, with limited resources, very creative ideas arise, such as using gloves under retroprojecteur, an old-fashioned overhead projector, or using just light from mobile phone as a "Chinese-shadows play". In this way participants were trained how to navigate a needle during the puncture under just monoplane fluoroscopy. Tips and tricks for evaluation of depth were given as the needle had to be targeted in two dimensions, with careful evaluation of the third (Venn et al. 2022; Voorhees et al. 2009).

Tract establishment on a watermelon model was found to be good as an initial model. It allows learning all the techniques of tract dilation (Alken metallic dilation, Amplatz sequential or one-step dilation, balloon dilation), insertion of a safety guidewire and it gives areal haptic feeling (Watson et al. 2022). Other vegetables can be used, pumpkin, winter squash, butternut, melon, eggplants…but it is better to choose one with hard skin to give the feeling of resistance and difficulty during dilation (World Health Organization 2015) (Fig. 3).

4 Instruments, Devices and Procedure Settings

For better understanding of the complexity urologists are facing in treating patients with kidney stones, we must be familiar with current status of medical care and equipment in LMICS. That is why, ideally, preparation of the operating theatre team is best done in the LMICs setting for the surgeon to learn in his own operative environment and resources. Also, the entire team and staff will learn simultaneously including the anesthesiology team, nursing staff and radiographer (Ziaee et al. 2010).

There is a large difference in LMICs health systems. There are countries with free public health service, which might be poor and not well organized, providing just the basic medical needs. Other countries have an elementary health system (Chandrasekera 2019; Cracco and Scoffone 2011), yet might be unreachable for many reasons, logistic, economic, cultural, religious… (Geraghty et al. 2023). Thus, the diagnosis of renal stones is mostly made in a late stage, with large and complex renal calculi.

Flexible ureteroscopes are expensive and with a short durability. The procedure also requires a laser for stone fragmentation along with disposables, including wires, baskets, access sheaths which are expensive. Also, ureteroscopy might need more ancillary procedures, including JJ stent placement and removal and more than one surgical session. All these needs usually cannot be offered to patients in developing countries with an imperative of treatment in a single session.

Under the described circumstances, PCNL may be selected as the treatment of choice even for small stones that would otherwise be treated by ESWL, flexible URS and laser fragmentation in developed countries. PCNL can be performed with rigid metallic instruments, nephroscopes, forceps, ballistic lithotripter, which are reusable and durable.

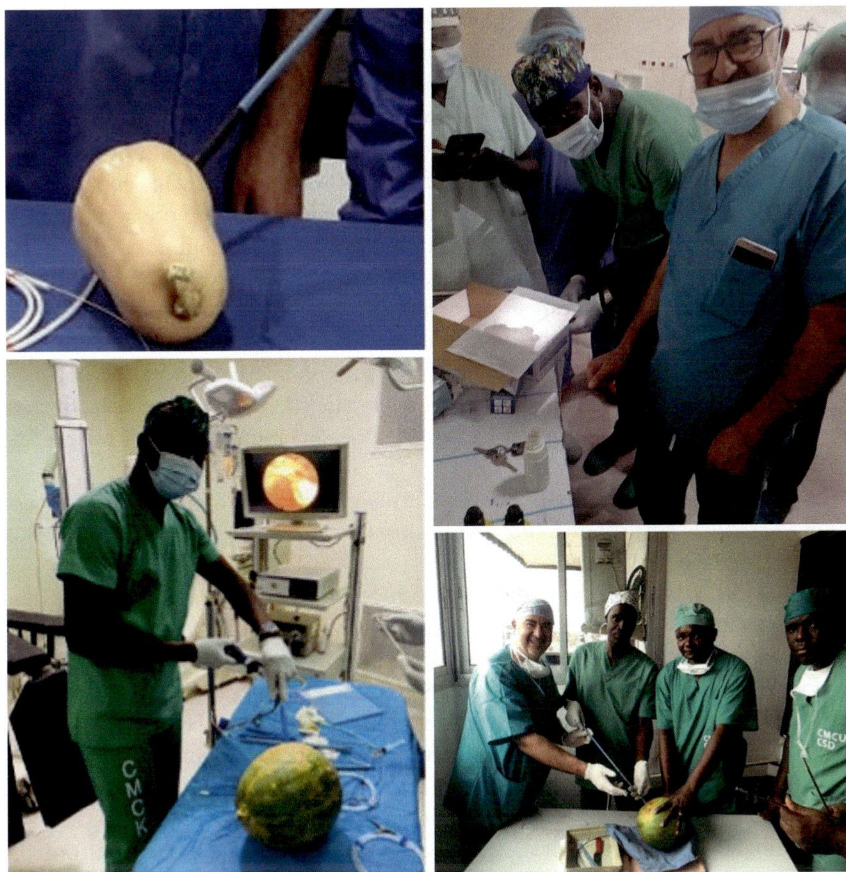

Fig. 3 Professor Mohammed Lezrek—training "made easier" and possible, available models and "Chinese-shadows play" used for experiencing needle navigation

As relates the technical aspect and setting of PCNL, limitations are present at every level—operating table, tower, camera, light source. Something urologists in developed countries do not even consider as a possible problem are irrigation fluids. Without fluid endoscopic procedures are impossible. PCNL needs at least 10–20 L of irrigant per case, and more in the case of large and complex stones.

As alternative, a cheap and isotonic saline solution is prepared from running water and 9 g/l of cooking salt, and stored in a 25-L reservoir specially developed. It is sterilized by ebullition with the reservoir built-in heat resistor. Filling the reservoir at 100 °C effectively sterilises the inside of the container, the tubing can be cleaned by immersion in Cidex, or equivalent, and the solution used operatively when it has cooled to body temperature. Beside the clear economic benefit, the system has proven preferable to using multiple 500 mL bottles as the flow is more consistent and, therefore, conducive to shorter operating times (Chandrasekera 2019). The use of the 25 L reservoir mentioned above helps ensure that the surgeon does not lose their endoscopic access when the irrigant stops. An audit of the safety of the reservoir in 213 patients in Benin showed that 32 patients had a transient fever after its use, but 19 patients had a positive preoperative urine culture. There were no cases of electrolyte disturbance as a consequence of this frugal innovation, and no deaths. The cost saving was proportional to the duration of surgery. When one considers the socioeconomic status of these patients these cost savings were more significant to the patient than the apparent risks of using the reservoir. Last but not the least this liquid has to be prepared a day before surgery is scheduled.

What is a minimum equipment necessary or obligatory for a safe PCNL procedure? This question can always be repeated, as access to modern technology can not eliminate the risk of the procedure. With endoscopic control of the puncture during Endoscopic Combined Intrarenal Surgery (ECIRS) control and visualization are increased, but even in developed countries this technique is not yet widely and routinely used (Zeng et al. 2022).

In developing countries, the surgeon is usually asked to choose (if lucky not to receive without asking) one set of PCNL instruments. Another key purchase decision are energy sources for lithotripsy.

During 1980s instruments specifically created for PCNL were introduced. These instruments were metallic, and according to the inventor, Professor Peter Alken were named Alken dilators. Dilatation was performed with use of serial metallic dilators, ending with indwelling of the Amplatz, then and now called Standard Maxi PCNL 30 Fr. In experienced hands this metallic dilators can be safely used, but are associated with few potential risks, harming the tissue, over advancement due to excessive force and many steps, especially when used by beginners. That's why these dilators were replaced with plastic, allowing smoother progression and less steps of tract formation. Plastic dilators are created for a single use and are unaffordable in developing countries for routine use. In these circumstances reusable (metallic) dilators are the best option, but this decision is followed with a need to make the use of these dilators in the gentlest way, forcing all steps of puncture to be done perfectly.

Size of the instruments and scopes is also question with more possible answers. Using just a Maxi PCNL size may result in limited accessibility to stones placed in small calices, or in cases of narrow infundibulum, making advancement of the instrument harmful. These situations are sometimes overcome by innovative ideas of the surgeons, combining different instruments, such as using the ureteroscope for a second access (Fig. 4).

5 How To Perform PCNL in LMICs

There are a number of technical challenges to establishing PCNL in LMICs.

The first test is the operating theatre and its environment.

In many countries in SSA the electrical supply is often inadequate, and power-cuts are a common event, something that has to be planned for (Chandrasekera 2019). It is

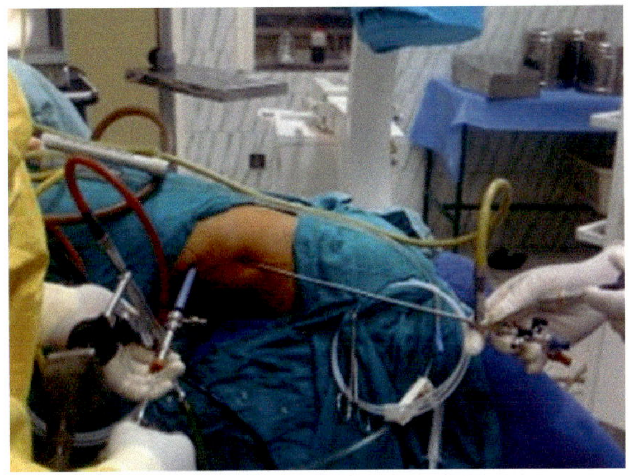

Fig. 4 Semirigid ureteroscope used for a second tract

also not unusual for multiple electrical items to malfunction if used synchronously; in one theatre the C-arm would not work when the patient monitoring was switched on. As one of the alternatives we can prepare to use a light from a mobile phone as a light source.

Operating table not optimal for fluoroscopy—large metallic border the patient is placed in the middle of the table?

The base and column are in fixed position in the middle of the table; the patient will be placed in the longest extremity, even with legs largely beyond the table, to allow the insertion of the C-arm. In the case of a completely radiopaque operating table, a wooden plank is fixed to the table top and the patient was placed outside the table during puncture.

If we should try recommend an example of the "one size fits all" idea of urologist practicing PCNL in developing countries with limited resources it would be to use:

Medium diameter Nephroscopes (Richard Wolf 20.8 Fr outer sheath and 18 Fr optical element. Storz: 22 Fr outer sheath and 19 Fr optical element) which are more versatile and allows two options; to work with the outer sheath with 22 or 24 Fr Amplatz sheath, or with only the optical element, as standalone, With 20 or 18 Fr Amplatz sheath. to pass down the ureter or a stenotic caliceal infundibulum, or allow more space between the nephroscope and Amplatz sheath for stone fragment spontaneous elimination.

As disposables are expensive, one or two reusable forceps including the tri-prong should be available.

This decision could be influenced by local stones characteristics, hardness and composition.

Coming to energy devices used for lithotripsy during PCNL, we have to emphasize that use of ballistic energy is still present in some countries, with extremely limited resources. Ballistic lithotripsy is the best single device for PCNL. There are many manufacturers proposing very cheap affordable devices (even less than 1000 € or $). It needs almost no maintenance; the handle and probes can be manufactured locally. It gives the quickest fragmentation in hard and large stone burden. However,

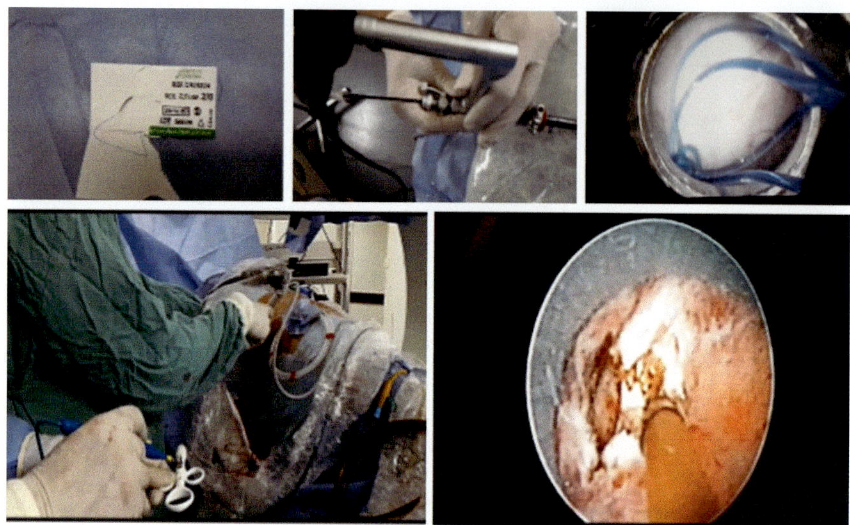

Fig. 5 Alternative tools and prevention of complications during PCNL. Baskets made from another material and cauterization of a tract bleeding vessel

it cannot be used with flexible scopes. It needs a good learning of stone extraction using forceps and baskets.

Use of ballistic devices can result in stone fragments migration to an inaccessible part of the collecting system. Urologists pushed to use this device still are also forced to think how to collect migrated fragments. From one position (use of ballistic device) another one is opened and search for solution is opened. Connecting the working channel to a vacuum devise, with short aspiration and prompt clamping, in aim to prevent bleeding is a way to solve this problem, if baskets and flexible scopes are unavailable. Baskets sometimes can be "handmade", such in this scenario, when monofilament/nylon suture was used to make a basket (Fig. 5).

6 Complications Prevention and Management

Complications following PCNL were and will remain one of the major issues when discussing this procedure. Bleeding and septic conditions are the most severe and their prevention is an integrative part of many PCNL focused sessions and meetings. Even in HICs with all improvements in term of downsized instruments and tract dilators, the percentage of these events did not decrease to an anticipated level.

Discussing complications in developing countries, we can emphasize the need for identification of risk factors. The main precautions for septic complications are sterilized instruments and fluid used. The lack of sterile and originally packed irrigation fluid opened a space for creating one from available resources. As mentioned above,

20–25 L irrigant reservoir is the most popular and available solution. In one of the series followed, many patients developed fever following procedure performed with this fluid, but we must emphasize that many of patients had previously detected and not adequately treated urinary tract infection. Even if it looks like an easily solved problem, the lack of irrigation fluid still impacts outcome of the PCNL significantly.

A risk of bleeding may be anticipated during the PCNL procedure. As interventional radiology is a rare possibility, the need of "possible intraoperative action" arises. If bleeding estimated during PCNL is considered as significant by surgeon, one of the possible ways to stop it is cauterization of tract at the end of or during surgery. With safety wire in place, amplatz and the nephroscope are retracted and the tract is visualized. As a tool for cauterization ureteral catheter with a steel mandarin stylet can be used, but also other available devices, disposables from other endoscopic procedures (Fig. 5).

Considering septic complications in setting where alternative irrigants were used, beside all other improvisations and circumstances, we can say that urologist must keep it in mind and consider to end the PCNL leaving nephrostomy tube in place. In this way infection cannot be prevented, but most severe septic complications may be mitigated.

7 Conclusion

Performing endoscopic procedures with limited resources is a challenge. Many frugal solutions are necessary to preform PCNL in LMICs at all. We could say as in candid camera—"Don't do this at home". But every home has its own rules. Probably many readers will be surprised with information presented in this chapter. For one wonder is others reality.

The best way to be aware of circumstances and plan future steps in establishing PCNL is to visit hospitals in LMICs, meet and understand challenges seeing them. Following a visit an education plan can be more realistically created. In the recent past, urologists from LMICs have applied for observerships or fellowships and were trained in European high volume PCNL centres. The next step was to invite experts from HIC and support LMICs urologists initial PCNLs in the local environment. After successfully performed surgeries, "local heroes" could proceed with independent work, organizing future training activities with volunteering presence of their tutors and trainers. That is why teaching activities, already well established in Europe under the umbrella of European School of Urology (ESU) should maintain its spread to developing countries. Involvement of local faculty should be mandatory. In this way the language barrier could be overcome. "Repetitio est mater studiorum"—practice in the home environment is essential to enable the technique to become a treatment standard! With the generosity of charitable organisations and hospitals, donations of old and/or not used, but correct reusable instruments from developed countries would be more than welcome. Under these circumstances, trained and encouraged local surgeons and available equipment, PCNL can become a viable part of local stone management.

At the end comes the answer on question from the beginning of the chapter.

With reality of using ballistic lithotriptors in LMICs stone fragments are still extracted, YES!

References

Akenroye OO, Adebona OT, Akenroye AT. Surgical care in the developing world-strategies and framework for improvement. J Public Health Afr. 2013;4(2):e20. Published 2013 Dec 3. https://doi.org/10.4081/jphia.2013.e20

Assimos D, Krambeck A, Miller NL, et al. Surgical management of stones: American urological association/endourological society guideline, Part II. J Urol. 2016;196:1161.

Bickler S, Ozgediz D, Gosselin R, et al. Key concepts for estimating the burden of surgical conditions and the unmet need for surgical care. World J Surg. 2010;34(3):374–80. https://doi.org/10.1007/s00268-009-0261-6.

Campain N, Mabedi C, Savopoulos V, Payne SR, MacDonagh R. Understanding cultural and logistical contexts for urologists in low-income countries. BJU Int. 2022;129(3):273–9. https://doi.org/10.1111/bju.15690.

Cassell A 3rd, Jalloh M, Ndoye M, et al. Surgical Management of Urolithiasis of the upper tract—current trend of endourology in Africa. Res Rep Urol. 2020;12:225–238. Published 2020 Jul 6. https://doi.org/10.2147/RRU.S25766

Chandrasekera S. The Sri Lankan magic box for endourology training. Instructional Course 11: Urologic Endoscopy in Resource Restricted Environments. 39th Congress of the SIU—Athens, Greece October 17–20 2019.

Cracco CM, Scoffone CM. ECIRS (Endoscopic Combined Intrarenal Surgery) in the Galdakao-modified supine Valdivia position: a new life for percutaneous surgery? World J Urol. 2011;29(6):821–7. https://doi.org/10.1007/s00345-011-0790-0.

Durutović O, Filipović A, Milićević K, et al. 3D imaging segmentation and 3D rendering process for a precise puncture strategy during PCNL—a pilot study. Front Surg. 2022;9:891596. Published 2022 May 3. https://doi.org/10.3389/fsurg.2022.891596

Fernström I, Johansson B. Percutaneous pyelolithotomy. A new extraction technique. Scand J Urol Nephrol. 1976;10(3):257–259. https://doi.org/10.1080/21681805.1976.11882084

Geraghty RM, Davis NF, Tzelves L, et al. Best practice in interventional management of urolithiasis: an update from the European Association of urology guidelines panel for urolithiasis 2022. Eur Urol Focus. 2023;9(1):199–208. https://doi.org/10.1016/j.euf.2022.06.014.

Lezrek M, Bentani N, Moudouni S, Sarf I, Tazi H, El Khadim R, Bazine K, Slimani A, Alami M. VID.51 smartphone torch-app "ShadowsPlay" for learning of calyx puncture without radiation exposure. Abstract SIU 2016a Buenos Aires, Argentina book. World J Urol. 2016a;34(Suppl 1):117. https://doi.org/10.1007/s00345-016-1931-2

Lezrek M, Mawfik H, Errai A, Tazi H, Bazine K, Slimani A, Qarro A, Ammani A, Beddouch A, Alami M. VID.52 percutaneous micro-nephroscopy training in a glove model abstract SIU 2016b Buenos aires, Argentina book. World J Urol. 2016b;34(Suppl 1):118. https://doi.org/10.1007/s00345-016-1931-2

Lezrek M, Tazi H, Moufid K, Saherh Y, El Yazami O, Slimani A, Bazine K1, Ziouziou I, Alami M, Ammani A. VID.45 percutaneous tract dilation training on a pumpkin. In: Abstracts from 38th Congress of the Société Internationale d'Urologie Seoul Dragon City, October 4–7, 2018. World J Urol 2018;36(Suppl 1):191.

Meara JG, Leather AJ, Hagander L, et al. Global surgery 2030: evidence and solutions for achieving health, welfare, and economic development. Lancet. 2015;386(9993):569–624. https://doi.org/10.1016/S0140-6736(15)60160-X.

Osman M, Wendt-Nordahl G, Heger K, Michel MS, Alken P, Knoll T. Percutaneous nephrolithotomy with ultrasonography-guided renal access: experience from over 300 cases. BJU Int. 2005;96(6):875–8. https://doi.org/10.1111/j.1464-410X.2005.05749.x.

Payne SR, Chalwe M. Understanding the needs of low-income countries: how urologists can help. BJU Int. 2022;129(1):9–16. https://doi.org/10.1111/bju.15628.

Sorokin I, Mamoulakis C, Miyazawa K, Rodgers A, Talati J, Lotan Y. Epidemiology of stone disease across the world. World J Urol. 2017;35(9):1301–20. https://doi.org/10.1007/s00345-017-2008-6.

Tanriverdi O, Boylu U, Kendirci M, Kadihasanoglu M, Horasanli K, Miroglu C. The learning curve in the training of percutaneous nephrolithotomy. Eur Urol. 2007;52(1):206–11. https://doi.org/10.1016/j.eururo.2007.01.001.

Tatanis V, Cracco CM, Liatsikos E. Advances in percutaneous renal puncture: a comprehensive review of the literature. Curr Opin Urol. 2023;33(2):116–21. https://doi.org/10.1097/MOU.0000000000001059.

Venn S, Mabedi C, Ngowi BN, Mbwambo OJ, Mteta KA, Payne SR. Disseminating surgical experience for sustainable benefits: the Urolink experience. BJU Int. 2022;129(6):661–7. https://doi.org/10.1111/bju.15733.

Voorhees JR, Tubbs RS, Nahed B, Cohen-Gadol AA. William S. Halsted and Harvey W. Cushing: reflections on their complex association. J Neurosurg. 2009;110(2):384–390. https://doi.org/10.3171/2008.4.17516

Watson G, Niang L, Chandresekhar S, Natchagande G, Payne SR. The feasibility of endourological surgery in low-resource settings. BJU Int. 2022;130(1):18–25. https://doi.org/10.1111/bju.15770.

World Health Organization. Compendium of innovative health technologies for low resources settings 2011–2014. Geneva: WHO; 2015.

Zeng G, Zhong W, Pearle M, et al. European association of urology section of urolithiasis and international alliance of urolithiasis joint consensus on percutaneous nephrolithotomy. Eur Urol Focus. 2022;8(2):588–97. https://doi.org/10.1016/j.euf.2021.03.008.

Ziaee SA, Sichani MM, Kashi AH, Samzadeh M. Evaluation of the learning curve for percutaneous nephrolithotomy. Urol J. 2010;7(4):226–31.

Complications of Percutaneous Nephrolithotomy

Hal D. Kominsky, Samuel F. Lieb, Thomas Knoll, and Margaret S. Pearle

Abstract Percutaneous nephrolithotomy (PCNL) is a common, albeit challenging, procedure for the treatment of large and complex stones. Although PCNL is the most effective of the minimally invasive stone procedures, the risks associated with the procedure are accordingly higher. Complications of PCNL include bleeding, infection, damage to surrounding organs, intrarenal or ureteral obstruction, fistulae and musculoskeletal and neurologic injuries associated with patient positioning. A thorough understanding of intrarenal and relational anatomy of the kidney is essential to diagnose, treat and prevent these complications. This chapter provides a comprehensive review of the diagnosis and management of the complications of PCNL.

Keywords Percutaneous nephrolithotomy · Nephrolithiasis · Complications · Injury · Hemorrhage · Sepsis

1 Introduction

Percutaneous nephrolithotomy (PCNL) is the preferred treatment for large (> 2 cm) and complex kidney stones due to its efficacy and favorable safety profile. However, compared to alternative minimally invasive therapies for upper urinary tract stones such as shock wave lithotripsy (SWL) and ureteroscopy (URS), the complication rate for PCNL is significantly higher. In most cases, complications are minor, and major complications occur rarely (Michel et al. 2007). While even experienced PCNL

H. D. Kominsky · M. S. Pearle
Department of Urology, University of Texas Southwestern Medical Center, 2001 Inwood Road, WCB3 4th Floor, Dallas, TX 75390-9110, USA
e-mail: Margaret.pearle@utsouthwestern.edu

S. F. Lieb · T. Knoll (✉)
Department of Urology, Sindelfingen-Boeblingen Medical Center, Sindelfingen, Germany
e-mail: t.knoll@klinikverbund-suedwest.de

© The Author(s), under exclusive license to Springer Nature Switzerland AG 2023
J. D. Denstedt and E. N. Liatsikos (eds.), *Percutaneous Renal Surgery*,
https://doi.org/10.1007/978-3-031-40542-6_28

surgeons will experience complications on occasion, prompt recognition and appropriate troubleshooting will minimize the impact. The following chapter will review the identification, management and prevention of complications of PCNL.

2   Hemorrhage

Despite its minimally invasive nature, there is a potential for bleeding with any of the steps of PCNL. Access technique, surgeon experience, operative time, preoperative anemia, diabetes, and tract size have all been implicated as risk factors for bleeding during percutaneous renal surgery (Stoller et al. 1994; Kukreja et al. 2004; Turna et al. 2007).

2.1   Pre-operative Considerations

The withholding of antiplatelet and anticoagulation medications perioperatively is typically left to the discretion of the surgeon. However, it is generally recommended that these agents be held prior to surgery if possible, although, recently, the continued use of low dose aspirin through the preoperative period was assessed and found to be safe (Otto et al. 2018; Leavitt et al. 2014). From a preventative standpoint, the preoperative use of tranexamic acid has been shown in randomized trials to reduce the risk of post-operative hemorrhage when administered routinely, or selectively in high-risk patients (Prasad et al. 2023; Lee et al. 2022). A recent systematic review and meta-analysis comprising 6 randomized trials and 1323 patients demonstrated a 67% lower likelihood of needing a blood transfusion in patients treated with tranexamic acid compared to those in the control group (OR 0.33, 95% CI 0.21 to 0.52, $p < 0.00001$) (Prasad et al. 2023).

2.2   Intraoperative Bleeding

Bleeding can occur at any step in the percutaneous procedure. During percutaneous access, the risk of bleeding is minimized when the puncture is performed through a posterior calyx, along the axis of the infundibulum, because it avoids injury to the interlobar vessels that run parallel to the infundibulum (Mahaffey et al. 1994). Although some authors have advocated for infundibular puncture, and no higher incidence of hemorrhage with infundibular compared to calyceal puncture in a randomized trial (Kallidonis et al. 2017a, 2017b; Pearle 2019), anatomic considerations would favor a calyceal puncture. When placing the access sheath, it is best to advance it just to the calyx, because advancement too far into the collecting system increases the risk of tearing the infundibulum, leading to bleeding (Stoller et al. 1994).

Tract size and dilation technique have both been evaluated for their potential impact on bleeding risk during PCNL, sometimes with conflicting results (Davidoff and Bellman 1997; Lam et al. 1992). Davidoff and Bellman reviewed 150 patients undergoing percutaneous renal procedures and compared rates of hemorrhage between those who underwent tract dilation with sequential dilators (n = 50) versus those undergoing balloon dilation (n = 100). They found a significantly higher rate of blood transfusion in the sequential dilator group compared to the balloon dilation group (25% vs. 10%, $p = 0.048$) (Davidoff and Bellman 1997). Likewise, Turna and colleagues reviewed 197 patients undergoing PCNL and found a greater reduction in hematocrit post-operatively in patients undergoing sequential dilation compared to those undergoing balloon dilation (9.1% vs. 6.1%, $p = 0.007$) (Turna et al. 2007). A large multi-institutional study comprising 5537 patients found no difference in rates of hemorrhage according to type of dilation although it did show an association between bleeding and increasing tract size (Yamaguchi et al. 2011).

The increasing popularity of mini-PCNL has in part been attributed to a purported lower risk of bleeding compared with standard PCNL. Indeed, multiple recent meta-analyses comparing outcomes of PCNL with different size working sheaths have, for the most part, demonstrated that patients undergoing PCNL with smaller caliber sheaths (≤ 22 F) tend to have lower transfusion rates and a greater decrease in post-operative hemoglobin compared to those undergoing standard PCNL (24–30F sheath) (Wan et al. 2022; Qin et al. 2022).

Bleeding can occur during the nephroscopy stage of PCNL, even with an optimally placed puncture, as a result of overmanipulating and/or torquing of the nephroscope and sheath, resulting in tearing of the urothelium and injury to the underlying vessels. Liberal use of flexible nephroscopy can prevent this complication.

Minor intraoperative bleeding rarely necessitates termination of the procedure as long as visibility is maintained. Simple repositioning of the working sheath can tamponade the site of bleeding, and increased irrigation pressure can improve visibility. However, high pressure irrigation should be used judiciously and for short periods of time to avoid fluid extravasation, volume overload and sepsis, and it is not a substitute for addressing the source of bleeding.

If bleeding is significant and precludes safe continuation of the procedure, the procedure should be terminated and a large bore nephrostomy tube (18F or greater) placed. If bleeding is due to a venous injury, the tamponade effect of the nephrostomy tube should be sufficient to slow or stop the rate of hemorrhage. However, when bleeding fails to respond to conservative measures and leads to hemodynamic instability, an arterial injury is likely and renal angiography with embolization should be promptly pursued.

Minor bleeding after removal of the working sheath is expected and is usually self-limited. However, brisk bleeding from the tract, even after placement of a nephrostomy tube, indicates renal parenchymal injury or direct vascular injury (Poudyal 2022). Several maneuvers have been described to reduce tract bleeding, including placement of a large caliber nephrostomy tube (Kessaris et al. 1995), manual flank or simultaneous flank and abdominal compression (Ganpule et al. 2014; Wollin and Preminger 2017) or clamping the nephrostomy tube for several hours to allow blood in the collecting system to clot and tamponade further bleeding (Ganpule et al. 2014; Lee and Stoller 2007). Specialized tamponade balloon catheters are reserved for cases in which bleeding fails to respond to any of these measures (Kerbl et al. 1994; Goldfischer et al. 1997). The use of hemostatic agents administered intravenously (e.g., tranexamic acid) or locally into the tract (e.g., gelatin-thrombin matrix) can be considered for minor bleeding, but are unlikely to resolve serious bleeding. If not already present and particularly if a nephrostomy tube was not left in place, a foley catheter should be placed to facilitate monitoring of the urine for blood I the post-operative period. If bleeding fails to abate despite all the previous measures, immediate transport to the interventional radiology suite for angiography and possible embolization is advised.

2.3 *Postoperative Bleeding*

Postoperative bleeding occurs in 0.8–7.6% of PCNL cases (Jinga et al. 2013). Intra-operative misadventures described above can lead to persistent bleeding postoper-atively (Kessaris et al. 1995). A number of studies have evaluated the impact of patient-related factors (gender, age, body mass index, diabetes, urinary tract infec-tions, renal function, abnormal anatomy), stone characteristics (size, composition, complexity), and intraoperative factors (positioning, site of access, technique of punc-ture, size and number of tracts, dilation technique, operative time, drainage) on risk of postoperative bleeding, with conflicting results (Poudyal 2022). For the purposes of this discussion, we distinguish between early (less than 24 h) and delayed (greater than 24 h) postoperative bleeding.

Subcapsular (Fig. 1a) or perinephric hemorrhage should be suspected in the face of declining hemoglobin, flank pain and clear urine. Often, the diagnosis is made incidentally at on post-operative imaging. In most cases, subcapsular or perinephric hematomas can be managed conservatively with bed rest and transfusion as needed (Wollin and Preminger 2017; Knoll et al. 2017). However, if the patient becomes unstable or if the hemoglobin continues to drop despite conservative measures, arteriogram with embolization should be pursued.

Delayed bleeding typically occurs within 2–3 weeks of the procedure but can occur as late as 6–8 weeks post-operatively (Srivastava et al. 2005). Patients often present with abrupt onset of intermittent or persistent gross hematuria, after having previously clear urine for days to weeks post-operatively. In most cases, hemorrhage is due to injury to the interlobar or segmental arteries (Kessaris et al. 1995; Srivas-tava et al. 2005). Because of the high pressure associated with arterial blood flow from the injured artery, communication with an adjacent vein can lead to arteriove-nous fistula. Communication with adjacent parenchyma leads to pseudoaneurysm formation (Cope and Zeit 1982).

Stable patients can initially be treated conservatively with bed rest, fluid resus-citation, hemostatic agents and Foley catheter drainage with or without continuous bladder irrigation. Close monitoring for signs of hemorrhagic shock, obtaining serial

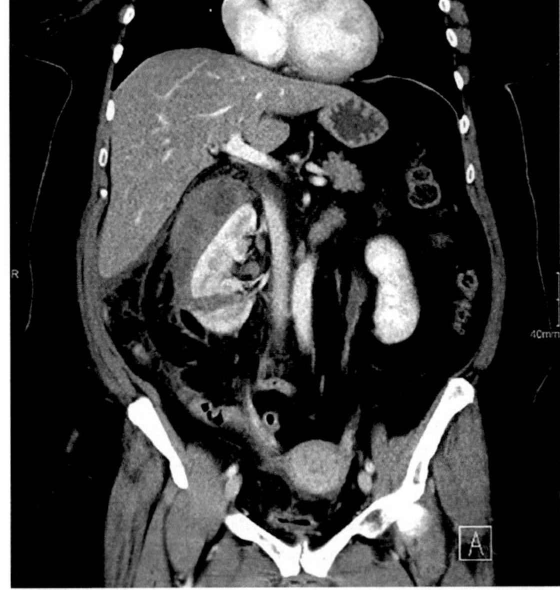

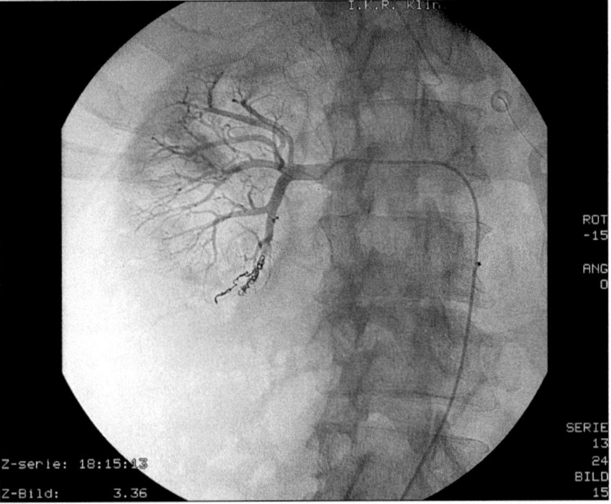

Fig. 1 **a** Patient with subcapsular hematoma due to bleeding from the nephrostomy tract 10 days after PCNL. **b+C.** Postoperative arteriovenous fistula before (top) and after placement of coils (bottom) (courtesy of A. Muslumanoglu, Istanbul, Turkey)

hematocrits (better indicator than hemoglobin), and classification of the degree of hematuria are essential to assess the need for more urgent invasive measures (Srivastava et al. 2005). Imaging such as sonography (including duplex sonography and color Doppler), CT angiography (CTA), and magnetic resonance angiography (MRA) can detect renal vascular lesions and inform the need for angioembolization. In particular, CTA has been recommended prior to arteriography to identify a vascular injury and potentially reduce the amount of contrast needed for angiography. However, there is little evidence to support that a negative CTA reliably predicts a negative arteriogram (Zhao et al. 2014; Yang et al. 2022). Consequently, arteriography with angioembolization is recommended for patients presenting with delayed bleeding after PCNL. Even if bleeding ceases, consultation with interventional radiology for arteriography should be pursued, as rebleeding is likely.

In patients with hemodynamic instability and a rapid, substantial decrease in hemoglobin, prompt intervention with angioembolization is essential (less than 1% of cases) (Jinga et al. 2013; Wollin and Preminger 2017; Mavili et al. 2009). During arteriography, a flush arteriogram is performed to localize the injured vessel and determine the site of optimal coil placement. Successful coil placement is confirmed with a repeat contrast run (Fig. 1b+c#). "Super-selective angioembolization" indicates embolization of a tertiary or quaternary branch of the renal artery, while "complete embolization" refers to occlusion of a main renal branch (Ganpule et al. 2014). In rare cases, primarily those with extensive renal parenchymal ischemia, postembolization syndrome comprised of flank pain, leukocytosis, nausea, vomiting, and fever has been described. Rare reports have described embolization coils migrating into the bloodstream, lungs or urinary tract (Jinga et al. 2013; Ganpule et al. 2014; Mavili et al. 2009). With a success rate over of 90% in experienced centers, percutaneous transarterial embolization is an effective, low-risk procedure that should be employed promptly in suspicious cases (Srivastava et al. 2005; Richstone et al. 2008).

3 Collecting System Injury

3.1 *Perforation*

Perforation of the collecting system can occur at any stage of the PCNL procedure, from tract dilation and sheath insertion to stone removal and placement of the nephrostomy tube. Lee and Smith estimated the rate of collecting system perforation to be 7% in a series of over 580 cases (Lee et al. 1987). More contemporary case series estimate the frequency of collecting system injury at 3–5% (Mousavi-Bahar et al. 2011; Rosette et al. 2011). Perforation of the collecting system is apparent when retroperitoneal structures or perirenal or sinus fat are encountered during nephroscopy or when contrast extravasation is observed fluoroscopically during antegrade nephrostogram. Large collecting system perforations can lead to the accumulation of fluid in the retroperitoneal or peritoneal space, although a distended abdomen may be difficult to appreciate if the patient is prone. Extravasation of large volumes of fluid into the abdomen can lead to difficulty ventilating, hemodynamic instability, acid base disturbances, and post operative ileus (Ghai et al. 2003; Taylor et al. 2012).

Collecting system perforation can be avoided by adhering to simple principles. Passage of dilators or balloons for tract dilation should be performed over a stiff guidewire with constant tension on the wire and intermittent monitoring with fluoroscopy or ultrasound to avoid buckling of the guidewire or over-advancement of the sheath beyond the calyx. In addition, passage of the working sheath just to the calyx and maintaining it there during nephroscopy is essential to prevent extravasation of fluid from the tract and avoid overdilation and splitting of the infundibulum. Extreme torque on the working sheath can lead also lead to perforation of the collecting system and fluid extravasation. Finally, careful passage of the nephrotomy tube over a guidewire under image-guidance assures that the nephrostomy tube is placed within the collecting system and does not perforate outside the collecting system.

While small collecting system perforations may be managed with slight advancement of the working sheath in some cases and/or quick completion of the procedure, large collecting system injuries should be managed with prompt termination of the procedure and placement of a nephrostomy tube with or without a ureteral stent to divert urine for a minimum of 3–7 days (Irby et al. 1999). For large collecting system injuries, confirmation of the absence of fluid extravasation with a nephrostogram may be advisable before removal of the tube.

3.2 Strictures of the Ureteropelvic Junction (UPJ) and Ureter

Strictures of the UPJ or ureter are significantly less common after PCNL than after URS (1.0% vs. 3.5%) (Wollin and Preminger 2017; Jonge et al. 2015). The most likely causes are injury to the urothelium from perforation, with extravasation of urine/stone leading to fibrosis, or stone impaction and associated inflammation/fibrosis (Roberts et al. 1998). Ureteral or UPJ strictures are usually identified on routine post-operative imaging or because of intermittent or persistent post-operative flank pain or infection. However, up to 20% of stenoses remain asymptomatic and thus may go undetected (Meretyk et al. 1992). To prevent asymptomatic loss of renal function, post-operative imaging (sonography or CT scan) should be performed within 6–12 weeks of the procedure (Seitz). UPJ or ureteral strictures can be temporized with nephrostomy or stent drainage until definitive intervention is performed. Since most of these strictures are non-ischemic and generally short, endoscopic management should be considered (Drain et al. 2021; Cotta and Buckley 2017). In cases of long strictures (> 2 cm), open or robotic surgery with ureteroureterostomy, buccal mucosal grafting, auto-transplantation, ileal substitution or ureteroneocystotomy (with or without psoas hitch and Boari flap) may be required (Drain et al. 2021).

3.3 Infundibular Stenosis

Mechanical or thermal damage during surgery of large or complex kidney stones can lead to scarring of an infundibulum, most often the infundibulum associated with the calyx of entry (Danilovic et al. 2021). In some cases, inflammation and fibrosis of the infundibulum due to an infected staghorn calculus may be the culprit. These strictures may be asymptomatic and discovered on post-operative imaging or incidentally at a later time (Danilovic et al. 2021). For this reason, the reported frequency varies widely from 2 to 26% (Danilovic et al. 2021; Parsons et al. 2002). Asymptomatic strictures can be managed conservatively with close follow-up to assure there is no continued loss of renal parenchyma. If imaging and laboratory studies are equivocal for obstruction, renal scintigraphy scan may be helpful (Parsons et al. 2002). In symptomatic patients, ureteroscopic or percutaneous endoinfundibulotomy should be performed (Danilovic et al. 2021; Walsh et al. 1679).

3.4 Retained Foreign Body

In rare cases foreign bodies, most commonly parts of the nephrostomy tube or suture, laser fiber or guide wire, may shear off or be retained in the collecting system, renal parenchyma or along the nephrostomy tract in the retroperitoneum (Wollin and Preminger 2017; Kaba et al. 2015). Likewise, stone fragments may migrate outside the renal collecting system into the retroperitoneum (Evans and Stoller 1993). Although most foreign bodies (FB) in the retroperitoneum are inert and cause no symptoms, patients should be informed of their presence as the FB will appear on subsequent imaging studies obtained for unrelated reasons. Rarely, a FB can migrate or cause infection (particularly with retained infection stones) and may require intervention (Kaba et al. 2015; Evans and Stoller 1993; Hennessey et al. 2012). FBs in the collecting system are more likely to cause obstruction, infection and hematuria and should therefore be removed ureteroscopically, percutaneously or even robotically (Hennessey et al. 2012; Alkan and Basar 2014; Chen et al. 1728). The size, shape, mobility, and location of the FB influence the choice of therapy, although generally, the least invasive therapy should be performed first (Chen et al. 1728).

4 Injury to Surrounding Organs

Because of the proximity of the kidney to lung, colon, bowel, liver and spleen, these organs are at risk of injury primarily during percutaneous access and establishment of the tract. While anomalous anatomy may increase the risk of injury as in the case of retrorenal colon, dilated colon, hyperinflated lungs and distorted body habitus, even normal relational anatomy poses a risk of surrounding organ injury depending on the location of the kidney in the retroperitoneum and the stone within the kidney. Fluoroscopic guidance is unable to identify surrounding structures, while ultrasound guidance can often detect these structures and provide a greater measure of safety during access.

4.1 Lung and Pleura

The lung, and more commonly the pleura, are the most common structures to be injured during PCNL. In most series, the rate of pleural injury ranges from less than 1 to 15% (Lang 1987; Roth and Beckmann 1988). Supra-costal access is associated with the highest risk of injury to the lung and pleura. In a review of CT images, Hopper and colleagues demonstrated that supa-11th rib access traverses lung and/or pleura in about 80% of patients, and supra-12th rib access in up to 30% of cases (Hopper and Yakes 1990). Of note, however, clinically significant lung and pleural injuries resulting in hydro- or pneumothorax occur less frequently than reported by Hopper and associates, with an incidence of 10–15% for supra-costal access (above either 11th or 12th rib), and 1.5–4.5% below the 12th rib (Lojanapiwat and Prasopsuk 2006; Munver et al. 2001). The use of a working sheath during PCNL can minimize the risk of immediate hydrothorax associated with transthoracic access, because much of the air and irrigation fluid are diverted away from the pleural cavity. However, once the working sheath is removed and a small nephrostomy tube or no nephrostomy tube is left, urine can traverse the tract into the pleural space resulting in a hydrothorax.

Prompt recognition of a hydrothorax can minimize patient morbidity and prevent a prolonged length of stay. Routine chest fluoroscopy at the conclusion of PCNL can detect a hydrothorax intraoperatively (Fig. 3a), allowing placement of a small-bore chest tube while the patient is still anesthetized (Fig. 3b). Ogan and Pearle determined that intraoperative chest fluoroscopy at the conclusion of PCNL is sufficient to detect pleural complications without the need for post-operative chest x-ray, although subsequent imaging with CT on post-operative day one can detect delayed hydrothoraces in stable patients without pulmonary symptoms (Ogan et al. 2003).

Small, asymptomatic hydrothoraces or pneumothoraces can be safely monitored without aggressive intervention, or with simple aspiration of pleural fluid or supplemental oxygen, respectively. However, larger or symptomatic hydrothoraces or pneumothoraces (Fig. 2) should be managed with tube thoracostomy. Benson and associates demonstrated that small bore chest tubes (8–12F) are as effective as large bore (32F) thoracostomy tubes because the pleural fluid is generally comprised of urine, not blood (Benson et al. 2013). In patients with known or suspected infection stones, the threshold for placing a chest tube should be low to avoid the occurrence of empyema. In the case of loculated, infected pleural fluid, visual-assisted thoracoscopic surgery (VATS procedure) may be required to lyse the loculations and remove the infected fluid, necessitating placement of a large bore thoracostomy tube and incurring additional hospital stay (Kumar et al. 2014; Maheshwari et al. 2009). Fortunately, these events are rare.

Along with pleural drainage, it is imperative to assure good antegrade drainage from the collecting system to the bladder. Evaluation for distal obstruction in the form of a retained ureteral stone, clot or ureteral edema should be undertaken with appropriate imaging. If antegrade drainage is equivocal or poor, a ureteral stent or a lower pole nephrostomy tube should be placed. If a stent is placed, bladder catheter drainage should be provided for at least a day or two to prevent reflux of urine into

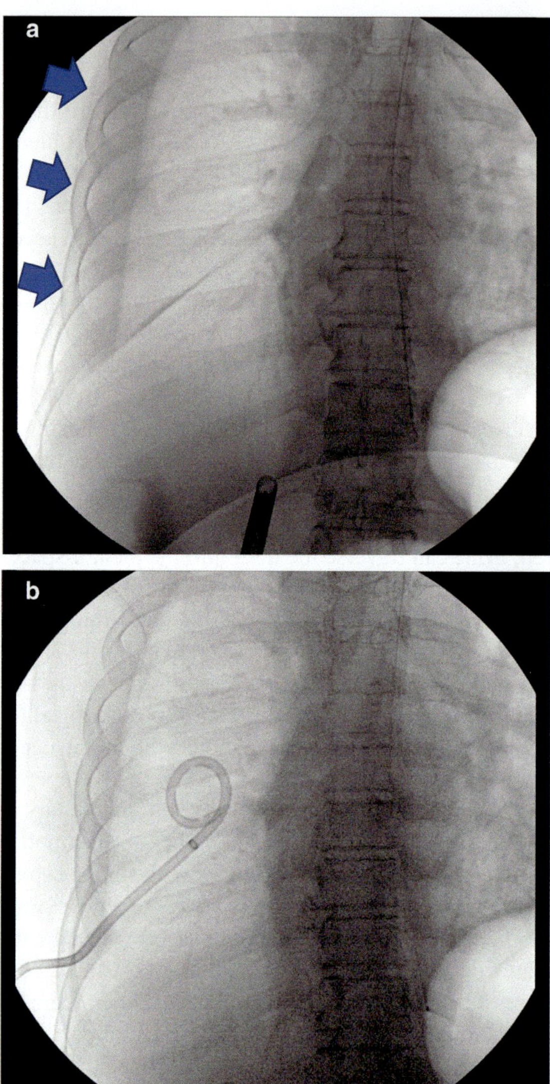

Fig. 2 **a** Intraoperative fluoroscopic chest image reveals hydrothorax (arrows denote dependent fluid collecting in pleural space). **b** Thoracostomy tube placement under fluoroscopic guidance to drain hydrothorax

the pleural space. Once chest tube output is minimal, the bladder catheter can be removed. If chest tube output remains low after discontinuing the bladder catheter, the chest tube can then be removed. Finally, the ureteral stent is removed 7–10 days later, presuming any ureteral obstruction has been addressed or resolved.

Nephropleural fistula, or persistent drainage of urine from the collecting system into the pleural space occurs in less than 1% of cases (Munver et al. 2001; Lallas et al. 2004). Most commonly occurring after an upper pole, often supracostal puncture, nephropleural fistula can occur up to several weeks following surgery (Bansal

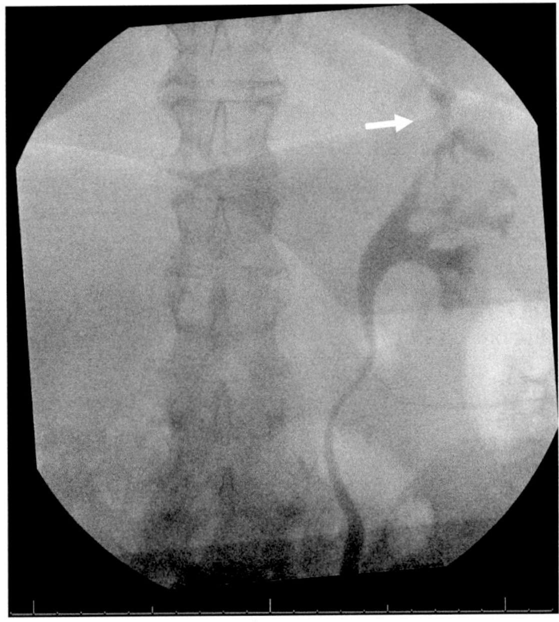

Fig. 3 Retrograde pyelogram in a patient with a nephropleural fistula. Contrast extravasation from upper pole into pleural cavity (white arrow)

et al. 2017). Persistent or new drainage from a previous thoracostomy tract is pathognomonic. Patients may also experience pulmonary symptoms, including shortness of breath and chest pain (Lallas et al. 2004; Kaler et al. 2016). Retrograde pyelography (Fig. 3), CT urogram or chest xray will demonstrate the communication between the collecting system and the pleural space or new hydrothorax. Nephropleural fistula most commonly occurs as a result of distal obstruction preventing proper antegrade urine drainage. Treatment is best approached with continuation of thoracostomy drainage along with renal drainage by way of either a ureteral stent or nephrostomy tube to assure proper antegrade drainage and reduce flow of urine into the pleural space (Lallas et al. 2004). CT of the urinary tract should be performed to exclude distal obstruction (due to stones, blood clot, strictures, or injuries), and if identified should be addressed (Kaler et al. 2016). The chest tube and stent/nephrostomy tube should be left in place until the drainage of pleural fluid ceases (Lallas et al. 2004). In case of a persistent fistula despite no distal obstruction, a thoracic surgeon should be consulted and further options such as video-assisted exploration, decortication or pleural sclerosis discussed (Lallas et al. 2004).

4.2 Colon

Colon injury during percutaneous access occurs in less than 1% of cases, primarily because retro-renal colon is relatively rare (Lee et al. 1987; El-Nahas et al. 2006;

Nouira et al. 2006; Vallancien et al. 1985). Hadar and Gadoth estimated that retro-renal colon occurs in only about 0.6% of the general population (Hadar and Gadoth 1984). Patients at higher risk of colon injury during PCNL include those with a horseshoe kidney, conditions that predispose to colonic distension and a history of extensive colon surgery, as well as those undergoing lower pole access or left-sided procedures (El-Nahas et al. 2006). Although supine PCNL has been theorized to increase the risk of colon injury (Öztürk 2014), most series have not shown a difference in rates of colon injury between supine and prone PCNL (Wu et al. 2011; Liu et al. 2010).

Early recognition of colonic perforation is vital to mitigate the consequences of the injury. Identification of colon injury during PCNL generally involves visualization of contrast within loops of large bowel during nephrostogram. Post-operatively, the finding of gas or feculent matter emanating from the nephrostomy tract, hematochezia, excessive diarrhea, or peritonitis should raise suspicion of colon injury (Noor Buchholz 2004; Hussain et al. 2003).

Colon injuries can generally be managed conservatively if the patient remains clinically stable. Classic teaching advises withdrawing the nephrostomy tube into the colon under fluoroscopic guidance and draining the kidney with a ureteral stent to separate the urine and fecal streams (Nouira et al. 2006). However, in many cases simple drainage of the kidney with a ureteral stent and removal of the nephrostomy tube will suffice. Broad spectrum antibiotics should be maintained for 7–14 days. While some authors recommend a low residue diet, others make no specific dietary recommendations (Öztürk 2014, 2015). If a colostomy tube is placed, a contrast study performed through the tube in 7–10 days assures no further communication with the kidney and allows for safe removal of the colostomy tube (Gerspach et al. 1997).

The occurrence of peritonitis, sepsis, or transperitoneal perforation in the context of a known colonic injury, although rare, should prompt consultation with a general surgeon. Open/robotic exploration and colostomy or repair of the colon injury may be required in rare cases.

Nephroeneteric fistulae, most commonly involving the colon, are rare. LeRoy and colleagues observed two in their first 1000 percutaneous procedures (LeRoy et al. 1985). These fistulae are best treated by separating the urine and fecal stream by withdrawing the nephrostomy tube into the colon (if there is still a nephrostomy tube) and placing a ureteral stent to promote antegrade flow of urine. After 4–6 weeks, ureteropyelography can be performed, and if there is no extravasation, the ureteral stent can be removed (Seitz et al. 2012). In case of failed conservative management, intraperitoneal colonic perforation, peritonitis, or sepsis, open/robotic surgical exploration with colotomy should be performed (Oztürk 2015; Traxer 2009).

4.3 Small Intestine

The second and third portions of the duodenum are in close enough proximity to the right kidney that they can be injured during PCNL, albeit rarely. Perforation of the renal pelvis during nephrostomy tract dilation or sheath placement can lead to anterior perforation and duodenal injury. Fluoroscopic monitoring during percutaneous renal access, dilation and placement of the working sheath should reduce the risk of perforation of hollow viscera. Small intestine injuries should be suspected when intestinal mucosa or succus is encountered. Antegrade nephrostogram may show contrast filling loops of small bowel.

Small bowel injury incurred during percutaneous nephrolithotomy is rare since the trajectory of the access into the kidney does not typically cross the small bowel (Saad et al. 2014; Al-Assiri et al. 2005). In the event of small bowel perforation, prompt exploration and repair with possible small bowel resection provides the best outcome (Fig. 4). Nephrostogram or CT urogram at 10–14 days should be performed to ensure no fistulous communication between the kidney and small bowel.

4.4 Liver, Gallbladder, Spleen

Injury to the liver is a rare complication of PCNL, occurring in less than 1% of cases. Hopper and Yakes evaluated CT images to determine the relational anatomy of the kidney with respect to percutaneous access and concluded that right sided supracostal access is theoretically associated with a 14% risk of injuring the liver (Hopper and Yakes 1990), although in reality the occurrence of liver injury under these conditions is decidedly less. The risk of liver injury can be mitigated by careful review of pre-operative CT images and noting hepatomegaly or other anomalies that might preclude safe fluoroscopic-guided percutaneous. In these situations, CT- or ultrasound-guided access may be advisable (Matlaga et al. 2003). In the event a liver injury is identified on post-operative CT imaging (Fig. 5), the nephrostomy tube should be left in place for 7–10 days to allow maturation of the tract and hemostasis, after which the tube can be removed with careful observation for signs of bleeding. Leaving a stent in place may reduce the risk of renobiliary fistula formation, which is nonetheless a rare event.

Injury to the spleen is also a very rare complication, typically encountered with left percutaneous access above the 11th rib (Hopper and Yakes 1990; Kondás et al. 1994). Splenic injuries are more likely than liver injuries to result in hemorrhage, leading to hypovolemic shock in the most severe cases. While conservative management with bedrest and close observation may be attempted if the patient is hemodynamically stable, some patients with splenic injury require splenectomy for hemodynamic instability (Öztürk 2014; Kondás et al. 1994).

Injury to the gallbladder is a rare complication of PCNL. Signs of gallbladder injury include drainage of bile from the nephrostomy tube, peritonitis or sepsis,

Fig. 4 CT showing nephrostomy tube (A, B) traversing small intestine (red arrows). Resected loop of small intestine (C) shows perforation from nephrostomy tube (black arrow)

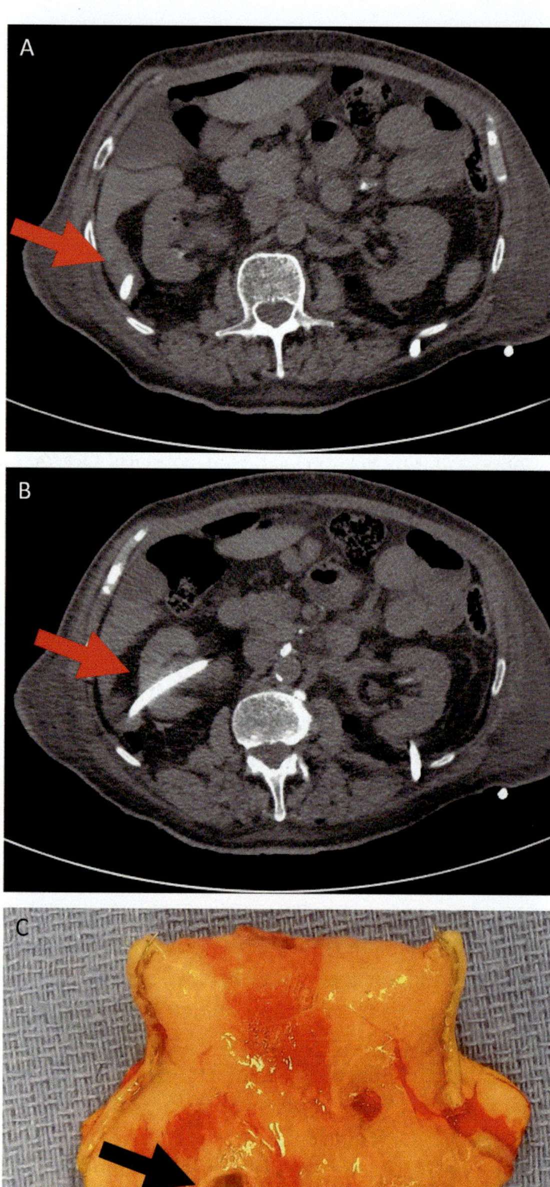

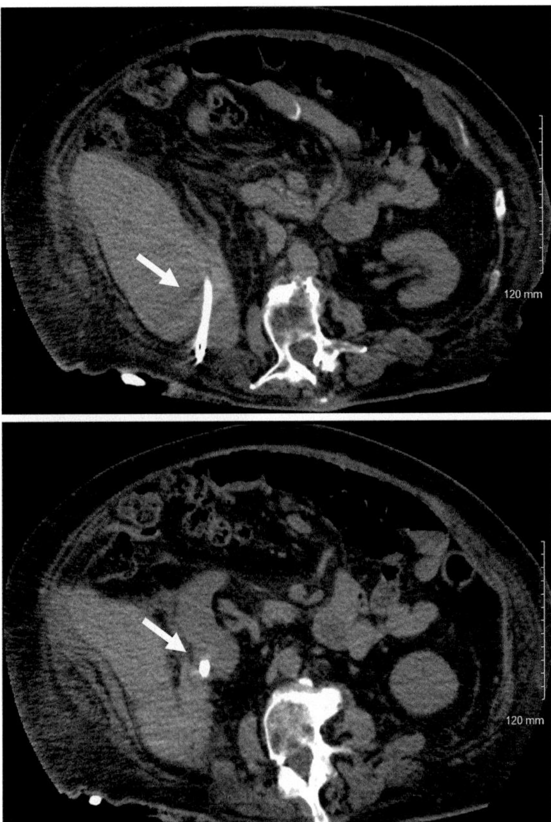

Fig. 5 CT showing nephrostomy tube traversing liver (top image) prior to entering right kidney (bottom image)

and the diagnosis is evident on CT imaging. General surgery consultation is recommended in these cases, and most patients will undergo cholecystectomy (Öztürk 2014; Fisher et al. 2004).

Nephrocutaneous Fistula

The nephrostomy tract can be expected to close within 6–12 h of surgery if no nephrostomy tube is left in place and within 24–48 h of nephrotomy tube removal if a tube had been left in place (Tefekli et al. 2007; Dirim et al. 2011; Kallidonis et al. 2016). Leakage from the tract beyond 24–48 h is generally rare, and persistent and prolonged drainage from the tract, i.e., nephrocutaneous fistula, occurs in less than 1% of cases (Tefekli et al. 2007; Liatsikos et al. 2005). Nephrocutaneous fistula is typically due to distal obstruction within the collecting system or ureter, by which antegrade flow of urine is precluded, and drainage from the tract persists. CT imaging should be obtained to identify distal obstruction from infundibular stenosis, ureteral edema, stricture, residual stone fragment or blood clot (Fig. 6) (Andonian et al. 1427). Temporary relief of the obstruction with a stent or nephrostomy tube and/or definitive treatment of the obstruction should allow resolution of the nephrocutaneous fistula (Goel et al. 2020). A short duration of an indwelling bladder drainage can also be helpful to promote optimal drainage of the urinary tract while the fistula tract closes.

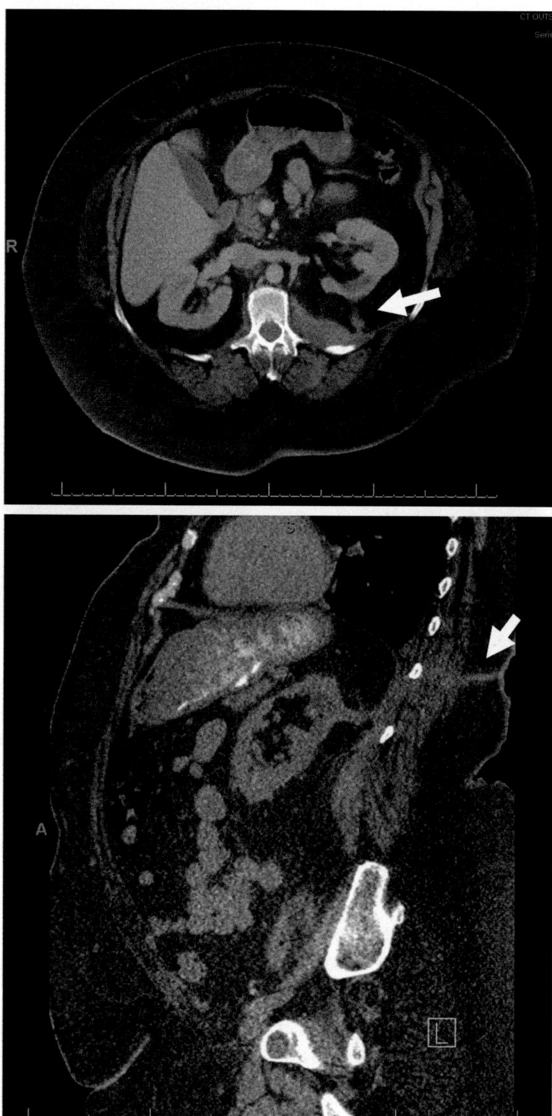

Fig. 6 CT scan showing nephrocutaneous fistula (white arrows). Patient experienced persistent drainage from nephrostomy site 6 months after surgery

5 Medical Complications

5.1 Infection and Sepsis

Infectious complications are among the most common and feared post-operative complications encountered in patients undergoing PCNL, occurring in 0.6–1.5% of cases (Roth and Beckmann 1988; Segura et al. 1985). Factors predictive of postoperative urinary sepsis include positive urine and stone cultures, greater stone burden, history of recurrent urinary tract infections, renal failure, longer operative time, and history of multi-drug resistant bacteria (Gao et al. 2020; Kreydin and Eisner 2013; Koras et al. 2015).

Treatment of patients with pre-operative positive urine cultures with antibiotics prior to PCNL is strongly supported by practice guidelines (Assimos et al. 2016; Türk et al. 2016). However, recommendations for pre-treatment with antibiotics in the face of sterile pre-operative urine is less clear. Historically, one week of peri-operative antibiotic therapy was recommended prior to PCNL (Wollin et al. 2017; Mariappan et al. 2006). However, this practice has recently been challenged by several prospective trials suggesting no advantage of preoperative antibiotic treatment in low risk patints (Chew et al. 2018; Sur et al. 2021; Bag et al. 2011; Doğan et al. 2002). Chew and colleagues found no increased risk of sepsis following PCNL in patients who received one week of preoperative antibiotics compared to those that did not (Chew et al. 2018). In this study, 86 patients with sterile preoperative urine cultures and no indwelling tubes were randomized to receive one week of nitrofurantoin (100 mg twice daily) or to a control arm receiving no pre-procedural antibiotics. Both groups received a combination of ampicillin and gentamicin intravenously at the time of surgery. They found no significant difference between groups regarding rates of postoperative sepsis (14% in the antibiotic group versus 12% in the control group, $p = 1.0$).

These same authors also evaluated the optimal duration of pre-operative antibiotics in a prospectively randomized high-risk group of patients who had either a positive pre-operative culture and/or an indwelling tube. In one arm of the study, 72 patients received 7 days of culture-specific antibiotics and in the other arm, 55 patients received 2 days of culture-specific antibiotics prior to undergoing PCNL. Although they found no significant difference in rates of sepsis between the 2 groups, multivariable analysis, after controlling for confounding factors, did show that two days of antibiotics was associated with an increased the risk of sepsis compared to seven days of treatment (OR 3.1, 95% CI 1.1–8.9, $p = 0.031$) (Sur et al. 2021).

Some patients undergoing PCNL experience postoperative infection and sepsis events despite a negative preoperative urine culture. One explanation is the release of endotoxins and tumor necrosis factor during surgery (Rao et al. 1991). However, several authors have demonstrated a lack of concordance in cultures collected from bladder and renal pelvis urine or from the stone (Benson et al. 2014; Margel et al. 2006; Walton-Diaz et al. 2017). In patients with a negative preoperative bladder urine culture, stone or renal pelvis urine cultures have been shown to be positive in 25–43%

of cases (Margel et al. 2006). Obtaining an intraoperative culture from renal pelvis urine or from the stone should be strongly considered in high risk patients.

Patients experiencing sepsis after PCNL may have fever or demonstrate hemodynamic instability, changes in mental status and alterations in laboratory values such as increased white blood cell count or lactate. While low-grade fever and mild leukocytosis are relatively common after surgery, greater elevations in temperature and white count should prompt further sepsis work-up (Cadeddu et al. 1998; Bozkurt et al. 2015). Repeat urine and blood cultures are recommended to increase the likelihood of identifying the offending organism. Empiric antibiotic therapy and aggressive fluid resuscitation should be initiated. Patients unresponsive to first line therapy may require pressor support and intensive care monitoring. CT imaging should be considered to identify other possible pathologies such as injuries to adjacent structures, urine leak or perinephric or subcapsular hematoma.

5.2 Fluid Overload

Fluid absorption during uncomplicated PCNL has been estimated at about half a liter (Kukreja et al. 2002). However, in the setting of significant collecting system perforation or venous injury, that volume can be substantially greater. As such, these injuries should prompt quick termination of the procedure and drainage of the collecting system. For small collecting perforations, the procedure can be continued if the irrigation pressure remains low and remaining operating time is brief. If the perforation is in the infundibulum associated with the calyx of entry, the working sheath can be gently advanced to prevent further fluid loss from the tract.

Careful monitoring by the operative team for discrepancy between fluid input and output can identify unrecognized collecting system perforation before significant fluid absorption occurs. Larger access sheaths can maximize drainage during the surgery and limit the absorption of fluid by maintaining low intrarenal pressure. For patients with signs of significant hypervolemia and cardiopulmonary compromise, diuresis may be warranted.

5.3 Hypothermia

At least some degree of hypothermia occurs in all patients during PNCL. Reduction in core body temperature is thought to be the result of a combination of factors including vasodilatory effects of anesthesia, exposed body surfaces, room temperature and irrigation fluid temperature. Prevention of hypothermia is an important consideration, as reduced core body temperature can impact coagulation profiles, enzymatic drug clearance, and tissue oxygen consumption (Roberts et al. 1994).

Roberts and colleagues found that when using room temperature irrigation fluid, patient core body temperature dropped on average 1 °C during the procedure (Roberts et al. 1994). Longer operative times and female gender predicted the greatest decline in core body temperature. Blood loss and advanced age did not appear to significantly impact the risk of hypothermia. Warmed irrigation fluid can reduce the risk of hypothermia compared to the use room temperature or cold irrigation fluid (Tekgul et al. 2015; Hosseini et al. 2019). While the use of fluid warmed in a fluid warmer is helpful, active and ongoing fluid warming by way of fluid management systems is more effective at maintaining body temperature. Use of warming drapes and placement of blankets under the sterile surgical drapes can also help preserve patient core body temperature.

5.4 Positioning-Related Injury

Patient positioning can be associated with a number of potential injuries, although the rate of injury has not been shown to differ between prone and supine PCNL (Zhang et al. 2014; Giusti and Lisa 2020; Perrella et al. 2022). Proper positioning and padding is essential to avoid nerve and musculoskeletal injuries and is the responsibility of the entire surgical and anesthesia team.

Several injuries are associated specifically with prone positioning. Brachial plexus injuries occur from inadequate shoulder flexion (greater than 90°. Perioperative visual loss due to ischemic optic neuropathy is a rare complication for which intraoperative hypotension and diabetes are risk factors. Meralgia paresthetica (lateral femoral cutaneous nerve neuropathy) occurs from direct compression by bolster pads/rolls on the anterior superior iliac spine impinging on the lateral femoral cutaneous nerve. Finally, pressure ulcers of the forehead and chin can occur despite the use of foam face pillows. Duration of surgery and obesity have been shown to be risk factors for this complication (DePasse et al. 2015).

Optimal prone positioning during percutaneous nephrolithotomy includes maintaining the upper arms at less than 90°from the shoulders, placing chest rolls to provide for chest excursion but avoiding compression of the nipples, flexing slightly at the knees, maintaining the ankles in a neutral position and providing padding under the forearms, thighs and knees.

Neuropraxia that develops as a result of poor positioning will typically resolve without intervention, although it is distressing to the patients. Some patients may benefit from a short course of physical therapy. Neurologic evaluation may be indicated for severe and refractory cases of neuropraxia.

Decline of Renal Function

Stone patients are at higher risk of renal failure due to recurrent stone formation, repeated surgeries, urinary tract obstruction and recurrent infection (Gambaro et al. 2001; Kurien et al. 2009). The risk of chronic kidney disease or end-stage renal disease is two-fold higher in recurrent stone formers than in the general population

(Gambaro et al. 2017). This risk is even greater in those who form cystine, uric acid, and struvite stones (Gambaro et al. 2017).

For patients undergoing PCNL, poor preoperative renal function, diabetes, hypertension, and multiple percutaneous tracts, have been shown to predispose to further decline in renal function post-operatively (Reeves et al. 2020). Surgical misadventures can additionally exacerbate renal impairment, although this is less common (less than 6% of cases) (Lechevallier et al. 1993).

An increase in serum creatinine and decrease in creatinine clearance and estimated glomerular filtration rate have been observed in the early post-operative period (up to 72 h) after PCNL (Mukherjee et al. 2019; Handa et al. 2006). This potential temporary reduction in renal function should be taken into account when ordering antibiotics and other medications and when considering diagnostic imaging utilizing intravenous contrast. Long-term studies (1–2 years) have shown stable or even significantly improved renal function postoperatively, even in patients with chronic kidney disease, likely due to relief of obstruction (Kurien et al. 2009; Yaycioglu et al. 2007).

6 Conclusions

PCNL is a safe, highly effective procedure that constitutes standard of care for the treatment of large and/or complex stones. While most complications associated with PCNL are minor (CD 1 + 2) and transient and can be treated conservatively, rare complications are severe, life-threatening and require further surgical intervention. Many of the complications of PCNL can be mitigated with careful pre-operative preparation and by following standard intraoperative principles. However, some complications are accepted consequences of the procedure and anatomy. In these cases, prompt recognition and management will minimize morbidity.

References

Al-Assiri M, Binsaleh S, Libman J, et al. Jejunal perforation during percutaneous nephrolithotrypsy. Sci World J. 2005;5:496.

Alkan E, Basar MM. Endourological treatment of foreign bodies in the urinary system. JSLS: J Soc Laparoendosc Surg. 2014;18.

Andonian S, Okhunov Z, Shapiro EY, et al. Diagnostic utility and clinical value of postpercutaneous nephrolithotomy nephrostogram. https://home.liebertpub.com/end. 2010;24:1427.

Assimos D, Krambeck A, Miller NL, et al. Surgical management of stones: American Urological Association/Endourological Society Guideline, PART I. J Urol. 2016;196:1153.

Bag S, Kumar S, Taneja N, et al. One week of nitrofurantoin before percutaneous nephrolithotomy significantly reduces upper tract infection and urosepsis: a prospective controlled study. Urology. 2011;77:45.

Bansal D, Nayak B, Singh P, et al. A rare case of persistent nephropleural fistula following percutaneous nephrolithotomy. BMJ Case Rep. 2017;2017.

Benson JS, Hart ST, Kadlec AO, et al. Small-bore catheter drainage of pleural injury after percutaneous nephrolithotomy: feasibility and outcome from a single large institution series. J Endourol. 2013;27:1440.

Benson AD, Juliano TM, Miller NL. Infectious outcomes of nephrostomy drainage before percutaneous nephrolithotomy compared to concurrent access. J Urol. 2014;192:770.

Bozkurt IH, Aydogdu O, Yonguc T, et al. Predictive value of leukocytosis for infectious complications after percutaneous nephrolithotomy. Urology. 2015;86:25.

Cadeddu JA, Chen R, Bishoff J, et al. Clinical significance of fever after percutaneous nephrolithotomy. Urology. 1998;52:48.

Chen BH, Chang TH, Chen M, et al. Retrieval of intrarenal coiled and ruptured guidewire by retrograde intrarenal surgery: a case report and literature review. Open medicine (Warsaw, Poland) 2021;16:1728.

Chew BH, Miller NL, Abbott JE, et al. A randomized controlled trial of preoperative prophylactic antibiotics prior to percutaneous nephrolithotomy in a low infectious risk population: a report from the EDGE consortium. J Urol. 2018;200:801.

Cope C, Zeit RM. Pseudoaneurysms after nephrostomy. AJR Am J Roentgenol. 1982;139:255.

Cotta BH, Buckley JC. Endoscopic treatment of urethral stenosis. Urol Clinics N Am. 2017;44:19.

Danilovic A, Torricelli FCM, Marchini GS, et al. Does previous standard percutaneous nephrolithotomy impair retrograde intrarenal surgery outcomes? Int Braz J Urol: Official J Braz Soc Urol. 2021;47:1198.

Davidoff R, Bellman GC. Influence of technique of percutaneous tract creation on incidence of renal hemorrhage. J Urol. 1997;157:1229.

de Jonge PKJD, Simaioforidis V, Geutjes PJ, et al. Recent advances in ureteral tissue engineering. Curr Urol Rep. 2015;16:1.

de la Rosette J, Assimos D, Desai M, et al. The clinical research office of the endourological society percutaneous nephrolithotomy global study: indications, complications, and outcomes in 5803 patients. J Endourol. 2011;25:11.

DePasse JM, Palumbo MA, Haque M, et al. Complications associated with prone positioning in elective spinal surgery. World J Orthop. 2015;6:351.

Dirim A, Turunc T, Kuzgunbay B, et al. Which factors may effect urinary leakage following percutaneous nephrolithotomy? World J Urol. 2011;29:761.

Doğan HS, Sahin A, Cetinkaya Y, et al. Antibiotic prophylaxis in percutaneous nephrolithotomy: prospective study in 81 patients. J Endourol. 2002;16:649.

Drain A, Jun MS, Zhao LC. Robotic ureteral reconstruction. Urol Clin North Am. 2021;48:91.

El-Nahas AR, Shokeir AA, El-Assmy AM, et al. Colonic perforation during percutaneous nephrolithotomy: study of risk factors. Urology. 2006;67:937.

Evans CP, Stoller ML. The fate of the iatrogenic retroperitoneal stone. J Urol. 1993;150:827.

Fisher MB, Bianco FJ, Carlin AM, et al. Biliary peritonitis complicating percutaneous nephrolithomy requiring laparoscopic cholecystectomy. J Urol. 2004;171:791.

Gambaro G, Favaro S, D'Angelo A. Risk for renal failure in nephrolithiasis. Am J Kidney Dis. 2001;37:233.

Gambaro G, Croppi E, Bushinsky D, et al. The risk of chronic kidney disease associated with urolithiasis and its urological treatments: a review. J Urol. 2017;198:268.

Ganpule AP, Shah DH, Desai MR. Postpercutaneous nephrolithotomy bleeding: Aetiology and management. Curr Opin Urol. 2014;24:189.

Gao X, Lu C, Xie F, et al. Risk factors for sepsis in patients with struvite stones following percutaneous nephrolithotomy. World J Urol. 2020;38:219.

Gerspach JM, Bellman GC, Stoller ML, et al. Conservative management of colon injury following percutaneous renal surgery. Urology. 1997;49:831.

Ghai B, Dureja GP, Arvind P. Massive intraabdominal extravasation of fluid: a life threatening complication following percutaneous nephrolithotomy. Int Urol Nephrol. 2003;35:315.

Giusti G, De Lisa A. PCNL in the prone position VS PCNL in the modified supine Double-S position: is there a better position? A prospective randomized trial. Urolithiasis. 2020;48:63.

Goel R, Nayak B, Singh P, et al. Percutaneous management of persistent urine leak after partial nephrectomy: sealing the leak site with glue. J Endourol Case Rep. 2020;6:472.

Goldfischer ER, Eiley DM, Smith AD. Novel hemostatic nephrostomy tube. J Endourol. 1997;11:405.

Hadar H, Gadoth N. Positional relations of colon and kidney determined by perirenal fat. AJR Am J Roentgenol. 1984;143:773.

Handa RK, Matlaga BR, Connors BA, et al. Acute effects of percutaneous tract dilation on renal function and structure. J Endourol. 2006;20:1030.

Hennessey, DB, Thomas AZ, Lynch TH, et al. Retained upper genitourinary gossypiboma can mimic renal neoplasms. A review of the literature. Internet J Urol. 2012;9.

Hopper KD, Yakes WF. The posterior intercostal approach for percutaneous renal procedures: risk of puncturing the lung, spleen, and liver as determined by CT. AJR Am J Roentgenol. 1990;154:115.

Hosseini SR, Mohseni MG, Aghamir SMK, et al. Effect of irrigation solution temperature on complication of percutaneous nephrolithotomy: a randomized clinical trial. Urol J. 2019;16:525.

Hussain M, Hamid R, Arya M, et al. Management of colonic injury following percutaneous nephrolithotomy. Int J Clin Pract. 2003;57:549.

Irby PB, Schwartz BF, Stoller ML. Percutaneous access techniques in renal surgery. Tech Urol. 1999;5:29.

Jinga V, Dorobat B, Youssef S, et al. Transarterial embolization of renal vascular lesions after percutaneous nephrolithotomy. Chirurgia (Bucharest, Romania: 1990) 2013;108:521.

Kaba M, Pirinççi N, Kaba S, et al. A rare complication observed during percutaneous nephrolithotomy: foreign body migration from the right kidney to the left lung. Eur J Pediatr Surg Rep. 2015;3:015.

Kaler KS, Cwikla D, Clayman RV. Delayed nephropleural fistula after percutaneous nephrolithotomy. J Endourol Case Rep. 2016;2:99.

Kallidonis P, Panagopoulos V, Kyriazis I, et al. Complications of percutaneous nephrolithotomy: classification, management, and prevention. Curr Opin Urol. 2016;26:88.

Kallidonis P, Kalogeropoulou C, Kyriazis I, et al. Percutaneous nephrolithotomy puncture and tract dilation: evidence on the safety of approaches to the infundibulum of the middle renal calyx. Urology 2017a;107:43.

Kallidonis P, Kyriazis I, Kotsiris D, et al. Papillary versus nonpapillary puncture in percutaneous nephrolithotomy: a prospective randomized trial. J Endourol. 2017b;31:S4.

Kerbl K, Picus DD, Clayman RV. Clinical experience with the Kaye nephrostomy tamponade catheter. Eur Urol. 1994;25:94.

Kessaris DN, Bellman GC, Pardalidis NP, et al. Management of hemorrhage after percutaneous renal surgery. J Urol. 1995;153:604.

Knoll T, Daels F, Desai J, et al. Percutaneous nephrolithotomy: technique. World J Urol. 2017;35:1361.

Kondás J, Szentgyörgyi E, Váczi L, et al. Splenic injury: a rare complication of percutaneous nephrolithotomy. Int Urol Nephrol. 1994;26:399.

Koras O, Bozkurt IH, Yonguc T, et al. Risk factors for postoperative infectious complications following percutaneous nephrolithotomy: a prospective clinical study. Urolithiasis. 2015;43:55.

Kreydin EI, Eisner BH. Risk factors for sepsis after percutaneous renal stone surgery. Nat Rev Urol. 2013;10:598.

Kukreja RA, Desai MR, Sabnis RB, et al. Fluid absorption during percutaneous nephrolithotomy: does it matter? J Endourol. 2002;16:221.

Kukreja R, Desai M, Patel S, et al. Factors affecting blood loss during percutaneous nephrolithotomy: prospective study. J Endourol. 2004;18:715.

Kumar S, Gautam S, Rai A. Chronic empyema thoracis after percutaneous nephrolithotomy. BMJ Case Rep. 2014;2014.

Kurien A, Baishya R, Mishra S, et al. The impact of percutaneous nephrolithotomy in patients with chronic kidney disease. J Endourol. 2009;23:1403.

Lallas CD, Delvecchio FC, Evans BR, et al. Management of nephropleural fistula after supracostal percutaneous nephrolithotomy. Urology. 2004;64:241.

Lam HS, Lingeman JE, Mosbaugh PG, et al. Evolution of the technique of combination therapy for staghorn calculi: a decreasing role for extracorporeal shock wave lithotripsy. J Urol. 1992;148:1058.

Lang EK. Percutaneous nephrostolithotomy and lithotripsy: a multi-institutional survey of complications. Radiology. 1987;162:25.

Leavitt DA, Theckumparampil N, Moreira DM, et al. Continuing aspirin therapy during percutaneous nephrolithotomy: unsafe or under-utilized? J Endourol. 2014;28:1399.

Lechevallier E, Siles S, Ortega JC, et al. Comparison by SPECT of renal scars after extracorporeal shock wave lithotripsy and percutaneous nephrolithotomy. J Endourol. 1993;7:465.

Lee KL, Stoller ML. Minimizing and managing bleeding after percutaneous nephrolithotomy. Curr Opin Urol. 2007;17:120.

Lee WJ, Smith AD, Cubelli V, et al. Complications of percutaneous nephrolithotomy. AJR Am J Roentgenol. 1987;148:177.

Lee MJ, Kim JK, Tang J, et al. The efficacy and safety of tranexamic acid in the management of perioperative bleeding after percutaneous nephrolithotomy: a systematic review and meta-analysis of comparative studies. J Endourol. 2022;36:303.

LeRoy AJ, Williams HJ, Bender CE, et al. Colon perforation following percutaneous nephrostomy and renal calculus removal. Radiology. 1985;155:83.

Liatsikos EN, Kapoor R, Lee B, et al. "Angular percutaneous renal access". Multiple tracts through a single incision for staghorn calculous treatment in a single session. Eur Urol. 2005;48:832.

Liu L, Zheng S, Xu Y, et al. Systematic review and meta-analysis of percutaneous nephrolithotomy for patients in the supine versus prone position. J Endourol. 2010;24:1941.

Lojanapiwat B, Prasopsuk S. Upper-pole access for percutaneous nephrolithotomy: comparison of supracostal and infracostal approaches. J Endourol. 2006;20:491.

Mahaffey KG, Bolton DM, Stoller ML. Urologist directed percutaneous nephrostomy tube placement. J Urol. 1994;152:1973.

Maheshwari PN, Mane DA, Pathak AB. Management of pleural injury after percutaneous renal surgery. J Endourol. 2009;23:1769.

Margel D, Ehrlich Y, Brown N, et al. Clinical implication of routine stone culture in percutaneous nephrolithotomy—a prospective study. Urology. 2006;67:26.

Mariappan P, Smith G, Moussa SA, et al. One week of ciprofloxacin before percutaneous nephrolithotomy significantly reduces upper tract infection and urosepsis: a prospective controlled study. BJU Int. 2006;98:1075.

Matlaga BR, Shah OD, Zagoria RJ, et al. Computerized tomography guided access for percutaneous nephrostolithotomy. J Urol. 2003;170:45.

Mavili E, Dönmez H, Özcan N, et al. Transarterial embolization for renal arterial bleeding. Diagnostic and Interventional Radiology (Ankara, Turkey), 2009;15:143.

Meretyk S, Albala DM, Clayman RV, et al. Endoureterotomy for treatment of ureteral strictures. J Urol. 1992;147:1502.

Michel MS, Trojan L, Rassweiler JJ. Complications in percutaneous nephrolithotomy {a figure is presented}. Eur Urol. 2007;51:899.

Mousavi-Bahar SH, Mehrabi S, Moslemi MK. Percutaneous nephrolithotomy complications in 671 consecutive patients: a single-center experience. Urol J. 2011;8:271.

Mukherjee S, Sinha RK, Jindal T, et al. Short-term alteration of renal function and electrolytes after percutaneous nephrolithotomy. Urol J. 2019;16:530.

Munver R, Delvecchio FC, Newman GE, et al. Critical analysis of supracostal access for percutaneous renal surgery. J Urol. 2001;166:1242.

Noor Buchholz NP. Colon perforation after percutaneous nephrolithotomy revisited. Urol Int. 2004;72:88.

Nouira Y, Nouira K, Kallel Y, et al. Colonic perforation complicating percutaneous nephrolithotomy. Surg Laparosc Endosc Percutan Tech. 2006;16:47.

Ogan K, Corwin TS, Smith T, et al. Sensitivity of chest fluoroscopy compared with chest CT and chest radiography for diagnosing hydropneumothorax in association with percutaneous nephrostolithotomy. Urology. 2003;62:988.

Otto BJ, Terry RS, Lutfi FG, et al. The effect of continued low dose aspirin therapy in patients undergoing percutaneous nephrolithotomy. J Urol. 2018;199:748.

Öztürk H. Gastrointestinal system complications in percutaneous nephrolithotomy: a systematic review. J Endourol. 2014;28:1256.

Öztürk H. Treatment of colonic injury during percutaneous nephrolithotomy. Rev Urol. 2015;17:194.

Parsons JK, Jarrett TW, Lancini V, et al. Infundibular stenosis after percutaneous nephrolithotomy. J Urol. 2002;167:35.

Pearle MS. Puncture for percutaneous surgery: is the papillary puncture a dogma? No! Curr Opin Urol. 2019;29:472.

Perrella R, Vicentini FC, Paro ED, et al. Supine versus prone percutaneous nephrolithotomy for complex stones: a multicenter randomized controlled trial. J Urol. 2022;207:647.

Poudyal S. Current insights on haemorrhagic complications in percutaneous nephrolithotomy. Asian J Urol. 2022;9:81.

Prasad S, Sharma G, Devana SK, et al. Is tranexamic acid associated with decreased need for blood transfusion in percutaneous nephrolithotomy: a systematic review and meta-analysis. Ann R Coll Surg Engl. 2023;105:99.

Qin P, Zhang D, Huang T, et al. Comparison of mini percutaneous nephrolithotomy and standard percutaneous nephrolithotomy for renal stones > 2 cm: a systematic review and meta-analysis. Int Braz J Urol. 2022;48:637.

Rao PN, Dube DA, Weightman NC, et al. Prediction of septicemia following endourological manipulation for stones in the upper urinary tract. J Urol. 1991;146:955.

Reeves T, Pietropaolo A, Gadzhiev N, et al. Role of endourological procedures (PCNL and URS) on renal function: a systematic review. Curr Urol Rep. 2020;21.

Richstone L, Reggio E, Ost MC, et al. First prize (tie): hemorrhage following percutaneous renal surgery: characterization of angiographic findings. J Endourol. 2008;22:1129.

Roberts S, Bolton DM, Stoller ML. Hypothermia associated with percutaneous nephrolithotomy. Urology. 1994;44:832.

Roberts WW, Cadeddu JA, Micali S, et al. Ureteral stricture formation after removal of impacted calculi. J Urol. 1998;159:723.

Roth RA, Beckmann CF. Complications of extracorporeal shock-wave lithotripsy and percutaneous nephrolithotomy. Urol Clin North Am. 1988;15:155.

Saad KS, Hanno A, El-Nahas AR. Injury of the ileum during percutaneous nephrolithotomy in a pediatric patient. Can Urol Assoc J. 2014;8:E204.

Segura JW, Patterson DE, LeRoy AJ, et al. Percutaneous removal of kidney stones: review of 1,000 cases. J Urol. 1985;134:1077.

Seitz C, Desai M, Häcker A, et al. Incidence, prevention, and management of complications following percutaneous nephrolitholapaxy. Eur Urol. 2012;61:146.

Seitz C. S2k-Leitlinie zur Diagnostik, Therapie und Metaphylaxe der Urolithiasis.

Srivastava A, Singh KJ, Suri A, et al. Vascular complications after percutaneous nephrolithotomy: are there any predictive factors? Urology. 2005;66:38.

Stoller ML, Wolf JS, St Lezin MA. Estimated blood loss and transfusion rates associated with percutaneous nephrolithotomy. J Urol. 1994;152:1977.

Sur RL, Krambeck AE, Large T, et al. A randomized controlled trial of preoperative prophylactic antibiotics for percutaneous nephrolithotomy in moderate to high infectious risk population: a report from the EDGE consortium. J Urol. 2021;205:1379.

Taylor E, Miller J, Chi T, et al. Complications associated with percutaneous nephrolithotomy. Transl Androl Urol. 2012;1:223.

Tefekli A, Altunrende F, Tepeler K, et al. Tubeless percutaneous nephrolithotomy in selected patients: a prospective randomized comparison. Int Urol Nephrol. 2007;39:57.

Tekgul ZT, Pektas S, Yildirim U, et al. A prospective randomized double-blind study on the effects of the temperature of irrigation solutions on thermoregulation and postoperative complications in percutaneous nephrolithotomy. J Anesth. 2015;29:165.

Traxer O. Management of injury to the bowel during percutaneous stone removal. J Endourol. 2009;23:1777.

Türk C, Petřík A, Sarica K, et al. EAU guidelines on interventional treatment for urolithiasis. Eur Urol. 2016;69:475.

Turna B, Nazli O, Demiryoguran S, et al. Percutaneous nephrolithotomy: variables that influence hemorrhage. Urology. 2007;69:603.

Vallancien G, Capdeville R, Veillon B, et al. Colonic perforation during percutaneous nephrolithotomy. J Urol. 1985;134:1185.

Walsh RM, Kelly CR, Gupta M. Percutaneous renal surgery: use of flexible nephroscopy and treatment of infundibular stenoses. https://home.liebertpub.com/end. 2009;23:1679.

Walton-Diaz A, Vinay JI, Barahona J, et al. Concordance of renal stone culture: PMUC, RPUC, RSC and post-PCNL sepsis-a non-randomized prospective observation cohort study. Int Urol Nephrol. 2017;49:31.

Wan C, Wang D, Xiang J, et al. Comparison of postoperative outcomes of mini percutaneous nephrolithotomy and standard percutaneous nephrolithotomy: a meta-analysis. Urolithiasis. 2022;50:523.

Wollin DA, Joyce AD, Gupta M, et al. Antibiotic use and the prevention and management of infectious complications in stone disease. World J Urol. 2017;35:1369.

Wollin DA, Preminger GM. Percutaneous nephrolithotomy: complications and how to deal with them. Urolithiasis 2017;46:1, 46:87, 2017.

Wu P, Wang L, Wang K. Supine versus prone position in percutaneous nephrolithotomy for kidney calculi: a meta-analysis. Int Urol Nephrol. 2011;43:67.

Yamaguchi A, Skolarikos A, Buchholz NP, et al. Operating times and bleeding complications in percutaneous nephrolithotomy: a comparison of tract dilation methods in 5537 patients in the clinical research office of the endourological society percutaneous nephrolithotomy global study. J Endourol. 2011;25:933.

Yang BB, Liu WZ, Ying JP, et al. Computed tomography angiography and three-dimensional reconstruction of renal arteries in diagnosing the bleedings after mini-percutaneous nephrolithotomy: a single-center experience of 7 years. Urology. 2022;169:47.

Yaycioglu O, Egilmez T, Gul U, et al. Percutaneous nephrolithotomy in patients with normal versus impaired renal function. Urol Res. 2007;35:101.

Zhang X, Xia L, Xu T, et al. Is the supine position superior to the prone position for percutaneous nephrolithotomy (PCNL)? Urolithiasis. 2014;42:87.

Zhao Y, Shen B, Zhong B, et al. Renal artery computed tomography angiography for the application of severe bleeding after PCNL. Zhonghua Yi Xue Za Zhi. 2014;94:2687.

Intra-renal Pressure

Eric Riedinger, Palle Jörn Sloth Osther, and Bodo Knudsen

Abstract Pressure generation via instillation of irrigation during percutaneous nephrolithotomy is necessary for procedural safety and efficacy; termed intra-renal pressure (IRP). As iatrogenic pressures rise above physiologic levels intra-renal reflux, or fluid transposition outside of the collecting system, can occur. This shift of fluid and endotoxins, if present, has implications on post-operative pain/recovery, infectious and inflammatory responses, and systemic fluid/electrolyte imbalances. Numerous *ex vivo* human and *in vivo* animal studies have evaluated pressure thresholds for the three subtypes of intrarenal reflux: pyelovenous backflow, pyelosinuous backflow and intra-renal backflow. Knowledge and mitigation of procedural factors that lead to pressure rise during PCNL allows Urologists to minimize complications associated with elevated IRP.

Keywords Intra-renal pressure · Renal pelvic pressure · Percutaneous nephrolithotomy · Intra-renal reflux · Pyelorenal backflow

1 Introduction

Endoscopic management of upper tract urologic pathologies, including nephrolithiasis, urothelial carcinoma, and ureteral strictures, through percutaneous access is dependent upon the generation of pressure within the collecting system. Pressure generation, through the instillation of irrigation, allows for distension of the urinary tract which creates appropriate working space, enhances visualization, and controls

E. Riedinger (✉) · B. Knudsen
Department of Urology, The Ohio State University Medical Center, 915 Olentangy River Road, Suite 3100, Columbus, OH 43215, USA
e-mail: ried23@osumc.edu

B. Knudsen
e-mail: bodo.knudsen@osumc.edu

P. J. S. Osther
Department of Urology, University of Southern Denmark, Vejle, Denmark
e-mail: Palle.Joern.Osther@rsyd.dk

© The Author(s), under exclusive license to Springer Nature Switzerland AG 2023
J. D. Denstedt and E. N. Liatsikos (eds.), *Percutaneous Renal Surgery*,
https://doi.org/10.1007/978-3-031-40542-6_29

"""

temperature when energy sources are utilized (Alsyouf et al. 2018; Yap et al. 2022). In essence, the generation of intra-renal pressure (IRP) during endoscopic urologic cases is integral for safety and efficacy. While appropriate IRP is necessary, a balance must be maintained to minimize risks associated with supra-physiologic renal pressures. A thorough understanding of renal physiology and factors that contribute to iatrogenic renal pelvic pressure is necessary for urologists to maintain procedural safety.

2 Background

The study of IRP, otherwise known as renal pelvic pressure (RPP), dates to the 1900's. Hinman et al. performed canine studies to define the association between elevated IRP on retrograde pyelography with intra-renal reflux, or the transposition of fluid outside of the collecting system (Hinman and Lee-Brown 1924). While this pre-dated the introduction of percutaneous nephrostomy procedures by Fernström and Johansson in 1976 and the multi-channel Storz rigid ureteroscope in 1980, it highlighted the underlying concerns associated with elevated iatrogenic renal pressures (Whitehurst and Somani 2018; Patel and Nakada 2015). Additionally, it sparked further evaluation of renal pressure in the setting of pathologic conditions in the urinary tract. In the 1960s, Whitaker developed an experiment to differentiate non-obstructive vs obstructive dilation of the renal collecting system utilizing renal pelvic pressure measurements (Johnston and Porter 2014). He theorized that obstructed renal units would have higher pressures at a constant flow. The test was conducted with antegrade access to the renal collecting system to allow for irrigant instillation at a controlled rate. Results demonstrated that non-obstructive kidneys maintained an IRP of <25 cm of water (cm H_2O) and a relative pressure of less than 15 cm H_2O (Johnston and Porter 2014). The application of this test mimics pressure generation during percutaneous nephrolithotomy today. Instillation of irrigant through percutaneous instruments generates pressure within the collecting system and this is offset by the ability of the irrigant to leave the system. Much in the same way that ureteral obstruction caused higher renal pressures during the Whitaker test, procedural factors that impede the ability of fluid to efflux will result in a similar rise in IRP.

3 Measurement of IRP

The measurement of IRP typically involves placement of an open-ended catheter into the renal pelvis either via a percutaneous or retrograde ureteral route. Historically, these catheters were connected to external manometers, which measure pressure through displacement of liquids such as mercury or water. The measurements were indirectly related to the density of the fluid (Saltzman et al. 1987). As a result, the units reported for IRP recordings are commonly in millimeters of mercury (mm Hg)

Fig. 1 (©Abbott): Pressure
sensing wire

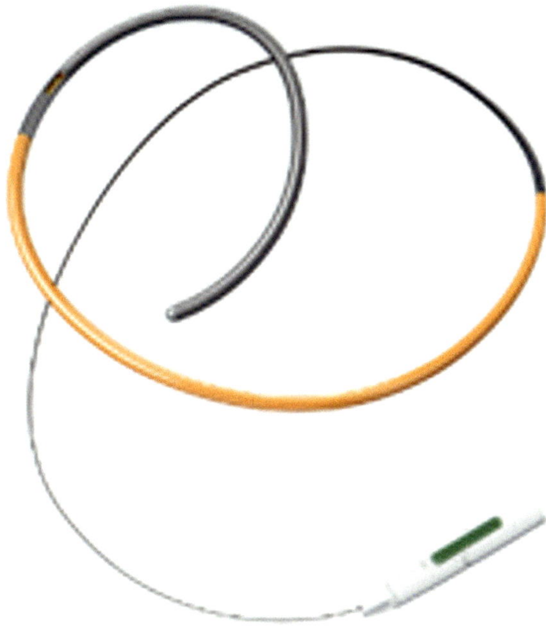

and centimeters of water (cm H_2O). The conversion rate between these units is 1 cm H_2O = 0.736 mm Hg (Croghan et al. 2022). For this chapter, all pressures reported in the literature have been converted to cm H_2O to allow for comparison of the study results.

As technology has advanced, pressure transducers have replaced traditional manometers. These devices convert pressure to an electrical signal which allows for extrinsic pressure display and monitoring (Deng et al. 2019; Wilson and Glenn 1990). Integration of pressure transducers into commonly used urologic devices such as guidewires (See Fig. 1) (PressureWire™ X Guidewire, Abbott, St. Paul, MN, USA) and percutaneous renal sheaths represent the latest development in IRP monitoring (Doizi et al. 2021a; Yang et al. 2016; Sierra et al. 2022). This integration makes continuous intra-operative pressure measurement feasible and has the potential to enable urologists to mitigate IRP rise during endoscopic surgeries in real-time.

4   Physiologic IRP

As highlighted by the Whitaker test, renal pelvic pressure will vary depending on intrinsic factors and pathologic conditions of the urinary tract (Johnston and Porter 2014). Physiologic renal pressures range from 0–15 cm H_2O in a non-obstructed system (Tokas et al. 2019a; Dean and Krambeck 2023; Walzak and Paquin 1961;

Jung and Osther 2015). High urine production and flow, such as during diuresis, can increase renal pressures upwards of 27.2 cm H_2O (Tokas et al. 2019a). Conditions resulting in obstruction will lead to further elevation, with the IRP in chronic renal obstruction reported as high as 68–69.52 cm H_2O (Tokas et al. 2019a; Walzak and Paquin 1961). The wide range of pressures within the urinary tract is explained by the physiology of urine propagation and fluid dynamics within the collecting system (Osther et al. 2016).

The propagation of urine under physiologic conditions requires the generation of both intra-renal and ureteral pressure. Calyceal, renal pelvic, and proximal ureteral contractions occur spontaneously and in a coordinated fashion by pacemaker cells (Hannappel et al. 1982). The coordination of signaling from the calyces to the pelvis and finally the ureter leads to a ureteral peristaltic contraction that occurs two to six times per minute. This intermittent contraction allows for the propagation of a discrete urine bolus down to the bladder (Hannappel et al. 1982).

Prior to this understanding of peristalsis, the flow of urine from the kidney to the bladder was thought to be dependent upon gravity (Jung et al. 2006). In this model, the flow of urine would be explained best by Poiseuille's law, which describes laminar flow of fluid along a rigid pipe: $V = \pi pr^4/8\ nl$. Where V is the flow rate, p is the pressure gradient between the two ends of a pipe (relative pressure), r is the radius of the pipe, l is the length of the pipe and n is the viscosity of the fluid (Pfitzner 1976). This implies that pressure within the urinary tract is directly related to the flow rate of urine. While this relationship between flow and pressure is apparent given the rise in IRP seen during diuresis; the relationship is not directly linear due to the compressible nature of the collecting system.

A better explanation of the flow to pressure relationship is explained by a porcine study that evaluated IRPs at varying flow rates, 0–20 mL/min (Mortensen and Djurhuus 1985). Four separate phases of fluid propagation down the ureter were identified depending on flow rate. During *phase 1*, with a flow rate of 0–4 mL/min, urine is transported as an isolated bolus from peristaltic contractions. The ureteropelvic junction remaining closed protects the renal pelvis from elevated pressures generated by the ureter and subsequently, IRP remains low even as flow increases. In *phase 2*, with a flow rate of 4–6 mL/min, there is a significant rise in IRP due to inhibition of passive filling of the ureter by the proximal peristaltic contraction. This leads to renal pelvic distension and thus IRP elevation. In *phase 3*, with a flow of 6 mL/min, the incremental rise in IRP decreases as urine flow passes between peristaltic contractions; outflow is continuous. Lastly, *phase 4* occurs when flow rises above 6 mL/min, the ureter functions as an open tube and there is a linear relationship between pressure and flow. At these high flow rates, the ureter functions much in the same way as Poiseuille's law describes (Jung et al. 2006; Mortensen and Djurhuus 1985).

While peristaltic contractions and the relative pressure from the renal pelvis to the bladder are primary drivers for urine propagation, Poiseuille's equation does not account for the impact of extrinsic compression on the collapsible ureter (Tokas et al. 2019a). As pressure is applied to the ureter extrinsically, increasing intrarenal or intra-ureteral pressures will be required to distend the urinary tract and allow for the flow of urine. This concept is explained by transmural pressure which is defined by the Laplace equation ($\Delta P = \gamma/r$). Transmural pressure (ΔP) is the tension per unit length where γ is the surface tension and r the radius of the cylinder. It reflects the pressure gradient across the ureteral wall, a balance of internal vs external forces. Tension within the urinary tract and radius of the ureter are impacted by inherent qualities specific to an individual including wall thickness, wall elasticity, and compliance (Satish et al. 2022). These factors affect resistance to extrinsic pressure and will determine the degree of pressure rise as the system distends. In an unobstructed system, the initial pressure rise will remain low during filling reflecting the compliance of the urinary tract (Tokas et al. 2019a). Chronic ureteral obstruction disrupts these subtle coordinating mechanisms that seem to be modulated by various receptors, including α-adrenergic, β-adrenergic, and parasympathetic receptors (Osther et al. 2016).

5   IRP in Percutaneous Nephrolithotomy

To evaluate the literature regarding iatrogenic intra-renal pressures during percutaneous nephrolithotomy, an understanding of procedural nomenclature and indications is required. The American Urologic Association recommends percutaneous nephrolithotomy (PCNL) as a first-line procedural intervention for total renal stone burdens above 2 cm and for lower pole renal stone burdens above 1 cm (Assimos et al. 2016). Additional indications can include aberrant or surgically altered urinary tracts (i.e., urinary diversions). PCNL allows for direct entry into the collecting system with a working sheath and larger instruments compared to retrograde renal surgery. This results in higher stone clearance, shorter procedural time, and decreased need for repeat intervention for larger renal stone burdens compared to retrograde intra-renal surgeries. Secondary to access for the procedure, PCNL carries risks of bleeding and injury to surrounding organs (Ganpule et al. 2016). Additionally, post-operative recovery can be more challenging for patients. The complications associated with PCNL have prompted innovation with the development of smaller renal access sheaths and operating scopes to reduce post-operative bleeding, pain, and hospital length of stay while still maintaining efficacy (Desai et al. 2011; Wright et al. 2016; Gui et al. 2022). This miniaturization has implications for elevated iatrogenic IRPs.

Percutaneous surgical interventions can be broken down into four categories depending on the size of the renal access sheath utilized. While no universal definition exists, Wright et al. standardized the nomenclature based on the size of the working renal sheath (Wright et al. 2016). Standard percutaneous nephrolithotomy: renal sheath 24 to 30 french (F). Mini percutaneous nephrolithotomy (mPCNL): renal sheath 14 to 20F. Ultra mini percutaneous nephrolithotomy (umPCNL): renal sheath 11 to 13F. Micro percutaneous nephrolithotomy (microPCNL): 4.85F renal sheath. An important distinction exists with microPCNL compared to the other three procedures with regard to renal pressure development: the smaller access sheath utilized in microPCNL does not permit placement of a nephroscope or ureteroscope into the

Table 1 Renal pressures for *in vivo*, human studies

Procedure	Average IRP	Maximum IRP
sPCNL (Alsyouf et al. 2018; Saltzman et al. 1987; Croghan 2022; Tokas et al. 2019a; Troxel and Low 2002; Tepeler et al. 2014; Wu et al. 2017)	6.5–41.21 cm H_2O	80 cm H_2O
mPCNL (Guohua et al. 2007, Zhong et al. 2008, Jung et al. 2022)	7.9–33.8 cm H_2O	> 40.8 cm H_2O
umPCNL (Shah et al. 2015)	5–10 cm H_2O	10 cm H_2O
microPCNL (Tepeler 2014)	41.2 cm H_2O	51.1 cm H_2O

collecting system. Instead, the 4.85F sheath is connected to a three-way adapter that allows for the placement of an optical fiber, laser, and irrigation inflow (Desai and Mishra 2012). This configuration limits passive drainage of irrigation from the renal working sheath that is common in sPCNL, mPCNL, and umPCNL.

As numerous factors determine iatrogenic pressures during percutaneous nephrolithotomy, IRPs exist over a wide range in the literature. Additionally, there are a limited number of *in vivo* human studies evaluating IRPs in umPCNL and microPCNL. As such, reported renal pressures, specifically in these two procedures, may not reflect the true ranges that develop clinically. Listed below are the average and maximum IRPs in *in vivo* human studies without the use of active irrigant evacuation (Table 1).

6 Implications of Elevated IRP

As previously noted, Hinman et al. demonstrated the relationship between pressure and intra-renal reflux (Hinman and Lee-Brown 1924). As pressure was increased in the collecting system via retrograde instillation of dyed irrigation, dye could be seen traversing the urothelium and entering the vascular system. This process of fluid leaving the collecting system is termed pyelorenal backflow. Subsequent studies further delineated the types of pyelorenal backflow based on the system the renal pelvic fluid/urine entered. Pyelovenous backflow refers to fluid entering the renal venous system. Pyelosinuous backflow refers to the shifting of fluid from the collecting system to the peri-pelvic sinus tissue. Lastly, intra-renal backflow refers to fluid shifting into the collecting ducts, tubules, or the renal interstitium (Tokas et al. 2019a).

7   Pyelovenous Backflow

Pyelovenous backflow has been analyzed in numerous *in vivo* animal studies and *ex vivo* human and animal renal units. In Hinman's canine model, the pyelovenous threshold was noted with IRPs of 40.77–47.57 cm H_2O (Hinman and Lee-Brown 1924). In 1988, Stenberg et al. performed an *in vivo* study within a rat model. Pyelovenous flow was noted with an intra-renal pressure as low as 13.59–27.18 cm H_2O (Stenberg et al. 1988). Within a human urinary tract, Boccafoscshi et al. performed retrograde instillation of dye diluted in saline in cadaveric and fresh human renal units (Boccafoschi and Lugnani 1985). Pyelovenous backflow began near 40 cm H_2O. However, with the simulation of arterial pressure, the threshold for pyelovenous backflow increased to 60 cm H_2O suggesting that renal blood flow may be protective.

8   Pyelosinuous Backflow

Pyelosinuous backflow occurs when a defect within the collecting system allows urine or irrigation to escape into the peri-pelvic space. This fluid is then able to be absorbed into systemic circulation. The most common site of extravasation occurs at a calyceal fornix, as this represents a weak point within the system. Lee et al. performed an *in vivo* porcine study to evaluate a pressure threshold for parenchymal injury. Instillation of irrigant via a ureteroscope resulted in forniceal rupture when IRP rose above 185 mm Hg (Lee et al. 2022). Thomsen et al. performed a similar study in an *in vivo* rabbit model (Thomsen et al. 1981). Forniceal rupture occurred within the urinary tract when pressures reached 81.6–95 cm H_2O. IRP cutoffs for forniceal rupture within the human urinary tract are not well established.

9   Intra-Renal Backflow

Intra-renal backflow, also termed pyelotubular and pyelointerstitial reflux, describes the phenomenon of the collecting system fluid entering the renal parenchyma (Tokas et al. 2019a). Within an *ex vivo*, human study of renal units, retrograde instillation of dye generated intra-renal backflow when IRP was as low as 15 cm H_2O (Boccafoschi and Lugnani 1985). With simulated renal blood flow, the intra-renal backflow threshold increased to an IRP of 40 cm H_2O. Like pyelovenous backflow, vascular pressure appears protective against pyelotubular reflux. *Ex vivo* porcine models demonstrate similar IRP pressure cutoffs for intra-renal backflow, in the 40.77–47.57 cm H_2O range (Thomsen et al. 1982; Thomsen and Larsen 1983).

The correlation between elevation of IRP and degree of intra-renal backflow is seen in both *ex vivo* human and animal studies (Boccafoschi and Lugnani 1985;

Thomsen et al. 1982). Loftus et al. simulated flexible ureteroscopy by retrograde instillation of dyed irrigation into porcine renal units at increasing pressures (Loftus et al. 2021). Renal units were then harvested and analyzed microscopically. At 68 cm H_2O of irrigation pressure, pyelotubular reflux reached 33.1% of the distance from the collecting system to the capsule. Increasing irrigation pressure to 272 cm H_2O resulted in irrigant traveling 99.3% of the way to the capsule. In addition to the depth of penetration, raising IRP also increases the frequency of intra-renal backflow. In an *ex vivo*, porcine urinary tract experiment performed by Thomsen et al. renal units subjected to low IRP (defined as less than 41–48 cm H_2O) were compared to those subjected to high IRPs (95–102 cm H_2O). Intra-renal backflow was seen in 33% of renal units exposed to the lower IRPs compared to 100% of the units exposed to the high IRPs (Thomsen et al. 1982). Using Gadolinium-enhanced MRI, intra-renal backflow was evaluated dynamically in an *in vivo* porcine model by Lildal et al. (2023). Retrograde instillation of gadolinium solution demonstrated that intra-renal backflow was dependent on both IRP and time. Visual backflow was demonstrated at pressures as low as 22 cm H_2O, which is considerably lower than previously assumed. Real-time MRI demonstrated backflow of Gadolinium into the renal cortex in all cases, with a mean intra-renal pressure of 58 cm H_2O and mean duration of irrigation at 70 min. On average, 66% of the renal cortex was involved. Thus, it seems that intrarenal backflow occurs as a continuous function of IRP increases rather than at a specific threshold. Furthermore, morphology of the renal papillae may affect intra-renal backflow. It has been shown that intra-renal backflow occurs at considerably lower levels of IRP in compound papillae (Ransley and Risdon 1979; Coulthard et al. 2002).

10 Pressure Injury

The application of elevated renal pressure to the collecting system is transmitted to the renal parenchyma and can impact renal architecture and function. This concept is well known in the setting of acute and chronic ureteral obstruction. Following complete occlusion of a ureter there is a rise of IRP. After an initial increase in renal blood flow (RBF), RBF decreases with a resultant drop in the glomerular filtration rate for the unit. Over time, chronic occlusion results in permanent loss of renal function and atrophy of the kidney (Wahlberg et al. 1984). With acute rises of IRP during endoscopic procedures, renal blood flow and renal architecture are similarly affected. In an *ex vivo*, porcine urinary tract Thomsen et al. found that exposing renal units to higher IRPs lead to a decrease in renal blood flow (Thomsen et al. 1982). Renal units subjected to low IRPs (41–48 cm H_2O) had a 16% reduction in RBF which further decreased to 57% in units exposed to high IRP (95–102 cm H_2O). This reduction of blood flow causes ischemia and can lead to renal tubular injury. Injury can occur when renal units are exposed to IRPs as low 20 cm H_2O for less than an hour (Fung and Atala 1998). Furthermore, the degree of injury directly correlates to blood flow reduction and degree of IRP elevation.

Histologic analysis of porcine renal units following *in vivo* simulated ureteroscopy at low vs high IRPs (122 vs 204 cm H_2O) demonstrates changes to normal renal architecture (Schwalb et al. 1993). In acutely harvested porcine urinary tracts, diffuse urothelial denudation and renal parenchymal submucosal edema was noted in the high IRP group. With delayed harvesting of renal units, 4–6 weeks after the procedure, 71% of specimens exposed to high IRP demonstrated focal parenchymal scarring compared to 0% in the low IRP subgroup.

While these studies demonstrate the potential impacts on RBF and imply that pressure can result in acute/chronic parenchymal injury, the data is mixed. In a separate *in vivo*, porcine urinary tract study simulating flexible ureteroscopy, Lee et al. exposed the renal unit to sustained IRP of 68, 136 and 204 cm H_2O. Following the simulated procedure, the pigs were euthanized, and the renal units analyzed microscopically. No histologic changes were noted in the study (Lee et al. 2022).

11 Clinical Pearls

In summary, elevated IRP has implications on fluid shift from within the urinary tract to surrounding systems (See Fig. 2). Additionally, increasing pressure applied to the renal parenchyma impacts renal blood flow which leads to transient ischemia and can cause parenchymal injury. Extrapolation of this information from *ex vivo* human and *in vivo* animal studies to clinical practice implies that if IRP is left uncontrolled during PCNL, it could lead to complications for patients. While the absolute cutoff for pyelorenal backflow during endoscopic procedures is unknown, inferring from the studies mentioned above, maintaining IRPs < 40 cm H_2O (30 mm Hg) is prudent to avoid potential complications (Tokas et al. 2019a; Dean and Krambeck 2023). Since patients with abnormal papillary morphology (compound papillae, medullary sponge kidney) may experience intra-renal backflow at lower pressures, such findings during endoscopy should give rise to extra vigilance regarding pressure increases during the procedure.

12 Clinical Manifestations of Elevated IRP

Intra-renal reflux allows for contents of the collecting system to enter systemic circulation. The clinical manifestations of this process can include increased fluid absorption, electrolyte disturbances, inflammatory reactions to endotoxins and the development of sepsis (Croghan 2022; Dean and Krambeck 2023; Tokas et al. 2019b). Additionally, increasing pressure applied to the urothelium and renal parenchyma can infer a pain response that impacts post-operative recovery (Alsyouf et al. 2018; Travaglini et al. 2004; Guo et al. 2008).

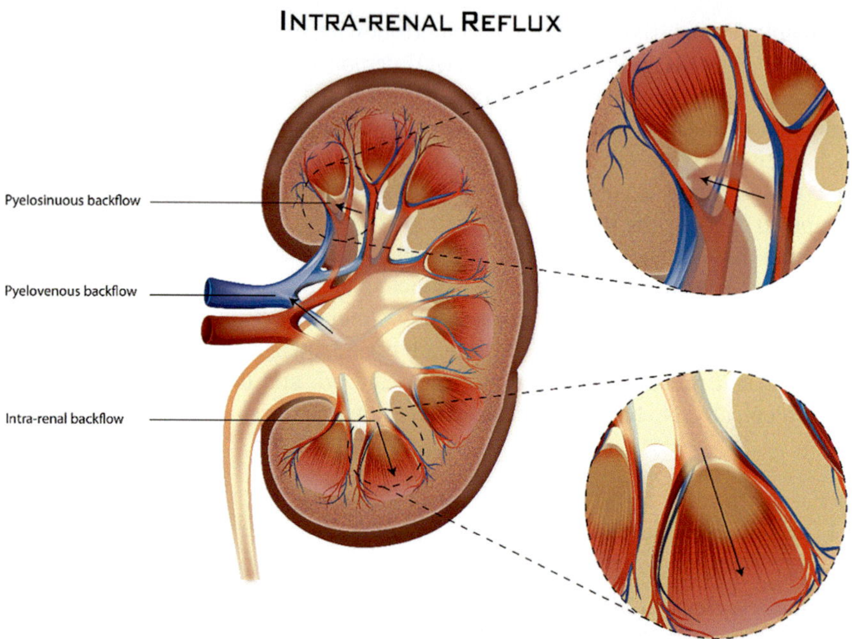

Fig. 2 Elevation of IRP allows irrigant to transit outside the collecting system into systemic venous circulation, peri-renal space, and the renal parenchyma

13 Fluid Absorption

Fluid absorption during percutaneous nephrolithotomy occurs via a multitude of pathways including exposed vessels, leakage of irrigant into the retroperitoneal space, and via intra-renal reflux (Ganpule et al. 2016; Kukreja et al. 2002). It can cause electrolyte disturbances, fluid overload, and cardiopulmonary distress in rare instances. The fluid absorption for sPCNL ranges widely; values between 13–1,916 mL have been reported (Kukreja et al. 2002; Malhotra et al. 2001; Guzelburc et al. 2016). There are a multitude of factors that will determine the amount of irrigant absorbed including duration of the procedure, amount of irrigation utilized, blood loss and perforation of the collecting system. Intra-renal pressure during surgery is also a driver. Kukreja et al. performed an *in vivo* sPCNL experiment evaluating systemic fluid absorption in low vs high pressured systems (Kukreja et al. 2002). Standard PCNL in the lower pressure system, performed with a working renal sheath, resulted in less systemic fluid absorption. The impact of elevated renal pressures was most notable when large volumes of irrigant were utilized, above 9 L, with the average fluid absorption in high pressure system vs low pressure system: 302 vs 205 mL.

14 Inflammatory/Infectious Response

Intrarenal reflux allows for endotoxins and bacteria, if present, to enter systemic circulation (Loftus et al. 2018). Clinically, this could result in the development of post-operative fever, systemic inflammatory response (SIRS), or sepsis. An *in vivo*, porcine study evaluating standard vs mini PCNL in an infected system demonstrates this concept (Loftus et al. 2018). After instilling *E. coli* bacteria into the urinary tract, simulated standard or mini PCNL was performed with real time renal pelvic pressure monitoring. Blood cultures were taken during the procedure and after completion, tissue cultures were obtained. The mini-PCNL arm was found to have higher average renal pelvic pressures and longer time spent above the pyelovenous cutoff of 40 cm H_2O. This correlated with increased positive blood cultures and higher rates of bacterial seeding to distant organs in the mPCNL arm implying that elevated IRPs can drive bacteria into the bloodstream. While this study highlights an association of distal bacterial seeding and elevated renal pressures, limitations exist. The mini-PCNL arm of the study was simulated with a semi-rigid ureteroscope which is smaller in caliber compared to mini-nephroscopes. Additionally, the simulated procedure only involved advancements of the scope three centimeters in and out of the sheath and thus does not reflect typical manipulation performed during PCNL.

In vivo, human studies are conflicting on the association of elevated IRP to post-operative fever and systemic inflammatory response. Omar et al., performed an *in vivo* sPCNL study comparing low irrigation pressure, 109 cm H_2O, to high irrigation pressure, 272 cm H_2O; irrigation pressure will directly correlate to IRP (Omar et al. 2016). This study demonstrated significant difference in SIRS development in the high-pressure group compared to the low-pressure group, 46 vs 11%. Conversely, an *in vivo*, human study in patients undergoing standard PCNL found that a single IRP pressure above 40 cm H_2O did not correlate with post-operative fever (Troxel and Low 2002). Similarly in the mPCNL literature, an *in vivo*, human study by Guohua et al. comparing the impact of mini-PCNL sheath sizes (14, 16, 18 and double 16F) on IRP and postoperative fever found no difference in fever rates between the arms (Guohua et al. 2007). This is despite higher average renal pelvic pressures and time above the pyelovenous threshold in the 14F renal sheath arm.

The discrepancy between these studies may be attributed to how renal pelvic pressure is analyzed and measured. While the pyelovenous threshold of 40 cm H_2O is generally accepted, the clinical impact of surpassing that threshold depends on the degree and duration of elevation. As such, single pressures rising above intra-renal reflux thresholds for short durations are unlikely to be clinically meaningful. Zhong et al., performed an *in vivo* mPCNL study in a similar fashion to Guoha et al. but evaluated renal pelvic pressure and its impact on post operative fever independent of access sheath size (Zhong et al. 2008). Average RPP remained below 40 cm H_2O in all arms of the study, although mean IRP rose as tract size decreased. A single recording of RPP > 40 cm H_2O did not correlate to the development of post operative fever. However, mean renal pelvic pressure $\geq$ 27 cm H_2O, regardless of access sheath size, increased the risk for post-operative fever: 57% vs 14%. Additionally, patients with IRP $\geq$ 40 mm Hg for $\geq$ 50 s during the operation had a significant increased risk of post operative fever: 39% vs 9%. Another study comparing renal pelvic pressure and postoperative fever in sPCNL (24F) and mPCNL (18F), had similar findings (Wu et al. 2017). In the mPCNL and sPCNL arms, patients with an average RPP $\geq$ 27 cm H_2O were significantly more likely to develop fever: 35 vs 15% (mPCNL), 24% vs 8% (sPCNL). In the mPCNL arm, RPP $\geq$ 40 cm H_2O for 60 s or longer was associated with higher risk of fever. The conflicting data in the literature may also in part be related by the huge heterogeneity regarding papillary morphology and consequently the degree of intra-renal backflow at a given pressure, explaining why no studies have been able to directly correlate level of IRP to infectious complications.

15   Post-Operative Recovery

Elevation of renal pressure during PCNL has implications for post operative pain and recovery from surgery. Distension of the collecting system can cause stretching of nociceptive nerve endings (mechanosensitive receptors) located in the submucosa of the renal capsule, renal pelvis, and ureter (Travaglini et al. 2004). Similarly, endoscopic interventions, such as PCNL, will cause mechanical stretching of nociceptive nerve endings due to distension of the collecting system. *In vivo* human studies on patients undergoing PCNL have demonstrated a direct relation between IRP and postoperative pain (Pedersen et al. 2012). *In vivo*, human sPCNL and mPCNL studies have demonstrated that average procedural IRP of > 40 cm H_2O or increased duration above the 40 cm H_2O threshold are associated with increased post operative pain scores and longer length of hospital stays (Alsyouf et al. 2018; Guo et al. 2008; Lai et al. 2020).

16   Clinical Pearls

In vivo human studies have demonstrated an association between elevated IRP and post-surgical pain scores for patients undergoing PCNL. The literature highlights that a solitary or short duration rise in IRP above the pyelorenal backflow (40 cm H_2O) threshold is unlikely to be of clinical significance. However, as the duration spent above this threshold increases, so do the risks. Further studies are needed to establish desired cutoffs to avoid these complications, however minimizing duration of time spent above the pyelorenal backflow thresholds should be the goal.

17 Procedural Factors Influencing IRP

Iatrogenic intra-renal pressures during percutaneous nephrolithotomy are influenced by a variety of procedural factors. Broadly, this is broken down into impacts on irrigation inflow and irrigation outflow (Dean and Krambeck 2023). Inflow is driven by irrigating pressure primarily. Irrigation outflow is affected by five components of percutaneous renal surgery including renal access sheath specifications, nephroscope size, ureteral cannulation, bladder filling and utilization of suction devices for active evacuation. Modification of these variables during surgery enables Urologists to mitigate elevation of IRP.

18 Irrigation Pressure

Irrigation pressure is a primary driver of IRP during surgery. Modalities of delivery include gravity drainage, mechanical pumping, and manual pumping (Landman et al. 2002). Regardless of delivery method, as irrigation pressures increases so do intra-renal pressures when controlling for other procedural factors. Manual irrigation tends to create the highest IRPs for endoscopic surgeries due to variability in applied pressure by the user (Noureldin et al. 2019). For most percutaneous procedures gravity or mechanical irrigation is employed due to the desire for continuous flow. In an *ex vivo*, cadaveric urinary tract model for standard PCNL, simulated sPCNL was performed with rising irrigation pressures (68 to 408 cm H_2O). Intra-renal pressures rose in a near linear fashion as the irrigating pressures increased. Max IRP with irrigation pressure at 408 cm H_2O surpassed the 40 cm H_2O threshold (Landman et al. 2002). Similarly, in synthetic and animal models, the linear relationship between irrigating pressure and IRP holds true (Yap et al. 2022; Doizi et al. 2021b; Mager et al. 2015).

19 Renal Access Sheath Size

Current procedural practice for percutaneous nephrolithotomy relies on the use of a working renal access sheath. The benefits of its utilization are multiple and include tamponade of bleeding, improved visibility from evacuation of debris/blood, and extraction of large stone fragments (Saltzman et al. 1987). Additionally, a working sheath allows outflow of irrigant and will lower renal pelvic pressure. *In vivo*, human sPCNL studies have shown a working renal sheath reduces average IRP by 50% compared to utilization of nephroscope alone (Saltzman et al. 1987).

As working renal sheaths decrease in size, renal pelvic pressures will rise due to decreased outflow. This is exemplified by comparative studies of sPCNL, mPCNL and umPCNL when controlling for irrigation pressures (Tepeler et al. 2014; Wu et al.

2017; Guohua et al. 2007; Zhong et al. 2008). In mPCNL, *in vivo* comparison of 18F, 16F and 14F renal sheaths showed the corresponding rise in average IRP as sheath size decreases, 15.9 vs 22.1 vs 33.8 cm H_2O. Additionally, the rise in average IRP correlated to increased time of IRP above the intra-renal reflux threshold. In the 14F access sheath arm, time above threshold was 316 s, significantly longer than the other sheath sizes evaluated (Guohua et al. 2007; Zhong et al. 2008). Similarly, in a comparison study of microPCNL and sPCNL, average IRPs are significantly higher for microPCNL than sPCNL (41.2 vs 27.3 cm H_2O) (Tepeler et al. 2014).

In addition to the size of the renal access tract, the utilization of a second access tract offers another avenue to decrease IRP by enhancing irrigation drainage. Comparison studies of mPCNL access sheath sizes demonstrate that double 16F access sheaths result in significantly lower IRP compared to 18F sheaths (7.9 vs 15.9 cm H_2O) (Guohua et al. 2007). Similarly, *in vivo,* porcine models in sPCNL demonstrate significant reduction in RPP with two separate renal access tracts during rigid nephroscopy (Abourbih et al. 2017).

20 Nephroscope Size

The relative size of the nephroscope to the renal sheath will directly affect the ability of irrigant to leave the collecting system. As the nephroscope and internal diameter of the renal working sheath approach each other in size, renal pressures will rise. *Ex vivo,* porcine studies utilizing a 26F rigid nephroscope in the setting of 30F vs 26F renal access sheath result in higher average IRPs in the 26F access sheath arm, 12.4 vs 7.8 cm H_2O (Yap et al. 2022). *In vivo,* porcine sPCNL comparison of rigid nephroscopy (26F) vs flexible nephroscopy (16F) in the setting of a 30F access sheath shows significant reduction in pressure in the flexible arm. Average IRP was 42.6 vs 15.1 cm H_2O favoring the flexible nephroscopy arm (Abourbih et al. 2017). Within an *in vivo* human sPCNL study (30F renal sheath), flexible nephroscopy (16F) results in significant lower mean IRPs compared to rigid nephroscopy (24F), 17.5 vs 41.2 cm H_2O (Alsyouf et al. 2018).

21 Positioning of Renal Sheath and Nephroscope

Changes in renal access sheath and nephroscope location during PCNL will alter iatrogenic IRPs. Incomplete positioning of the access sheath into the collecting system will impair drainage and leads to elevated renal pressures (Troxel and Low 2002). This specific scenario is equivalent to performing the procedure without a working sheath. Access into a calyx with a narrowed infundibulum will also impact IRPs. When the nephroscope is advanced through the infundibulum into the renal pelvis, the infundibulum will function as a constriction point, inhibiting the flow of irrigant back into the renal access sheath (See Fig. 3). Within a sPCNL, *in vivo* human

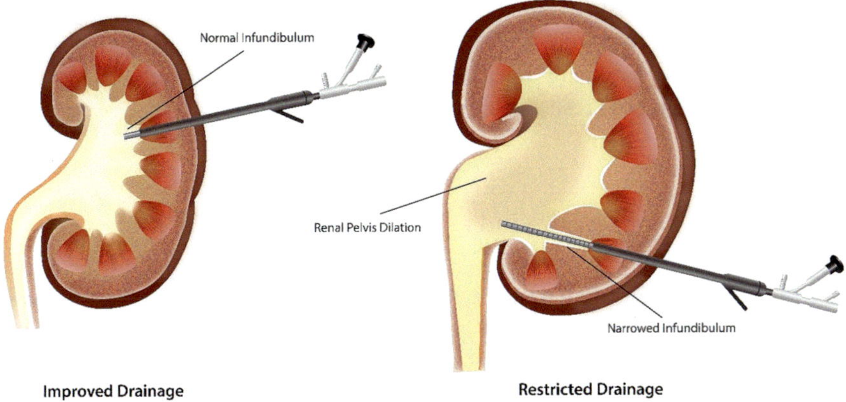

Fig. 3 A narrowed infundibulum restricts drainage through the nephrostomy sheath leading to elevated in IRP

study these two clinical scenarios resulted in elevated of IRP above the pyelovenous threshold (Saltzman et al. 1987; Troxel and Low 2002).

The relative positioning of the scope to the access sheath alters irrigation outflow and thus pressure. *In vivo*, mPCNL studies demonstrate that pressure generation is highest with the nephroscope positioned in the renal pelvis while the access sheath is in the calyx. Pressure will decrease if the sheath is advanced into the renal pelvis. Mean pressures from these two positions are 35.3 cm H_2O and 22.5 cm H_2O respectively. IRPs also remain lower when the scope is within the working sheath whether the sheath is in a calyx or renal pelvis, 17.4 cm H_2O and 19.6 cm H_2O respectively (Gokce et al. 2021).

22 Ureteral Cannulation

While efflux of irrigant via renal access sheath is the primary route for standard PCNL, as access sheath sizes decreases ureteral drainage becomes important. Enhancing ureteral drainage via cannulation provides another means for providers to mitigate rise in IRP. Secondary benefits of ureteral cannulation include increasing irrigation flow leading to better visibility (Landman et al. 2002). This is of particular importance in micro PCNL as irrigant is unable to leave via the 4.5F access needle (Tepeler et al. 2014). An *ex vivo*, human urinary tract study in sPCNL comparing the use of ureteral access sheaths, 6F open ended ureteral catheters, or empty ureter at increasing irrigation pressures demonstrates this relationship well. The utilization of 10/12F or 12/14F ureteral access sheaths resulted in mean IRPs below the pyelovenous threshold even as irrigation pressures were increased to 408 cm H_2O. The mean IRP at 408 cm H_2O of irrigation pressure in the ureteral access sheath arms were both near 20 cm H_2O. Interestingly, utilization of a 6F open ended catheter increased mean renal pelvic pressures compared to an empty ureter. This is likely due to obstruction of ureteral outflow with the 6F open ended catheter. At 300 mm Hg of irrigation pressure, mean IRP for the 6F open ended catheter and empty ureter arms were 50 cm H_2O and 40 cm H_2O respectively (Landman et al. 2002).

23 Bladder Decompression

As irrigant travels down the ureter during PCNL, bladder filling will result unless evacuation via foley catheterization is in place. Drainage from the renal pelvis to the bladder is partially determined by the pressure gradient between the two, thus it stands to reason that bladder fullness would limit ureteral drainage and result in higher renal pressures (Schwalb et al. 1993). *In vivo*, rat models comparing renal and bladder pressures in obstructed and non-obstructed renal units found that bladder pressure directly impacts renal pelvic pressure. In non-obstructed renal units, renal pelvic pressure increased from 2.12 H_2O to 9.75 cm H_2O when the bladder was decompressed and full, respectively (Fichtner et al. 1994). During percutaneous nephrolithotomy, continuous bladder decompression via urethral catheterization should be utilized to enhance ureteral drainage and lower renal pressures.

24 Active Irrigant Evacuation

The previous factors mentioned that affect outflow of irrigant are passive in nature. The pressure gradient from the renal pelvis to the external environment via the renal sheath or to the bladder via the ureter drives irrigation to leave the system. A way to enhance drainage is to utilize suction devices to actively evacuate irrigant. A balance must be maintained with suction to ensure distension of the system required for visibility and working space. Additionally, collapsing the collecting system may result in mucosal bleeding.

Vaccuum assisted percutaneous procedures include suction through ureteral instrumentation, integrated vacuum renal access sheaths and working instruments in the urinary tract (Alsyouf et al. 2018; Gokce et al. 2021; Zanetti et al. 2021; Alsmadi et al. 2018). For sPCNL, implementation of suction is common with use of an ultrasonic lithotripter. This device generates high frequency ultrasonic waves to break urinary tract calculi. A hollow component of the device allows for active suction implementation which leads to the evacuation of small stone fragments and fluid (Matlaga and 2009). An *in vivo*, human study of patients undergoing standard PCNL compared the impact of suction on IRP. Rigid nephroscopy with a suction lithotripter resulted in a significant reduction in mean RPP, 3.7 cm H_2O, vs without suction, 41.1 cm H_2O (Alsyouf et al. 2018).

For mPCNL, umPCNL and micro-PCNL ultrasonic lithotripter use is limited by the size of working channels. These procedures typically use laser or pneumatic lithotripsy for stone fragmentation and active evacuation is limited to integrated access sheaths or ureteral instrumentation. In a comparison, *in vivo* human study of mPCNL vs vacuum assisted mPCNL, active aspiration prevented renal pressures from rising above the pyelovenous threshold (Gokce et al. 2021) (See Fig. 4). Without active aspiration, RPP commonly rose above the pyelovenous threshold with maximum pressure reaching 54 cm H_2O, despite the placement of a 9.5/11.5F ureteral access sheath. This highlights that active aspiration should be considered in addition to maximizing ureteral drainage in procedures with smaller renal sheaths. Larger *in vivo*, mPCNL and umPCNL studies evaluating the implementation of suction integrated access sheaths demonstrate excellent control of iatrogenic renal pressures (Lai et al. 2020). Average renal pressures in vacuum assisted mPCNL are reported at 15.3 cm H_2O, with median time above pyelovenous threshold limited to 28.52 s (Zanetti et al. 2021). In vacuum assisted umPCNL average renal pressure was 26.5 cm H_2O, with median time above pyelovenous threshold of 55 seconds (Alsmadi et al. 2018).

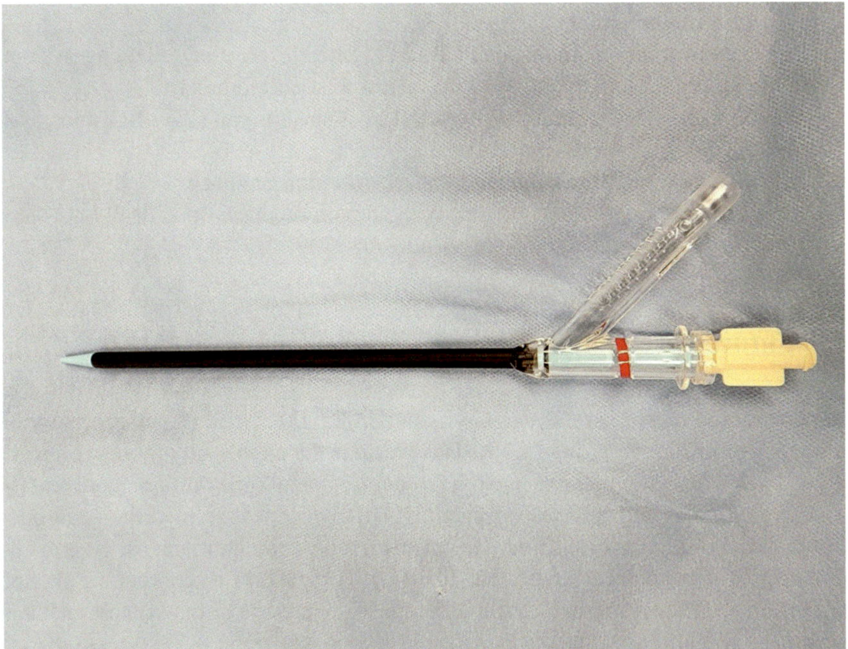

Fig. 4 ClearPetra nephrostomy sheath (Micro-Tech Endoscopy, Ann Arbor, MI, USA). Allows for continuous suction to connect to the accessory arm of the sheath

25 Clinical Pearls

Iatrogrenic IRP during PCNL is determined by factors that impact irrigation inflow and irrigation outflow. IRP commonly rises above the pyelorenal backflow threshold during percutaneous nephrolithotomy especially when miniaturized tracts are utilized. While there is a lack of robust data to guide practice, for each procedural factor discussed, general recommendations to mitigate degree and duration of elevated IRPs include:

- Use the minimum irrigation pressure needed for procedural safety. In sPCNL and mPCNL, gravity irrigation at a height of 80 cm H_2O or less tends to keep IRPs below the pyelovenous threshold (Mager et al. 2015).
- Use of larger renal access sheaths or multiple access tracts will reduce IRP and can be considered by proceduralists. This must be balanced against risks associated with larger or multiple access tracts.
- Utilization of small endoscopes relative to sheath size will enhance irrigation outflow and reduce IRP.
- Ensure appropriate position of renal access sheath into the collecting system. Where possible, avoid access sites via a narrowed infundibulum.
- Enhancing ureteral drainage via ureteral access sheaths can lower IRP. Increased importance with miniaturized tracts.
- Maintain bladder decompression to enhance ureteral drainage.
- Utilize active evacuation of irrigant with suction devices. Specifically consider when using miniaturized tracts.

26 Future Directions

The integration of pressure sensors into endourologic devices allows for real time evaluation of pressures during PCNL. This presents the opportunity for development of integrated platforms that manage renal pressure in real time through modification of irrigation inflow or outflow, via suction. This concept is termed the source-to-source principle, meaning use the IRP measurements to control the source of the pressure rise (Rawandale-Patil et al. 2019). In comparison to continuous suction devices, intermittent suction may allow for better distension of the urinary tract and visualization. Three separate platforms have been tested in the PCNL literature, one reliant on modification of irrigating pressure with the other two on modulation of suction pressures. A safe pressure range is pre-set within the system below the intra-renal backflow threshold. As IRP rises towards the maximum tolerated pressure, the system will modulate the source parameter.

A small *in vivo*, human study of five patients undergoing mPCNL with laser lithotripsy evaluated the implementation of a novel IRP monitoring/irrigation system. This system utilized real time IRPs to modulate mechanical irrigation pressures during the procedure. IRP measurements were performed via ureteric catheter connected to an extrinsic pressure sensor. Maximum tolerated IRP was set to 25 cm of H_2O. For all 5 patients, maximum pressures during the procedure never exceeded the 25 cm H_2O cutoff (Rawandale-Patil et al. 2019).

An *in vivo*, human study evaluated sixty patients undergoing vacuum assisted mPCNL for staghorn renal calculi with a novel IRP monitoring, suctioning system (Yang et al. 2016). The mPCNL renal sheath was integrated with a pressure sensor for real time monitoring and allowed for suction through the sheath. In the study, the maximum IRP was set to 40 cm H_2O for all patients. As IRP increased towards the maximum pressure, suction pressure would increase to improve fluid evacuation. IRP ranged from -16.3 to 2.7 cm H_2O in all patients, well below the pyelovenous threshold. In a similar *in vivo*, human study of 63 patients, a separate novel IRP monitoring, suction system maintained low IRPs even with increasing irrigation flow rates/pressure (Deng et al. 2019).

27 Conclusions

Generation of IRP is a necessity for PCNL efficacy and safety. A balance must be maintained to minimize risks associated with elevation of IRP. IRPs above 40 cm H_2O result in intra-renal reflux and pressure injury to the renal parenchyma. Clinically, this can impact volume status, inflammatory response, infectious response, and post-operative recovery. Procedural specific aspects directly impact IRP and thoughtful modification of factors where available should be considered to avoid consequences of elevated IRP. Further *in vivo* human studies will elucidate IRP dynamics and cutoffs that directly impact clinical outcomes (Croghan 2022). Such studies should try to embrace the huge heterogeneity of papillary morphology and renal anatomy among kidney stone patients, since these aspects will influence relation between IRP and intrarenal backflow, and consequently the resulting adverse events.

Acknowledgements Appreciation to Pradeep Sharma for his assistance in medical illustration for this chapter.

References

Abourbih S, et al. Renal pelvic pressure in percutaneous nephrolithotomy: the effect of multiple tracts. J Endourol. 2017;31(10):1079–83.

Alsmadi J, et al. The influence of super-mini percutaneous nephrolithotomy on renal pelvic pressure in vivo. J Endourol. 2018;32(9):819–23.

Alsyouf M, et al. Elevated renal pelvic pressures during percutaneous nephrolithotomy risk higher postoperative pain and longer hospital stay. J Urol. 2018;199(1):193–9.

Assimos D, et al. Surgical management of stones: American urological association/endourological society guideline PART II. J Urol. 2016;196(4):1161–9.

Boccafoschi C, Lugnani F. Intra-renal reflux. Urol Res. 1985;13(5):253–8.

Coulthard MG, et al. Renal scarring caused by vesicoureteric reflux and urinary infection: a study in pigs. Pediatr Nephrol. 2002;17(7):481–4.

Croghan SM et al. Upper urinary tract pressures in endourology: a systematic review of range, variables and implications. BJU Int 2022.

Dean NS, Krambeck AE. Endourologic procedures of the upper urinary tract and the effects on intrarenal pressure and temperature. J Endourol. 2023;37(2):191–8.

Deng X, et al. A novel technique to intelligently monitor and control renal pelvic pressure during minimally invasive percutaneous nephrolithotomy. Urol Int. 2019;103(3):331–6.

Desai M, Mishra S. Microperc' micro percutaneous nephrolithotomy: evidence to practice. Curr Opin Urol. 2012;22(2):134–8.

Desai MR, et al. Single-step percutaneous nephrolithotomy (microperc): the initial clinical report. J Urol. 2011;186(1):140–5.

Doizi S, et al. Continuous monitoring of intrapelvic pressure during flexible ureteroscopy using a sensor wire: a pilot study. World J Urol. 2021;39(2):555–61.

Doizi S, et al. Comparison of intrapelvic pressures during flexible ureteroscopy, mini-percutaneous nephrolithotomy, standard percutaneous nephrolithotomy, and endoscopic combined intrarenal surgery in a kidney model. World J Urol. 2021b;39(7):2709–17.

Fichtner J, et al. Congenital unilateral hydronephrosis in a rat model: continuous renal pelvic and bladder pressures. J Urol. 1994;152(2 Pt 2):652–7.

Fung LC, Atala A. Constant elevation in renal pelvic pressure induces an increase in urinary N-acetyl-beta-D-glucosaminidase in a nonobstructive porcine model. J Urol. 1998;159(1):212–6.

Ganpule AP, et al. Percutaneous nephrolithotomy (PCNL) a critical review. Int J Surg. 2016;36(Pt D):660–4.

Gokce MI, et al. Effect of active aspiration and sheath location on intrapelvic pressure during miniaturized percutaneous nephrolithotomy. Urology. 2021;153:101–6.

Gui H, et al. Mini-percutaneous nephrolithotomy with an endoscopic surgical monitoring system for the management of renal stones: a retrospective evaluation. Front Surg. 2022;9: 773270.

Guo HQ, et al. Relationship between the intrapelvic perfusion pressure in minimally invasive percutaneous nephrolithotomy and postoperative recovery. Zhonghua Wai Ke Za Zhi. 2008;46(1):52–4.

Guohua Z, et al. The influence of minimally invasive percutaneous nephrolithotomy on renal pelvic pressure in vivo. Surg Laparosc Endosc Percutan Tech. 2007;17(4):307–10.

Guzelburc V, et al. Comparison of absorbed irrigation fluid volumes during retrograde intrarenal surgery and percutaneous nephrolithotomy for the treatment of kidney stones larger than 2 cm. Springerplus. 2016;5(1):1707.

Hannappel J, et al. Pacemaker process of ureteral peristalsis in multicalyceal kidneys. Urol Int. 1982;37(4):240–6.

Hinman F, Lee-Brown RK. Pyelovenous back flow: its relation to pelvic reabsorption, to hydronephrosis and to accidents of pyelography. J Amer Med Assoc 1924;82(8):607–613.

Johnston RB, Porter C. The Whitaker test. Urol J. 2014;11(3):1727–30.

Jung H, Osther PJ. Intraluminal pressure profiles during flexible ureterorenoscopy. Springerplus. 2015;4:373.

Jung HU, et al. Pharmacological effect on pyeloureteric dynamics with a clinical perspective: a review of the literature. Urol Res. 2006;34(6):341–50.

Jung G, et al. Surgical parameters related to excessive intrarenal pressure during minimally invasive percutaneous nephrolithotomy in the supine position: a prospective observational clinical study. Biomed Res Int. 2022;1199052.

Kukreja RA, et al. Fluid absorption during percutaneous nephrolithotomy: does it matter? J Endourol. 2002;16(4):221–4.

Lai D, et al. Use of a novel vacuum-assisted access sheath in minimally invasive percutaneous nephrolithotomy: a feasibility study. J Endourol. 2020;34(3):339–44.

Landman J, et al. Comparison of intrarenal pressure and irrigant flow during percutaneous nephroscopy with an indwelling ureteral catheter, ureteral occlusion balloon, and ureteral access sheath. Urology. 2002;60(4):584–7.

Lee MS, et al. Determining the threshold of acute renal parenchymal damage for intrarenal pressure during flexible ureteroscopy using an *in vivo* pig model. World J Urol. 2022;40(11):2675–81.

Lildal SK, et al. Gadolinium-enhanced MRI visualizing backflow at increasing intra-renal pressure in a porcine model. PLoS ONE. 2023;18(2): e0281676.

Loftus CJ, et al. Mini versus standard percutaneous nephrolithotomy: the impact of sheath size on intrarenal pelvic pressure and infectious complications in a porcine model. J Endourol. 2018;32(4):350–3.

Loftus C, Byrne M, Monga M. High pressure endoscopic irrigation: impact on renal histology. Int Braz J Urol. 2021;47(2):350–6.

Mager R, et al. Introducing a novel in vitro model to characterize hydrodynamic effects of percutaneous nephrolithotomy systems. J Endourol. 2015;29(8):929–32.

Malhotra SK, et al. Monitoring of irrigation fluid absorption during percutaneous nephrolithotripsy: the use of 1% ethanol as a marker. Anaesthesia. 2001;56(11):1090–115.

Matlaga BR, American Board of U. Contemporary surgical management of upper urinary tract calculi. J Urol. 2009;181(5):2152–6.

Mortensen J, Djurhuus JC. Hydrodynamics of the normal multicalyceal pyeloureter in pigs: the pelvic pressure response to increasing flow rates, its normal ranges and intra-individual variations. J Urol. 1985;133(4):704–8.

Noureldin YA et al. The effect of irrigation power and ureteral access sheath diameter on the maximal intra-pelvic pressure during ureteroscopy: in vivo experimental study in a live anesthetized pig. J Endourol. 2019;33(9):725–729.

Omar M, et al. Systemic inflammatory response syndrome after percutaneous nephrolithotomy: a randomized single-blind clinical trial evaluating the impact of irrigation pressure. J Urol. 2016;196(1):109–14.

Osther PJ, et al. Pathophysiological aspects of ureterorenoscopic management of upper urinary tract calculi. Curr Opin Urol. 2016;26(1):63–9.

Patel SR, Nakada SY. The modern history and evolution of percutaneous nephrolithotomy. J Endourol. 2015;29(2):153–7.

Pedersen KV, et al. Distension of the renal pelvis in kidney stone patients: sensory and biomechanical responses. Urol Res. 2012;40(4):305–16.

Pfitzner J. Poiseuille and his law. Anaesthesia. 1976;31(2):273–5.

Ransley PG, Risdon RA. The pathogenesis of reflux nephropathy. Contrib Nephrol. 1979;16:90–7.

Rawandale-Patil AV, Ganpule AP, Patni LG. Development of an innovative intrarenal pressure regulation system for mini-PCNL: a preliminary study. Indian J Urol. 2019;35(3):197–201.

Saltzman B, Khasidy LR, Smith AD. Measurement of renal pelvis pressures during endourologic procedures. Urology. 1987;30(5):472–4.

Satish M, Tadi P. Physiology, vascular. *StatPearls*. 2022: Treasure Island (FL).

Schwalb DM, et al. Morphological and physiological changes in the urinary tract associated with ureteral dilation and ureteropyeloscopy: an experimental study. J Urol. 1993;149(6):1576–85.

Shah AK, et al. Implementation of ultramini percutaneous nephrolithotomy for treatment of 2–3 cm kidney stones: a preliminary report. J Endourol. 2015;29(11):1231–6.

Sierra A et al. Real time intrarenal pressure control during flexible ureterorrenscopy using a vascular pressurewire: pilot study. J Clin Med. 2022;12(1).

Stenberg A, et al. Back-leak of pelvic urine to the bloodstream. Acta Physiol Scand. 1988;134(2):223–34.

Tepeler A, et al. Comparison of intrarenal pelvic pressure during micro-percutaneous nephrolithotomy and conventional percutaneous nephrolithotomy. Urolithiasis. 2014;42(3):275–9.

Thomsen HS, Dorph S, Olsen S. Pyelorenal backflow in normal and ischemic rabbit kidneys. Invest Radiol. 1981;16(3):206–14.

Thomsen HS, Larsen S. Intrarenal backflow during retrograde pyelography with graded intrapelvic pressure. A pathoanatomic study. Acta Pathol Microbiol Immunol Scand A 1983;91(4):245–52.

Thomsen HS, Talner LB, Higgins CB. Intrarenal backflow during retrograde pyelography with graded intrapelvic pressure. A radiologic study. Invest Radiol 1982;17(6):593–603.

Tokas T, et al. Pressure matters: intrarenal pressures during normal and pathological conditions, and impact of increased values to renal physiology. World J Urol. 2019a;37(1):125–31.

Tokas T, et al. Pressure matters 2: intrarenal pressure ranges during upper-tract endourological procedures. World J Urol. 2019;37(1):133–42.

Travaglini F, et al. Pathophysiology of reno-ureteral colic. Urol Int. 2004;72(Suppl 1):20–3.

Troxel SA, Low RK. Renal intrapelvic pressure during percutaneous nephrolithotomy and its correlation with the development of postoperative fever. J Urol. 2002;168(4 Pt 1):1348–51.

Wahlberg J, Karlberg L, Persson AE. Total and regional renal blood flow during complete unilateral ureteral obstruction. Acta Physiol Scand. 1984;121(2):111–8.

Walzak MP, Paquin AJ. Renal pelvic pressure levels in management of nephrostomy. J Urol 1961;85:697–702.

Whitehurst LA, Somani BK. Semi-rigid ureteroscopy: indications, tips, and tricks. Urolithiasis. 2018;46(1):39–45.

Wilson WTP, Glenn M. Intrarenal pressures generated during flexible deflectable ureterorenoscopy. J Endourol. 1990;4(2):135–41.

Wright A, et al. Mini, ultra, micro'—nomenclature and cost of these new minimally invasive percutaneous nephrolithotomy (PCNL) techniques. Ther Adv Urol. 2016;8(2):142–6.

Wu C, et al. Comparison of renal pelvic pressure and postoperative fever incidence between standard- and mini-tract percutaneous nephrolithotomy. Kaohsiung J Med Sci. 2017;33(1):36–43.

Yang Z, et al. The new generation mini-PCNL system—monitoring and controlling of renal pelvic pressure by suctioning device for efficient and safe PCNL in managing renal staghorn calculi. Urol Int. 2016;97(1):61–6.

Yap LC, et al. Intrarenal pressures during percutaneous nephrolithotomy: a porcine kidney model. Scand J Urol. 2022;56(3):251–4.

Zanetti SP, et al. Vacuum-assisted mini-percutaneous nephrolithotomy: a new perspective in fragments clearance and intrarenal pressure control. World J Urol. 2021;39(6):1717–23.

Zhong W, et al. Does a smaller tract in percutaneous nephrolithotomy contribute to high renal pelvic pressure and postoperative fever? J Endourol. 2008;22(9):2147–51.

Percutaneous Management of Upper Tract Urothelial Carcinoma

Gregory Mullen, Tareq Aro, and Zeph Okeke

Abstract Upper tract urothelial carcinoma (UTUC) is a rare malignancy. The European Association of Urology stratifies patients with UTUC as either low-risk or high-risk for disease progression. High-risk patients should be managed with radical nephroureterectomy and low-risk patients should be offered kidney-sparing surgery including percutaneous management. Percutaneous management of UTUC allows the use of larger caliber instruments, which remove bulky tumor more efficiently and may provide more accurate staging. Newer adjuvant topical agents aim to reduce the high rate of recurrence often seen with kidney-sparing surgeries for UTUC. Oncologic outcomes of patients treated with percutaneous management are similar to outcomes for radical nephroureterectomy for patients with low-risk disease. Patients with imperative indications to avoid nephroureterectomy can be treated with percutaneous management of UTUC with high renal preservation rates. Lifelong surveillance is needed for patients treated with percutaneous management given high recurrence rates that can occur years after the initial diagnosis.

Keywords Upper tract urothelial carcinoma · Percutaneous renal surgery

1 Introduction

Upper tract urothelial carcinoma (UTUC) is a rare malignancy, with an incidence of roughly 2 cases per 100,000 person-years in the United States, which has slowly increased over the past 30 years (Raman et al. 2011). An analysis of the National

G. Mullen · T. Aro · Z. Okeke (✉)
The Smith Institute for Urology, Northwell Health, Zucker School of Medicine at Hofstra/Northwell, 450 Lakeville Road, Lake Success, NY 11042, USA
e-mail: zokeke@northwell.edu

G. Mullen
e-mail: gmullen1@northwell.edu

T. Aro
e-mail: taro@northwell.edu

© The Author(s), under exclusive license to Springer Nature Switzerland AG 2023
J. D. Denstedt and E. N. Liatsikos (eds.), *Percutaneous Renal Surgery*,
https://doi.org/10.1007/978-3-031-40542-6_30

Cancer Database (NCDB) found that the median age at diagnosis is 72 years old, with 60.3% of cases occurring in men. 26.4% of UTUC was found to be low grade, 56.1% of UTUC was found to be high grade, and the remaining 17.5% of cases were unknown or unable to be graded. Renal pelvis tumors accounted for 57.6% cases of UTUC, with the remaining 42.4% of tumors located in the ureter (Browne et al. 2018). Despite the similarities to bladder cancer, UTUC is a distinct disease arising from unique genetic mutations leading to differences in presentation, staging, and treatment options. UTUC accounts for 5 to 10% of urothelial cancers and typically presents at a higher grade and stage disease than does bladder cancer (Green et al. 2013; Stewart et al. 2005).

The European Association of Urology (EAU) guidelines on UTUC stratify patients as either low-risk or high-risk for disease progression. Patients are considered low-risk if all the following criteria are met: unifocal disease, tumor size < 2 cm, no high-grade cytology, low-grade biopsy, and no evidence of invasion on imaging. Patients are considered high-risk if any of the following criteria are met: multifocal disease, tumor size > 2 cm, high grade cytology, high-grade biopsy, evidence of local invasion on imaging, hydronephrosis, prior radical cystectomy for high-grade bladder cancer, or any variant histology. Figure 1. Open radical nephroureterectomy with bladder cuff excision is considered the gold standard treatment for the management of high-risk UTUC, whereas kidney-sparing surgeries are preferred for low-risk UTUC as they decrease morbidity without compromising oncologic outcomes (Guidelines 2022; Seisen et al. 2016). Kidney-sparing surgeries include ureteroscopic ablation, percutaneous resection, and segmental ureteral resection.

The first reported cases of percutaneous management of UTUC were by Orihuela, Crowley, and Smith at the 1986 American Urological Association meeting (Orihuela et al. 1986). Not long after, Streem and Pontes published the first paper on percutaneous management of UTUC in the Journal of Urology in 1986 (Streem and Pontes

Fig. 1 Risk for tumor progression

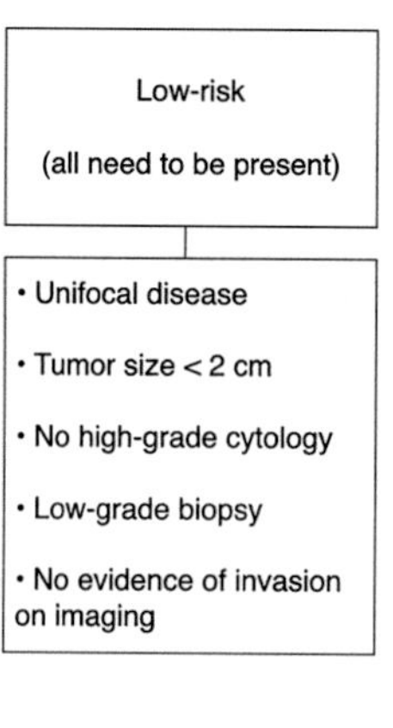

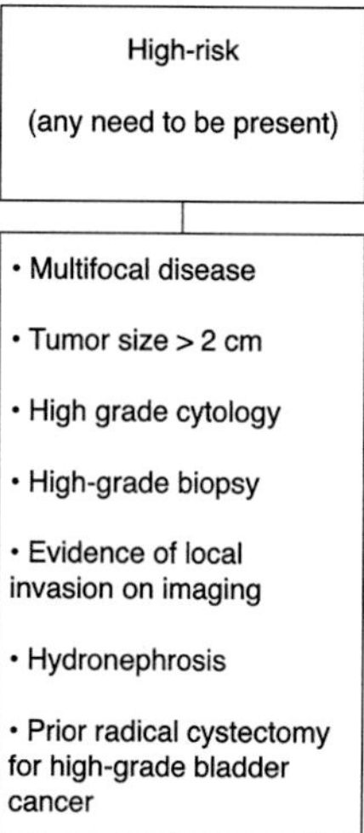

1986). The initial utilization of percutaneous management for UTUC was typically for patients with imperative indications to avoid radical nephroureterectomy, such as anatomically or functionally solitary kidneys, baseline renal insufficiency, bilateral disease, or in patients unwilling or unfit to undergo radical surgery.

2 Indications and Contraindications

Given the imperative indications to avoid radical nephroureterectomy, one of the main rationales for kidney-sparing surgery is renal preservation. Although radical nephroureterectomy was shown in one study to decrease mean estimated glomerular filtration rate (eGFR) by only 8 ml/min/1.73 m^2, this decline resulted in 25% of patients having a new eGFR below 60 ml/min/1.73 m^2 and 15% of patients having a new eGFR below 45 ml/min/1.73 m^2 (Raman et al. 2014). These eGFR cutoffs are typically used to determine eligibility for adjuvant chemotherapy and the choice of chemotherapy agent used. More importantly, chronic kidney disease is a known risk factor for increased cardiovascular morbidity and mortality, as well as overall mortality (Lamprea-Montealegre et al. 2021). In a single-institution study spanning 30-years, Motamedinia et al. found that percutaneous management of UTUC resulted in a renal preservation rate of 87% with a median follow up of 66 months (Motamedinia et al. 2016).

In addition to the imperative indications to avoid radial nephroureterectomy, kidney-sparing surgeries are the primary treatment options for patients with low-risk UTUC (Guidelines 2022). Percutaneous management of UTUC, specifically, is best utilized for patients with large volume (>1.5 cm), low grade, non-invasive tumors located in the calyces, renal pelvis, and proximal ureter (Farrow et al. 2021). It is also the preferred management for patients with urinary diversions. The percutaneous approach permits the use of larger caliber instruments than does the ureteroscopic approach, which allows for resection of a higher volume disease in a more efficient manner. Additionally, biopsies obtained from the percutaneous approach are usually deeper than biopsies obtained from the ureteroscopic approach, which may provide more accurate staging.

Despite the EAU risk stratification and treatment recommendations, an analysis of the NCDB found that 51% of patients with low-grade UTUC underwent radical nephroureterectomy. However, the rate of radical nephroureterectomy decreased from 59.6 to 56.7% over the 10-year study period (Browne et al. 2018). Similarly, data from the Clinical Research Office of the Endourological Society (CROES) Global UTUC registry showed that 60.1% of patients were treated with radical nephroureterectomy. Kidney-sparing surgeries were performed in 54% of patients, of which only 0.8% of patients had percutaneous management (Baard et al. 2021). While radical nephroureterectomy remains the gold standard treatment for patients with high-risk UTUC, its utilization has slowly decreased over time as more patients are offered kidney-sparing surgeries.

Patients with high-risk UTUC should not typically be offered kidney-sparing surgeries unless they have imperative indications to avoid radical nephroureterectomy. Other contraindications to percutaneous management of UTUC include active infection, bleeding diathesis or coagulopathy. Obesity does not preclude percutaneous management, but does necessitate use of longer instruments. Patients who are unwilling or unable to undergo long-term surveillance should also not be offered kidney-sparing surgery.

3 Preoperative Evaluation

According to the CROES UTUC registry, 53% of patients evaluated for UTUC had symptoms, whereas 14.8% were incidentally noted to have abnormalities on imaging studies. The most common symptom was macroscopic hematuria, found in 58.3% of patients, followed by pain in 19.2% of patients (Baard et al. 2021). Once the diagnosis of UTUC is suspected, a key component to the workup includes cross-sectional abdominal and pelvic imaging. Computed tomography (CT) urography is the gold standard non-invasive imaging modality for UTUC, with a sensitivity of 92% and specificity of 95% (Janisch et al. 2020). Lesions are typically identified as filling defects in the affected kidney or ureter. For patients with allergies to iodinated contrast dye or with renal insufficiency, magnetic resonance (MR) urography is an acceptable alternative with a sensitivity of 70% and specificity of 97% (Takahashi et al. 2010). While invasive, retrograde pyelography can also be performed with a sensitivity of 96% and specificity of 97% (Cowan et al. 2007).

In addition to radiologic studies, cystoscopy should be performed to rule out any bladder lesions. Selective cytology from the upper tracts can also be obtained. The presence of abnormal or high-grade urine cytology is highly suggestive of UTUC. Before proceeding with percutaneous management, retrograde ureteroscopy can be performed to determine the volume and location of tumor, as well as to obtain tissue samples for grading and staging.

Patients selected to undergo percutaneous management of UTUC should be counseled regarding the risks of the procedure including pain, bleeding, infection, and damage to surrounding organs. The risk of tumor seeding is rare and has only been reported in a few case reports (Huang et al. 1995). Patients must also be counseled regarding the need for strict follow up due to the likelihood of recurrence. To minimize the risk of bleeding, anticoagulants should be discontinued prior to surgery in consultation with the patient's primary care physician. All bleeding diatheses should be corrected and urinary tract infections should be treated with culture appropriate antibiotics. Preoperative evaluation should be performed to ensure that the patient's cardiac and pulmonary status is optimized.

4 Operative Details

Either the supine or prone approach can be utilized. The prone approach is preferred at our institution due to the ability to more easily obtain upper pole access as well as more easily access multiple calyces, if necessary. In this case, general anesthesia is induced with endotracheal tube on a stretcher. The patient is then repositioned onto the operating room table in the prone surrender position with chest rolls and all pressure points padded. The flank and back are prepped with chlorhexidine and the genitalia prepped with betadine solution. The patient is draped in the usual standard sterile fashion.

Flexible cystoscopy is performed to evaluate for the presence of any bladder tumors. The ipsilateral ureteral orifice is identified and cannulated with a guidewire, which is passed into the kidney under fluoroscopic control. A 5 or 6 French (Fr) open ended ureteral catheter is advanced over the guidewire into the renal pelvis and the guidewire is removed. Urine for cytology is obtained. Retrograde pyelogram is then performed, which combined with the preoperative cross-sectional imaging helps to delineate calyceal anatomy and plan for renal puncture. The calyx containing tumor is the ideal access site as this facilitates maximal tumor resection. Posterior upper pole or interpolar access is preferred for tumors located in the renal pelvis as these access sites reduce the amount of torque required to reach the renal pelvis and ureter.

After selecting the calyx of entry, an 18-gauge diamond-tip needle is inserted into the collecting system under biplanar fluoroscopy. Ultrasound-guided percutaneous renal access can also be performed if the surgeon is comfortable with this approach. However, calyces filled with tumor may be difficult to discern on ultrasound potentially limiting this approach. Once access is obtained, a guidewire is advanced into the cannula of the needle and either coiled in the collecting system or, preferably, advanced down the ureter into the bladder. The tract is dilated to 30Fr using either a balloon or with Amplatz dilators. The 30Fr sheath is advanced over the dilator into the collecting system, with care taken to ensure that the sheath remains within the collecting system to reduce the potential risk of tumor seeding.

Rigid nephroscopy is performed with a 26Fr offset-lens rigid nephroscope. The cup biopsy forceps is the preferred instrument to debulk and resect tissue as it minimizes thermal artifact to the specimen and also minimizes the risk of deep resection into renal parenchyma and large vessels. The base of the tumor is biopsied and sent separately from the rest of the specimen to aid the pathologist in correctly staging the patient. Once all visible tumor is resected, the base is cauterized with either electrocautery or laser. Cautery should be limited near infundibuli and the ureteropelvic junction to minimize the risk of stenosis. The remainder of the collecting system is inspected with either a rigid or flexible nephroscope to ensure there is no residual tumor in these areas. Once confirmed, the sheath is removed and a nephrostomy tube is placed over the access tract guidewire to help tamponade any tract bleeding, maintain adequate renal drainage, and provide access for a possible second stage procedure or instillation of topical agent, if indicated. Second stage procedures are needed if visibility is limited during the first stage due to bleeding, which prevents complete resection of tumor or inspection of the collecting system (Samson et al. 2018).

5　Topical Agents

Guidelines for non-muscle invasive bladder cancer recommend the instillation of adjuvant topical immuno- or chemotherapeutic agents in order to reduce disease recurrence and progression (Referenced with permission from the NCCN Clinical Practice Guidelines in Oncology 2023). Given the success in bladder cancer, similar topical agents have been used in hopes of preventing disease recurrence and progression in patients with UTUC that have undergone kidney-sparing surgeries. The most commonly used agents are Bacillus Calmette–Guérin (BCG) and mitomycin. Treatments are typically given in six weekly instillations. Method of delivery depends on patient and provider preference. Options include double J ureteral stent placement with intravesical instillation of the agent and reliance on vesicoureteral reflux to the upper tract, instillation via a retrograde ureteral catheter, or instillation via an antegrade nephrostomy tube.

Despite early optimism regarding the efficacy of adjuvant topical therapies, a meta-analysis assessing the oncologic outcomes of patients with UTUC treated with kidney-sparing surgery and adjuvant topical agents found no difference in disease recurrence when compared to similar patients who did not receive adjuvant topical agents. Furthermore, the meta-analysis found that there was no difference in disease recurrence, progression, cancer-specific survival, or overall survival between any of the different delivery methods of these agents (Foerster et al. 2019). This is likely due, in part, to the absence of storage capacity of the upper urinary tract and the continuous flow of urine, which limit the contact time of these topical agents, thus limiting their therapeutic efficacy.

Due to the limited contact time of these topical agents, a mitomycin-containing reverse thermal gel (UGN-101) was developed. The properties of the gel allow for administration of the medication as a cold liquid, which converts into a semi-solid gel upon warming in the upper urinary tract. The gel subsequently dissolves with normal urine flow and exposes the upper urinary tract to mitomycin for four to six hours. An open-label, single-arm, phase 3 trial evaluated 71 patients with low-risk UTUC treated with six weekly instillations of UGN-101 via a retrograde ureteral catheter. Complete response, defined as negative endoscopic exam, negative cytology, and negative for-cause biopsy four to six weeks after completion of therapy, was seen in 42 patients (59%) (Kleinmann et al. 2020). Of the patients who had complete response, 41 patients were available for follow up at 12 months, of which 23 patients (56%) remained in complete response (Matin et al. 2022). Ureteric stenosis—defined as a discrete narrowing of the ureter during ureteroscopy or a discrete narrowing of the ureter identified on retrograde pyelogram at the time of ureteroscopy, that required dilation or stenting to pass a ureteroscope for proximal visualization—was the most common complication in the initial trial, occurring in 31 patients (44%).

The study authors hypothesize this may be related to the repeated ureteric manipulation and instrumentation with ureteral catheters that are less pliable than traditional polyurethane catheters (Kleinmann et al. 2020). Subsequent studies evaluating the antegrade administration of UGN-101 through nephrostomy tubes have shown similar complete response rates and significantly lower ureteric stenosis rates (Rose et al. 2022).

At our institution, we typically offer patients with low-risk disease adjuvant topical agents, most commonly UGN-101. Given the ureteric stenosis rates seen, we tend to avoid the medication in patients with solitary kidneys and typically administer the drug via a nephrostomy tube.

6 Outcomes

To date, there are no randomized trials comparing kidney-sparing surgeries to radical nephroureterectomy for the treatment of UTUC. Furthermore, most studies examining outcomes after percutaneous management for UTUC are small and retrospective in nature. A systematic review published in 2012 examined 11 studies of percutaneous management for UTUC with a minimum of 10 patients. All of the included studies evaluated less than 40 patients, with one exception from Long Island Jewish Medical Center, which examined 89 patients at the time. 288 patients treated with percutaneous management of UTUC were included with follow up ranging from 19 to 64 months. Despite concerns regarding selection bias, the review found comparable outcomes with ureteroscopic ablation of UTUC. Recurrence in the upper tract occurred in 37% of patients treated with percutaneous management compared to 52% of patients treated with ureteroscopic ablation. Recurrence in the bladder occurred in 24% of patients treated with percutaneous management compared to 34% of patient treated with ureteroscopic ablation. 78% of patients treated with percutaneous management avoided radical nephroureterectomy compared to 81% of patients treated with ureteroscopic ablation. Lastly, disease specific survival was 89% for patients treated with percutaneous management compared to 91% for patients treated with ureteroscopic ablation (Cutress et al. 2012).

A systematic review published by the EAU in 2016 examined the oncologic outcomes of kidney-sparing surgeries compared to radical nephroureterectomy. Despite similar selection bias concerns, the authors determined that survival outcomes after percutaneous management of UTUC were similar to survival outcomes after radical nephroureterectomy, albeit at the expense of increased tumor recurrence. However, the authors specified that these survival similarities were only for patients with low-grade and noninvasive UTUC (Seisen et al. 2016).

The largest series evaluating percutaneous management of UTUC is the most recently published study from the Long Island Jewish Medical Center, which contains 141 patients with a median follow-up of 66 months. Recurrence occurred in 37% of patients with low-grade disease and 63% of patients with high-grade disease. Median time to recurrence was 71.4 months for patients with low-grade disease and 36.4 months for patients with high-grade disease. Grade was the only predictor of recurrence (HR 2.12, p = 0.018). The longest time to develop recurrence was 116 months after the initial diagnosis of UTUC. Multifocal disease was not found to increase the risk of recurrence, progression, or death. On multivariate analysis, age, imperative indication to avoid radical nephroureterectomy, and history of bladder cancer were the only negative predictors of overall survival. 87% of patients treated with percutaneous management avoided radical nephroureterectomy. Based on these findings, the authors advocate that percutaneous management of UTUC should be offered to patients with advanced age, imperative indications to avoid radical nephroureterectomy, or a history of bladder cancer, even if they have high-grade disease (Motamedinia et al. 2016).

7 Complications

Percutaneous management of UTUC is fairly well tolerated. Risks including pain, bleeding, infection, and damage to surrounding organs must be discussed with patients. The 2012 systematic review found a 17% transfusion rate, however, this rate has most likely decreased since then as techniques have been mastered and technologies improved (Cutress et al. 2012). Significant hemorrhage can be caused by vascular injury during percutaneous renal access and dilation, or from tumor resection. Bleeding caused by the access and dilation can typically be addressed by maneuvering the Amplatz sheath to tamponade the offending vessels. If this is unsuccessful, the procedure should be abandoned and a large bore nephrostomy should be placed. If bleeding resolves the procedure can resume several days later, however, if bleeding persists, super-selective angioembolization may be required, though this is necessary in less than 1% of cases (Cutress et al. 2012). Bleeding from tumor resection can be controlled with complete tumor resection and fulguration of the tumor base.

Rare complications include injury to surrounding organs such as the lung, colon, liver, and spleen. With the increased utilization of ultrasound-guided percutaneous renal access, these structures can be identified and avoided if possible. Infundibular and ureteropelvic junction strictures can occur due to cautery, however, tumor recurrence must also be excluded. Tumor seeding the percutaneous tract is even rarer with only a few case reports (Huang et al. 1995).

8 Surveillance

Given the high rates of recurrence in both the bladder and upper tract after percutaneous management of UTUC, surveillance is necessary for early detection and treatment (Cutress et al. 2012). Most recurrences occur within the first three years of initial therapy, but can be seen as many as 116 months after initial diagnosis, highlighting the need for lifelong surveillance (Motamedinia et al. 2016). For the first year after initial treatment, surveillance is performed every 3 months, which includes cystoscopy and ipsilateral ureteroscopy. Even if no visible tumors are identified, cytology should be obtained during each survey. For the second year, surveillance is performed every 6 months, after which surveillance is performed annually. CT urography or alternative cross-sectional imaging should be performed yearly. If any recurrence is found, the surveillance schedule restarts. For patients who recur frequently and require repeated surveillance and treatment, incision of the ureterovesical junction has been described to facilitate ureteroscopy without the need for wires or dilation (Kerbl and Clayman 1993).

9 Conclusions

Kidney-sparing surgeries are preferred for the management of low-risk patients with UTUC. Patients with imperative indications to avoid nephroureterectomy can also be offered kidney-sparing surgeries to avoid the morbidity of radical nephroureterectomy while also having comparable oncologic outcomes. Although percutaneous management of UTUC is infrequently used, it remains an important treatment option for select patients. Renal preservation rates are high even for patients with high-grade disease. The development of novel topical agents to decrease the risk of recurrence may further the trend towards kidney-sparing surgeries and away from radical nephroureterectomy.

References

Baard J, Cormio L, Cavadas V, Alcaraz A, Shariat SF, de la Rosette J, Laguna MP. Contemporary patterns of presentation, diagnostics and management of upper tract urothelial cancer in 101 centres: the clinical research office of the Endourological society global upper tract urothelial carcinoma registry. Curr Opin Urol. 2021;31(4):354–62.

Browne BM, Stensland KD, Moynihan MJ, Canes D. An analysis of staging and treatment trends for upper tract urothelial carcinoma in the national cancer database. Clin Genitourin Cancer. 2018;16(4):e743–50.

Cowan NC, Turney BW, Taylor NJ, McCarthy CL, Crew JP. Multidetector computed tomography urography for diagnosing upper urinary tract urothelial tumour. BJU Int. 2007;99(6):1363–70.

Cutress ML, Stewart GD, Zakikhani P, Phipps S, Thomas BG, Tolley DA. Ureteroscopic and percutaneous management of upper tract urothelial carcinoma (UTUC): systematic review. BJU Int. 2012;110(5):614–28.

Farrow JM, Kern SQ, Gryzinski GM, Sundaram CP. Nephron-sparing management of upper tract urothelial carcinoma. Investig Clin Urol. 2021;62(4):389–98.

Foerster B, D'Andrea D, Abufaraj M, Broenimann S, Karakiewicz PI, Rouprêt M, Gontero P, Lerner SP, Shariat SF, Soria F. Endocavitary treatment for upper tract urothelial carcinoma: a meta-analysis of the current literature. Urol Oncol. 2019;37(7):430–6.

Green DA, Rink M, Xylinas E, Matin SF, Stenzl A, Roupret M, Karakiewicz PI, Scherr DS, Shariat SF. Urothelial carcinoma of the bladder and the upper tract: disparate twins. J Urol. 2013;189(4):1214–21.

EAU Guidelines. Edn. presented at the EAU Annual Congress, Amsterdam: 2022. ISBN 978-94-92671-16-5

Huang A, Low RK, deVere WR. Nephrostomy tract tumor seeding following percutaneous manipulation of a ureteral carcinoma. J Urol. 1995;153(3 Pt 2):1041–2.

Janisch F, Shariat SF, Baltzer P, Fajkovic H, Kimura S, Iwata T, Korn P, Yang L, Glybochko PV, Rink M, Abufaraj M. Diagnostic performance of multidetector computed tomographic (MDCTU) in upper tract urothelial carcinoma (UTUC): a systematic review and meta-analysis. World J Urol. 2020;38(5):1165–75.

Kerbl K, Clayman RV. Incision of the ureterovesical junction for endoscopic surveillance of transitional cell cancer of the upper urinary tract. J Urol. 1993;150(5 Pt 1):1440–3.

Kleinmann N, Matin SF, Pierorazio PM, Gore JL, Shabsigh A, Hu B, Chamie K, Godoy G, Hubosky S, Rivera M, O'Donnell M, Quek M, Raman JD, Knoedler JJ, Scherr D, Stern J, Weight C, Weizer A, Woods M, Kaimakliotis H, Smith AB, Linehan J, Coleman J, Humphreys MR, Pak R, Lifshitz D, Verni M, Adibi M, Amin MB, Seltzer E, Klein I, Konorty M, Strauss-Ayali D, Hakim G, Schoenberg M, Lerner SP. Primary chemoablation of low-grade upper tract urothelial carcinoma using UGN-101, a mitomycin-containing reverse thermal gel (OLYMPUS): an open-label, single-arm, phase 3 trial. Lancet Oncol. 2020;21(6):776–85.

Lamprea-Montealegre JA, Shlipak MG, Estrella MM. Chronic kidney disease detection, staging and treatment in cardiovascular disease prevention. Heart. 2021;107(16):1282–8.

Matin SF, Pierorazio PM, Kleinmann N, et al. Durability of response to primary chemoablation of low-grade upper tract urothelial carcinoma Using UGN-101, a Mitomycin-containing reverse thermal gel: OLYMPUS trial final report. J Urol. 2022;207(4):779–88.

Motamedinia P, Keheila M, Leavitt DA, Rastinehad AR, Okeke Z, Smith AD. The expanded use of percutaneous resection for upper tract urothelial carcinoma: a 30-year comprehensive experience. J Endourol. 2016;30(3):262–7.

Orihuela E, Crowley AR, Smith AD. Percutaneous management of renal pelvic transitional cell carcinoma (TCCA). J Urol. 1986 part 2;135:164A, abstract 244.

Raman JD, Messer J, Sielatycki JA, Hollenbeak CS. Incidence and survival of patients with carcinoma of the ureter and renal pelvis in the USA, 1973–2005. BJU Int. 2011;107(7):1059–64.

Raman JD, Lin YK, Kaag M, Atkinson T, Crispen P, Wille M, Smith N, Hockenberry M, Guzzo T, Peyronnet B, Bensalah K, Simhan J, Kutikov A, Cha E, Herman M, Scherr D, Shariat SF, Boorjian SA. High rates of advanced disease, complications, and decline of renal function after radical nephroureterectomy. Urol Oncol. 2014;32(1):47.e9-14.

Referenced with permission from the NCCN Clinical Practice Guidelines in Oncology (NCCN Guidelines®) for Bladder Cancer V.1.2023. © National Comprehensive Cancer Network, Inc. 2023. All rights reserved. To view the most recent and complete version of the guideline, go online to NCCN.org.

Rose KM, Narang G, Rosen G, et al. Antegrade administration of mitomycin gel for upper tract urothelial carcinoma via percutaneous nephrostomy tube: a multi-institutional retrospective cohort study [published online ahead of print, 2022 Oct 26]. BJU Int. 2022.

Samson P, Smith AD, Hoenig D, Okeke Z. Endoscopic management of upper urinary tract urothelial carcinoma. J Endourol. 2018;32(S1):S10–6.

Seisen T, Peyronnet B, Dominguez-Escrig JL, Bruins HM, Yuan CY, Babjuk M, Böhle A, Burger M, Compérat EM, Cowan NC, Kaasinen E, Palou J, van Rhijn BW, Sylvester RJ, Zigeuner R, Shariat SF, Rouprêt M. Oncologic outcomes of kidney-sparing surgery versus radical Nephroureterectomy for upper tract urothelial carcinoma: a systematic review by the EAU non-muscle invasive bladder cancer guidelines panel. Eur Urol. 2016;70(6):1052–68.

Stewart GD, Bariol SV, Grigor KM, Tolley DA, McNeill SA. A comparison of the pathology of transitional cell carcinoma of the bladder and upper urinary tract. BJU Int. 2005;95(6):791–3.

Streem SB, Pontes EJ. Percutaneous management of upper tract transitional cell carcinoma. J Urol. 1986;135(4):773–5.

Takahashi N, Glockner JF, Hartman RP, King BF, Leibovich BC, Stanley DW, Fitz-Gibbon PD, Kawashima A. Gadolinium enhanced magnetic resonance urography for upper urinary tract malignancy. J Urol. 2010;183(4):1330–65.

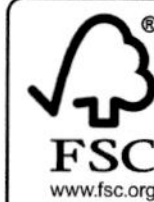

MIX
Papier aus verantwortungsvollen Quellen
Paper from responsible sources
FSC® C105338

If you have any concerns about our products,
you can contact us on
ProductSafety@springernature.com

In case Publisher is established outside the EU,
the EU authorized representative is:
**Springer Nature Customer Service Center GmbH
Europaplatz 3, 69115 Heidelberg, Germany**

Printed by Libri Plureos GmbH
in Hamburg, Germany